SO-AWC-504

Pharmacology for Pharmacy Technicians

THIRD EDITION

Kathy Moscou, RPh, MPH, PhD

Adjunct Professor, Faculty of Education
Brandon University
Brandon, Manitoba, CANADA
Fellow
WHO Collaborating Centre for Governance, Accountability and Transparency in the Pharmaceutical Sector
Leslie Dan Faculty of Pharmacy University of Toronto
Toronto, CANADA
Partial-load Professor, Workforce Development
Niagara College Canada
Welland, CANADA

Karen R. Snipe, CPhT, MAEd

Pharmacy Technician Clinical Coordinator
Trident Technical College
Charleston, South Carolina

ELSEVIER

PHARMACOLOGY FOR PHARMACY TECHNICIANS, THIRD EDITION   ISBN: 978-0-323-49722-0

Copyright © 2019 by Elsevier, Inc. All rights reserved.

No part of this publication may be reproduced or transmitted in any form or by any means, electronic or mechanical, including photocopying, recording, or any information storage and retrieval system, without permission in writing from the publisher. Details on how to seek permission, further information about the Publisher's permissions policies and our arrangements with organizations such as the Copyright Clearance Center and the Copyright Licensing Agency, can be found at our website: www.elsevier.com/permissions.

This book and the individual contributions contained in it are protected under copyright by the Publisher (other than as may be noted herein).

Notice

Practitioners and researchers must always rely on their own experience and knowledge in evaluating and using any information, methods, compounds or experiments described herein. Because of rapid advances in the medical sciences, in particular, independent verification of diagnoses and drug dosages should be made. To the fullest extent of the law, no responsibility is assumed by Elsevier, authors, editors or contributors for any injury and/or damage to persons or property as a matter of products liability, negligence or otherwise, or from any use or operation of any methods, products, instructions, or ideas contained in the material herein.

Previous editions copyrighted 2013 and 2009.

Drug photos provided by Clinical Pharmacology.

Library of Congress Control Number: 2018961754

Director, Private Sector Education Content: Kristin Wilhelm
Content Development Manager: Lisa Newton
Senior Content Development Specialist: Laura Selkirk
Publishing Services Manager: Julie Eddy
Project Manager: Abigail Bradberry
Design Direction: Patrick Ferguson

Printed in Canada

Last digit is the print number: 9   8   7   6   5   4   3   2

ELSEVIER

3251 Riverport Lane
St. Louis, Missouri 63043

Working together
to grow libraries in
developing countries

www.elsevier.com • www.bookaid.org

Reviewers

Technical Reviewer

Ashlee Mattingly, PharmD
Abilities Lab Pharmacist and Technician Training Coordinator
Department of Pharmacy Practice and Science
University of Maryland School of Pharmacy
Baltimore, Maryland

Reviewers

Melissa Ballard, CPhT
Assistant Professor, Pharmacy Technology
Mountwest Community and Technical College
Huntington, West Virginia

Katrina Brasuell, BS, CPhT, TR Ph
Pharmacy Technician Coordinator/Instructor
Vernon College
Wichita Falls, Texas

Thera Celestine, Associate Degree of Science in Liberal Arts
Pharmacy Technology Program Director
Health Science and Workforce Division
Lamar State College - Orange
Orange, Texas

Mary Leigh Curtis, PharmD
Health Technology
Germanna Community College
Fredericksburg, Virginia

Lindsay Elcure, CLS, CPhT
Secondary Health Science Educator
Career and Technology Education - Health Science
Clear Creek High School
League City, Texas

Anthony Guerra, M.HCI, PharmD, RPh
Professor, Chemistry/Pharmacology
Des Moines Area Community College
Ankeny, Iowa

Adam R. Hasty, BS, CPhT
Program Director/Instructor
Pharmacy Technician Program
Tennessee College of Applied Technology - Murfreesboro
Murfreesboro, Tennessee

Elena Bablenis Haveles, BS Pharmacy, PharmD, RPh
Adjunct Associate Professor of Pharmacology
Old Dominion University, Schools of Dental Hygiene and Nursing
Norfolk, Virginia
Adjunct Professor of Pharmacology
Stratford University, Health Sciences
Virginia Beach, Virginia

Lisa R. Jones, EdS, MHA, BSHCS, AAT, CPhT
Pharmacy Technician Academic Program Coordinator
Allied Health Sciences
Aiken Technical College
Graniteville, South Carolina

Joshua J. Neumiller, Pharm D, CDE, FASCP
Vice-Chair and Associate Professor, Department of Pharmacotherapy
Director of Experiential Services
Editor-in-Chief, *Diabetes Spectrum*
Washington State University, College of Pharmacy
Pullman, Washington

Bobbi Steelman, CPhT, BS ED, MAEd,
Director of Education, Pharmacy Technician Program Director
Academics
Daymar College
Bowling Green, Kentucky

Preface

The pharmacy technician profession has been growing by leaps and bounds because of the increase in the number of prescriptions written, the aging of the population, and the increasing number of new pharmacies. The role of the pharmacy technician has expanded to address the growing need for pharmaceutical services, coupled with increasing requirements for pharmacists to provide cognitive services and direct patient care. It does not matter in which type of pharmacy setting one is employed, a basic understanding of pharmacology is needed to assist the pharmacist effectively in the dispensing of medications and education of the clients of the pharmacy. To this end, *Pharmacology for Pharmacy Technicians* seeks to provide a body of knowledge that will enable the pharmacy technician to understand the principles of pharmacology and apply them to the daily activities and challenges presented in all pharmacy practice settings.

Background

This book was conceived and developed by both a pharmacist and pharmacy technician who saw the need for a comprehensive pharmacology text that would provide knowledge and applications for students in the field of pharmacy practice. The authors have extensive experience training pharmacy technicians and more than 40 years combined experience working with pharmacy technicians in community pharmacy and hospital practice settings in the United States and Canada.

Who Will Benefit from This Book?

Pharmacology for Pharmacy Technicians provides students with comprehensive coverage of pharmacology and also gives the instructor the tools necessary to present this information effectively. Today's pharmacy technicians are increasingly called on to perform highly technical tasks that were previously the responsibility of the pharmacist. In all practice settings, pharmacy technicians are required to perform their duties and maintain accuracy and professionalism. Knowledge of pharmacology will increase the pharmacy technician's brand and generic name recognition. Moreover, the study of pharmacology will help pharmacy technicians identify duplicate drugs and speed the process of identifying the drug requested for refill when the patient can't remember the drug name. Given the volume of medication doses currently dispensed, pharmacy technicians need to understand the general principles of pharmacology to be able to assist the pharmacist in spotting medication errors and drug interactions.

Why Is This Book Important to the Profession?

In addition to basic pharmacology, this textbook provides current drug information, tools to enhance learning, and Tech Alerts and Tech Notes that are important aids for pharmacy technicians and other health professionals to prevent medication errors. The material is presented in a format and language that is easily understood and grasped by the reader.

Organization

Pharmacology for Pharmacy Technicians provides an integrated approach to the understanding of pharmacology and pharmacotherapy. Unit I includes content on pharmaceutics, pharmacokinetics, and pharmacodynamics. The unit presents the basic foundation for understanding pharmacology. Unit II through Unit XI are organized according to body systems—the nervous system, musculoskeletal system, ophthalmic and otic systems, cardiovascular system, gastrointestinal system, respiratory system, reproductive system, endocrine system, and integumentary system. An overview of common disorders of each body system is described, including symptoms. This will help students understand why a given medication is useful for treatment of the condition. The mechanism of action for drugs is also presented. It builds on basic information presented in Unit I and aids in understanding pharmacotherapeutics. Duplicate entries of some drugs are found throughout the text for those that are prescribed for the treatment of more than one medical condition as the rationale for usage may differ according to the medical condition being treated. Each chapter contains a list of basic terminology, key points, review questions, and critical thinking exercises. Common endings of drug classifications are provided to aid in memorizing drugs and their use.

Distinctive Features

Pharmacology for Pharmacy Technicians makes extensive use of tables and figures to enhance learning. U.S. and Canadian brand names are provided for each generic name product. Available strengths and dosage forms are placed in tables along with photographs of many of the top 200 selling drugs to aid in product identification.

Additional unique features include common endings of drug classifications, warning labels for every drug, Tech Alerts for drug look-alike and sound-alike issues, and Tech Notes for important information and precautions. As compared with other pharmacology texts, *Pharmacology for Pharmacy Technicians* is comprehensive and contains descriptions of hundreds of pharmaceuticals.

Learning Aids

A variety of pedagogical features are included in the book to aid in learning:
- **Learning Objectives.** These are listed at the beginning of each chapter and clearly outline what students are expected to learn from the chapter materials.
- A list of **Key Terms** follows the Learning Objectives, that identifies new terminology, and makes it easier for students to

learn the new vocabulary. Learning this new terminology is vital to success on the job.

- **Tech Alerts** are found throughout the text and alert the student to drug look-alike and sound-alike issues.
- Helpful **Tech Notes** are presented throughout the chapters and provide critical, need to know information regarding dispensing concerns and interesting points about pharmacology.
- **Mini drug monographs** with pill photos are provided for every body system and in every drug classification chapter. These include generic and trade names, strength of medication, route of administration, dosage form, dosing schedule, and warning labels.
- **Key Points** are found at the end of each chapter that summarizes the key concepts of the chapter.
- **Review Questions** further enhance student review and retention of chapter content by testing them on the key content within the chapter.
- The **Technician's Corner** provides critical thinking exercises that help students prepare for on the job experiences by challenging them to pull together a collection of facts and information to reach a conclusion.
- The **Bibliography** provides a list of sources that students and instructors can use for additional information on the chapter's topic.

Ancillaries

For the Instructor

Evolve

We are offering several assets on Evolve (http://evolve.elsevier.com/Moscou/pharmacology) to aid instructors:

- **Test Bank:** An ExamView test bank of over 1,000 questions that features rationales, learning objectives, cognitive levels, and page number references to the text. This can be used as a review in class or for test development.
- **PowerPoint Presentations:** One PowerPoint presentation per chapter. These can be used as is or as a template to prepare lectures.
- **Image Collection:** All the images from the book are available in JPEG format and can be downloaded into PowerPoint presentations. These can be used during lectures to illustrate important concepts.
- **Text Answer Key:** All the answers to the Review Questions and Technician's Corner questions from the text.

- **Workbook Answer Key:** All the answers to the Workbook exercises.
- **TEACH:** Provides instructors with customizable lesson plans based on learning objectives. With these valuable resources, instructors will save valuable preparation time and can create a learning environment that fully engages students in classroom preparation. The lesson plans are keyed chapter by chapter and are divided into logical lessons to aid in classroom planning.

For the Student

Student Workbook

The student workbook includes:

- Fill-in-the-blank exercises, multiple-choice questions, matching questions, and true-false questions reinforce the concepts presented in the textbook.
- Research activities and Case Studies teach students how to keep current with an ever-changing industry.
- Critical thinking exercises help students apply the knowledge that they learn in class to real-life scenarios, including testing their knowledge of pharmacy calculations.

Evolve

The student resources on Evolve include:

- Two comprehensive practice exams, which includes more than 200 questions, to check students' knowledge and comprehension.
- Access to *Clinical Pharmacology*.

Note to the Student

Pharmacology for Pharmacy Technicians was created to provide pharmacy technicians with a strong foundation in pharmacology. As you proceed through this text, you will notice that key concepts are repeated to reinforce learning. Review the key terms before you begin to read the chapter; this will help you understand the chapter better. The chapter summary provides a synopsis of key concepts in each chapter. You will want to refer often to the tables of brand and generic names as this knowledge of brand and generic names is critical for your profession. The drug photos will help you learn to identify commonly prescribed medicines; familiarity with product appearance helps reduce medication errors. You may also find this text useful in other pharmacy technician courses.

Acknowledgments and Dedication

The education of pharmacy technicians to assume ever-expanding professional responsibilities has been the focus of much of my professional career. This book is dedicated to all my former students at North Seattle Community College, whom I have challenged and hopefully inspired to achieve their best, for themselves and the profession. I dedicate this book to my husband, Gervan Fearon, who has supported me throughout the arduous process of writing this textbook, and my children, Gyasi and Chi Moscou-Jackson, who have started their own professional careers. Finally, I would like to thank my co-author, Karen Snipe, for her enthusiasm and motivation throughout the writing of this book, and the Pharmacy Technician Educators Council and other organizations for encouraging the development of instructional materials for pharmacy technicians.

— *Kathy Moscou*

The pharmacy technician's role in pharmacy practice has evolved to a point where the knowledge and understanding of pharmacology is vital to patient care. Students will be challenged when learning about all of the aspects of pharmacology and its role in healthcare. Being a pharmacy technician for 25 years has shown me that our role is ever expanding, and pharmacists have come to appreciate our knowledge of pharmaceuticals. I would like to thank my family especially my husband Roy; without their continuous support, I would not have pursued this project. And I'd like to say thank you to my writing partner, Kathy, whose encouragement and support was priceless throughout this project. I dedicate this text to my pharmacy technician students who have inspired me to write teaching materials that are relevant and pertinent to their training.

— *Karen Snipe*

Contents

Introduction to Pharmacology

The aim of drug therapy is to diagnose, treat, cure, or lessen the symptoms of disease. The study of pharmacology applies knowledge of properties of drugs, mechanism of drug action, anatomy and physiology, and pathology. It is essential to the accurate, effective, and efficient performance of pharmacy technician duties who, possessing a substantial knowledge of pharmacology, are able to reduce dispensing errors associated with look-alike or sound-alike drugs, as well as recognize drug interactions, incorrect drugs and strengths, incorrect dosage form, improper dosing schedule, therapeutic duplication and drug interactions, and excessive drug alerts screened by the computer before dispensing to patients and hospital medical personnel. Medication errors can be avoided by becoming familiar with trade/generic drug names, their strengths, dosage forms, and dosing frequencies. Pharmacy technicians can also assist patients who do not remember drug names.

In Unit I, pharmacology, pharmacokinetics and pharmacodynamics of medicines are described. Pharmacokinetics (drug movement) involves 4 phases: *absorption, distribution, metabolism,* and *elimination* (ADME). These pharmacokinetic phases control the intensity of the drug's effect and the duration of the drug action. Pharmacodynamics looks at patient-related factors that affect how the body responds to drugs that are administered. Age, gender, disease, pregnancy, weight, and genetics are patient-related factors that influence drug response. Psychological factors can also affect drug response, and adherence to drug therapy is influenced by patient belief that the therapy will be beneficial. In Unit I, drug classifications, such as legend (requiring a prescription) or OTC (over the counter) are introduced. Product formulations for administration by mouth (enteral) or injection (parenteral), such as intramuscularly, intravenously, or subcutaneously, inhalation, or topical application, are described.

Pharmacy technicians who understand the aspects of pharmacology, pharmacokinetics, pharmacodynamics, the mechanisms of drug action, and strategies to reduce medication errors will be of great benefit to both pharmacists and the patients they serve.

1

Fundamentals of Pharmacology

LEARNING OBJECTIVES

1. Explain why the study of pharmacology is necessary for pharmacy technicians.
2. Illustrate global contributions to the knowledge of pharmaceuticals.
3. Identify key legislation responsible for protecting public health and regulating drug distribution.
4. Describe the drug approval process.
5. Describe commonly dispensed dosage forms.
6. Compare and contrast routes of drug administration.
7. Learn the terminology associated with the fundamentals of pharmacology.

KEY TERMS

Bioavailability The portion of the administered drug dose that enters the systemic circulation and is available to produce drug effect.

Biopharmaceuticals Pharmaceuticals derived from biological sources (e.g., proteins, gene sequences) and manufactured using biotechnology methods such as recombinant DNA technology.

Controlled substance Drug whose possession and distribution is restricted because of its potential for abuse as determined by federal or state law. Controlled substances are placed in schedules according to their abuse potential and effects if abused.

Dosage form Drug formulation (e.g., capsule, tablet, solution).

Dose Amount of a drug required for one application or administration.

Dosing schedule How frequently a drug dose is administered (e.g., "four times a day").

Drug Substance used to diagnose, treat, cure, prevent, or mitigate disease in humans or other animals (US Food and Drug Administration, 2017).

Drug delivery system Dosage form or device designed to release a specific amount of drug.

Enteral Drug dosage form that is administered orally that passes through the gastrointestinal tract.

Homeopathic medicine Drugs that are administered in minute quantities to stimulate natural body healing systems.

Legend drugs Drugs that are required by state or federal law to be dispensed by a prescription only. Prescriptions must be written for a legitimate medical condition and issued by a practitioner authorized to prescribe.

Over-the-counter (OTC) drugs Drugs that may be obtained without a prescription.

Parenteral Drug dosage form that is administered by injection or infusion.

Pharmacognosy Science dealing with the biological, biochemical features of natural drugs and their constituents. It is the study of drugs of plant and animal origins.

Pharmacology Study of drugs and their interactions with living systems, including chemical and physical properties, toxicology, and therapeutics.

Pharmacotherapy Use of drugs in the treatment of disease.

Toxicology: Science dealing with the study of poisons.

Pharmacology

Pharmacology is the study of drugs and their interactions with living systems, including chemical and physical properties, *toxicology*, and therapeutics. Knowledge of *pharmacology* is essential to the accurate, effective, and efficient performance of the responsibilities of pharmacy technicians. Pharmacy technicians educated in pharmacology have the skills to properly identify the drug from a patient's profile when refills are requested and the patient does not remember the drug name. Less time is spent searching for drugs when pharmacy technicians have good brand and generic name recognition. Pharmacy technicians possessing substantial knowledge of pharmacology may be able to reduce dispensing errors associated with look-alike or sound-alike drugs, incorrect drug or strength, incorrect dosage form, and improper dosing schedule. Knowledge of pharmacology facilitates selection of warning labels for drugs dispensed. Pharmacy technicians who possess a good knowledge of pharmacology understand the importance of recognizing drug interactions, therapeutic duplication, and excessive dose alerts screened by the computer. Overall, pharmacy technicians who have a working knowledge of pharmacology can perform duties within their scope of practice with greater independence.

History of Medicines and Their Use

Plants have been collected, cultivated, and harvested for their healing properties and used in the treatment of illness for centuries. Contributors to the current knowledge about drugs span the globe. Records dating as early as 3000 BC document the pharmacological knowledge by the people of ancient Egypt, Mesopotamia, India, and China. Papyrus Ebers (1550 BC), which was found in Egypt and describes more than 700 medical compounds and lists more than 811 prescriptions, is thought to be a copy of an ancient manuscript that dates to 3000 BC. More than 800 clay tablets have been unearthed describing more than 500 remedies in Mesopotamia (Persian Gulf 2500 BC), and Emperor Shen Nung is credited with writing the *Pen T'sao Ching* (2750 BC) in which more than 1000 medicinal compounds are described and 11,000 prescription remedies are listed. The *Dravyaguna* (2500 BC) is an ancient Ayurvedic manuscript (India) of **materia medica** (medicinal materials) and includes sources, descriptions, criteria for identification, properties, methods for preparation, and therapeutic uses of hundreds of medicinal herbs. Some of the medicinal compounds described in these ancient manuscripts are still used today for essentially the same purposes. For example, castor oil and tincture opii were described in *Papyrus Ebers*.

Theophrastus (300 BC), the "father of botany," was a Greek physician known for his accurate observation of medicinal plants. By the first century, Dioscorides, another Greek physician, known as the "father of pharmacology," described approximately 600 medicinal plants in *De Materia Medica*. Aloe, belladonna, ergot, and opium are a few of the medicines described in the manuscript that are still in use today.

Since the 20th century, research into medicines and the introduction of new drugs and vaccines have grown exponentially. Antiinfective agents, the discovery of insulin and its use for the treatment of diabetes, and antiretroviral drugs for the treatment of HIV/AIDS have all been discovered since the 1930s. The Human Genome Project, a study of human genes, has provided data useful in understanding diseases that are caused by genetic defects or linked to heredity. The study of genes has enabled scientists to develop new genetically modified drugs, such as human insulin. Bioengineering is the process used to produce *biopharmaceuticals*.

A pharmacology timeline is shown in Box 1.1.

Origin of Drugs

Pharmacognosy, a term derived from the Greek words *pharmakon* ("drug") and *gnosis* ("knowledge"), is the branch of science dealing with the study of the natural origin of drugs. Pharmacognosy is the study of the constituents of natural drugs that are responsible for their effects. A *drug* is a substance that affects the normal function or structure of humans or animals and may be used to diagnose, treat, mitigate, cure, or prevent disease. Drugs may come from natural or synthetic origins. Natural drugs may be derived from plants (e.g., digitalis, quinine), animals (e.g., thyroid USP, pepsin), or minerals (e.g., silver nitrate). Some natural drugs are administered in their crude form; however, most frequently, the chief active ingredient(s) are extracted from the crude source.

> **TECH NOTE!**
>
> Some common beverages and foods are natural drugs. Coffee and tea contain the drug caffeine. Ginger and peppermint contain ingredients that can reduce nausea.

Synthetic drugs may be a chemical modification of a natural drug or manufactured entirely from chemical ingredients unrelated to the natural drug. The synthetic drug may be equally potent or more potent. Fentanyl is a synthetically manufactured analgesic that is more potent than the natural drug, morphine (a naturally occurring analgesic derived from the opium poppy). Drugs may also be produced via the process of bioengineering. Erythropoietin and human insulin are examples of biopharmaceuticals. Table 1.1 details common origins of selected drugs.

What Is Pharmacology?

Pharmacognosy and pharmacology are both sciences that involve the study of medicinal substances. However, the science of pharmacology involves the action of drugs on humans and animals. The aim of drug therapy is to diagnose, treat, cure, or lessen the symptoms of disease. The study of pharmacology applies knowledge of properties of drugs, mechanism of drug action, anatomy and

TABLE 1.1	Drugs and Their Sources		
Classification	**Source**	**Generic Name**	**Use**
Plant	Foxglove Cinchona Opium poppy	Digitalis Quinine Morphine	Heart failure (CHF) Malaria Pain
Animal	Thyroid gland Pancreas	Thyroid, USP Pancreatin	Hypothyroidism Digestive aid
Mineral	Silver Gold	Silver sulfadiazine Auranofin	Burns (antiinfective) Arthritis
Synthetic	Synthetic opioid Red azo dye	Fentanyl Sulfonamides	Pain Infection
Bioengineering (recombinant DNA technology)	Isolated DNA + *Escherichia coli* bacteria	Hepatitis B vaccine[a] Human insulin[b]	Hepatitis B prevention Diabetes mellitus

[a]Source of hepatitis B vaccine is viral DNA copied into a yeast cell.
[b]Source of human insulin is isolated DNA + *Escherichia coli* bacteria.

• BOX 1.1   Pharmacology Timeline

3000 BC
- Imhotep, Egyptian god of medicine

2750 BC
- Emperor Shen Nung (China) is credited with writing the *Pen T'sao Ching*. More than 1000 medicinal compounds are described, and 11,000 prescription remedies are listed.

2500 BC
- The *Dravyaguna*, an ancient Ayurvedic manuscript of medicinal materials, sources, descriptions, criteria for identification, properties, methods for preparation, and therapeutic uses of hundreds of medicinal herbs, is written in India.

1550 BC
- *Papyrus Ebers*, thought to be a copy of an ancient Egyptian manuscript that dates back to 3000 BC, describes more than 700 medical compounds and lists more than 811 prescriptions.

1000 BC
- Charaka described more than 2000 medicinal substances (including mercury compounds, e.g., merthiolate), methods to improve palatability, and metrology (measurements and dosages).

400 BC
- Hippocrates, the "father of medicine"

300 BC
- Theophrastus, the "father of botany," was a Greek physician known for his accurate observation of medicinal plants.

AD 100
- Dioscorides, the "father of pharmacology," a botanist and pharmacologist, authored *Dioscorides Herbal*.

AD 120 to 200
- Galen, the "father of pharmacotherapy," promoted Humoral theory, the dominant theory of disease and treatment for more than 1500 years. This theory states that illness is caused by an imbalance of "humors" and is treated with Simples, Composites, and Entities.

AD 1000
- Avicenna Ibn Sina, known as the "Persian Galen," whose writings unified pharmaceutical and medicinal knowledge of his time and whose teachings were accepted in the West until the 17th century.

AD 1500s
- Paracelsus, the "father of the pharmaceutical revolution," promoted the concept that disease is a chemical abnormality treated with chemicals. Introduced laudanum, a drug derived from opium that deadens pain.
- Indians of the Americas had pharmacological knowledge of up to 1200 plants, including:
  - West Indies: guaiacum (evergreen tree)
  - South America: cocaine (cocoa leaves), curare
  - Mexico: jalap (laxative)

- Peru: quinine (cinchona)
- Brazil: balsam Tolu (expectorant)

AD 1700s
- William Withering (United Kingdom) isolated digitalis from foxglove.
- Edward Jenner (United Kingdom) developed the vaccine against cowpox. His research led to the development of the smallpox vaccine.
- Bernard Courtois (France) discovered iodine, used to treat goiter and to decrease mucus (mucolytic).
- Joseph Caventou and Pierre Pelletier (France) discovered quinine, which is used to treat malaria.
- Johannes Buchner (Germany) identified salicin from willow bark (ASA) and nicotine in tobacco (niacin).
- Emil von Behring (Germany) worked with antitoxins, resulting in diphtheria and tetanus vaccine.
- Gregor Mendel (Austria), a famous scientist and monk, discovered the basis of genetics and how genes are woven into heredity.

1800s
- Friedrich Sertürner (Germany) extracted morphine from opium.
- Louis Pasteur's experiments showing that microorganisms can cause disease and heat can kill them became the basis of "germ theory."

1900s
- Frederick Banting and Charles Best (Canada) discovered that insulin lowers blood sugar levels and can be used to treat diabetes.
- Gerhardt Domagk (Germany) introduced the sulfonamide Prontosil, the first antiinfective agent.
- Alexander Fleming (United States) discovered penicillin, a chemical produced by a fungus.
- Beyer (United States) was instrumental in the development of thiazide diuretics, derivatives of sulfonamides, and other drugs.

2000s
- With the mapping of the human genome and new gene editing technology, precision therapies have been developed such as Ivacaftor (Kalydeco)—a new therapy for the treatment of cystic fibrosis (CF) that was approved for use in patients who have a specific mutation in the CF gene.
- Immunobiologic therapies such as monoclonal antibody immunomodulators, monoclonal (e.g., basiliximab, daclizumab, and muromonab) and mTor inhibitors (e.g., everolimus and sirolimus) were introduced.
- Vaccines to prevent HPV (e.g., Gardasil®) and new antiviral therapy for the HAART treatment of HIV/AIDS (e.g., Triumeq®—abacavir, dolutegravir, lamivudine) and hepatitis C (e.g., Harvoni®—ledipasvir/sofosbuvir) were introduced.
- New mechanisms of action for antiviral therapy such as Nonstructural Protein 5A (NS5A) Replication Complex Inhibitors were introduced (e.g., Daklinza—daclatasvir).
- New advances have been made in cellular and gene therapies (e.g., Hemacord—HPC cord blood).

physiology, and pathology. Selection of the appropriate drug for a patient in the proper *dose* and *dosage form*, administered at an appropriate dosing schedule, requires knowledge of pharmacology. The drug dose is the amount of drug units given for a single administration (e.g., two tablets, one teaspoonful). The *dosing schedule* is the number of times the drug dose is administered per day.

What Is Pharmacotherapy?

Pharmacotherapy is defined as the use of drugs in the treatment of disease. Contrasting philosophies about pharmacotherapy exist. Allopathic medicine, sometimes called Western medicine, is a system of medical practice in which the goal of pharmacotherapy is to fight disease by using drugs or surgery that produces effects different

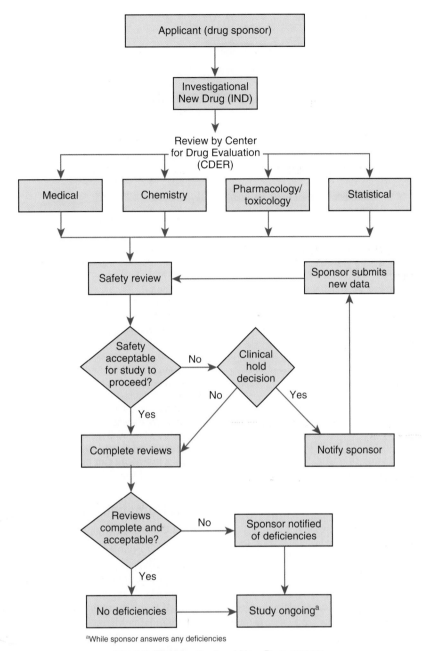

• **Fig. 1.1** The Investigational New Drug process.

from or incompatible with those produced by the disease being treated. In *homeopathic medicine* drugs are administered in minute quantities to produce effects similar to the disease in healthy persons, yet stimulate the body's natural healing systems in individuals with disease.

Research and Development

In 1906, the Pure Food and Drug Act was passed to protect the public from ineffective and harmful drugs. This act was expanded in 1938, and standards for allowing new drugs onto the market were set. Today, it can take several years to move a new drug from the idea phase to making it available to the public. Thousands of chemical compounds may be tested before one is discovered that can produce the desired effects with an acceptable level of adverse effects.

There are many steps in the drug development process (Fig. 1.1). The steps from the test tube to production and distribution of a new drug involve preclinical research, clinical studies, new drug application (NDA) process, and review. Manufacturers of new drugs must submit data showing that their drug is reasonably safe before a preliminary small-scale clinical study is approved. Preclinical research is conducted to determine a pharmacological profile for the drug and acute toxicity of the drug in at least two species of animals. Upon completion of the preclinical phase, drug manufacturers file an Investigational New Drug (IND) application. Only approved INDs move to the clinical study phase.

There are three clinical study phases (Fig. 1.2). In phase 1 clinical trials, the drug is administered to a small number of healthy volunteers who are enrolled in the clinical study. Preliminary information about the drug's pharmacology, mechanism of action, and efficacy (effectiveness in humans in a controlled clinical trial)

• **Fig. 1.2** The preclinical and clinical phases of the new drug development process. *FDA,* US Food and Drug Administration; *IND,* investigational new drug. (From The New Drug Development Process, Food and Drug Administration: The new drug development process; From the US Food and Drug Administration [FDA]: *New drug development and review process,* updated 02.11.15. http://www.fda.gov/Drugs/DevelopmentApprovalProcess/SmallBusinessAssistance/ucm053131.htm.)

is gathered in phase 1. If appropriate, the drug enters phase 2 clinical studies. Phase 2 studies are controlled trials with a limited number of patients with the condition to be treated. During this phase, data are collected to determine the drug's efficacy and the drug's side effects in patients with the disease. Phase 3 clinical studies involve hundreds to a few thousand patients. Drug safety is evaluated, and the benefit of taking the drug is compared with the risks associated with taking the drug. If safety and efficacy are shown, the drug begins the new drug application process and then moves on to review. An accelerated process exists to speed drug development and review when the drug provides significant benefit over existing therapies or a life-threatening illness is present. Additional safety information is collected in the postmarketing phase. Phase 4 trials are studies that are conducted after the drug is marketed to the public to determine safety and effectiveness when the drug is used in "real-world" conditions.

In 1992, the Prescription Drug User Fees Act (PDUFA) was passed to allow companies to pay a fee to the US Food and Drug Administration (FDA) in return for a faster review period. The PDUFA was renewed in 2012 (PDUFA V). On July 9, 2012, the Food and Drug Administration Safety and Innovation Act (FDASIA) was signed into law. This law includes the reauthorization of PDUFA V through September 2017 and sets performance goals for the speed in which new drug and biologic license applications are reviewed.

The FDA Amendments Act permits PDUFA user fees to be used for risk management and communication, increasing the FDA's responsibility to adopt a more proactive approach to pharmacovigilance, and set guidelines for postmarket clinical studies.

Drug approval and marketing of new drugs are also regulated in Canada. The Therapeutic Products Directorate reviews scientific information, premarket clinical trial applications and investigational testing applications. The TPD also monitors drug safety issues by review of adverse drug reaction reports. Approves prescription drugs in Canada, and the Marketed Health Products Directorate is responsible for monitoring postmarket drug safety and

communicating risks to the public. Preclinical and phase I to IV clinical studies are also required in Canada. A Notice of Compliance (NOC) or NOC/c (approval with conditions) must be issued before a new drug can be marketed in Canada. Prescription drugs are issued a Drug Identification Number (DIN).

Drug Nomenclature

All drugs are identified by a generic name, a chemical name, and a proprietary name. The name of a new drug is made according to standards set by the Center for Drug Evaluation and Research (CDER). The standards published in the CDER Data Standards Manual (DSM) are used by the Drug Product Reference File (DPRF) and the Drug Registration and Listing System (DRLS). (The CDER Data Standards Manual is available at http://www.fda.gov/Drugs/DevelopmentApprovalProcess/FormsSubmissionRequirements/ElectronicSubmissions/DataStandardsManualmonographs/default.htm.)

> **⊙ TECH NOTE!**
>
> Every drug has a generic name; however, the drug cannot be manufactured by a generic manufacturer until the patent expires.

Official drug names are nonproprietary names that are selected by the US Adopted Name (USAN) Council and must be approved by the FDA. The USAN and International Nonproprietary Name (INN) designated by the World Health Organization is usually identical. The drug name that is published in an official compendium like the United States Pharmacopoeia is the official name. If a drug contains more than one active ingredient, all official drug names must be listed. The ending of the official name of many drugs indicates the pharmacological class to which the drug belongs (Table 1.2). For example, many local anesthetics have the common ending "-caine."

TABLE 1.2 Examples of Common Endings to Official Drug Names

Classification	Common Ending	Prototypical Drug
Benzodiazepine	-zepam -zolam	Diazepam Alprazolam
Corticosteroid	-sone -lone	Prednisone Prednisolone
Nonsteroidal antiinflammatory drug (NSAID)	-profen -olac	Ibuprofen Ketorolac
β-Adrenergic blocking drug (β-blocker)	-olol	Propranolol
H₂ receptor antagonist	-tidine	Cimetidine
Proton pump inhibitor	-prazole	Omeprazole
Calcium channel blockers (dihydropyridines)	-dipine	Nifedipine
Macrolide antiinfective	-thromycin	Erythromycin

TABLE 1.3 Examples of Chemical, Generic, and Proprietary Names

Generic Name	Chemical Name	Brand Name
fluoxetine HCl	N-methyl-3-phenyl-3-[4-(trifluoromethyl)phenoxy]propan-1-amine	Prozac
acetaminophen	N-(4-Hydroxyphenyl)acetamide	Tylenol
ibuprofen	2-[4-(2-methylpropyl)phenyl]propanoic acid	Motrin

The generic name is the official or unofficial nonproprietary name commonly used to designate the drug. The chemical name describes the molecular structure of the drug. The chemical structure of the drug determines its activity and side effects.

The proprietary name, or brand name, is assigned by the drug manufacturer according to nomenclature guidelines and must be approved by the CDER. Factors considered when selecting a suitable proprietary name are risk for medication errors caused by existing "look-alike" and "sound-alike" names and ease of association with the generic name or active ingredient name (Table 1.3).

TECH NOTE!
Whereas brand name or proprietary drugs are commonly written beginning with a capital letter, generic or nonproprietary drugs begin with a lowercase letter.

Comparisons Between Brand Name Drugs and Generic Drugs and Biosimilars

The innovator of a new drug may apply for patent protection. If awarded, the manufacturer is given up to 20 years' exclusive rights to manufacture and distribute the new drug. The manufacturer selects a brand name for the drug according to CDER recommendations. When the drug is off patent, other drug companies may manufacture a generic equivalent. Generic drugs contain the same active ingredient as the original manufacturer's drug in the same strength and in the same dosage form. Generic drugs may contain different inactive ingredients. Occasionally, these inactive

ingredients result in slight differences between brand name and generic products that affect how much of the drug is available to produce drug action or how quickly drug effect is produced. Generic drugs that are not significantly different from the innovator's product receive an "A" rating from the FDA and may be substituted for the brand name product according to state and federal product substitution laws.

Generic drugs are always less expensive than brand name drugs. In many states and provinces, pharmacists routinely dispense generic drugs. Most prescription drug insurance plans require that generic drugs be dispensed; brand name drugs are only dispensed when the prescriber insists that a brand name drug is necessary. A biosimilar is a biopharmaceutical or biologic that is designed to have active properties similar to a biologic that has previously been approved. An example is infliximab (Remicade®), a biologic used to treat Crohn's disease, ulcerative colitis and psoriatic arthritis. Biosimilars are: infliximab-DYYB (Inflectra®), infliximab-QBTX (Ixifi®), and infliximab-ABDA (Renflexis®).

TECH NOTE!
Technicians must concentrate on memorizing each drug's generic name and brand name. Medication errors can also be avoided by arranging drugs on the pharmacy shelves according to the generic names.

TECH NOTE!
Many drugs look and sound alike. Technicians should become familiar with the Institute for Safe Medication Practices' (ISMP) list of lookalike/soundalike drug names. See list at https://www.ismp.org/tools/confuseddrugnames.pdf.

Drug Legislation

The Pure Food and Drug Act (1906) was the first significant legislation passed to protect the public from harmful and ineffective drugs in the United States. Over the years, many more laws have been passed that regulate drug manufacture and distribution. The Durham-Humphrey Amendment (1951) established the distinction between *legend drugs* and drugs that could safely be used by the public without supervision by a health care provider. Legend drugs can only be obtained by prescription, whereas *over-the-counter (OTC) drugs* do not require a prescription. "Rx only" (United States) and "Pr" (Canada) must be printed on the manufacturer's product label for all legend drugs (prescription only). The Kefauver-Harris Amendment (1962) requires that all drugs be safe and effective before they are made available to the public. INDs are limited to drug study participants until clinical studies have shown them to be safe and effective. The Drug Price Competition Act and Patent Restoration Act (1984) encouraged the creation of generic drugs by streamlining the drug approval process for drugs no longer patented. A patent gives exclusive production rights to manufacturers of proprietary drugs for up to 20 years. When a patent has expired, manufacturers of generic drugs may produce and market the drug. Generic manufacturers are not required to conduct additional studies to prove safety and effectiveness but instead are permitted to rely on safety data submitted by the manufacturer of the proprietary drug. There is a transitional status between Rx only and OTC drugs known as behind-the-counter (BTC) drugs in the United States and Canada. BTC drugs are classified in National Association of Pharmacy Regulatory Authority (NAPRA) Schedule II in Canada. BTC drugs may be sold without prescription, but access is restricted and pharmacist intervention is required to ensure safe, appropriate use and to monitor misuse, abuse, chronic use, and the need for

TABLE 1.4   Controlled Substances (United States): Schedules, Classification, Dispensing Rules, and Examples

Schedule	Classification	Dispensing Rules	Examples
C-I	The drug has a high potential for abuse. The drug has no currently accepted medical use in treatment in the United States.	Only with approved protocol or investigational use	Ecstasy, heroin, LSD, marijuana, PCP
C-II	The drug has a high potential for abuse. Abuse of the drug may lead to severe psychological or physical dependence. The drug has an accepted medical use in treatment in the United States.	Written prescription (if called in or faxed in, a written prescription must follow within 72 hours) No refills allowed	Methylphenidate, codeine, meperidine, oxycodone, secobarbital, hydromorphone, amphetamine
C-III	The drug has a potential for abuse less than that of C-II drugs. Abuse may lead to moderate or low physical dependence or high psychological dependence. The drug has an accepted medical use in treatment in the United States.	Written, oral, or faxed prescription Prescription expires within 6 months Refillable (no more than five refills within 6 months)	Codeine with acetaminophen, hydrocodone with acetaminophen, methyltestosterone, phendimetrazine, buprenorphine
C-IV	The drug has a potential for abuse less than that of C-III drugs. Abuse may lead to limited physical dependence or psychological dependence relative to the C-III drugs. The drug has an accepted medical use in treatment in the United States.	Written, oral, or faxed prescription Prescription expires within 6 months Refillable (no more than five refills within 6 months)	Alprazolam, butorphanol, diazepam, diethylpropion, pentazocine plus naloxone, phentermine, triazolam, carisoprodol
C-V	The drug has a potential for abuse less than that of C-IV drugs. Abuse may lead to limited physical dependence or psychological dependence relative to C-IV drugs. The drug has an accepted medical use in treatment in the United States.	*Prescription:* Written, oral, or faxed prescription Prescription expires within 6 months Refillable (no more than five refills within 6 months) *OTC:* Rules vary for each state	Diphenoxylate plus atropine, lacosamide

LSD, Lysergic acid diethylamide; *OTC,* over the counter; *PCP,* phencyclidine.

physician referral. Examples of BTC Schedule II drugs include iron supplements, insulin, lice treatments (e.g., pyrethrins), aspirin for pediatric use, nitroglycerin, and exempt narcotics (e.g., Tylenol with codeine 8 mg) and Plan B. In Canada, Plan B is classified as Schedule II (BTC) and Schedule III (OTC). Where the product is stocked depends on directions for use found on the package labeling. In the United States, Plan B One-Step is found in the feminine care aisle at many retail stores. It is available without a prescription or ID, and with no age restriction.

In the United States, the Combat Methamphetamine Epidemic Act of 2005 (CMEA) was passed to curb the illegal manufacture and use of "crystal meth." The CMEA was signed into law on March 6, 2006, to regulate, among other things, retail OTC sales of ephedrine, pseudoephedrine, and phenylpropanolamine products used to manufacture crystal meth. Purchase limits, placement of product out of direct customer access, sales logbooks, customer ID verification, employee training, and self-certification of regulated sellers are required provisions of the CMEA.

The Comprehensive Drug Abuse Prevention and Control Act, also known as the Controlled Substance Act (CSA), was passed by Congress in 1970. It regulates drugs that have a history for abuse in the United States. Access to *controlled substances* is more restrictive than access to legend drugs. Controlled substances are placed in Schedule C-I, C-II, C-III, C-IV, or C-V categories according to their abuse potential and effects if abused (Table 1.4). Controlled substance schedules are determined by federal and state laws.

Canada, similar to the United States, has passed legislation to limit the access to drugs with a potential for abuse. Narcotics, controlled drugs, and benzodiazepines and targeted substances regulations are found in the Controlled Drug and Substances Act. Controlled drugs are identified by a ⬦ symbol on the product label. Narcotics are identified by an Ⓝ symbol on the product label, and the symbol used to identify benzodiazepines and targeted substances is ⊠. Examples of narcotics, controlled substances, and benzodiazepines are given in Table 1.5.

> ● **TECH NOTE!**
>
> It is important to know the drug schedule and dispensing requirements for prescription and BTC drugs.

Drug Dosage Forms and Delivery Systems

Drugs are formulated for delivery by mouth (oral), injection (parenteral), inhalation, or topical application to skin or a mucous membrane. Factors influencing the choice for drug formulation are chemical properties of the drug and human physiology. Chemical

TABLE 1.5 Examples of Narcotics, Controlled Substances, and Benzodiazepines and Targeted Substances (Canada)

	Examples	Dispensing Rules
Narcotics	Codeine, meperidine, hydromorphone, morphine, oxycodone	Written or faxed prescription only No refills permitted Part fills allowed
Verbal narcotics	Narcotic preparations containing two or more non-narcotic ingredients (e.g., codeine + acetaminophen and caffeine)	Written, faxed, or verbal prescription No refills permitted Part fills allowed
Controlled substances	Amphetamines (e.g., Dexedrine), methylphenidate, (part I, schedule G), barbiturates (e.g., secobarbital) (part II), anabolic steroids (e.g., testosterone) (part III)	Written, faxed, or verbal prescription Refills permitted for part I controlled substances only when written on prescription Verbal refills permitted on part II and III controlled substances Part fills allowed
Benzodiazepines and targeted substances	Diazepam, clonazepam	Written, faxed, or verbal prescription Refills may be dispensed when authorized if <1 year has elapsed since the original prescription was issued

properties of the drug influence absorption, distribution, metabolism, and elimination of the drug in the body. Normal physiological processes can affect the effectiveness of the drug. For example, drugs formulated for transdermal administration must have sufficient lipid solubility to enable the drug to pass through the cell membranes of skin and get to the site of action. Insulin is formulated for subcutaneous injection because it is composed of two amino acid strands and, if formulated for oral delivery, would be destroyed by the digestive enzymes that break down protein foods.

> ● **TECH NOTE!**
> The Latin abbreviation for by mouth is PO (per os). It can be easily remembered as per oral.

Dosage Forms for Oral (Enteral) Administration

Oral administration is safe, easy, and generally more economical than parenteral administration. Common oral formulations include tablets, capsules, solutions, emulsions, syrups, suspensions, and elixirs.

Tablets

Tablets are solid dosage forms containing one or more active ingredients plus binders and fillers. Binders are added to aid in compressing the drug into a tablet shape. Fillers make up the required bulk and help bind the tablet. Binders and fillers are inactive ingredients but may influence the rate of drug absorption. Tablets are formulated to deliver their contents immediately or over time. Types of tablets are listed below:

Repeat-action tablets are layered. The outer layer rapidly disintegrates in the stomach, and the inner layer dissolves in the small intestine.
Delayed-action tablets slow the release of drug to avoid stomach upset, improve absorption, or prevent drug destruction in the stomach.
Enteric-coated tablets are a type of delayed-action tablet (Fig. 1.3). Enteric-coated tablets do not dissolve in the stomach. They release their contents in the small intestine.

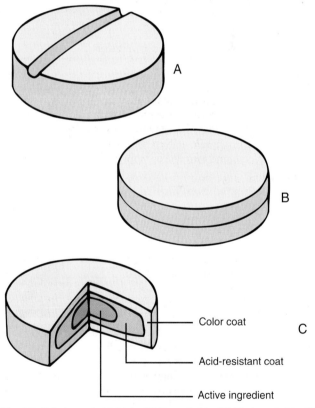

● **Fig. 1.3** Enteric-coated tablets. (A) Scored side. (B) Unscored side. (C) Interior of tablet. (From Clayton BD, Willihnganz MJ: *Basic pharmacology for nurses*, ed 17, St. Louis, 2017, Elsevier.)

Sustained-release and *time-release tablets* deliver their contents over time. Some drugs are formulated to deliver their contents over 24 hours and only need to be taken once a day. Sustained-release drugs should be swallowed whole; crushing may cause the contents to be released immediately. Sustained release and time release are patented processes.
Film coating and *sugar coating* tablets make them easier to swallow and improves taste.

Chewable tablets are formulated for people who have difficulty swallowing pills. Many children's medicines are available in a chewable dosage form.

Sublingual tablets and *buccal tablets* dissolve in the mouth. Sublingual tablets are dissolved under the tongue, and buccal tablets are dissolved in the cheek pouch. Many blood vessels are located in the mouth. Drugs that are destroyed by stomach acids or need to get into the bloodstream rapidly (e.g., nitroglycerin) may be formulated for sublingual or buccal administration.

Oral disintegrating tablets (ODTs) or *orodispersible tablets (ODTs)* are similar to sublingual tablets, but they disintegrate more rapidly (in <60 seconds) when placed on the tongue.

Pastilles are solid medicated preparations designed to dissolve slowly in the mouth. They are softer than lozenges and their bases are either glycerol and gelatin, or acacia and sugar.

Troches and *lozenges* are dissolved in the mouth.

Thin film includes a thin layer of film that disintegrates or dissolves to release the drug and is applied to sublingual tablets (dissolves on the tongue), buccal tablets (absorption in the mouth), and extended-release tablets.

> ● **TECH NOTE!**
>
> Pharmacy technicians must carefully read the labels of medications available for immediate release, sustained release, and delayed release to avoid errors. Many are available in the same strength.

Capsules

Capsules are solid dosage forms containing one or more active ingredient plus binders and fillers (Fig. 1.4). Capsules are formulated to deliver their contents immediately or over time. An osmotic controlled-release capsule delivers the drug through a rigid water-permeable membrane with one or more small holes. As the capsule passes through the body, the osmotic pressure of water entering the capsule pushes the active drug through the opening in the capsule.

Oral Liquids

Oral liquids include suspensions, solutions, syrups, elixirs, tinctures, and emulsions (explained below). Typically, they are water based. Drugs formulated in liquids are easy to swallow. Liquid medicines work more rapidly than tablets or capsules.

Suspensions contain small drug particles (solute) suspended in a solvent (Fig. 1.5). Drug particles settle to the bottom of the bottle when suspensions are left standing. Suspensions may be administered orally, topically, or rectally. *Solutions* are dosage forms in which drug particles completely dissolve in the liquid. Solutions remain clear.

Syrups contain a high concentration of sucrose or other sugar.

Elixirs contain between 5% and 40% alcohol.

Tinctures may contain as little 17% alcohol or as much as 80% alcohol.

Emulsions are similar to suspensions. Drugs suspended in oil may be dispersed in water (O/W) or drugs suspended in water may be dispersed in oil (W/O).

> ● **TECH NOTE!**
>
> When suspensions are dispensed, a SHAKE WELL auxiliary label should be placed on the prescription bottle.

● **Fig. 1.4** Capsules. (From Clayton BD, Willihnganz MJ: *Basic pharmacology for nurses*, ed 17, St. Louis, 2017, Elsevier.)

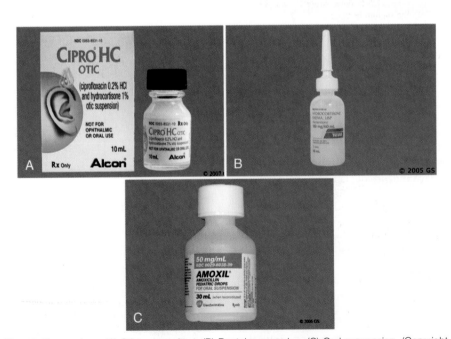

● **Fig. 1.5** Suspensions. (A) Otic suspensions. (B) Rectal suspension. (C) Oral suspension. (Copyright © Gold Standard, Inc., 2007.)

Dosage Forms for Topical Administration

Solutions, suspensions, and emulsions are also formulated for topical application to the skin, eye, ear, and mucous membranes of the rectum and vagina. Topical dosage forms not previously described include ointments, creams, and suppositories.

> **● TECH NOTE!**
>
> Eye drops (sterile) may be placed in the ear, but ear drops (nonsterile) should not be used in the eye.

Dusting powders are free-flowing very fine powders for external use.

Ointments are semisolid preparations containing petrolatum or another oily base (lanolin, wool fat). They soften dry, scaly skin and protect the skin by forming a barrier between the skin and harmful substances.

Creams are semisolid emulsions. Vanishing creams have high water content (O/W); cold cream is an oil-in-water emulsion (W/O).

Hydrogels contain up to 99% water and are a controlled-release *drug delivery system*. They are used in transdermal implants (e.g., histrelin) and wound dressings (e.g., Microcyn Skin and Wound Hydrogel).

Suppositories are solid or semisolid dosage forms intended to be inserted into a body orifice. They are shaped for vaginal, urethral, or rectal insertion. Suppositories melt at body temperature, dispersing the medicine (Fig. 1.6).

> **● TECH NOTE!**
>
> The auxiliary label FOR TOPICAL USE ONLY should be applied to topical products that are dispensed.

> **● TECH NOTE!**
>
> Patients should be advised to remove the foil or outer wrapper from the suppository before inserting it into the rectum or vagina.

Transdermal Drug Delivery Systems (Patches)

Transdermal patches are controlled-release devices that deliver medication across skin membranes into the general circulation (Fig. 1.7). They produce systemic effects (throughout the body)

in addition to local effects. Medicines formulated for transdermal application are used to treat angina (e.g., nitroglycerin), male hypogonadism (e.g., testosterone), menopause (e.g., estrogen), pain (e.g., fentanyl), ADHD (methylphenidate), and Alzheimer disease (rivastigmine).

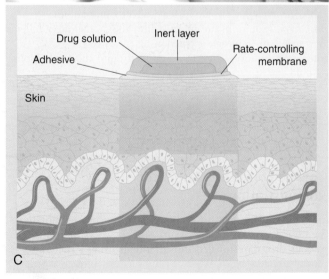

• **Fig. 1.7** Transdermal patches. A and B, Examples of transdermal patches. C, Distribution of drug applied as a transdermal patch across skin membranes to blood vessels. (A and B, Courtesy Rick Brady Riva, MD. From Lilley LL, Collins SR, Snyder JS: *Pharmacology and the nursing process*, ed 8, St. Louis, 2017, Elsevier. C, From Page C, Hoffman B, Curtis M, et al: *Integrated pharmacology*, ed 3, Philadelphia, 2006, Mosby.)

• **Fig. 1.6** Typical shapes of suppositories. (From Clayton BD, Willihnganz MJ: *Basic pharmacology for nurses*, ed 17, St. Louis, 2017, Elsevier.)

• **Fig. 1.8** Typical containers for parenteral medications. A, Syringes. B, Ampules. C, Vials. (From Potter PA, et al: *Essentials for nursing practice*, ed 8, St Louis, 2015, Elsevier.)

Dosage Forms for Parenteral Administration

Parenteral drugs are injected or infused (slowly injected) directly into a blood vessel, muscle, skin, or joint (Fig. 1.8). Parenterally administered drugs enter the bloodstream, often producing rapid action. In the bloodstream, the side effects cannot be easily stopped. To avoid introducing contaminants that are harmful if injected into a patient, pharmacy technicians prepare parenterally administered drugs using aseptic technique in a sterile environment. The following are examples of parenteral drugs:

Intravenous (IV) solutions are injected or infused directly into a vein and go immediately into the bloodstream.

Intramuscular (IM) solutions and suspensions are injected deep into a skeletal muscle.

Subcutaneous (subcut) solutions and suspensions are injected just beneath the skin.

Intraarticular solutions are injected directly into a joint.

Intradermal solutions are injected into the dermal layer (allergy tests or tuberculosis vaccinations).

Intrathecal solutions are injected directly into the cerebrospinal fluid.

> ■ **TECH NOTE!**
> To avoid drug contamination, aseptic technique must always be followed when preparing drugs for parenteral administration.

Dosage Forms for Respiratory Tract Administration

Solutions and suspensions are applied to mucous membranes of the nose as sprays or drops. Micro-fine powders, solutions, and gaseous drugs are inhaled into the lungs using a metered-dose aerosol inhaler (Fig. 1.9) or a nebulizer. A nebulizer is a device that turns solutions into vapors that can be inhaled.

Routes of Administration

The formulation of a drug is largely controlled by the chemical properties of the drug and human physiology. The method of drug

• **Fig. 1.9** (A) Proper use of an inhaler. (B) Inhaler with spacer (also known as an aerochamber). (C) Accuhaler. (A and B, From Potter PA, Perry AG, Stockert P, Hall A: *Fundamentals of nursing*, ed 9, St. Louis, 2017, Elsevier. C, From Clayton BD, Willihnganz MJ: *Basic pharmacology for nurses*, ed 17, St. Louis, 2017, Elsevier.)

administration is determined by drug dosage form. When a drug is available for administration via more than one route, the selection of one route of administration over another is made according to the properties of the drug (e.g., lipid solubility, ionization), ease of administration, pathophysiology (e.g., kidney or liver disease), and therapeutic objectives (e.g., need for rapid onset or long duration of action).

The major routes of drug administration are *enteral* (oral), *parenteral* (IV, IM, subcut), inhalation, and topical. Enteral, parenteral, and inhalation routes typically produce systemic effects. Systemic effects extend beyond the area of drug application or administration. Drugs that are applied topically usually produce a local effect. Local effects occur predominantly at or near the site of application. These are general rules. Some drugs that are administered orally produce a local effect (e.g., antacids, neomycin), and some drugs administered by injection produce a local effect (e.g., local anesthetics). Transdermal patches produce systemic effects.

Enteral Drug Administration

Oral administration is safe and easy compared with parenteral administration. No special techniques are required for administration and, if needed, the drug can be removed from the body via vomiting (emesis) or binding with activated charcoal. Drugs available for oral administration are generally less expensive than their parenteral dosage form. All orally administered drugs must disintegrate and dissolve into solution before they can be absorbed and distributed. This process is the pharmaceutical phase of drug disposition. Tablets and capsules contain binders and fillers that can influence the rate and extent of disintegration and dissolution.

Disadvantages of oral administration are variable absorption and decreased bioavailability. *Bioavailability* is the fraction of the administered drug dose that enters the systemic circulation and is available to produce drug effect. The extent to which a drug is absorbed and distributed to the site of action may be influenced by the presence of food in the stomach, which can delay the absorption of some drugs and aid the absorption of others. The first-pass effect, a process whereby the liver metabolizes a fraction of an administered dose of drug before it passes into the general circulation, also reduces bioavailability (see Chapter 2).

> ● *TECH NOTE!*
> It is important to apply warning labels to medications that inform the patient to TAKE WITH FOOD or TAKE ON AN EMPTY STOMACH.

There are other disadvantages to oral administration. Drugs that are swallowed must pass through the gastrointestinal (GI) tract. Stomach contents contain powerful acids and digestive enzymes. These acids and enzymes can significantly decrease the amount of drug to be absorbed or inactivate some drugs (e.g., penicillin G, insulin).

Parenteral Drug Administration

Parenteral administration is preferred when the patient is unable to swallow (e.g., unconscious) or is experiencing nausea and vomiting or the drug is poorly absorbed via an oral route. Medicines that are administered parenterally bypass the GI tract. Drugs administered parenterally directly enter the general circulation and therefore are not subject to degradation by GI and liver enzymes. The bioavailability of parenterally administered drugs is greater than that of orally administered drugs. An advantage of parenteral administration is the rapid onset of action. The amount of drug delivered parenterally can be carefully controlled by managing flow rates. The exact amount of drug circulating throughout the body cannot be controlled when drugs are administered orally. There are disadvantages to parenteral administration of drugs. Aseptic

TABLE 1.6	Summary of Potential Advantages and Disadvantages of Oral Versus Parenteral Administration	
Oral	**Intravascular**
Self-administration easy	Self-administration difficult
Safer; recall by emesis	No recall
Absorption slower	Absorption faster
Less expensive	Relatively expensive
Bioavailability lower	Bioavailability higher
Degraded by gastrointestinal enzymes	Not degraded by gastrointestinal enzymes
Subject to the "first-pass effect"	Not subject to the "first-pass effect"
Sterile preparation not critical	Aseptic product preparation critical

technique must be used when preparing drugs for parenteral administration to avoid introducing life-threatening contaminants into the patient's bloodstream. After a drug has been administered parentally, it cannot be recalled through vomiting. Table 1.6 compares the advantages and disadvantages of oral and parenteral administration.

> ● *TECH NOTE!*
> Pharmacy technicians must carefully read the labels of medications to avoid dispensing errors. Many drugs are available for immediate release and slow depot release. Many are available in the same strength.

Parenteral drugs must be administered using specialized techniques. Proper injection procedures must be followed to avoid harm to the patient (Fig. 1.10). When a large volume of a drug is to be administered intravenously (injected into a vein), it must be injected slowly to avoid the destruction of red blood cells (hemolysis). Drugs formulated for IM administration (injected into a muscle) may produce a rapid onset or a slow onset of action. Rapid-onset formulations are typically prepared in water-soluble solutions. Slow-onset, prolonged-duration-of-action formulations are suspended in oil or other nonaqueous vehicles (solvent). As the vehicle diffuses out of the muscle into which it has been injected, the drug is slowly deposited. The drug is slowly released from the muscle depot.

> ● *TECH NOTE!*
> Make sure to double-check your calculations for parenteral medications. After being administered, the drug cannot be recalled from the body.

Drugs intended for subcutaneous injection pose fewer risks than intravascular administration; however, aseptic technique must still be followed, and the site of injection must be rotated to avoid complications.

• **Fig. 1.10** Forms of injection: intradermal injection, subcutaneous injection, and intramuscular injection. (From McCuistion LE, DiMaggio K, Winton MB, et al: *Pharmacology: a patient-centered nursing process approach*, ed 9, St. Louis, 2018, Elsevier.)

Inhalation

Inhalation is one of the most effective ways to rapidly deliver drugs locally to cells of the respiratory tract and into the general circulation. Absorption problems that are encountered with oral administration are avoided. Some of the side effects associated with oral or parenteral administration are minimized. Inhalation is an effective method for the delivery of medications used to treat asthma and other respiratory disorders. Some medicines used to produce general anesthesia are administered by inhalation.

Transdermal Drug Administration

Drugs that are formulated for transdermal administration are applied to the skin to produce systemic effects. Drugs such as nitroglycerin, estrogen, and testosterone, methylphenidate, nicoderm, and scopolamine are available for transdermal administration. Patients may experience systemic side effects and local side effects from drugs applied as transdermal patches. Local side effects such as skin irritation are often associated with the adhesives used to affix the patch to the skin and can be minimized by rotating the site where the patch is applied.

Topical

Topically administered drugs typically produce a local effect. For example, hydrocortisone cream applied to the skin will reduce itchiness and redness associated with rashes without the systemic side effects associated with oral administration of the drug unless the drug is applied to a large percentage of body surface area. Side effects associated with topical administration are usually localized to the site of application. Topical administration is not exclusively used to produce a local effect. Nitroglycerin cream, a drug used to in the treatment of angina, is an example of topically administered drug used for its systemic effects.

TECHNICIAN'S CORNER

1. The Kefauver-Harris Amendment (1962) requires all drugs to be safe and effective before they are made available to the public. Exactly what is involved in making a drug "safe and effective" for public use?
2. How would you explain to a client that a generic drug works just as well as a brand name drug?

Key Points

- Knowledge of pharmacology is essential to the accurate, effective, and efficient performance of pharmacy technician responsibilities.
- Pharmacy technicians possessing a substantial knowledge of pharmacology may be able to reduce dispensing errors.
- Less time is spent searching for drugs when pharmacy technicians have good brand and generic name recognition and can perform their duties with greater independence.
- Knowledge of pharmacology facilitates selection of warning labels for drugs dispensed.
- Pharmacy technicians who possess a good understanding of pharmacology understand the importance of recognizing drug interactions, therapeutic duplication, and excessive dose alerts screened by the computer.
- People from around the globe have contributed to the knowledge of drugs.
- Drugs may come from natural or synthetic origins.

- Plants have been collected, cultivated, and harvested for their healing properties and used in the treatment of illness for centuries.
- Pharmacognosy is the study of the constituents of natural drugs that are responsible for their effects.
- Natural drugs may be derived from plants, animals, or minerals.
- Synthetic drugs may be a chemical modification of a natural drug or manufactured entirely from chemical ingredients unrelated to the natural drug.
- Drugs may also be produced by the process of bioengineering. Drugs produced by bioengineering are called *biopharmaceuticals*.
- Pharmacology is the study of the action of drugs on humans and animals.
- The new drug application process takes years to complete and includes preclinical research; clinical studies; phase 1, phase 2, and phase 3 drug trials; and phase 4 postmarket studies.

- The FDA regulates the new drug and IND process in the United States. The Therapeutic Products Directorate and the Marketed Health Products Directorate regulate new drugs in Canada.
- The name of a new drug is made according to standards set by the CDER.
- The generic name is the official or unofficial, nonproprietary drug name.
- The chemical name describes the molecular structure of the drug.
- The proprietary name, or brand name, is assigned by the drug manufacturer. Factors considered when selecting a suitable proprietary name are existing "look-alike" and "sound-alike" names and ease of association with the generic name or active ingredient name.
- Patent holders for new drugs are given up to 20 years of exclusive right to manufacture and distribute the new drug.
- Generic drugs contain the same active ingredient as the original manufacturer's drug in the same strength and in the same dosage form.
- Generic drugs may contain different inactive ingredients.
- Generic drugs are less expensive than brand name drugs.
- The Durham-Humphrey Amendment established the distinction between legend drugs and OTC drugs.
- The Kefauver-Harris Amendment requires all drugs be safe and effective before they are made available to the public.
- The Drug Price Competition Act and Patent Restoration Act encouraged the creation of generic drugs.
- Access to controlled substances is more restrictive than access to legend drugs because controlled substances may cause physical or psychological dependence.
- BTC drugs may be sold without a prescription, but access is restricted, and pharmacist intervention is required.
- Drugs are formulated for delivery by mouth, injection, inhalation, or topical application to skin or a mucous membrane. Factors influencing the choice for drug formulation are chemical properties of the drug and human physiology.
- The formulation of a drug is largely controlled by the chemical properties of the drug and human physiology.
- When a drug is available for administration by more than one route, the selection of one route of administration over another is made according to the properties of the drug, ease of administration, therapeutic objectives, and whether the patient has a preexisting disease.

- The major routes of drug administration are enteral (oral), parenteral (IV, IM, subcut), inhalation, and topical.
- The enteral, parenteral, and inhalation routes typically produce systemic effects.
- Topical administration is typically used to produce local effects but may be administered for systemic effects.
- Orally administered drugs must disintegrate and dissolve into solution before they can be absorbed and distributed. This process is called the pharmaceutical phase.
- Drugs that are swallowed must pass through the GI tract. Acids in the stomach and digestive enzymes can inactivate some drugs (e.g., penicillin G).
- Medicines that are administered parenterally bypass the GI tract. Drugs administered parenterally directly enter the general circulation and therefore are not subject to the degradation by GI and liver enzymes.
- An advantage to parenteral administration is the rapid onset of action.
- Aseptic technique must be used when preparing drugs for parenteral administration to avoid introducing life-threatening contaminants into the patient's bloodstream.
- When a large volume of a drug is to be administered intravenously (injected into a vein) it must be injected slowly to avoid destruction of red blood cells (hemolysis).
- Drugs formulated for IM administration (injected into a muscle) may produce a rapid onset or a slow onset of action. Rapid-onset formulations are typically prepared in water-soluble solutions, and slow-onset, prolonged duration of action formulations are suspended in oil or other nonaqueous vehicles (solvent).
- Inhalation is one of the most effective ways to rapidly deliver drugs locally to cells of the respiratory tract and into the general circulation. Inhalation is an effective method for delivery of medications used to treat asthma, other respiratory disorders, and general anesthetics.
- Drugs such as nitroglycerin, estrogen, and testosterone are formulated for transdermal administration (applied to the skin) but produce systemic effects.
- Transdermal patches may cause skin irritation, which is associated with the adhesive. Rotating the site of patch application can reduce risk of skin irritation.

Review Questions

1. Who was called the "father of pharmacology" and was a Greek physician known for his accurate observation of medicinal plants?
   a. Dioscorides
   b. Theophrastus
   c. Hippocrates
   d. Shen Nung
2. What is the study of the constituents of natural drugs that are responsible for their effects?
   a. Pharmacology
   b. Pharmacogenomics
   c. Pharmacognosy
   d. Pharmacokinetics

3. In 1906, what law was passed to protect the public from ineffective and harmful drugs?
   a. Pure Food and Drug Act
   b. Harrison Narcotic Act
   c. Pure Food Drug and Cosmetic Act
   d. None of the above
4. Which of the following drugs is *not* made from a plant?
   a. Morphine
   b. Fentanyl
   c. Quinine
   d. Digitalis
5. The study of pharmacology applies knowledge of
   a. Properties of drugs
   b. Mechanism of drug action
   c. Anatomy, physiology, and pathology
   d. All of the above

6. Which of the following is **not** a step in developing and receiving approval for a new drug?
   a. Preclinical research
   b. Clinical studies
   c. Marketing
   d. New drug application process and review

7. The official, nonproprietary name of the drug is the
   a. Generic name
   b. Trade name
   c. Brand name
   d. Chemical name

8. Which drugs can be obtained **only** by prescription?
   a. Herbal remedies
   b. Legend
   c. Compounded
   d. All of the above

9. Which of the following is **not** an oral formulation?
   a. Tablet
   b. Capsule
   c. Suspension
   d. Suppository

10. Parenterally administered drugs must be prepared using
   a. Aseptic technique in sterile environment
   b. Countertops cleaned with alcohol
   c. Patient carts in nursing units
   d. None of the above

Bibliography

Basch E, Ulbricht C: *Natural standard herb & supplement handbook: the clinical bottom line*, St Louis, 2005, Mosby.

Food and Drug Administration (2017). CDER data standards manual. Retrieved from https://www.fda.gov/Drugs/DevelopmentApprovalProcess/FormsSubmissionRequirements/ElectronicSubmissions/DataStandardsManualmonographs/ucm071748.htm. (Accessed 6 October 2017).

Food and Drug Administration (2015). PDUFA Legislation and Background. Retrieved October 6, 2017, from https://www.fda.gov/ForIndustry/UserFees/PrescriptionDrugUserFee/ucm144411.htm.

Food and Drug Administration (2017). Development & Approval Process (Drugs). Retrieved October 6, 2017, from https://www.fda.gov/Drugs/DevelopmentApprovalProcess/default.htm.

Food and Drug Administration (2017). Drugs@FDA Glossary of Terms. Retrieved October 6, 2017, from http://www.fda.gov/Drugs/InformationOnDrugs/ucm079436.htm?utm_campaign=Google2&utm_source=fdaSearch&utm_medium=website&utm_term=glossary&utm_content=1.

Goodman L, Gilman A: *The pharmacological basis of therapeutics*, ed 5, New York, 1975, Macmillan, pp 1–8.

Haas LF: Neurological stamp: Papyrus of Ebers and Smith, *J Neurol Neurosurg Psychiatry* 67:578, 1999.

Jennifer LE (2017). The Merck Manual Consumer Version. Introduction to Administration and Kinetics of Drugs. Retrieved October 6, 2017 from http://www.merck.com/mmhe/sec02/ch010/ch010a.html.

National Library of Medicine, History of Medicine Division: Classics of traditional Chinese medicine. https://www.nlm.nih.gov/exhibition/chinesemedicine/emperors.html.

Shargel L, Mutnick A, Souney P, et al: *Comprehensive pharmacy review*, ed 4, Philadelphia, 2001, Lippincott Williams & Wilkins, pp 28–66.

Tyler V, Brady L, Robbers J: *Pharmacognosy*, ed 9, Philadelphia, 1988, Lea & Febiger, pp 1–6.

United States Drug Enforcement Administration: Title 21: food and drugs, chapter 13: drug abuse prevention and control. https://www.deadiversion.usdoj.gov/21cfr/21usc/index.html.

Wiktorowicz ME, Lexchin J, Moscou K, et al: *Keeping an eye on prescription drugs, keeping Canadians safe. Active monitoring systems for drug safety and effectiveness in Canada and internationally*, Toronto, 2010, Health Council of Canada. http://publications.gc.ca/collections/collection_2011/ccs-hcc/H174-21-2010-eng.pdf.

2

Principles of Pharmacology

LEARNING OBJECTIVES

1. Give a definition for each pharmacokinetic phase.
2. Describe factors that influence each pharmacokinetic phase.
3. Explain the importance of the first-pass effect.
4. Describe the function of the blood-brain barrier.
5. List major routes of drug elimination.
6. Describe elimination half-life.
7. Explain the importance of bioavailability to generic drug substitution.
8. Learn the terminology associated with the principles of pharmacology.

KEY TERMS

Absorption Process involving the movement of drug molecules from the site of administration into the circulatory system.

Anion Negatively charged particle.

Bicarbonate Substance used as a buffer to maintain the normal levels of acidity (pH) in blood and other fluids in the body.

Bioavailability The fraction of an administered dose that enters the systemic circulation in an unchanged form and is available to produce its effects.

Bioequivalent drug Drug that shows no statistical differences in the rate and extent of absorption when it is administered in the same strength, dosage form, and route of administration as the brand name product.

Biotransformation Process of drug metabolism in the body that transforms a drug to a more active, equally active, or inactive metabolite.

Colloids Proteins or other large molecules that remain suspended in the blood for a long period of time and are too large to cross membranes.

Crystalloids Intravenous solutions that contain electrolytes in concentrations similar to those of plasma.

Electrolytes Small charged molecules essential for homeostasis that play an important role in body chemistry.

Diffusion Passive movement of molecules across cell membranes from an area of high drug concentration to lower concentration.

Distribution Process of movement of the drug from the circulatory system across barrier membranes to the site of drug action.

Duration of action Time between the onset of action and discontinuation of drug action.

Elimination Process that results in the removal of drug from the body.

Enzyme Protein capable of causing a chemical reaction. Enzymes are involved in the metabolism of some drugs.

First-pass effect Process whereby only a fraction of an orally administered drug reaches systemic circulation because much of the drug is metabolized in the liver to an inactive metabolite before entering the general circulation.

Half-life (t$^{1/2}$) Length of time it takes for the plasma concentration of an administered drug to be reduced by half.

Hydrophilic Having a strong affinity for water; water loving. Able to dissolve in and absorb water.

Hydrophobic Lacking an affinity for water; water hating. Resistant to wetting.

Ionization Chemical process involving the gain or release of a proton (H$^+$). Ionized drug molecules may have a positive or negative charge.

Lipid Fatlike substance.

Lipophilic Having an affinity for lipids; lipid loving.

Metabolism Biochemical process involving transformation of active drugs to a compound that can be easily eliminated, or the conversion of prodrugs to active drugs.

Metabolite Product of drug metabolism. Metabolites may be inactivated drugs or active drugs with equal or greater activity than the parent drug.

Microvilli Brushlike border of each villus in the small intestine; increases the surface area for absorption.

Onset of action Time it takes for drug action to begin.

Osmosis The movement of water across a semipermeable membrane from a higher to lower concentration.

Peak effect Maximum drug effect produced by a given dose of drug after the drug has reached its maximum concentration in body.

Pharmaceutical alternative Drug that contains the same active ingredient as the brand name drug; however, the strength and dosage form may be different.

Pharmaceutical equivalent Drug that contains identical amount of active ingredient as brand name drug but may have different inactive ingredients, be manufactured in a different dosage form, and exhibit different rates of absorption.

Pharmacokinetics Science dealing with what the body does to a drug, which includes the study of absorption, distribution, metabolism, and elimination.

Prodrug Drug administered in an inactive form that is metabolized in the body to an active form.

Therapeutic alternative Drug that contains different active ingredient(s) than the brand name drug yet produces the same desired therapeutic outcome.

Pharmacokinetics

The word *pharmacokinetics* is derived from the Greek words pharmaco ("drug") and kinesis ("movement"). There are four pharmacokinetic phases. They are absorption, distribution, metabolism, and elimination (ADME). Drugs that are administered must be absorbed into the bloodstream and distributed to their site of action before they can begin to produce their effect. The body metabolizes the drug, and then it is eliminated. As a drug moves throughout the body, it undergoes changes that may increase or decrease its absorption, distribution, metabolism, or elimination. These pharmacokinetic phases control the intensity of the drug's effect and the duration of the drug action (Fig. 2.1).

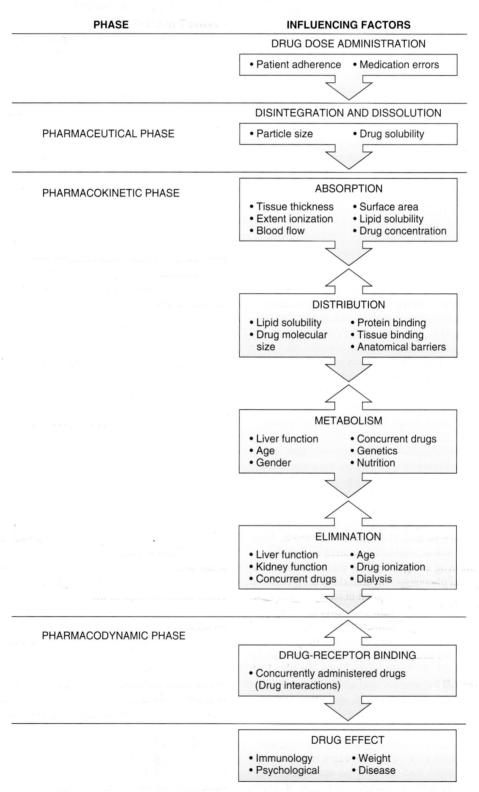

PHASE	INFLUENCING FACTORS
	DRUG DOSE ADMINISTRATION
	• Patient adherence • Medication errors
PHARMACEUTICAL PHASE	**DISINTEGRATION AND DISSOLUTION**
	• Particle size • Drug solubility
PHARMACOKINETIC PHASE	**ABSORPTION**
	• Tissue thickness • Surface area • Extent ionization • Lipid solubility • Blood flow • Drug concentration
	DISTRIBUTION
	• Lipid solubility • Protein binding • Drug molecular size • Tissue binding • Anatomical barriers
	METABOLISM
	• Liver function • Concurrent drugs • Age • Genetics • Gender • Nutrition
	ELIMINATION
	• Liver function • Age • Kidney function • Drug ionization • Concurrent drugs • Dialysis
PHARMACODYNAMIC PHASE	**DRUG-RECEPTOR BINDING**
	• Concurrently administered drugs (Drug interactions)
	DRUG EFFECT
	• Immunology • Weight • Psychological • Disease

• **Fig. 2.1** Phases of drug distribution.

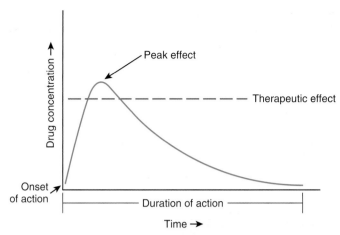

• **Fig. 2.2** Onset of action, peak effect, duration of action, and therapeutic effect.

> **● *TECH NOTE!***
>
> A good way to remember the order of the pharmacokinetic phases is to use the acronym ADME.

The length of time it takes for drug action to begin after a dose is administered is called the *onset of action*. The onset of action is not achieved until the drug reaches the minimum concentration in the body needed to produce drug action. The maximum drug effect, or *peak effect*, occurs after the maximum drug concentration of the drug is reached in the body. The *duration of action* is the time between the onset of action and discontinuation of drug action. The duration of action is the amount of time the drug concentration remains within the therapeutic range (Fig. 2.2).

Pharmacokinetic Phases

Absorption

Absorption is the first pharmacokinetic phase. Absorption is the process that involves the movement of drug molecules from the site of administration, across cell membranes, and into the circulatory system of the body (blood or lymphatic system). Absorption may occur across the skin or cells that line blood vessels. How quickly or slowly a drug is absorbed is determined by the characteristics of the drug, the drug dosage form, the route of administration, human anatomy, and physiology. The amount of drug absorbed is also influenced by many factors. Absorption of tablets and capsules that have been swallowed does not begin until after the drug goes into solution, so factors effecting disintegration or dissolution of the drug (pharmaceutical phase) can decrease absorption (see Chapter 1). Absorption of drugs taken by mouth may also be delayed when food is present in the stomach. The ease with which the drug is able to cross cell membranes is a factor with how readily the drug is absorbed via oral, rectal, vaginal, and other routes of administration.

Cell Membrane

Drug movement from the site of administration into the circulatory system depends on the ability of the drug to move across cell membranes. The cell membrane is a complex structure of *lipids,* protein, and water-filled channels (Fig. 2.3). Movement across the cell membrane is restricted unless the drug can pass through the lipid layers of the cell membrane or is small enough to pass through the small water-filled (aqueous) channels. A lipid-soluble drug can move easily across the cell membrane. Caffeine, vitamin C (ascorbic acid), vitamin B_3 (niacin), and ephedrine are examples of drugs that pass through aqueous channels in the cell membrane.

Drug Transport Mechanisms

Passive Transport

Drug absorption across the cell membrane may occur via passive or active transport mechanisms. Drugs that are absorbed by passive diffusion move from a region of greater concentration to a region of lesser concentration. When the drug first enters the body, the concentration at the administration site is greater than in the bloodstream. Lipid-soluble drugs readily diffuse across the cell membrane of the blood vessel into the bloodstream. Lipid-soluble drugs are *lipophilic* (lipid loving) and *hydrophobic*, or water hating. Water-soluble drugs are *hydrophilic*, or water loving, and move through the small water channels in the cell membrane. Most drugs are transported via passive transport.

Active Transport

Active transport mechanisms permit the drug to move across cell membranes without regard to concentration. A drug can move from an area where drug concentration is low to an area where the concentration is high. Active transport takes energy and requires special carrier proteins or pumps to "carry the drug" across the cell membrane.

Factors Influencing Absorption

Effect of pH on Drug Absorption

Most drugs are either weak acids or weak bases. In solution, weak acids and weak bases exist between the ionized and the nonionized state. In solution, weak acids (HA) disassociate, releasing a proton (H^+) and negatively charged *anion* (A^-).

$$HA \rightleftarrows H^+ + A^-$$

Weak bases also release a proton when they are in solution; however, when the proton is released, the resulting drug molecule is nonionized (uncharged).

$$B^+H \rightleftarrows B + H^+$$

Weakly acidic drugs are more ionized when they are in basic solutions. When the drugs are in an acidic solution, they are less ionized. Weakly basic drugs are more ionized when they are in acidic solution and less ionized in basic solution. This is important because as the drug travels throughout the body, it passes through acidic solutions (e.g., in the stomach) and basic solutions (e.g., in the small intestine). The ability of a drug to diffuse across the cell membrane depends on properties of the drug and the pH of the body fluid in which it is dissolved. The pH is a measure of how acidic or alkaline (basic) a solution is. A pH of 1 is very acidic (e.g., stomach acids [HCl]). A pH of 7 is neutral. Plasma has a pH between the range of 7.35 and 7.45. A pH of greater than 7 is alkaline. Intravenous solutions that contain *electrolytes* in concentrations similar to those of plasma are called *crystalloids*.

Diffusion across the cell membrane is greatest when the drug is lipid soluble and nonionized. When a weakly acidic drug such as phenobarbital is in the stomach, it is less ionized and can readily cross the cell membranes. Absorption is high. When the drug moves into the small intestine, ionization increases and absorption is reduced. *Osmosis* is the movement of water across a

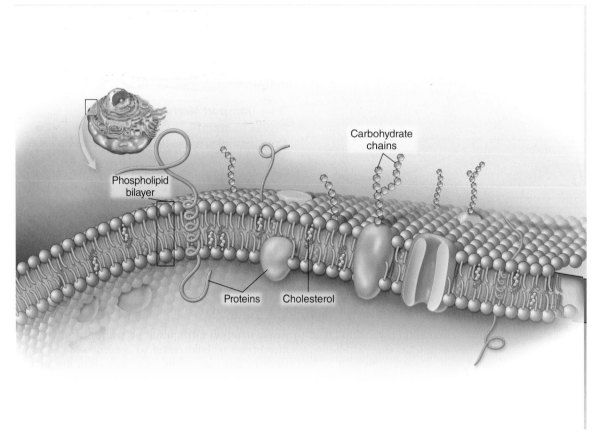

• **Fig. 2.3** Plasma membrane. (From Patton KT, Thibodeau GA: *The human body in health and disease,* ed 7, St. Louis, 2018, Elsevier.)

semipermeable membrane from a higher to lower concentration. Electrolytes are more concentrated inside than outside the cells, and the water outside the cells is less concentrated, or dilute, because it contains fewer electrolytes.

Effect of Blood Flow on Drug Absorption

Absorption is greatest in areas of the body that have a good blood supply. Medications administered sublingually have good absorption because many blood vessels are located under the tongue. Absorption of orally administered drugs is greatest in the small intestine. The structure of the intestine is designed to perform the specialized job of absorption. Thousands of *microvilli* line the walls of the small intestine. The microvilli are filled with blood vessels. As the drug passes through the cell membrane of the microvilli, it is quickly absorbed into the bloodstream. Absorption of drugs that are injected intramuscularly or subcutaneously is increased when the patient applies heat to the muscle, exercises, or does some other activity to stimulate blood flow to the site of administration.

Effect of Surface Area on Drug Absorption

Microvilli also increase the surface area of the small intestine, making it the largest absorbing surface in the body (Fig. 2.4). The area for absorption in the small intestine is approximately 1000 times greater than in the stomach.

Effect of Contact Time at the Absorption Surface

Drug absorption increases the longer the drug is in contact with the absorbing surface. Drug absorption is decreased if the patient has diarrhea because of the rapid passage of contents through the gastrointestinal (GI) tract. Absorption of delayed-release drugs can be increased when a drug is taken with food because of delayed gastric emptying.

Effect of Tissue Thickness on Absorption

Drug absorption is greater across single cell membranes than multiple cell layers because some drugs may become trapped in cell layers. As tissue thickness increases, the portion of the drug trapped in the cell layers increases.

Distribution

Distribution is the process of movement of the drug from the circulatory system across barrier membranes to the site of drug action (Fig. 2.5). It is the second pharmacokinetic phase. The volume of drug that is distributed is influenced by the properties of the drug, the extent of drug binding to blood proteins or tissue, the blood supply to the region, and the ability of the drug to cross natural body barriers. The drug may be distributed to water compartments of the body or to fat cells or proteins. Water compartments include plasma, extracellular fluid, and total body water.

Body Fluid Compartments and Electrolytes

Extracellular fluid consists mainly of the plasma found in the blood vessels and the interstitial fluid that surrounds the cells. Intracellular fluid refers to the water inside the cells.

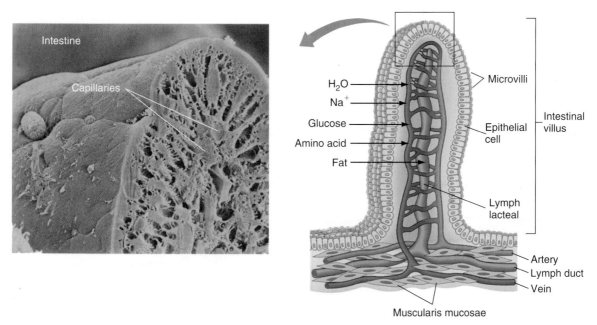

• **Fig. 2.4** Intestinal villi showing absorbing surfaces. (From Patton KT, Thibodeau GA: *Anatomy and physiology*, ed 9, St. Louis, 2016, Elsevier.)

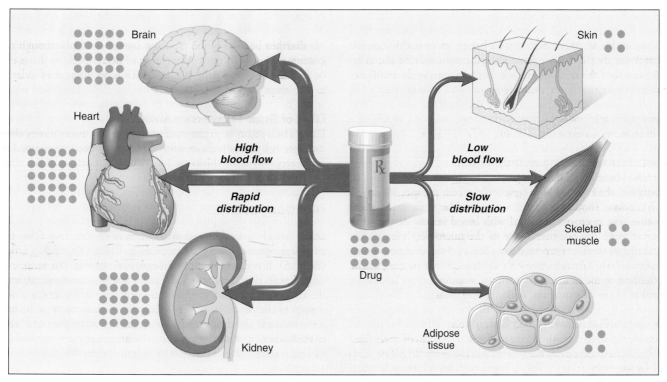

• **Fig. 2.5** Distribution. (From Raffa RB, Rawls SM, Beyzarov EP: *Netter's illustrated pharmacology*, Philadelphia, 2005, WB Saunders.)

Sodium, potassium and chloride are major electrolytes found in the body. Sodium is the major positive ion in extracellular fluid. Sodium regulates the total amount of water in the body and the transmission of sodium into and out of individual cells. It plays a role in critical processes in the brain, nervous system, and muscles that require electrical signals for communication.

Potassium is the other major cation found inside of cells. The proper level of potassium is essential for normal cell function. Regulation of the heartbeat and muscle contraction are two important functions of potassium.

Chloride is the major anion (negatively charged ion) found in the fluid outside of cells and in blood.

> **TECH NOTE!**
>
> 0.9% sodium chloride (NaCl) is also known as normal saline (NS) because it is the same concentration (isotonic) as in the body.

> **TECH NOTE!**
>
> Water follows sodium ions when they are moved through the cell membrane. Lots of sodium in the body means that water stays inside (instead of leaving through kidney cells and then the bladder), which means that there is more blood volume and blood pressure is higher.

Factors Influencing Distribution

Effect of Drug Properties on Distribution

The distribution of a drug across the blood vessel cell membrane and transport to its site of action are influenced by the chemical nature of the drug, such as lipid solubility. Drugs that are lipid soluble, nonionized, or size small enough to pass through slit junctions in the capillary wall are readily distributed. Slit junctions located in the capillaries vary in size. Slit junctions in the capillaries of the brain are so tight that drugs cannot pass through them. On the other hand, slit junctions in the capillaries of the liver and spleen are larger, and the size of the drug molecule is less of a limiting factor to drug distribution.

Effect of Protein Binding on Distribution

The blood contains albumin, a plasma protein. Many drugs have an affinity for albumin and bind (reversible) to the protein. When the drug is bound to plasma proteins, it is unable to move out of the blood vessels to get to the site of drug action. *Colloids*, proteins, or other large molecules that are too large to cross membranes remain suspended in the blood for a long period of time. Plasma proteins act like a drug reservoir for the bound drug trapped within the blood vessels. As the concentration of unbound or "free" drug decreases in the bloodstream, the drug that is bound to the plasma protein is released and transported to the site of action. When two drugs are administered that both have an affinity for plasma albumin, the drug with the greatest affinity will competitively bind to the protein. Albumin has the greatest affinity for weak acids and hydrophobic drugs. This competition for albumin binding can result in the release of bound drug, enabling it to get to its site of action. Severe burns can decrease plasma protein levels (hypoalbuminemia), which may alter the level of "free drug." Competitive protein binding represents a mechanism for drug interactions (Fig. 2.6).

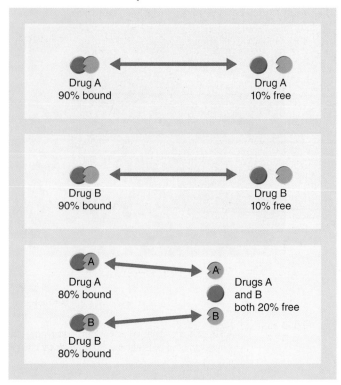

• **Fig. 2.6** Protein binding and free fraction of drugs. (From Page C, Hoffman B, Curtis M, et al: *Integrated pharmacology*, ed 3, Philadelphia, 2006, Mosby.)

Anatomic Barriers to Distribution

Natural body barriers may limit access to the site of drug action. The anatomic structures that selectively limit drug access are the blood-brain barrier, blood-placenta barrier, and blood-testicular barrier.

The blood-brain barrier is composed of cells lining the capillaries of the brain that form tight junctions (Fig. 2.7). The blood vessels in the brain are also surrounded by fatty structures called *glial feet* (also known as *astrocyte foot processes*). These structures limit the passage of ions between the capillaries and brain tissue. They permit passage of lipid-soluble, hydrophobic drugs into the brain and limit access of ionized hydrophilic drugs.

The blood-placenta barrier limits access of drugs taken by a pregnant woman to the fetus; however, many drugs are able to cross the blood-placenta barrier, so it is important for pregnant women to ask their physicians or pharmacists about potential safety issues before taking a drug. Prior to 2015, drugs were classified in five pregnancy safety categories (A, B, C, D, and X). Drugs classified in pregnancy safety category A were shown to be safe when taken during pregnancy. Fetal abnormalities were reported in drugs listed in category X. In 2015, the FDA replaced this system of classification. New rules require manufacturers to include a summary of the drugs risks if taken during pregnancy and lactation, description of data supporting the drug summary, information to aid in counseling of pregnant women, and health care provider prescribing.

Metabolism

Few drugs that are administered are eliminated unchanged. Most drugs are transformed by *enzymes* to a *metabolite(s)*.

TABLE 2.1	Products of Metabolism		
Parent Drug	**Example**	**Metabolite**	**Example**
Active drug	6-Mercaptopurine	Inactive drug	6-Mercapturic acid
Active drug	Prednisolone Imipramine	Equally active drug	Prednisone Desipramine
Active drug	Diazepam Codeine	More active drug	Oxazepam Morphine
Inactive drug	Fosamprenavir Levodopa Fosinopril	Active drug	Amprenavir Dopamine Fosinoprilat

• **Fig. 2.7** Barriers. (A, Courtesy Marie Simar Couldwell, MD, and Maiken Nedergaard. In Patton KT, Thibodeau GA: *Anatomy of physiology*, ed 9, St. Louis, 2016, Elsevier. B and C, From Patton KT, Thibodeau GA: *Anatomy and physiology*, ed 9, St. Louis, 2016, Elsevier.)

Biotransformation is the process of drug metabolism in the body that transforms a drug to a more active, equally active, or inactive metabolite. The primary site of biotransformation is the liver; however, metabolism may occur in the intestines, lung, kidney, or other cells in the body. Microsomal enzymes in the liver are responsible for transforming lipophilic drugs to compounds that can be more easily eliminated by the kidney. The cytochrome P-450 (CYP450) system is frequently involved in this process. Drugs that interfere with the enzymes of the CYP450 system can enhance or inhibit the metabolism of other drugs that are taken concurrently. Phenobarbital, a drug used in the treatment of epilepsy, increases metabolic enzyme activity of other antiseizure medications (phenytoin, valproic acid), resulting in increased elimination of the drugs. This decreases their effectiveness. CYP450 activity is also found in the mucous membranes of the nose. Metabolic enzymes are found in saliva and are secreted by bacteria in the intestines.

Not all drugs are metabolized to inactive metabolites. Table 2.2 shows the potential products of metabolism.

Latanoprost is a drug that is used to treat glaucoma. It is an example of a drug that is metabolized in the eye rather than in the liver. It is also a good example of a prodrug. *Prodrugs* are drugs that are administered in an inactive form and must be metabolized to their active form. Drugs may be formulated as prodrugs to avoid side effects or to increase distribution to the site of action. Levodopa is a prodrug that is metabolized to dopamine in the brain. The drug is used to treat Parkinson disease. Levodopa is able to cross the blood-brain barrier better than dopamine. Administration of the prodrug increases the volume of drug distributed into the brain. Adding the drug carbidopa to levodopa further increases the amount of drug that is converted to dopamine, because carbidopa interrupts levodopa metabolism outside the brain.

"First-Pass Effect"

Orally administered drugs must pass into the hepatoportal circulation (liver) before entering the general circulation. The *first-pass effect* is a process whereby only a fraction of an orally administered drug reaches systemic circulation. Much of the drug is metabolized in the liver to an inactive metabolite before passing into the general circulation (Fig. 2.8). Orally administered nitroglycerin is approximately 90% cleared during a single pass through the liver. Sublingual administration avoids the first-pass effect because drugs administered by this route can pass directly into the general circulation, through the many blood vessels located under the tongue, before passing through the liver. Morphine is also subject to the first-pass effect.

Factors Influencing Metabolism

When metabolism is increased, the duration of effect of many drugs is reduced except prodrugs, for which the onset of drug action begins with metabolism.

Effect of Liver Function on Metabolism

The liver is the primary site for metabolism. If the liver is functioning below capacity, metabolism is decreased. Drug doses are often be reduced in the presence of liver dysfunction.

Effect of Disease on Metabolism

Diseases such as hepatitis decrease the metabolic capacity of the liver. Lung disease and kidney disease can also reduce the ability of the body to metabolize drugs. Heart failure decreases blood flow to the liver, altering the extent of drug metabolism.

Effect of Age on Metabolism

Metabolism in the liver is decreased in elderly adults and in infants. Age-related changes in the liver decrease metabolic enzyme function in elderly adults. Metabolizing enzyme systems (CYP450) are not fully developed in infants; therefore their ability to metabolize drugs is decreased. Infants and elderly adults generally require lower doses of drug to produce therapeutic effects.

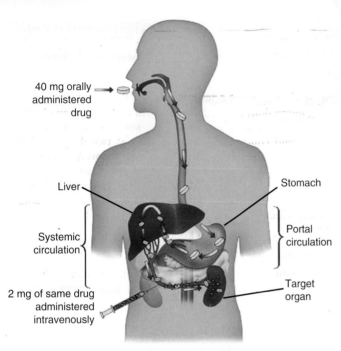

40 mg orally administered drug

Liver

Systemic circulation

2 mg of same drug administered intravenously

Stomach

Portal circulation

Target organ

• **Fig. 2.8** The first-pass effect. (From Lilley LL, Aucker RS: *Pharmacology and the nursing process*, ed 3, St. Louis, 2001, Mosby.)

Effect of Concurrent Administration of Drugs (Interactions)

Administration of two or more drugs that both use the same metabolic pathways can alter the metabolism of each other. CYP450 isoform substrates are a large group of metabolic enzymes. The metabolism of many drugs is altered by the coadministration of CYP450 substrate inducers or inhibitors. Enzyme inducer–substrate binding increases metabolic enzyme activity, and enzyme inhibitor–substrate binding decreases metabolic enzyme activity. For example, the metabolism of phenytoin is decreased when it is administered concurrently with the antifungal agents ketoconazole and fluconazole, which are metabolic enzyme inducers.

Cigarette smoke contains ingredients that can stimulate the activity of metabolic enzymes. These enzymes increase the metabolism and clearance of theophylline, a drug used to treat asthma.

Effect of Genetics on Metabolism

A genetic deficiency of a metabolic enzyme can reduce the body's ability to metabolize drugs that use the enzyme. NutraSweet (aspartame) is a common sweetener found in diet foods and beverages. It is a derivative of the amino acid phenylalanine. People diagnosed with the disorder phenylketonuria lack the enzyme needed to metabolize the amino acid phenylalanine to tyrosine. If they consume products containing aspartame, then they may build up toxic levels of phenylalanine.

Effect of Nutrition on Metabolism

Metabolism is decreased when nutritional status is severely depressed, as in starvation. Low-protein diets and diets deficient in essential fatty acids can reduce the synthesis of drug-metabolizing enzymes and decrease metabolism. Deficiencies of vitamins and minerals can affect metabolism because they catalyze biochemical reactions in the body. For example, vitamin B_2 catalyzes oxidation-reduction reactions. Oxidation and reduction are metabolic processes that result in drug inactivation.

Foods can influence metabolism of drugs. Many drug interactions are linked to consumption of grapefruit juice. Grapefruit juice is

TABLE 2.3	Routes of Drug Elimination
Routes	**Eliminated in**
Major	
Kidney	Urine
Lung	Expired air
Bowel	Feces
Minor	
Liver	Bile
Skin	Sweat
Eyes	Tears
Mouth	Saliva
Nose	Mucus
Penis	Semen
Breast	Breast milk

an inhibitor of metabolic enzyme CYP3A4. When drugs that have a CYP3A4 substrate, such as the anticholesterol drug lovastatin and the antiretroviral drug saquinavir, are taken with grapefruit juice, metabolism is reduced, and blood levels of the drugs can increase, along with drug effects.

> **◦ TECH NOTE!**
>
> Be sure to apply the warning label stating: "DO NOT TAKE WITH GRAPEFRUIT JUICE" when appropriate.

Effect of Gender on Metabolism

The rate of metabolism of some drugs varies between men and women, suggesting the sex hormones may influence metabolism. Men metabolize propranolol (a heart drug) faster than do women. Women metabolize acetaminophen (an analgesic) slightly faster than do men.

Elimination

Elimination is the final pharmacokinetic phase. Elimination results in removal of the drug from the body and discontinuation of drug action. The three major routes of drug elimination are the kidney, lung, and bowel (Table 2.3).

The normal function of the kidney is to filter the blood and remove things that are foreign or harmful. This job is done by the nephrons of the kidney (Fig. 2.9). Free drug (not bound to albumin) is transported to Bowman capsule, where it is filtered by the glomerulus. As the drug moves through the nephron to the distal convoluted tubule, its concentration increases. If the drug is nonionized, it may diffuse out of the nephron back into the systemic circulation and continue to produce drug action. When the drug is ionized, elimination in the urine is increased.

Factors Influencing Elimination

Effect of Kidney Function on Elimination

Kidney dysfunction can have a profound effect on elimination of drugs from the body. Decreased kidney function decreases the extent of drug cleared and the rate of clearance. This can cause a buildup of drug in the body and produce toxic drug effects. Drugs that are highly eliminated via the kidneys require a reduction in dose to avoid toxicity when kidney function is impaired. When kidney function is critically impaired, dialysis is needed. Dialysis mechanically filters the blood and can increase drug elimination.

Effect of Drug Ionization on Elimination
Changes in the acidity of the urine can influence the rate in which a drug is cleared from the body. Weakly acidic drugs are less ionized in acidic urine. As the pH of the urine becomes more basic, the *ionization* of acidic drugs increases. Weak bases are more ionized when the urine is acidic and less ionized when the urine is basic. Drugs that are ionized are eliminated in the urine. Nonionized drugs are reabsorbed back into the circulatory system to continue their drug action.

Effect of Disease on Elimination
Lung, kidney, and bowel disease decrease the body's capacity to eliminate drugs and their metabolites. Bowel disease may increase or decrease elimination. Crohn disease causes excessive diarrhea,

which speeds the elimination of drugs. When movement of contents of the bowel is slowed, drug elimination is delayed. Lung diseases such as chronic obstructive pulmonary disease decrease elimination in expired air.

Effect of Concurrent Administration of Drugs (Interactions)
Drug interactions can result in increased or decreased elimination of drugs. Pharmacists and health care providers may purposefully recommend concurrent administration of two drugs to delay elimination and prolong drug action or to speed elimination. Urinary buffers may be administered to adjust the level of acidity in the urine that affects the degree of ionization. Urinary acidifiers (e.g., vitamin C) decrease the elimination of acidic drugs. Urinary alkalinizers (e.g., *bicarbonate*) decrease the elimination of basic drugs.

Elimination Half-Life ($t^{1/2}$)
Elimination *half-life ($t^{1/2}$)* refers to the time it takes for 50% of a drug to be cleared from the bloodstream. It takes approximately

Renal corpuscle — Bowman capsule
Glomerulus
Efferent arteriole
Juxtaglomerular (JG) apparatus
Afferent arteriole
Distal convoluted tubule (DCT)
Artery and vein
Peritubular capillaries
Ascending limb of Henle loop
Descending limb of Henle loop

Proximal convoluted tubule (PCT)
Peritubular capillaries
Collecting duct (CD)

• **Fig. 2.9** Nephron. (From Patton KT, Thibodeau GA: *The human body in health and disease,* ed 7, St. Louis, 2018, Elsevier.)

eight half-lives to entirely eliminate a drug from the body. Every drug has a unique half-life that is dependent on characteristics of the drug (e.g., active metabolites). Knowledge of elimination half-life is important; it is an indicator of how long a drug will produce effects in the body. The half-life of a drug can be as short as a few minutes (e.g., drugs used to produce general anesthesia) or as long as several days (e.g., levothyroxine, a drug used to treat hypothyroidism). Drugs with long half-lives are dosed less frequently than are drugs with very short half-lives.

Bioavailability and Bioequivalence of Drugs

Bioavailability is defined as the rate and extent to which the active ingredient of an administered drug enters the systemic circulation, reaches the site of action, and is available to produce its effect. The bioavailability of a drug is influenced by drug absorption, the first-pass effect, and distribution to the site of action. The bioavailability of generic drugs is compared with the innovator's product to determine if the generic is bioequivalent. Tests are conducted to measure maximum concentration (C_{max}) of the drug in the bloodstream after a single dose is administered. The time it takes to reach maximum concentration (T_{max}) is also measured. Bioavailability tests are conducted to determine if the generic drug achieves the same maximum blood concentration in the same time as the brand name drug. The generic is bioequivalent if no statistical differences are found in the rate and extent of absorption when the drug is administered in the same strength, dosage form, and route of administration as the brand name product.

Pharmaceutical Equivalents and Pharmaceutical Alternatives

Pharmaceutical equivalents differ from bioequivalents. *Bioequivalent drugs* and pharmaceutical equivalent drugs both contain the same active ingredient in the same strength as the innovator's drug (brand name). *Pharmaceutical equivalents* may have different inactive ingredients, be manufactured in a different dosage form, and exhibit different rates of absorption than the brand name. *Pharmaceutical alternatives* contain the same active ingredient as the brand name product; however, the strength and dosage form may be different. A *therapeutic alternative* may contain different active ingredients yet produce the same desired therapeutic outcome.

> **TECH NOTE!**
>
> Product substitution laws regulate the dispensing of generic drugs. Only generics that are bioequivalent can be substituted and dispensed when brand name drugs are prescribed.

> **TECHNICIAN'S CORNER**
>
> 1. What is the difference between bioavailability and bioequivalence?

Key Points

- There are four pharmacokinetic phases: absorption, distribution, metabolism, and elimination.
- As a drug moves throughout the body, it undergoes changes that may increase or decrease its absorption, distribution, metabolism, or elimination.
- Pharmacokinetic phases control the intensity of the drug's effect and the duration of the drug action.
- The onset of drug action begins once the drug reaches the minimum concentration necessary to produce a therapeutic effect.
- The peak effect occurs when the maximum concentration of the drug is reached in the body.
- Duration of action is the time between the onset of action and discontinuation of drug action.
- The pharmaceutical phase of drug disposition involves drug disintegration and dissolution.
- Drugs administered parenterally enter directly into the general circulation; therefore they are not subject to the first-pass effect and are not degraded by GI enzymes.
- The bioavailability of parenterally administered drugs is greater than orally administered drugs.
- Absorption is the process that involves the movement of drug molecules from the site of administration, across cell membranes, into the circulatory system of the body (blood or lymphatic system).
- Drugs are absorbed across cell membranes via active and passive transport mechanisms.
- Factors influencing absorption are chemical nature of the drug, pH, blood flow, surface area, and tissue thickness.
- Distribution is the process of movement of the drug from the circulatory system across barrier membranes to the site of drug action.
- Factors influencing distribution are the chemical nature of the drug, protein and tissue binding, and ability to move across anatomical barriers.
- Metabolism is a biochemical process involving enzymes that convert the administered drug to metabolites that are more active or less active than the original drug.
- Drugs that interfere with the enzymes of the CYP450 can enhance or inhibit the metabolism of other drugs that are taken concurrently.
- First-pass metabolism describes a process whereby only a fraction of an orally administered drug reaches systemic circulation because the drug is metabolized in the liver to an inactive metabolite before passing into the general circulation.
- Factors influencing metabolism are liver function, diseases, age, drug interactions, genetics, nutrition, and gender.
- Elimination results in removal of the drug from the body and discontinuation of drug action.
- Factors influencing elimination are kidney function, diseases, drug ionization, and drug interactions.
- Elimination half-life ($t^{1/2}$) refers to the time it takes for 50% of a drug to be cleared from the bloodstream. It takes approximately eight half-lives to eliminate a drug from the body.
- Bioavailability is the rate and extent to which the active ingredient of an administered drug enters the systemic circulation, reaches the site of action, and is available to produce its effect.

- A generic drug is bioequivalent if no statistical differences are found in the rate and extent of absorption when the drug is administered in the same strength, dosage form, and route of administration as the brand name product.
- Pharmaceutical equivalents may have different inactive ingredients, be manufactured in a different dosage form, and exhibit different rates of absorption than the brand name.
- Pharmaceutical alternatives contain the same active ingredient as the brand name drug; however, the strength and dosage form may be different.
- A therapeutic alternative may contain different active ingredients yet produce the same desired therapeutic outcome.

Review Questions

1. Name the four phases of pharmacokinetics.
   a. absorption, dissolution, catabolism, elimination
   b. absorption, distribution, metabolism, elimination
   c. assimilation, dissolution, metabolism, excretion
   d. assimilation, distribution, anabolism, excretion
2. Lipid-soluble drugs are _____.
   a. hydrophobic
   b. lipophobic
   c. lipophilic
   d. a and c
3. A process whereby the liver clears a portion of an administered dose of drug before it passes into the general circulation is known as the:
   a. first-pass effect
   b. dissolution effect
   c. metabolite effect
   d. liver-pass effect
4. A drug that contains different active ingredient(s) than the brand name drug yet produces the same desired therapeutic outcome is called a therapeutic _____.
   a. equivalent
   b. alternative
   c. substitution
   d. replacement
5. The process that involves the movement of drug molecules from the site of administration, across cell membranes into the circulatory system of the body is known as:
   a. distribution
   b. metabolism
   c. absorption
   d. elimination
6. Which factors might the pharmacist NOT consider when counseling a woman about the risks and benefits of taking a drug during pregnancy?
   a. The summary of drug risks described in the product packaging
   b. Data supporting the summary of potential risks listed in the package insert
   c. Anecdotal stories provided by friends, family, or found on websites
   d. Peer reviewed literature (journal articles)
7. The metabolism of drugs via biochemical processes involving enzymes to metabolites is termed:
   a. bioequivalence
   b. biotransformation
   c. bioavailability
   d. bioeffect
8. A drug that is administered in an inactive form and must be metabolized to its active form is called a(an):
   a. investigational drug
   b. metabolite
   c. prodrug
   d. none of the above
9. Which body organ serves as the primary site of the metabolism of drugs?
   a. kidney
   b. lungs
   c. stomach
   d. liver
10. The time it takes for 50% of the drug to be cleared from the bloodstream is termed the
   a. distribution half-life ($t^{1/2}$)
   b. elimination half-life ($t^{1/2}$)
   c. metabolism half-life ($t^{1/2}$)
   d. absorption half-life ($t^{1/2}$)

Bibliography

DiPiro JT, Talbert RL, Yee GC, et al: *Pharmacotherapy: A pathophysiologic approach*, ed 9, 2014, McGraw Hill.

Fulcher E, Soto C, Fulcher R: *Pharmacology: Principles and applications. A worktext for allied health professionals*, Philadelphia, 2003, WB Saunders, pp 21–22, 60–65, 83.

Indiana University School of Medicine: Flockhart Table ™ - Cytochrome P450 Drug Interaction Table, 2016. From http://medicine.iupui.edu/clinpharm/ddis/main-table.

Page CP, Hoffman BB, Curtis MJ, et al: *Integrated pharmacology*, Philadelphia, 2005, Elsevier Mosby, pp 57–70.

Raffa RB, Rawls SM, Beyzarov EP: *Netter's illustrated pharmacology*, Philadelphia, 2005, WB Saunders, pp 10–11, 25–27.

Shargel L, Mutnick A, Souney P, et al: *Comprehensive pharmacy review*, ed 4, Baltimore, 2001, Lippincott Williams & Wilkins, pp 78–84, 42–65, 131–132.

3

Pharmacodynamics

LEARNING OBJECTIVES

1. Explain the drug-receptor theory.
2. Compare and contrast agonists, antagonists, and partial agonists.
3. Illustrate the relationship between drug effectiveness and potency.
4. Discuss the importance of pharmacodynamics to drug action.
5. Discuss the factors influencing patient response to drug therapy.
6. List ways to improve patient adherence to drug therapy.
7. Learn terminology associated with pharmacodynamics and drug action.

KEY TERMS

Affinity Attraction that the receptor site has for the drug.
Agonist Drug that binds to its receptor site and stimulates a cellular response.
Antagonist Drug that binds to the receptor site and does not produce an action. An antagonist prevents another drug or natural body chemical from binding and activating the receptor site.
Efficacy Measure of a drug's effectiveness.
Idiosyncratic reaction Unexpected drug reaction.
Inverse agonist Drug that has affinity and activity at the receptor site. The drug can turn "off" a receptor that is activated or turn "on" a receptor that is not currently active.
Mechanism of action Manner in which a drug produces its effect.
Noncompetitive antagonist Drug that binds to an alternative receptor site that prevents the agonist from binding to and producing its desired action.

Partial agonist Drug that behaves like an agonist under some conditions and acts like an antagonist under different conditions.
Pharmacodynamics Study of drugs and their action on the living organism.
Pharmacotherapeutics Use of drugs in the treatment of disease. It is the study of factors that influence patient response to drugs.
Potency Measure of the amount of drug required to produce a response. It is the effective dose concentration.
Receptor site Location of drug-cell binding.
Therapeutic index (TI) Ratio of the effective dose to the lethal dose.

Pharmacodynamics

The previous chapter looked at how a drug is altered as it travels throughout the compartments of the body. *Pharmacodynamics* is the study of drugs and their action on a living organism. Pharmacodynamics looks at how the body responds to drugs that are administered. The *mechanism of action* (MOA) describes how the drug produces its effect. An understanding of pathophysiology and a drug's MOA can aid decision making about the best drug to treat a patient's medical condition. Pathophysiology is the study of disease in the body.

Drug-Receptor Interactions

According to *drug-receptor theory*, drugs interact or bind with targeted cells in the body to produce pharmacologic action. Most drugs bind with specific proteins in the body; however, they may also bind to carbohydrates, lipids, or enzymes. The location of drug-cell binding is called the *receptor site*. Drug-receptor binding is similar to the action of a lock and key (Fig. 3.1). The drug is the key, and the receptor site is the lock. The more similar the drug is to the shape of the receptor site, the greater the *affinity*, or attraction, that the receptor site has for the drug. When two or more drugs are administered, the receptor site will preferentially bind with the drug for which it has the greatest affinity (the drug that best fits the lock). Drug binding to the receptor is usually reversible. Most drugs spontaneously bind and disassociate with the receptor site.

Some drugs do not produce their actions by directly binding to a receptor site on the cell. They are able to produce a change in cell membrane stability or excitability through nonspecific mechanisms. Some general anesthetic gases produce their effects via nonspecific interactions.

Second Messengers

Drug response does not always occur by stimulation of the primary drug receptor. In some cases, stimulation of the primary receptor causes a second receptor to be activated, and it is only after the release of the second messenger that the desired drug effect is produced.

Types of Drug-Receptor Interactions

A drug may be classified as an agonist, partial agonist, antagonist, inverse agonist competitive antagonist, or noncompetitive antagonist, based on its effect at the receptor site (Table 3.1).

Agonists

An *agonist* is a drug that binds to and activates the receptor site, eliciting a cellular response (Fig. 3.2). Agonist binding may activate a receptor that was resting or turn off a receptor that was activated. *Inverse agonists* are drugs that have affinity at the receptor site but produce opposite actions (turn "off" a receptor that is activated or turn "on" a receptor that is not currently active). When two or more agonists are administered together, a competition for drug-receptor binding sites occurs. The drug with the greatest affinity will bind to the receptor site. The result of agonist binding may mimic the effects produced by binding of normal body chemicals to their target receptor. An example is the binding of barbiturates to their drug-receptor site. This mimics the effects produced by the neurotransmitter γ-aminobutyric acid (GABA), a chemical messenger of the nervous system, when it binds to its receptor site. Drug-receptor binding may also stimulate the release of a normal biologic chemical. For example, when the drug amantadine is administered, it stimulates the release of the neurotransmitter dopamine. An increase in dopamine levels reduces the symptoms associated with Parkinson disease. It is not necessary for all drug-receptor sites to be occupied before the maximum drug effect is achieved.

Antagonists

Antagonists bind to the receptor site and do not activate the receptor. They prevent another drug or natural body chemical from binding by occupying or inactivating the receptor site. Antagonists block the actions of agonists, inverse agonists, and partial agonists.

Naloxone is an example of a pure antagonist. Administration reverses the effects of opioids (e.g., fentanyl) by occupying the receptor site and preventing the fentanyl from binding.

Noncompetitive antagonists bind to an alternative site than the agonist to prevent the agonist from binding the receptor. Noncompetitive antagonist binding results in inactivation of the receptor site.

Partial Agonists

A *partial agonist* behaves like an agonist under some conditions and acts like an antagonist under different conditions. Buprenorphine is an example of a partial agonist. It behaves like an antagonist in patients who are under the influence of a high concentration of an agonist or when administered after recent exposure to high

• **Fig. 3.1** Drug-receptor interactions. (From Clayton BD, Willihnganz MJ: *Basic pharmacology for nurses*, ed 17, St. Louis, 2017, Elsevier.)

TABLE 3.1	Summary of Effects of Drug-Receptor Binding	
Interaction Term	**Definition**
Agonist	Drug binds to a receptor, and there is a response.
Partial agonist	Drug binds to a receptor, and there is a diminished response compared with that elicited by the agonist.
Antagonist	Drug binds to receptor, but there is no response. Drug prevents binding of agonists.
Competitive antagonist *Narcan*	Drug competes with the agonist for binding to receptor. If it binds, there is no response.
Noncompetitive antagonist	Drug combines with different parts of receptor and inactivates it, so agonist has no effect.

From Lilley LL, Collins SR, Snyder JS: *Pharmacology and the nursing process*, ed 8, St. Louis, 2017, Elsevier.

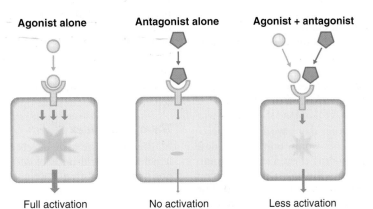

Agonist alone · Antagonist alone · Agonist + antagonist

Full activation · No activation · Less activation

• **Fig. 3.2** Effect of agonist and antagonist binding. Agonists are drugs that occupy receptors and activate them. Antagonists are drugs that occupy receptors but do not activate them. Antagonists block receptor activation by agonists.

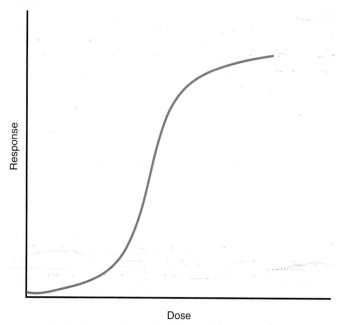

• **Fig. 3.3** Dose-response curve.

• **Fig. 3.4** Efficacy.

• **Fig. 3.5** Potency.

concentrations of an agonist but acts like an agonist in opioid-naïve patients that have not had any recent exposure to opioids.

Dose-Response Relationship

Typically, increasing the drug dose will increase the cellular response and a drug's effect. Many other factors may also influence the strength of the response to a dose of administered drug such as pharmacokinetic factors (absorption, distribution, metabolism, and elimination) and individual properties of a drug also influence drug response. A dose-response curve shows the relationship between the effect(s) of a drug and the administered dose. The effects produced by a given drug dose can be quantified and graphed. The graph is called a dose-response curve. The dose-response curve shows the drug's relative efficacy and potency (Fig. 3.3). A steep dose-response curve indicates that a small change in drug dose will produce a large change in the drug response. A flatter dose-response curve shows that a large increase in the dose of the drug administered is needed to produce a greater drug response.

Efficacy

Efficacy is a measure of the drug's effectiveness under controlled conditions, as opposed to real-world conditions (Fig. 3.4). The efficacy of an antagonist is measured by the extent to which it interferes with the effect of an agonist. Efficacy can be measured for each effect produced by a drug.

Potency

Efficacy and *potency* are related. Drugs that have a high efficacy at a low dose are very potent. In other words, only a small dose is required to produce the maximum drug effect. Drugs that must be administered in very high doses to produce a minimal effect have low potency. In Fig. 3.5, drug A is more potent than drug B and drug C because a lower dose produces an equal response.

Efficacy is more important than potency when determining usefulness of a drug, unless the dose that is required to produce the therapeutic effect is so large that it is impractical to administer.

When choosing between two equally effective drugs, pharmacokinetic factors, the disease, and the ability of the patient to tolerate the side effects of the drug become more important than the dose that is required to produce an effect.

Ceiling Effect

In Fig. 3.3 the dose-response curve shows that as the drug dose increases, the drug effect increases. Drug effects increase up to a ceiling. This ceiling effect may be reached when all drug receptors are saturated or when the maximum possible effect that could be produced is reached. For example, the ceiling effect for opioid analgesics is reached at the point when no more pain relief is achieved even if additional opioid is administered.

Therapeutic Index

All drugs produce toxic effects that can lead to death. When the lethal dose of a drug is close to the effective dose, the drug is not very safe. The safest drugs have a wide margin between the lethal dose and the effective dose. The *therapeutic index (TI)* is the ratio of the effective dose to the lethal dose; the formula is shown as follows. ED_{50} represents the effective dose for 50% of a population, and LD_{50} is the lethal dose for 50% of a population.

$$\text{Therapeutic index (TI)} = \frac{\text{Lethal dose (LD}_{50})}{\text{Effective dose (ED}_{50})}$$

Digoxin, a drug used to treat heart disease, has a narrow TI. The drug dose needed to increase the force of heart contractions is similar to the drug dose that can cause the heart to stop beating. Another drug with a small TI is warfarin. The dose required to prolong blood clotting time is near the dose that causes hemorrhage and death. Patients respond differently to different doses of drug. Variation in patient response to a drug can become critical when the TI is narrow.

■ TECH NOTE!

The pharmacy should consider the therapeutic index when making product substitution decisions, especially for drugs with a narrow therapeutic index (e.g., digoxin) or bioequivalency problems (e.g., phenytoin).

Factors Influencing Pharmacotherapeutics

Pharmacotherapeutics is the process of using drugs for the treatment of disease. Factors that influence patient response to drugs range from pharmacokinetics to patient-specific factors. A variety of patient-related factors ranging from the presence of chronic disease, drug allergies, age, obesity, or gender to the patient's belief that the therapy will be beneficial can affect the success of pharmacotherapy. Drug response is heightened if the patient has had a prior exposure to the drug that produced an allergic reaction and decreased if the patient has developed tolerance to the effects of the drug. The patient's response to a drug is not always predictable. Drug doses and dosing schedules should be modified to control for known factors that influence patient drug response.

Patient Physiologic Factors

Humans are unique, and individual variability influences the outcome of drug therapy. Physiologic factors that may affect drug response are described in this section. Desired therapeutic effects are achieved when optimum drug doses are administered. Doses that are too low result in subtherapeutic effects. Doses that are too high result in toxic effects.

Age

The human body undergoes physiologic and hormonal changes between birth and death. Age-related changes influence how effectively the body is able to handle drugs. Neonates and infants have an underdeveloped capacity to absorb, distribute, metabolize, and eliminate drugs. The ability of the lungs, liver, and kidneys to process and eliminate drugs declines as humans age. Elderly adults and infants require lower drug doses.

Weight

Drug doses for children are often calculated according to the child's weight; however, dose calculations based on body surface area are more accurate than those based on weight. Dose adjustments may need to be considered for obese or severely underweight adults. Drug doses must be increased in obese patients to produce therapeutic effects. Doses are decreased in severely underweight or emaciated adults and children to avoid toxic side effects.

Gender

Gender may influence drug distribution and metabolism. The fat-to-muscle ratio varies between women and men and may influence the volume of drug distribution. In addition, the rate of metabolism of some drugs varies between men and women, suggesting the sex hormones may influence metabolism.

Genetics

Genetics influences enzyme and protein production in the body. Absence of certain enzymes can produce deadly side effects in people who take drugs that require the enzyme for metabolism and elimination.

Disease

The presence of disease can significantly influence pharmacotherapeutics. More severe drug reactions can occur in patients with kidney disease, liver disease, or lung disease because their ability to distribute, metabolize, and eliminate drugs may be compromised. The effects of a drug may diminish because the disease itself becomes more debilitating over time. Parkinson disease is linked to progressive destruction of dopamine-releasing nerve cells in the body. The ability of anti–Parkinson disease drugs to improve patient symptoms decreases as the disease progresses.

Pregnancy

Drug response may be altered during pregnancy because of pregnancy-related physiologic changes. Gastrointestinal motility slows, which can increase drug absorption and drug effects. Pregnancy-related increases in blood volume, urination, and vomiting may alter drug absorption, distribution, and elimination that result in decreased drug response.

Immunologic Factors

Hypersensitivity reactions are extreme allergic reactions and can occur after a single dose of the drug or after multiple exposures to the drug. The reaction occurs because the patient develops antibodies to the drug. The presence of antibodies causes the release of histamine and other body chemicals that produce allergic symptoms. Symptoms may range from a mild rash to anaphylactic shock.

Desensitization

Repeated exposures to a drug may result in a decreased drug response. Desensitization is caused by changes to drug receptors (especially proteins) that decrease drug-receptor binding or reduce receptor site activation when binding occurs. When desensitization occurs, the effects can be limited to a single receptor or may influence multiple receptors. When drug-receptor binding involves a second messenger, the result may be desensitization to the effects that would have been produced by binding to multiple receptors (i.e., all of the receptors normally activated by binding of the drug to its primary receptor). Desensitization may be used therapeutically to minimize allergic reactions (e.g., allergy shots).

Idiosyncratic Reactions

Sometimes the response to a drug cannot be predicted. Unexpected drug reactions are known as *idiosyncratic reactions*.

Psychologic Factors

Drug therapy is influenced by the patient's belief that the therapy will be beneficial. Studies have shown that sugar pills can produce the desired effect if the patient believes they will be effective. This is known as the placebo effect. Double-blind clinical studies are conducted to control for the placebo effect. In a double-blind study, some of the people in the study receive a drug containing active ingredient, and others receive a drug look-alike that does not contain active ingredients. Neither the people taking the drugs nor their care providers know who is receiving the real drug. This reduces the risk that drug effects reported are caused by placebo effect. This also decreases the likelihood that care providers will treat their patient differently because they know they are receiving the active drug. Increased attention can also improve patient outcomes.

Adverse Drug Reactions

Few drugs are so specific that they produce only their desired therapeutic effect. Drugs may additionally produce undesired effects. Undesired effects are called adverse reactions. Approximately 10% of people who receive health care in industrialized countries will experience a preventable adverse drug reaction (ADR).

ADRs have an impact on patients, family members, employers, pharmacies, health care facilities, and society. ADRs can cause or prolong hospitalization, missed school or work, and even death. ADRs are estimated to cost more than $30 billion annually in the United States and nearly $36 million annually in Canada, with nearly 80% of drug-related costs due to hospitalization.

Some populations are at greater risk for ADRs than others. The elderly have an increased risk for ADRs because they are more likely to be on multiple-drug therapy and their capacity to metabolize and eliminate drugs is less than that of younger adults. Multiple-drug therapy (polypharmacy) is also a risk factor for hospitalized patients. The average patient in the hospital is prescribed up to 10 drugs. The risk for drug side effects and drug interactions increases with the number of medications a person is administered.

ADRs may be localized and only occur at the site where the drug was administered. Other adverse reactions are widespread and occur throughout the body. Adverse effects may cause minor discomfort such as a rash, or they may be life threatening (e.g., coma and death).

Common adverse effects that occur in the central nervous system are drowsiness, dizziness, stimulation, or confusion. Life-threatening central nervous system effects include respiratory depression, coma, and death. Hepatotoxicity is a toxic adverse reaction that occurs in the liver. Some common drugs that can produce hepatotoxicity are acetaminophen and isoniazid (a drug used to treat tuberculosis). Nephrotoxicity is a serious adverse effect that occurs in the kidney. Nonsteroidal antiinflammatory drugs such as ibuprofen and naproxen can produce nephrotoxicity.

ADRs also occur as a result of nonsterile drug preparation. Intravenous fluids and other parenterals must be prepared using aseptic technique. Failure to use aseptic technique can result in the introduction of contaminants, pathogens, and fever-causing

agents into the solution. Prolonged illness or death may occur if the contaminated solution is injected into a patient.

Teratogenicity

ADRs that produce harm to a developing fetus are called teratogenic effects. To reduce possible harm to the fetus, pregnant women and their health care providers must weigh the risks versus the benefit of taking drugs during pregnancy. To assist in their decision making, the FDA requires manufacturers to include a summary of the drugs risks if taken during pregnancy and lactation, and a description of data supporting the drug summary, in drug product package labeling.

Carcinogenicity

Drugs and natural products that stimulate the growth of cancers are classified as carcinogens. Carcinogenic drugs interact with DNA and produce permanent genetic mutations. Many of the drugs used to treat one type of cancer are capable of producing cancers in other areas. Drugs used to treat ovarian cancer, such as melphalan, increase the risk for acute nonlymphocytic leukemia (ANLL). The synthetic estrogen diethylstilbestrol (DES) is no longer prescribed to women to prevent miscarriage because it increases the risks for breast and uterine cancer. The drug is still prescribed for the treatment of prostate cancer. Sassafras tea was widely used as a cleansing tea or tonic until it was discovered to be carcinogenic in the 1960s.

Dependence and Tolerance

Patients taking controlled substances may develop dependence or tolerance to the drug's effects. Drugs are placed in controlled substance schedules according to their likelihood to produce physiologic or psychological dependence. Patients who have developed dependence to a drug must continue to take the drug to prevent the onset of withdrawal symptoms. Once tolerance to a drug has developed, the patient must take increasing doses of the drug to produce the same effects as was previously produced by a lower dose. Tolerance may occur to the therapeutic effect or side effects. Tolerance develops to the sedation produced by some antiseizure drugs such as clonazepam before tolerance develops to the desired antiseizure effects.

Improving Adherence to Drug Therapy

Drug therapy is strongly influenced by whether the patient takes the medication as prescribed or whether medication is taken at all. Adherence to drug therapy is defined as taking the prescribed medication in the correct dose, at the right time, and without missed doses. It is currently recognized that patients and their caregivers must be actively involved in making decisions about drug therapy. Patients who recognize the importance of the drug therapy and are involved in decisions regarding the medication that is best suited for their individual needs are more likely to adhere to therapy.

Factors Influencing Adherence to Drug Therapy

Lack of adherence to drug therapy is associated with poor health outcomes. Understanding why medications are not taken as prescribed is important for the design of strategies to improve adherence. Strategies for improving adherence must be targeted at patients, caregivers, pharmacists, pharmacy technicians, clinicians, and other health care providers.

> ◆ **TECH NOTE!**
>
> USP 797 is the current regulation establishing standards to reduce contamination when compounding sterile products. Once implemented, USP Chapter 800 standards will increase protections for personnel and other health care workers who compound hazardous drugs, including all the antineoplastic and other hazardous drugs on the National Institute for Occupational Safety and Health (NIOSH) list.

Belief That Therapy Is Beneficial

Adherence to the prescribed drug therapy is increased when patients believe therapy is beneficial. This is particularly important when the medication has substantial adverse effects. Hypertension is known as the silent killer because often no symptoms are present. Medications to treat hypertension may cause dizziness, upset stomach, impotence, or even depression, causing many patients to discontinue drug therapy. Adherence to drug therapy can avoid many of the complications associated with untreated hypertension.

Adverse Drug Reactions

An ADR is an undesired side effect of a drug. An ADR may be mild (e.g., sedation and nausea) or severe (e.g., hepatotoxicity and seizures). ADRs are a principal cause of discontinuation of drug therapy. Even fear of potential adverse reactions is a sufficient disincentive for some patients to avoid taking their medications. Many drug formulations have been developed to minimize drug side effects. Enteric-coated formulations reduce the risk of stomach upset. GI side effects are avoided by use of drugs formulated for transdermal application.

Pharmacy technicians can assist pharmacists in reducing patients' anxiety about adverse reactions by alerting the pharmacists when patients have questions about their drug therapy and making certain patients receive pharmacist counseling for new medicines. Pharmacy technicians can also play a key role in helping patients limit adverse reactions by distributing patient drug information leaflets and affixing warning labels, also called auxiliary labels, to prescription vials, which are intended to ensure that the maximum benefits of drug therapy are achieved with minimum side effects. For example, taking medication with food or a glass of water can decrease the risk for upset stomach. Acting within their scope of practice, pharmacy technicians can assist pharmacists in providing drug information that may reduce the risk for drug side effects and increase adherence to prescribed drug therapy.

> ### • TECH NOTE!
> Many pharmacy computer systems now print auxiliary labels directly onto prescription labels using a different color for identification purposes.

Lack of Any Medication Administration Routine

Adherence is improved when patients develop a regular routine for taking medicine. The pharmacist and pharmacy technician can work with patients to develop a routine for taking medications that fits the patient's lifestyle. Some pharmacies sell devices that prompt the patient to remember to take medicines.

Understanding Dosing Schedule

Dosing schedules must be convenient and understandable if patients are to avoid missed doses or taking double doses. Adherence to drug therapy becomes more difficult as the number of medications prescribed increases. Selection of drug formulations that are taken once a day may improve adherence. The pharmacy may also dispense the medicine in compliance blister packs.

> ### • TECH NOTE!
> Extended-release (ER) medications promote patient adherence. Instead of taking medications three or four times a day, an ER, sustained-release (SR), or controlled-dose (CD) tablet may be taken once daily.

Ability to Afford Drug Therapy

People with low socioeconomic status are at increased risk for low adherence. Poverty decreases the ability to afford medications and decreases access to health care when adverse events are experienced. When drug therapy is expensive, prescriptions may not be filled. When prescriptions are filled, patients may take less than the dose prescribed to make the prescription last longer. Pharmacy personnel can work with prescribers to ensure that effective and affordable drugs (e.g., generics) are prescribed and dispensed when appropriate. Pharmacy technicians can also contact insurance companies to obtain approval for nonformulary medicines.

Reporting Adverse Drug Reactions

ADRs are reported to the US Food and Drug Administration (FDA) by drug manufacturers, health care professionals, and consumers using the Medwatch FDA Voluntary Reporting Form 3500 (Fig. 3.6). The ADR reports are compiled into a computerized information database called the Adverse Event Reporting System (AERS). Vaccine adverse events are reported to the Vaccine Event Reporting System (VAERS). The reports are analyzed and mined for signals of safety issues. The information is used to issue safety alerts for drugs, biologics, devices, and dietary supplements, update product labeling, send out a "Dear Health Care Professional" letter, or even reevaluate the drug approval decision. If reevaluation results in a decision to withdraw drug approval, then a recall will be issued. Patient and consumer information sheets are also available from the FDA. In Canada, ADRs are also reported by drug manufacturers, consumers, and health professionals. ADRs are reported to the Canada Vigilance Program. ADR reporting forms can be obtained from the MedEffect Canada website (http://www.hc-sc.gc.ca/dhp-mps/medeff/report-declaration/index-eng.php).

> ### TECHNICIAN'S CORNER
> 1. How can pharmacy technicians assist patients in reducing anxiety about adverse reactions?
> 2. Explain how people with low socioeconomic status are at an increased risk for adverse reactions.

U.S. Department of Health and Human Services

MedWatch

The FDA Safety Information and Adverse Event Reporting Program

For VOLUNTARY reporting of adverse events, product problems and product use errors

Form Approved: OMB No. 0910-0291, Expires: 9/30/2018
See PRA statement on reverse.

FDA USE ONLY

Triage unit sequence #

FDA Rec. Date

Note: For date prompts of "dd-mmm-yyyy" please use 2-digit day, 3-letter month abbreviation, and 4-digit year; for example, 01-Jul-2015.

A. PATIENT INFORMATION

1. Patient Identifier
2. Age
   - ☐ Year(s)   ☐ Month(s)
   - ☐ Week(s)   ☐ Days(s)
   - or Date of Birth (e.g., 08 Feb 1925)
   In Confidence
3. Sex
   - ☐ Female
   - ☐ Male
4. Weight
   - ☐ lb
   - ☐ kg

5.a. **Ethnicity** (Check single best answer)
- ☐ Hispanic/Latino
- ☐ Not Hispanic/Latino

5.b. **Race** (Check all that apply)
- ☐ Asian   ☐ American Indian or Alaskan Native
- ☐ Black or African American   ☐ White
- ☐ Native Hawaiian or Other Pacific Islander

B. ADVERSE EVENT, PRODUCT PROBLEM

1. **Check all that apply**
- ☐ Adverse Event   ☐ Product Problem (e.g., defects/malfunctions)
- ☐ Product Use Error   ☐ Problem with Different Manufacturer of Same Medicine

2. **Outcome Attributed to Adverse Event** (Check all that apply)
- ☐ Death   Include date (dd-mmm-yyyy):
- ☐ Life-threatening
- ☐ Hospitalization – initial or prolonged
- ☐ Other Serious (Important Medical Events)
- ☐ Required Intervention to Prevent Permanent Impairment/Damage (Devices)
- ☐ Disability or Permanent Damage
- ☐ Congenital Anomaly/Birth Defects

3. **Date of Event** (dd-mmm-yyyy)
4. **Date of this Report** (dd-mmm-yyyy)

5. **Describe Event, Problem or Product Use Error**

6. **Relevant Tests/Laboratory Data, Including Dates**

7. **Other Relevant History, Including Preexisting Medical Conditions** (e.g., allergies, pregnancy, smoking and alcohol use, liver/kidney problems, etc.)

C. PRODUCT AVAILABILITY

2. **Product Available for Evaluation?** (Do not send product to FDA)
- ☐ Yes   ☐ No   ☐ Returned to Manufacturer on (dd-mmm-yyyy)

D. SUSPECT PRODUCTS

1. **Name, Manufacturer/Compounder, Strength** (from product label)

#1 – Name and Strength	#1 – NDC # or Unique ID
#1 – Manufacturer/Compounder	#1 – Lot #
#2 – Name and Strength	#2 – NDC # or Unique ID
#2 – Manufacturer/Compounder	#2 – Lot #

FORM FDA 3500 (10/15)   Submission of a report does not constitute an admission that medical personnel or the product caused or contributed to the event.

3. **Dose or Amount   Frequency   Route**
- #1
- #2

4. **Dates of Use** (From/To for each) (If unknown, give duration, or best estimate) (dd-mmm-yyyy)
- #1
- #2

5. **Diagnosis or Reason for Use** (indication)
- #1
- #2

6. **Is the Product Compounded?**
- #1 ☐ Yes   ☐ No
- #2 ☐ Yes   ☐ No

7. **Is the Product Over-the-Counter?**
- #1 ☐ Yes   ☐ No
- #2 ☐ Yes   ☐ No

8. **Expiration Date** (dd-mmm-yyyy)
- #1
- #2

9. **Event Abated After Use Stopped or Dose Reduced?**
- #1 ☐ Yes   ☐ No   ☐ Doesn't apply
- #2 ☐ Yes   ☐ No   ☐ Doesn't apply

10. **Event Reappeared After Reintroduction?**
- #1 ☐ Yes   ☐ No   ☐ Doesn't apply
- #2 ☐ Yes   ☐ No   ☐ Doesn't apply

E. SUSPECT MEDICAL DEVICE

1. **Brand Name**
2. **Common Device Name**   2b. **Procode**
3. **Manufacturer Name, City and State**

4. Model #	Lot #	5. Operator of Device
Catalog #	Expiration Date (dd-mmm-yyyy)	☐ Health Professional
Serial #	Unique Identifier (UDI) #	☐ Lay User/Patient ☐ Other

6. **If Implanted, Give Date** (dd-mmm-yyyy)
7. **If Explanted, Give Date** (dd-mmm-yyyy)

8. **Is this a single-use device that was reprocessed and reused on a patient?**   ☐ Yes   ☐ No

9. **If Yes to Item 8, Enter Name and Address of Reprocessor**

F. OTHER (CONCOMITANT) MEDICAL PRODUCTS

Product names and therapy dates (Exclude treatment of event)

G. REPORTER (See confidentiality section on back)

1. **Name and Address**

Last Name: First Name:
Address:
City: State/Province/Region:
Country: ZIP/Postal Code:
Phone #:   Email:

2. **Health Professional?**   ☐ Yes   ☐ No
3. **Occupation**
4. **Also Reported to:**
- ☐ Manufacturer/Compounder
- ☐ User Facility
- ☐ Distributor/Importer

5. **If you do NOT want your identity disclosed to the manufacturer, please mark this box:** ☐

PLEASE TYPE OR USE BLACK INK

• **Fig. 3.6** Food and Drug Administration voluntary reporting form 3500. (Courtesy U.S. Food and Drug Administration, Rockville, MD.)

Key Points

- Pharmacodynamics looks at how the body responds to drugs that are administered.
- Drugs interact or bind with targeted cells in the body to produce pharmacological action.
- Drug-receptor binding is similar to a lock and key. The more similar the drug is to the shape of the receptor site, the greater is the affinity the receptor site has for the drug.
- Drug-receptor binding enhances or inhibits normal biologic processes.
- An agonist (e.g., fentanyl) is a drug that binds to its receptor site and stimulates a cellular response. Agonist binding may activate a receptor that was resting or turn off a receptor that was activated.
- Antagonists (e.g., naloxone) bind to the receptor site and prevent an agonist from activating the receptor. They prevent another drug or natural body chemical from binding by occupying or inactivating the receptor site. Binding may reverse the action of a currently administered drug.
- Partial agonists (e.g., Suboxone®) behave like antagonists in the presence of a high concentration of a full agonist or when administered after recent exposure to high concentrations of an agonist.
- Efficacy is a measure of the drug's effectiveness under controlled conditions rather than "real-world" conditions.
- Drugs that are administered in very low doses yet produce a maximum effect have high potency.
- The dose-response curve shows a drug's relative efficacy and potency. A steep dose-response curve indicates that a small change in drug dose will produce a big change in the drug response.
- The TI is the ratio of the effective dose to the lethal dose. Safe drugs have a wide margin between the lethal dose and the effective dose.

- Successful drug therapy is influenced by a variety of factors. The patient's response to a drug is not always predictable.
- Age, gender, disease, pregnancy, weight, and genetics are patient-related factors that influence drug response.
- Drug allergies cause a heightened response to drugs and can occur after one or more exposures to a drug.
- Patients may become desensitized to the effects of drugs.
- Idiosyncratic reactions are unpredictable.
- Psychological factors can influence drug response. The placebo effect demonstrates that patients can experience drug effects even when no active drug has been administered.
- Drugs produce desired effects (therapeutic effects) and undesired effects. Undesired effects are called adverse reactions.
- Multiple-drug therapy increases risks for ADRs. Elderly adults have increased risks for ADRs because they typically take several drugs.
- ADRs can be mild or severe. Effects range from rash, upset stomach, and sedation to hepatotoxicity, teratogenicity, and anaphylactic shock.
- Dependence and tolerance are adverse reactions associated with controlled substances. When tolerance develops, the patient must take increasing doses of the drug to get the desired effect. When dependence has developed, patients must continue to take the drug to prevent withdrawal symptoms.
- Patients, caregivers, pharmacists, pharmacy technicians, clinicians, and other health care providers must work as a team to improve adherence to drug therapy.
- Adherence to drug therapy is influenced by patient belief that the therapy will be beneficial.
- Selection of effective, affordable medicines that have few side effects and that are dosed in convenient schedules improves adherence to drug therapy.

Review Questions

1. An _____ is a drug that binds to a receptor site and elicits cellular response.
   - a. agonist
   - b. antagonist
   - c. alternative
   - d. antimetabolite
2. All drugs produce toxic effects that can lead to death. The therapeutic _____ is the ratio of the effective dose to the lethal dose.
   - a. equivalence
   - b. derivative
   - c. index
   - d. window
3. The process of using drugs in the treatment of disease is called _____.
   - a. pharmacodynamics
   - b. pharmacotherapeutics
   - c. pharmacokinetics
   - d. pharmacognosy
4. What is the measure of a drug's effectiveness called?
   - a. availability
   - b. bioequivalence
   - c. efficacy
   - d. potency

5. Humans are unique, and individual variability influences the outcome of drug therapy. Name some physiologic factors that influence drug therapy.
   - a. age, weight, and gender
   - b. genetics, disease, and pregnancy
   - c. allergies, hypersensitivities, and desensitization
   - d. both a and b
6. Toxic adverse reactions that cause hepatotoxicity occur in the _____, and toxic adverse reactions that cause nephrotoxicity occur in the _____.
   - a. liver, lungs
   - b. liver, kidneys
   - c. kidneys, bladder
   - d. kidneys, nephrons
7. _____ and _____ are associated with the use of controlled substances.
   - a. Hypersensitivities and dependence
   - b. Tolerance and toxicity
   - c. Dependence and tolerance
   - d. Toxicity and anaphylaxis
8. To which government agency are adverse reactions reported in the United States?
   - a. DEA
   - b. TJC
   - c. CMS
   - d. FDA

9. An adverse effect produced by drugs on fetuses is called _____.

    a. carcinogenic

    b. teratogenic

    c. pathogenic

    d. toxic

10. One drug that has a narrow therapeutic index is _____.

    a. acetaminophen

    b. penicillin

    c. digoxin

    d. melphalan

Bibliography

Baker GR, Norton PG, Flintolf V, et al: The Canadian Adverse Events Study: the incidence of adverse events among hospital patients in Canada, *Can Med Assoc J* 170:1678–1686, 2004.

Canadian Institutes for Health Information: Adverse Drug Reaction–Related Hospitalizations Among Seniors, 2006 to 2011, 2013. Retrieved September 5, 2017, from www.cihi.ca.

DiPiro JT, Talbert R, Yee CG, et al: *Pharmacotherapy A pathophysiologic approach*, ed 9, 2014, McGraw Hill.

Edwards IR: The WHO World Alliance for Patient Safety: a new challenge or an old one neglected? *Drug Saf* 28:379–386, 2005.

Page C, Curtis M, Sutter M, et al: *Integrated pharmacology*, Philadelphia, 2005, Elsevier Mosby, pp 57–70, 314.

Passarelli M, Jacob-Filho W, Figueras A: Adverse drug reactions in an elderly hospitalised population: inappropriate prescription is a leading cause, *Drugs Aging* 22:767–777, 2005.

Raffa RB, Rawls SM, Beyzarov EP: *Netter's illustrated pharmacology*, Philadelphia, 2005, WB Saunders, pp 10–11, 21–23.

Ratajczak H: Drug-induced hypersensitivity: role in drug development, *Toxicol Rev* 23:265–280, 2004.

Sorensen L, Stokes J, Purdie D, et al: Medication management at home: medication-related risk factors associated with poor health outcomes, *Age Ageing* 34:626–632, 2005.

Sultana J, Cutroneo P, Trifirò G: Clinical and economic burden of adverse drug reactions, *J Pharmacol Pharmacother* 4(Suppl 1):S72–S77, 2013. doi:10.4103/0976-500X.120957.

Tyler V, Brady L, Robbers J: *Pharmacognosy*, ed 9, Philadelphia, 1988, Lea & Febiger, p 486.

U.S. Food and Drug Administration: Adverse Event Reporting System. Retrieved from http://www.fda.gov/cder/aers/default.htm. (Accessed 19 June 2016).

U.S. Food and Drug Administration: Pregnancy, Lactation, and Reproductive Potential: Labeling for Human Prescription Drug and Biological Products—Content and Format Guidance for Industry, 2014. From https://www.fda.gov/drugs/developmentapprovalprocess/developmentresources/labeling/ucm093307.htm.

USP: FAQs: <800> Hazardous Drugs—Handling in Healthcare Settings, August 18, 2017. Retrieved September 7, 2017, from http://www.usp.org/frequently-asked-questions/hazardous-drugs-handling-healthcare-settings.

Wu WK, Pantaleo N: Evaluation of outpatient adverse drug reactions leading to hospitalization, *Am J Health Syst Pharm* 60:253–259, 2003.

4

Drug Interactions and Medication Errors

LEARNING OBJECTIVES

1. Learn the terminology associated with drug interactions and medication errors.
2. Give examples of drug-drug interactions, drug-food interactions, and drug-disease contraindications.
3. Describe several mechanisms for drug interactions.
4. List ways to avoid drug interactions.
5. Categorize medication errors.
6. Identify medication errors made by pharmacists and pharmacy technicians.
7. Describe techniques used to avoid medication errors in the pharmacy.

KEY TERMS

Additive effect Concurrent administration of two drugs enhances the effects produced by the individual drugs.

Antagonism A drug-drug interaction or drug-food interaction that decreases or blocks the effect of another drug.

Drug-disease contraindication Drug administration should be avoided because it may worsen the patient's medical condition.

Drug-drug interaction Effect that occurs when two or more drugs are administered at the same time.

Drug-food interaction Altered drug response that occurs when a drug is administered with certain foods.

Medication error Error made in the process of prescribing, preparing, dispensing, or administering drug therapy.

Potentiation Process where one drug, acting at a separate site or via a different mechanism of action, increases the effect of another drug. The drug produces no effect when administered alone. Food can also potentiate the effects of a drug.

Synergistic effects Drug-drug or drug-food interaction that produces an effect that is greater than would be produced if either drug were administered alone.

Therapeutic duplication Administration of two drugs that produce similar effects and side effects. These drugs may belong to the same therapeutic class.

Drug Interactions

Drug effects are influenced by concurrent administration with foods and other drugs. The more drugs that are administered to a patient, the more likely it is that interactions will occur. Drug-drug interactions and drug-food interactions can increase or decrease the intended drug effects. They may also increase or decrease drug side effects. Drug interactions may produce life-threatening or minor undesired effects, or they may enhance the desired drug effect. Low doses of antidepressant drugs such as amitriptyline are administered along with pain medications such as hydrocodone to enhance pain relief. By administering these two drugs together, less hydrocodone is needed, and the patient's risk for development of tolerance and dependence from the hydrocodone is reduced. The study of pharmacology is important because it enables the prediction of the likelihood that a drug interaction may occur.

Drug-Drug Interactions

An interaction that occurs between two or more drugs administered at the same time is called a *drug-drug interaction*. Drug-drug interactions may increase or decrease the effect or side effects of the drug. Tetracycline and penicillin both treat infections. If the drugs are administered together, the infection-fighting ability of penicillin is reduced by the tetracycline. The antifungal action of ketoconazole is reduced if the drug is taken with antacids. Antiulcer drugs such as cimetidine increase the effects of alcohol. Amoxicillin reduces the effectiveness of oral contraceptives.

> ### ● TECH NOTE!
>
> The pharmacy technician should alert the pharmacist to drug interactions that are identified by prescription-filling software when they are inputting new or refill prescription data.

Drug-Food Interactions

Foods may contain enzymes, vitamins, or minerals that enhance or interfere with drug effects. An interaction between an administered drug and food(s) consumed at the same time is called a *drug-food interaction*. The interaction may influence side effects too. A classic example is the interaction between dairy products and the antiinfective tetracycline. Tetracycline binds with the calcium in milk or cheese, decreasing the drug's effectiveness. The effectiveness of levothyroxine, a synthetic thyroid hormone, is decreased when iron supplements are taken concurrently. Grapefruit juice inhibits the metabolism of the cholesterol-lowering drug atorvastatin, thereby increasing the drug's effects and side effects.

Additive Effects

Additive effects may occur when two drugs are administered concurrently. The increased effect is equal to the sum of the individual effects produced by each of the drugs alone. Many drug interactions produce additive effects. The sleeping pill temazepam is administered to promote drowsiness. Alcoholic beverages also cause drowsiness. When alcoholic beverages are consumed together with temazepam, additional drowsiness is caused. The sedation caused by temazepam adds to the sedation caused by alcohol.

Additive effects can be described using the equation

$$1 + 1 = 2$$

Synergistic Effects

Drug-drug interactions and drug-food interactions may produce synergistic effects. *Synergistic effects* result when two drugs administered together produce effects that are greater than would be produced if either drug were administered alone or would be seen with additive effects. Bleeding is a potential side effect of warfarin and aspirin. When warfarin and aspirin are administered together, excessive bleeding may occur.

Synergistic effects can be described using the equation

$$1 + 1 = 3$$

Potentiation

The process whereby one drug, or a food, increases the effects of another drug, yet does not produce any effect when administered alone, is called *potentiation*. Carbidopa exhibits no anti–Parkinson disease activity when administered alone but can increase the anti–Parkinson disease effects of levodopa. Carbidopa decreases the destruction of levodopa in the gastrointestinal tract, thereby increasing the amount of levodopa that can get to its site of action in the brain. Grapefruit juice increases the effects of some antihypertensive drugs (e.g., diltiazem) because it inhibits metabolic enzymes. The action of the antifungal griseofulvin is increased when it is taken with fatty foods because food increases the absorption of the drug.

Potentiation can be described using the equation:

$$1 + 0 = 2$$

Antagonism

Antagonism is a drug-drug interaction or drug-food interaction that blocks drug effects. Naloxone is administered to block the respiratory depression produced by opioids (e.g., fentanyl, morphine, and heroin). Vitamin K is an antidote for the drug warfarin. It is administered to stop bleeding caused by an excessive dose of warfarin.

Antagonism can be described using the equation:

$$1 + 1 = 0$$

TECH NOTE!

Grapefruit juice is implicated in many drug-food interactions. When grapefruit juice is known to affect a drug's action, an auxiliary label is placed on the medication vial to let the patient know to avoid drinking grapefruit juice when taking the medication.

Mechanisms of Drug Interactions

Drug-drug interactions and drug-food interactions occur via many different mechanisms. Coadministration of drugs or drug with food can increase absorption, distribution, metabolism, or elimination and result in increased or decreased drug action or side effects. Epinephrine is added to local anesthetics to constrict blood vessels at the site of injection and thereby augment the local anesthetic effects at the injection site. Absorption of a drug can also be increased by administration of a second drug that speeds or slows movement within the gastrointestinal system. Prokinetic drugs such as metoclopramide stimulate movement through the stomach and increase the absorption of drugs that are primarily absorbed in the small intestine and decrease absorption of drugs that are absorbed in the stomach. Drugs that decrease the rate of gastric emptying or movement through the intestines, such as codeine and loperamide, can increase the absorption and effects of drugs (Fig. 4.1).

Drugs that are weak acids and weak bases are involved in many drug interactions. The absorption of cimetidine (H2 receptor antagonist) is decreased when taken with antacids, because antacids make the pH more alkaline and cimetidine is a weak acid. Absorption of cimetidine is greatest in an acidic pH. Intravenous solutions of acids and bases are incompatible and, when combined, form solid particles (precipitate). For example, if calcium gluconate is added to a solution of floxacillin sodium 2 g in normal saline, thick white clumps form. The resulting intravenous solution is not usable.

Displacement from protein binding sites is a mechanism for drug interactions that influences the distribution of a drug. Displacement increases the amount of drug that is free to get to its site of action and produce effects (see Fig. 2.6). Warfarin is a drug that is highly protein bound. Even a small change in the percent of

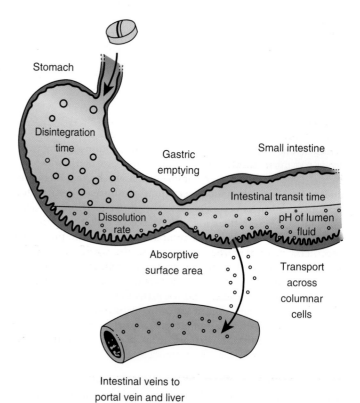

• **Fig. 4.1** Factors involved in gastrointestinal drug interactions. (From Kalant H, Grant DM, Mitchell J: *Principles of medical pharmacology*, ed 7, Philadelphia, 2007, Elsevier.)

"free" drug, drug that not bound to protein and able to get to the binding site, can increase warfarin's effects and risk for hemorrhage. Sulfonamides are a class of antiinfectives that are also strongly protein bound. When a sulfonamide and warfarin are both administered, displacement occurs.

Interactions that alter the rate of drug metabolism are caused by induction or inhibition of metabolic enzymes. Barbiturates such as phenobarbital stimulate metabolic enzymes of other antiseizure medications (phenytoin, valproic acid). Grapefruit juice is a powerful inhibitor of metabolic enzyme CYP3A4 and potentiates the effect of anticholesterol drugs such as atorvastatin. H2 receptor antagonists alter the metabolism of alcohol. When drugs such as cimetidine and ranitidine are taken with alcohol, the effects of alcohol may be increased and may last longer.

Some drug interactions influence elimination of drugs. Altering the pH of the urine can increase the elimination of a drug or enhance its reabsorption. Elimination of acidic drugs is increased when drugs that make the urine alkaline are administered. Elimination of alkaline drugs is increased when drugs that make the urine more acidic are administered.

Drug interactions that involve competition for a common transport system in the kidney can affect the elimination of some drugs. This describes the drug-drug interaction between penicillin and probenecid. When the drugs are administered together, elimination of penicillin is decreased.

Avoiding Undesired Drug Interactions

Studies indicate that between 7% and 22% of adverse drug reactions (ADRs) are caused by drug-drug interactions. Drug interactions that produce undesired effects should be avoided. Undesired drug interactions can result in cancellation of desired drug effect or reduced drug effect. At the opposite extreme, a drug interaction can produce toxic or harmful effects (Table 4.1). Failure to recognize drug interactions can harm the patient or prolong patient illness. It is the responsibility of pharmacists and pharmacy technicians to screen all prescriptions for potential drug interactions before dispensing the medication. Pharmacy technicians play a significant role in the screening process.

Pharmacy technicians play a key role in entering patient data into the pharmacy's prescription-filling software. Data entered into the computer must be complete and accurate if screening for drug interactions is to be effective. *Drug-disease contraindications* can be avoided by maintaining an up-to-date patient history of chronic and acute medical conditions. Computers prospectively screen for drug interactions so that adjustments can be made to the patient drug therapy before the drug is dispensed. When a drug-disease contradiction is identified by computer software, the pharmacy technician must alert the pharmacist so the significance of the computer-screened drug-disease contraindication can be evaluated. Drug-drug interactions can also be avoided by maintenance of an up-to-date patient profile. Pharmacy technicians and pharmacists should query patients about current nonprescription drug use, as well as prescription drug use. Information about prescriptions filled at other pharmacies should be obtained, if possible, and entered into the pharmacy's computer system.

TABLE 4.1	Summary of Selected Drug and Food Interactions	
Drug	Effects or Side Effects are Increased by:	Effects or Side Effects are Decreased by:
tetracycline		penicillin antacids dairy products
ketoconazole		antacids
alcoholic beverage (ethanol)	cimetidine	
oral contraceptives		amoxicillin
levothyroxine		iron supplements
triazolam	alcoholic beverages	
warfarin	NSAIDS (e.g., aspirin, ibuprofen)	vitamin K
levodopa	carbidopa	
verapamil	grapefruit juice	
griseofulvin	fatty foods	
morphine		naloxone
lidocaine	epinephrine	
cimetidine		antacids
phenobarbital		phenytoin sodium bicarbonate
penicillin	probenecid	

Pharmacy technicians must also be knowledgeable of intravenous drug incompatibilities. Combining acidic intravenous solutions and alkaline solutions causes precipitation of the drug out of the solution. Intravenous solutions that contain precipitates cannot be used and must be destroyed.

Drug-food interactions can be avoided by counseling patients to avoid consuming foods that interact with their medications. Spacing the time between food consumption and medication administration is often sufficient to avoid an undesired interaction. Pharmacy technicians can play an active role in ensuring that appropriate warning labels are affixed to prescription containers, when this task is within their scope of practice.

Medication Errors

The National Coordinating Council for Medication Error Reporting and Prevention defines a *medication error* as "any preventable event that may cause or lead to inappropriate medication use or patient harm while the medication is in the control of the health care professional, patient, or consumer. Such events may be related to professional practice, health care products, procedures, and systems, including prescribing; communicating drug orders; product labeling, packaging, and nomenclature; compounding; dispensing; distribution; administration; education; monitoring; and use." Medication errors harm approximately 1.3 million people in the United States annually and cause at least one death each day.

● TECH NOTE!

When taking a patient's medication history, ask the following: "Are you taking any over-the-counter medications? Are you taking any herbal supplements or vitamins? What other prescription drugs are you taking?"

Medication mishaps such as prescribing, repackaging, dispensing, administering, or monitoring can occur anywhere in the distribution system. Common causes of such errors include poor communication, inappropriate directions for medication use, look-alike and sound-alike product names, medical abbreviations, and poor handwriting by prescribers. Directions for use of medications can be confusing, leading to misuse by patients. Poor aseptic technique and procedures for medication preparation can also contribute to the problem. In addition to the previous points, job stress, a lack of knowledge and training in use or preparation of the products, and similar labeling or packaging of a product may be the cause of, or contribute to, actual or potential errors.

Medication errors are made by physicians, pharmacists, nurses, and pharmacy technicians in the health care setting. Medication errors typically occur in the process of ordering, transcribing, dispensing, and administering medications. Adverse drug events result from prescribing inappropriate medicines for patients, translating prescription orders, improper preparation or selection of drug to dispense, and improper drug administration. Medication errors may also be made by patients. Patient errors typically involve taking the wrong dose or forgetting to take a dose.

Medication Errors Made by Health Care Providers Who Prescribe Medication

Medication errors that are made by health care providers in hospital and ambulatory care settings account for 70% of medication errors that can potentially result in adverse effects to patients. As many as 4 in 1000 prescription errors are made when medications are ordered by physicians, nurse practitioners, pharmacists, dentists, and other health professionals legally able to prescribe medicines. Medication errors associated with prescribers are often a result of miscommunication or misinformation.

Miscommunication

Miscommunication of the drug ordered may involve poor handwriting, confusion between drugs with similar names, misuse of zeros and decimal points, confusion of metric and other dosing units, or inappropriate abbreviations.

Poor Handwriting

Many jokes have been made about physicians' poor handwriting (often called "chicken scratch"); however, medication errors that are made because prescriptions were not decipherable are no laughing matter. When prescriptions are illegible, there may be confusion between drugs with similar names. Electronic prescribing has been shown to eliminate medications errors caused by illegible handwriting and result in a sevenfold decrease in overall medication errors compared with handwritten prescriptions.

Confusion Between Drugs With Similar Names

Although the Center for Drug Evaluation and Research (CDER) tries to avoid assigning names to new drugs that are similar to existing drugs, sometimes this happens. Drugs with similar looking or sounding names are referred to as "look-alike/sound-alike drugs." According to the US Food and Drug Administration (FDA) MedWatch, medication errors have been made involving ZyrTEC and Zantac, VinCRIStine and VinBLAStine, GlipiZIDE and GlyBURIDE, LamMICtal and LamISIL, Zyprexa and CeleXA, and Serzone and SEROquel. When prescribers fail to write legibly, confusion about the drug to dispense arises (Table 4.2).

TABLE 4.2	Selected FDA, ISMP, and The Joint Commission List of Confused Drug Names
Drug Name	**Confused With Drug Name**
acetaZOLAMIDE	acetoHEXAMIDE
Aciphex	Aricept
Advair	Advicor
ALPRAZolam	LORazepam
Alora	Aldara
buPROPion	busPIRone
carBAMazepine	OXcarbazepine
CeleBREX	CeleXA, Cerebyx
DAUNOrubicin	DOXOrubicin, IDArubicin
Darvocet	Percocet
Diabeta	Zebeta
Effexor	Effexor XR
cycloSERINE	cycloSPORINE
glyBURIDE	glipiZIDE
ePHEDrine	EPINEPHrine
fentaNYL	SUFentanil
FLUoxetine	DULoxetine/PARoxetine
FluPHENAzine	fluvoxaMINE
HumaLOG	HumuLIN
hydrALAZINE	hydrOXYzine
HYDROcodone	oxyCODONE
HYDROmorphone	morphine
LaMICtal	LamISIL
NIFEdipine	niCARdipine
NovoLOG	NovoLIN, HumaLOG
OxyCODONE	HYDROcodone
PROzac	PriLOSEC
predniSONE	prednisoLONE
Retrovir	ritonavir
quiNIDine	quiNINE
Tobrex	Tobradex
traMADol	traZODone
vinBLAStine	vinCRIStine
Wellbutrin SR	Wellbutrin XL
Zantac	Xanax, ZyrTEC
ZyrPREXA	CeleXA

FDA, US Food and Drug Administration.
Adapted from Institute for Safe Medication Practices. ISMP's list of confused drug names, 2015. (http://www.ismp.org/Tools/confuseddrugnames.pdf and Institute for Safe Medication Practices) and FDA and ISMP Lists of look-alike drug names with recommended tall man letters, 2016. (http://www.ismp.org/Tools/tallmanletters.pdf).

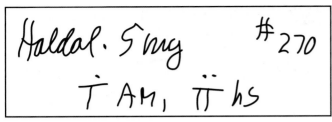

• **Fig. 4.2** Decimal point error example.

Misuse of Zeroes and Decimal Points

Orders for medication may be incorrect because the strength is written incorrectly or is illegible. Haloperidol is a drug used to treat schizophrenia. It is available as a 0.5-mg tablet and as a 5-mg tablet. If the decimal point to the left is illegible or the zero is omitted, there may be confusion about which strength to dispense. On the other hand, if the 5-mg tablet was ordered and the prescription was written as 5.0 mg, it could be confused with 50 mg. In both cases, if the error is not caught, the patient receives 10 times the desired dose (Fig. 4.2).

> **TECH NOTE!**
>
> To avoid medication errors, always place a zero in front of the decimal when calculating and recording doses that are less than 1 mL or 1 mg.

Confusion of Metric and Other Dosing Units or Inappropriate Abbreviations

Prescriptions may be written using metric units or apothecary units. Medication errors have been caused by improper conversion between the two systems of measurement. For example, the apothecary symbol for 1 dram (℈i) has been interpreted as 3 mL, 4 mL, and 5 mL. Most pharmacists and pharmacy technicians interpret ℈i = 5 mL = 1 teaspoonful. Prescribers unfamiliar with apothecary symbols may confuse the symbol for ounce (℥) and dram (℈), causing toxic or subtherapeutic effects.

Misinformation

Medication errors made by prescribers may also occur because of lack of information or misinformation. Limited information about the patient occurs when no medical or drug history was taken or insufficient information was collected from the patient. Studies have shown that more than 25% of the prescribing errors made in hospitals are associated with incomplete medication histories being obtained at the time of admission. A complete history is needed of patients' allergies, other medicines they are taking, previous diagnoses, and laboratory results to prevent medication errors.

Errors of Omission

An error of omission occurs when information is not collected or recorded in the patient's medical history. Studies have shown a 67% error rate in obtaining prescription medication histories. Medication histories taken by physicians were less accurate than histories taken by pharmacists. An incomplete drug history may be a cause for prescribing a drug similar to one currently being administered. This is called *therapeutic duplication*. Therapeutic duplication may increase or decrease desired effects. If both drugs compete for the same drug receptor binding sites or the same transport systems, the drug with the greatest affinity will bind. If the drug bound to the receptor is less potent, it decreases the desired drug effect. Therapeutic duplication may increase adverse reactions. Omission of drug allergy information could result in a prescription written and filled for a medicine that may cause extreme harm to the patient. Prescriptions written for drugs that are contraindicated often occur because of patient's disease state or allergies have not been recorded in the patient profile. An example of a drug-disease contraindication is the administration of the antidepressant bupropion to patients with a history of seizures. Patients can reduce their risk for drug interactions caused by errors of omission by filling all prescriptions at a single pharmacy that has the patient's complete medication history. Patients should also provide the pharmacy with a list of all regularly taken nonprescription drugs such as aspirin.

> **TECH NOTE!**
>
> Pharmacy technicians may encounter the abbreviations: NKDA (no known drug allergies) or NDA (no drug allergies).

Errors of Commission

Commission errors result when a previously discontinued drug is accidentally restarted or a nonprescribed drug is accidentally added to the patient's medication history. This can occur when inaccurate drug histories are collected from caregivers (when the patient is too ill to provide his or her own drug history) or from patient confusion. When this occurs, unneeded drugs are taken, and the patient is at risk for adverse reactions.

Prescriptions written for the wrong strength or wrong dosing schedule are medication errors that are not specifically errors of omission or commission but do involve prescribers. This type of error occurs when the prescriber lacks familiarity with the drug that is being prescribed. The error may occur when drug dose and dosing frequency are determined according to patient weight and inaccurate weight information is given in the medical history.

Medication Errors Made by Health Care Providers Who Dispense Medication

Pharmacists, pharmacy technicians, and pharmacy assistants make preventable medication errors too! Medication errors made by pharmacy personnel usually involve transcribing errors, incorrect interpretation of prescription contents, improper product preparation, lack of prescription monitoring, product labeling, and inaccurate dispensing. Some dispensing errors are caused by distractions in the pharmacy. The pharmacist or pharmacy technician filling a medication order may become distracted when his or her workflow is interrupted by the telephone ringing or by questions from a patient at the pharmacy counter.

> **TECH NOTE!**
>
> Always check the original prescription against the prescription label and the NDC number or DIN on the stock bottle to ensure accuracy.

Confusion of Metric and Other Dosing Units or Inappropriate Abbreviations

Serious medication errors have been caused by confusing abbreviations. This problem is so serious that The Joint Commission and the National Coordinating Council for Medication Error Reporting and Prevention have recommended abolishment of the use of certain abbreviations (Table 4.3).

> **TECH NOTE!**
>
> When in doubt about what is written on a prescription, always get a second opinion. Never guess at what the medication might be. Ask for help to verify the drug in question.

TABLE 4.3	Dangerous Abbreviations*	
Do Not Use	**Potential Problem**	**Use Instead**
AU, AS, AD	Misinterpreted as "OU" (both eyes), "OS" (left eye), "OD" (right eye)	Write, "both ears", "left ear", "right ear"
OU, OS, OD	Misinterpreted as "OU" (both ears), "OS" (left ear), "OD" (right ear or once daily)	Write, "both eyes", "left eye", "right eye"
U (unit)	Mistaken for "0" (zero), the number "4" (four), or "cc"	Write "unit"
IU (International Unit)	Mistaken for IV (intravenous) or the number 10 (ten)	Write "International Unit"
μg	Mistaken for mg (milligrams) resulting in 1000-fold overdose	Write "mcg" or "micrograms"
Q.D., QD, q.d., qd, (Latin abbreviation for every day)	Period after the Q mistaken for "I" and misinterpreted as QID (four times a day). In Canada, once daily is abbreviated OD which may be misinterpreted as every other day or right eye.	Write "daily"
Q.O.D., QOD, q.o.d, qod (Latin abbreviation for every other day)	Period after the Q mistaken for "I" and the "O" mistaken for "I". Misinterpreted as once daily or four times a day.	Write "every other day"
SC or SQ	Mistaken as SL (sublingual)	Write subcutaneous
TIW	Misinterpreted as three times a day or twice a week	Write as three times a week
D/C	Patients medications have been prematurely discontinued because D/C can be interpreted as either discharge or discontinue	Do not abbreviate
cc	Mistaken for U (units) when poorly written	Write "mL" or "milliliters"
HS	Latin for hour of sleep, the abbreviation may be misinterpreted as half-strength	Do not abbreviate
MS, MSO₄ and MgSO₄	Can mean morphine sulfate or magnesium sulfate; confused for one another	Write "morphine sulfate"
Trailing zero (X.0 mg)ª	Decimal point is missed	Write X mg
Lack of leading zero (.X mg)	Decimal point is missed	Write 0.X mg
Additional Abbreviations, Acronyms, and Symbols to consider avoiding		
< (greater than) and > (less than)	Misinterpreted as the number "7" (seven) or the letter "L"; confused for each other	Write "greater than" and "less than"
Apothecary units	Unfamiliar to many practitioners; confused with metric units	Use metric units
@	Mistaken for the number "2" (two)	Write "at"

*Applies to all orders and all medication-related documentation that is handwritten (including free-text computer entry) or on preprinted forms.
ªException: A "trailing zero" may be used only when required to demonstrate the level of precision of the value being reported, such as for laboratory results, imaging studies that report size of lesions, or catheter or tube sizes. It may not be used in medication orders or other medication-related documentation.
Adapted from National Coordinating Council for Medication Error Reporting and Prevention. (2017) and Dangerous Abbreviations and The Joint Commission. (2017). Facts about the Official "Do Not Use" List of Abbreviations.

Inaccurate Transcribing

Poor handwriting is responsible for many transcription errors. Medication orders received by the pharmacy must be translated and entered into the computer. If the order is illegible, the pharmacy must verify the order to prevent incorrect selection of the drug and strength ordered. Medication orders received by telephone or left on a computer messaging system are also subject to transcription errors. Verbal medication orders must be written down accurately, or medication errors may result.

Insufficient Monitoring of Drug Therapy

Medication errors occur when a pharmacy fails to carefully monitor drug therapy. An important role of the pharmacist is to monitor the appropriateness of drug therapy. Pharmacy technicians assist the pharmacist with this task. Together they review each prescription to determine whether the medication ordered, dose, and dosing frequency are appropriate for the patient. Pharmacy technicians also help the pharmacist screen for drug interactions, drug-disease contraindications, and drug allergies. Monitoring drug therapy also reduces therapeutic duplication. Pharmacy technicians and pharmacists work together to alert the prescriber when they see that two therapeutically equivalent drugs are ordered for the patient. Monitoring also prevents refills of discontinued medication.

Improper Medication Preparation

Another medication error made by pharmacy staff is improper sterile and nonsterile compounding. Medications for parenteral administration must be prepared using aseptic technique. Medication errors associated with incorrect calculations also occur. Combining incompatible drugs is another source of medication errors.

> **● TECH NOTE!**
>
> It is vitally important to adopt an "aseptic attitude" when preparing parenteral medications. Handwashing, hood cleaning, dose calculating, and proper aseptic technique ensure that the sterile products are not contaminated or inaccurate.

• **Fig. 4.3** Example of look-alike packaging. (Courtesy Institute for Safe Medication Practices [ISMP]).

Improper Labeling

Several medication errors involve improper labeling of drugs to be dispensed. A labeling error has occurred when the correct drug is selected but the container is labeled with the wrong drug name, dosage form, strength, or quantity. Putting the wrong patient's name on the label is another labeling error. Incorrect or incomplete directions typed on the label are other preventable label errors.

Product Selection Errors

Selection of the wrong drug to dispense is a preventable error. This type of error most often occurs when drugs have similar names or similar packaging (Fig. 4.3). Other product selection errors include dispensing the wrong strength or wrong dosage form.

Bagging Errors

Placing the correct prescription in the wrong patient's bag is a bagging error. Placing additional prescriptions into a patient's bag or omitting a prescription from the bag are also bagging errors.

Miscellaneous Dispensing Errors

A properly filled prescription that is dispensed to the wrong patient is a medication error. This may occur when two customers have similar names. The pharmacy staff may incorrectly hear the name of the person who wants to pick up his or her prescription. The patient may incorrectly hear the name of the person the pharmacy staff has announced. This error is preventable. Always verify the name and identification of the person picking up a prescription.

Medication Errors Made by Health Care Providers Who Administer Medication

Medication errors are made by health care providers and caregivers who administer medications. One error associated with drug administration can result in a drug being given to the wrong patient. Sometimes the correct drug is given to the right patient; however, the drug strength, dosing frequency, and dosage form are incorrect. This is also a medication error.

Medication Errors Made by Patients

Medication errors are made by patients too! Pharmacists, pharmacy technicians, and other health care providers can help patients prevent medication errors. Patients are often confused by generic and trade names. Their medicines may be labeled using the generic name in the hospital. The community pharmacy may label the same drug with the brand name. The patient may not realize the drugs are the same and take a double dose. A similar situation occurs when two similar medicines are prescribed by different physicians. The patient is unaware that taking both medicines is therapeutic duplication. Confusion is one reason why patients refill medications that have been discontinued by their health care provider.

Two other medication errors are important to note. They are (1) taking too much medicine and (2) taking too little medicine. Some patients believe the saying, "If one pill is good, then two pills are better." Others do not realize the importance of taking medicines without missing doses. They do not realize that a chronic illness becomes worse or drug resistance can develop when doses are skipped. For some patients, the medication is too expensive, and they take less than the prescribed dose to try to "stretch" the prescription and make it last longer. Regardless of the reason, taking too little or too much medicine can negatively influence drug therapy outcomes.

Avoiding Medication Errors

Pharmacy technicians can play an important role in preventing medication errors. Some tips for preventing medication errors are:

- Always verify prescriptions with similar drug names. Verify spelling and strength.
- Always verify unfamiliar abbreviations or abbreviations published in The Joint Commission's "do not use" list or the National Coordinating Council for Medication Error Reporting and Prevention dangerous abbreviation list.
- Always confirm the drug, strength, and dosing schedule when prescriptions are written and the handwriting is illegible. Never guess.
- Avoid product selection errors by using the pull–dispense–review (PDR) system. Verify the drug name and NDC number or DIN when selecting (pulling) the drug from the shelf. Check the drug name, strength, and dosage form against medication order. Confirm the drug a third time when returning the medicine to the shelf.
- Become familiar with the brand and generic names of commonly dispensed drugs.
- Become familiar with the strengths, dosage forms, and dosing frequencies of commonly dispensed drugs.
- Alert the pharmacist of all drug interactions and therapeutic duplications.
- Develop a routine to avoid errors associated with distractions.
- Check the identification of each person picking up prescriptions.
- Dispense patient information sheets as required.
- Affix warning labels to prescription vials as required.
- Verify all calculations.
- Check all labels for accuracy.

TECHNICIAN'S CORNER

1. Look-alike/sound-alike drugs are responsible for dispensing errors. How might dispensing errors be avoided?
2. What should a pharmacy technician do if he or she is unsure about the name of a medication handwritten on a prescription?

Key Points

- Drug-drug interactions and drug-food interactions can increase or decrease intended drug effects.
- The more drugs that are administered to a patient, the more likely it is that interactions will occur.
- Drug-drug interactions may increase or decrease side effects of drugs.
- Foods may contain enzymes, vitamins, or minerals that enhance or interfere with drug effects.
- Additive effects are said to occur when the coadministration of two drugs results in increased side effects.
- Synergistic effects result when two drugs administered together produce effects that are greater than would be produced if either drug were administered alone.
- The process during which one drug or a food increases the effects of another drug yet does not produce any effect when administered alone is called potentiation.
- Antagonism is a drug-drug interaction or drug-food interaction that causes decreased drug effects.
- Interactions that induce or inhibit of metabolic enzymes can alter the rate of drug metabolism.
- Interactions that involve competition for a common transport system in the kidney can affect the elimination of some drugs.
- It is the responsibility of the pharmacy technician to alert the pharmacist when the pharmacy software identifies a potential drug interaction.
- Drug-disease contradictions and drug-drug interactions can be avoided by maintaining an up-to-date history of each patients' chronic and acute medical conditions.
- Pharmacy technicians must be knowledgeable of intravenous drug incompatibilities. Combining acidic intravenous solutions and alkaline solutions causes the precipitation of drug out of the solution.

- Medication errors in the health care setting typically occur in the process of ordering, transcribing, dispensing, and administering medications.
- Poor handwriting is responsible for many medication errors. When prescriptions are illegible, there may be confusion between drugs with similar names.
- Medication errors occur because of misplacement of zeros and decimal points.
- Medication errors have been caused by improper conversion between systems of measurement.
- Medication errors occur when pharmacists, pharmacy technicians, physicians, and other health care workers lack familiarity with the drug that is being prescribed.
- Medication errors made by pharmacy personnel usually involve transcribing errors, incorrect interpretation of prescription contents, improper product preparation, lack of prescription monitoring, product labeling, and inaccurate dispensing.
- Some dispensing errors are caused by distractions in the pharmacy.
- Medication errors made by patients can be minimized by proper education.
- Medication errors can be avoided by verifying prescriptions with similar drug names and unfamiliar abbreviations.
- Avoid product selection errors by using the PDR system and checking all labels for accuracy.
- Prevent medication errors by becoming familiar with brand and generic names and the strengths, dosage forms, and dosing frequencies of commonly dispensed drugs.
- Medication errors can be minimized by verifying all calculations.

Review Questions

1. State whether the following statement is true or false: Drug-drug interactions may increase or decrease the effect or side effects of the drug.
   a. true
   b. false
2. When the coadministration of two drugs results in increased side effects, the interaction is described as _____.
   a. Antagonistic
   b. Additive
   c. Adverse
   d. Absorption
3. When warfarin and aspirin are administered together, excessive bleeding occurs. This type of effect is _____.
   a. antagonistic
   b. idiosyncratic
   c. both a and b
   d. synergistic
4. Whose responsibility is it to watch for potential drug interactions during the prescription filling process?
   a. pharmacist
   b. technician
   c. pharmacist and technician
   d. pharmacy manager

5. Medication errors made by pharmacy personnel typically occur in the process of
   a. prescribing medications
   b. transcribing medications
   c. administering medications
   d. a, b, and c
6. Orders for medication may be incorrect because the strength is written incorrectly or is illegible. Which of the following is the correct way of writing the dose for digoxin?
   a. digoxin 0.25 mg
   b. digoxin 25 mg
   c. digoxin .25 mg
   d. digoxin 025 mg
7. All of the following are "checks" to ensure that the right medication is pulled from the pharmacy shelf when preparing a prescription EXCEPT_____
   a. Compare the NDC number or DIN on the bottle with the computer-generated pharmacy label.
   b. Check with the pharmacy assistant every time a prescription is filled.
   c. Check the drug name against the medication order.
   d. Check the drug strength and dosage form against the medication order.

8. To which federal agency should medication errors be reported to using the MedWatch program?
   a. DEA (Drug Enforcement Agency)
   b. FDA (Food and Drug Administration)
   c. TJC (The Joint Commission)
   d. ISMP (Institute for Safe Medication Practices Canada)
9. Which agency developed a "do not use" abbreviation list to avoid medication errors?
   a. Food and Drug Administration
   b. Drug Enforcement Agency
   c. Health Canada
   d. The Joint Commission
10. Dispensing errors can be avoided by _____:
   a. Verifying the name of the person picking up the medication
   b. Verifying that the medication is placed in the correct patient's bag
   c. Being alert for patients with similar names
   d. All of the above

Bibliography

Adubofour K, Keenan C, Daftary A, et al: Strategies to reduce medication errors in ambulatory practice, *J Natl Med Assoc* 96:1558, 2004.

Corbett AH, Dana WJ, et al: *Drug information handbook*, ed 24, Hudson, OH, 2015, APhA Lexi-Comp.

Institute for Safe Medication Practices. (2016). FDA and ISMP Lists of Look-Alike Drug Names with Recommended Tall Man Letters. From: https://www.ismp.org/recommendations/tall-man-letters-list.

Institute for Safe Medication Practices. (2015). List of Confused Drugs. From: https://www.ismp.org/tools/confuseddrugnames.pdf. Retrieved 9 September 2017.

National Coordinating Council for Medication Error Reporting and Prevention. (2017). Dangerous Abbreviations. From: http://nccmerp.org/dangerous-abbreviations. Retrieved 9 September 2017.

Page C, Curtis M, Sutter M, et al: *Integrated pharmacology*, Philadelphia, 2005, Elsevier Mosby, pp 57–70.

Passarelli M, Jacob-Filho W, Figueras A: Adverse drug reactions in an elderly hospitalised population: inappropriate prescription is a leading cause, *Drugs Aging* 22:767–777, 2005.

Shargel L, Mutnick A, Souney P, et al: *Comprehensive pharmacy review*, ed 4, Baltimore, 2001, Lippincott Williams & Wilkins, pp 78–84, 42–65, 131–132.

Tam V, Knowles S, Cornish P, et al: Frequency, type and clinical importance of medication history errors at admission to hospital: a systematic review, *CMAJ* 173(5):2005.

The Joint Commission. (2017). Facts about the Official "Do Not Use" List of Abbreviations. From: https://www.jointcommission.org/facts_about_do_not_use_list/. Retrieved 9 September 2017.

U.S. Food and Drug Administration. (2017). Medication Errors Related to Drugs. From: https://www.fda.gov/drugs/drugsafety/medicationerrors/default.htm. Retrieved 9 September 2017.

U.S. Food and Drug Administration. (2015). Strategies to Reduce Medication Errors: Working to Improve Medication Safety. From: https://www.fda.gov/drugs/resourcesforyou/consumers/ucm143553.htm. Retrieved 9 September 2017.

Velo GP, Minuz P: Medication errors: prescribing faults and prescription errors, *Br J Clin Pharmacol* 67(6):624–628, 2009. doi:10.1111/j.1365-2125.2009.03425.x.

UNIT II

Drugs Affecting the Autonomic Nervous System and Central Nervous System

The nervous system is made up of the central nervous system (CNS) (brain and spinal cord), and the peripheral nervous system (PNS). The central nervous system integrates sensory input and motor output. The peripheral nervous system is comprised of the autonomic and somatic systems. The autonomic nervous system (ANS) is divided into the parasympathetic and sympathetic systems. The parasympathetic nervous system regulates involuntary actions such as the heartbeat, smooth muscle contraction, and glandular secretions. The sympathetic nervous system predominates whenever the body is undergoing physical or psychological stress initiating a "fight or flight" response. The nervous system transmits information very rapidly by nerve impulses conducted from one area of the body to another, communicating changes in the body's internal and external environment, and responding by initiating changes in muscles and glands. A healthy nervous system is vitally important for normal physiological function. There are more than 600 diseases of the nervous system. Many of the drugs that act on the brain and nervous system relieve symptoms such as pain, insomnia, and anxiety or treat mood disorders.

In Unit II, the pharmacotherapy for anxiety, depression, psychosis (e.g., schizophrenia), Parkinson's disease, Huntington's disease seizures, pain, migraine headache, Alzheimer's, sleep disorders, and attention-deficit hyperactivity disorder (ADHD) are described. A brief description of each disorder is provided, followed by a description of the drugs indicated for treatment that includes mechanisms of action, adverse reactions, strength(s) and dosage forms.

5

Treatment of Anxiety

LEARNING OBJECTIVES

1. Learn the terminology associated with anxiety and its treatment.
2. List and describe the function of neurotransmitters associated with symptoms of anxiety.
3. Classify medications used to treat anxiety.
4. Describe the mechanism of action for each class of drugs used to treat anxiety.
5. Identify significant drug look-alike/sound-alike issues.
6. Identify warning labels and precautionary messages associated with medications used to treat anxiety.

KEY TERMS

Anxiety Condition associated with tension, apprehension, fear, or panic.

Anxiolytic Drug used to treat anxiety.

Drug dependence Person taking the drug must continue to take the drug in order to avoid the onset of physical or psychological withdrawal symptoms (or both).

Generalized anxiety disorder Condition that is associated with excessive worrying and tension that is experienced daily for more than 6 months.

Obsessive-compulsive disorder A condition associated with an inability to control or stop repeated unwanted thoughts or behaviors.

Panic disorder Condition associated with repeated sudden onset of feelings of terror.

Phobia Irrational fear of things or situations that produce symptoms of intense anxiety.

Posttraumatic stress disorder Stress disorder that develops in persons who have participated in, witnessed, or been a victim of a terrifying event.

Tolerance Increasing doses of a drug are required to achieve the same effects as were achieved previously at lower doses.

Overview

Anxiety disorder is the leading mental health illness and affects more than 40 million US adults, according to Anxiety Disorders Association of America. In any 12-month period, approximately 18% of US adults have excessive anxiety. Nearly 3 million Canadians 18 years of age and older (11.6% of the population) have an anxiety disorder, according to the Public Health Agency of Canada (2014). The cause of anxiety disorders may be environmental, biologic, developmental, associated with socioeconomic conditions, or a combination of several of these individual factors. Anxiety disorders can interfere with routine daily activities, work, school, and/or social relationships.

There are four major types of anxiety disorders—generalized anxiety disorder (GAD), panic disorder, obsessive-compulsive disorder (OCD), and posttraumatic stress disorder (PTSD). Individuals diagnosed with anxiety disorders experience intense fear, apprehension, tension, or panic out of proportion to the actual threat or danger.

Certain physiologic symptoms are diagnostic for individual anxiety disorders; however, some symptoms are common to all anxiety disorders. Common physiologic symptoms include increased heart rate, palpitations, shortness of breath, rapid breathing, nausea, sweating, and dry mouth. All of these symptoms are associated with hyperactivity of the autonomic nervous system. More specifically, the physiologic symptoms produced by anxiety are related to stimulation of the sympathetic nervous system and the parasympathetic nervous system.

Generalized Anxiety Disorder

Although most adults will experience anxiety at one point in their lives, excessive worrying and tension that are experienced daily for longer than 6 months is an indication of *generalized anxiety disorder*. It may produce restlessness, difficulty concentrating, sleep problems, and irritability. It is the most common type of anxiety disorder. In any given year, 6.8 million Americans (3.1% of the adult population) are affected, according to Anxiety Disorders Association of America. GAD affects approximately 3% of Canadian adult population in any given year. Women are more likely to have GAD than are men, according to Statistics Canada (2015).

Panic Disorder

Panic disorder affects approximately 6 million American adults in any given year. The 12-month prevalence in Canada is 1.6% of the adult population. It occurs twice as frequently in women than in men. It may be accompanied by major depression. Signs and symptoms of panic disorder include a sudden onset of terror, shortness of breath, increased heart rate, trembling, and nausea. The person may feel paralyzed by fear and unable to perform routine daily activities. Most symptoms of panic disorder last for only a few minutes.

Panic attacks may be triggered by a phobia. A *phobia* is an irrational fear of things or situations that produce symptoms of intense anxiety. Phobias cause the person to try to avoid the thing that is feared. Agoraphobia is a condition in which people become so fearful of situations that may produce "panicky feelings" that they isolate themselves or severely restrict their activities. Other common phobias are claustrophobia (fear of being in confined spaces), aviophobia (fear of flying), and acrophobia (fear of heights). Nearly 15 million Americans are affected by social phobias. In any given year, 6.7% of Canadian adults experience a social phobia. Social phobias cause affected individuals to shy away from social situations where they fear embarrassment or humiliation. Fear of public speaking or asking questions in a public forum is often associated with a social phobia. Approximately 8% of the populations of the United States and Canada have some type of phobia.

Obsessive-Compulsive Disorder

Obsessive-compulsive disorder is a condition associated with an inability to control or stop repeated unwanted thoughts or behaviors. Individuals create rituals, which they perform repeatedly, to lessen anxieties about the things they fear. A person who fears germs may wash his or her hands excessively. The prevalence of OCD is 1.8% of the Canadian population between the ages of 15 and 64 years, according to the Public Health Agency of Canada Report on Mental Illness in Canada (2002). More than 2 million Americans (1% of the adult population) are affected by OCD in any given year. The lifetime incidence of OCD worldwide is 1.7% to 4%.

Posttraumatic Stress Disorder

Posttraumatic stress disorder may develop in persons who have participated in, witnessed, or been a victim of a terrifying event. According to National Institutes of Mental Health, nearly 3.5% of the adult population in the United States have experience PTSD. PTSD may occur in soldiers who have committed atrocities or witnessed horrific events during wartime. Up to 67% of the people exposed to mass violence develop PTSD. Women, men, and children who have been sexually assaulted may develop PTSD. Up to 65% of men and 45.9% of women who have been sexually assaulted have PTSD. PTSD is likely to develop at some point in the lifetimes of children who have been sexually abused. Some people develop PTSD after a natural disaster such as an earthquake, flood or human disasters such as an airplane crash. Depression, substance abuse, and anxiety disorders may accompany PTSD.

Neurochemistry of Anxiety

There are four major classes of medicines used for the treatment of anxiety. They are selective serotonin reuptake inhibitors (SSRIs) (e.g., citalopram, fluoxetine, and sertraline), serotonin-norepinephrine (SNRI) reuptake inhibitors (e.g., venlafaxine and duloxetine), tricyclic antidepressants (TCAs) (e.g., amitriptyline and nortriptyline), and benzodiazepines (e.g., alprazolam and lorazepam). The drugs act on the neurotransmitters γ-aminobutyric acid (GABA), serotonin (5-hydroxytryptamine [5-HT]), and norepinephrine (NE).

Role of γ-Aminobutyric Acid

The mechanism of action for most drugs used to treat anxiety, is to potentiate the effects of GABA (γ-Aminobutyric Acid), a neurotransmitter. GABA decreases neuronal excitability and nerve impulse transmission.

Role of Serotonin

5-HT is another neurotransmitter that plays a role in the treatment of anxiety. Numerous 5-HT receptors have been identified. Most are located in the pons and midbrain. Activation of the 5-HT_{1A} autoreceptors in the raphe region of the brain decreases firing of serotonergic neurons that are linked to anxiety-like behavior.

Role of Norepinephrine

NE is an important neurotransmitter for the sympathetic nervous system. It is responsible for mediating some of the adrenergic-related symptoms of anxiety (e.g., increased heart rate).

Drugs Used to Treat Anxiety

Anxiety disorder is treated by the administration of anxiolytics and psychotherapy, including cognitive behavioral therapy. An *anxiolytic* is a drug that reduces symptoms of anxiety.

Benzodiazepines

Benzodiazepines are indicated for short-term treatment of anxiety (Table 5.1). They reduce anxiety even when taken in low doses. Other indications for benzodiazepines are panic attack, insomnia, seizure disorder, and muscle relaxation. These additional indications are listed under the description of individual benzodiazepines.

> ● *TECH NOTE!*
>
> Two common endings for drugs that are classified as benzodiazepines are *-epam* and *-olam*.

Mechanism of Action

Benzodiazepines bind to receptor sites on the $GABA_A$ complex. They promote relaxation and reduce physical symptoms of anxiety, including muscular tension (Fig. 5.1).

Pharmacokinetics

Benzodiazepines readily cross the blood-brain barrier. The duration of action varies from one benzodiazepine to another and may influence the selection of one benzodiazepine over another. A benzodiazepine that has a long duration of action may have long-lasting, unwanted side effects. The effects of some benzodiazepines may persist for up to 3 days.

The benzodiazepines are fully metabolized, and some agents are metabolized to active metabolites (see Chapter 2). The half-life ($t^{1/2}$) of the active metabolites can be several days which accounts for the long duration of action of some anxiolytics such as diazepam.

Adverse Reactions

Certain side effects are common to all benzodiazepines, but others are drug specific. All benzodiazepines produce some degree of sedation, ataxia, confusion, and reduced motor performance. Benzodiazepines can also interfere with cognitive functions and

TABLE 5.1	Benzodiazepines Used in the Treatment of Anxiety	
Generic Name	US Brand Name(s) Canadian Brand(s)	Dosage Forms and Strengths
alprazolam[a]	Xanax, Xanax XR	**Solution (concentrate):** 1 mg/mL
	Xanax	**Tablets (Xanax):** 0.25 mg, 0.5 mg, 1 mg, 2 mg
		Tablets, triscored: 2 mg
		Tablets, extended release (Xanax XR): 0.5 mg, 1 mg, 2 mg, 3 mg
		Tablets, disintegrating: 0.25 mg, 0.5 mg, 1 mg, 2 mg
clonazepam[a]	Klonopin	**Tablets:** 0.25 mg[b], 0.5 mg, 1 mg, 2 mg
	Rivotril	**Tablets, disintegrating**[c]**:** 0.125 mg, 0.25 mg, 0.5 mg, 1 mg, 2 mg
clorazepate[a]	Gen-xene, Tranxene	**Tablets:** 3.75 mg, 7.5 mg, 15 mg
	Tranxene	
diazepam[a]	Diastat, Diazepam Intensol, Valium	**Rectal gel (Diastat):** 5 mg/mL, 10 mg/2 mL[c], and 2.5 mg/0.5 mL[c] prefilled syringe, 20 mg prefilled syringes[b]
	Diastat, Valium	**Injection, IM:** 5 mg/mL
		Oral, solution: 1 mg/1 mL
		Oral concentrate (Diazepam Intensol)[c]**:** 5 mg/mL
		Tablets (Valium): 2 mg, 5 mg, 10 mg
lorazepam[a]	Ativan	**Injection, solution (Ativan):** 2 mg/mL[c]; 4 mg/mL
	Ativan	**Solution, oral concentrate**[c]**:** 2 mg/mL
		Tablets (Ativan): 0.5 mg, 1 mg, 2 mg
midazolam[a]	Generic	**Injection, solution:** 1 mg/mL and 5 mg/mL
	Generic	**Syrup**[c]**:** 2 mg/mL
oxazepam[a]	Generic	**Capsules**[c]**:** 10 mg, 15 mg, 30 mg
	Generic	**Tablets**[b]**:** 10 mg, 15 mg, 30 mg

[a]Generic available.
[b]Available in Canada only.
[c]Available in the United States only.
IM, Intramuscular.

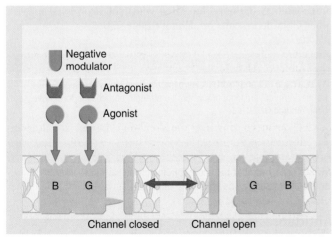

Mechanism of action of

G = GABA receptor site

B = benzodiazepine binding site

• **Fig. 5.1** Anxiolytic agents. (From Page C, Curtis M, Sutter M, et al: *Integrated pharmacology*, ed 3, Philadelphia, 2006, Mosby.)

memory because they produce a type of amnesia. This side effect is sometimes used purposefully, such as when benzodiazepines are used to reduce anxiety associated with dental or medical procedures. The person receiving the drug "forgets" the procedure, so anxiety associated with future procedures is reduced. Adverse reactions are dose dependent, and side effects increase as the dose increases. The therapeutic index for benzodiazepines is high. The lethal dose is approximately 1000 times greater than the typical therapeutic dose.

Tolerance and Dependence

All benzodiazepines are capable of producing tolerance and dependence, which is why they are classified as class IV controlled substances in the United States. Benzodiazepines are categorized as a targeted substance in Canada and listed in schedule IV of the Canadian Controlled Drugs and Substances Act.

Tolerance to a drug is said to have developed when the patient must take increasing doses to achieve the same effects as were achieved previously at lower doses. Tolerance to benzodiazepines can develop in as little as 14 days. Benzodiazepines are also known to produce *drug dependence*. When drug dependence has developed, the person taking the drug must continue to take the drug to avoid the onset of physical or psychological withdrawal symptoms (or both). Sudden cessation of benzodiazepines can bring on the onset of withdrawal symptoms such as tremors, anxiety, insomnia, agitation, and confusion. Onset of withdrawal symptoms is drug specific. Withdrawal symptoms develop soon after discontinuation of benzodiazepines with short half-lives. The onset of withdrawal symptoms is delayed after abrupt discontinuation of benzodiazepines that have long half-lives. The risk of developing withdrawal symptoms is minimized when benzodiazepines are discontinued slowly.

> ### ● TECH NOTE!
> Class IV drugs produce less risk for physical and psychological addiction than do class I, II, and III drugs.

Precautions

Benzodiazepines potentiate the sedative effects of other central nervous system (CNS) depressants. They also should be used cautiously in patients who have liver disease. When midazolam is administered, respiratory resuscitation equipment should be readily available. There is a drug interaction between midazolam and cimetidine that results in increased midazolam levels.

> ### ● TECH ALERT!
> Xanax, Zantac, and ZyrTEC have look-alike/sound-alike issues. Immediate release and extended release also have look-alike/sound-alike issues!

> ### ● TECH ALERT!
> Clorazepate immediate release and sustained release have look-alike/ sound-alike issues.

> ### ● TECH ALERT!
> ClomiPRAMINE, chlorpromazine, and clomiPHENE have look-alike/ sound-alike issues.

> ### ● TECH ALERT!
> Diazepam oral solution and oral concentrate have look-alike/sound-alike issues.

> ### ● TECH ALERT!
> Lorazepam and alprazolam have look-alike/sound-alike issues. Ativan and Atarax have look-alike/sound-alike issues.

Azapirones

Buspirone is currently the only azapirone drug. Azapirones are effective in management of anxiety disorders (Table 5.2) and have a benefit over benzodiazepines because they do not produce tolerance or dependence.

TABLE 5.2	Azapirones Used in the Treatment of Anxiety	
Generic Name	US Brand Name(s) / Canadian Brand(s)	Dosage Forms and Strengths
buspirone[a]	Generics	**Tablets:** 5 mg[b], 7.5 mg[b], 10 mg, 15 mg[b], 30 mg[b]
	Generics	

[a]Generic available.
[b]Available in the United States only.

buspar (handwritten)

Mechanism of Action

The action produced by azapirones is believed to be caused by binding at dopamine (DA2) and 5-HT (5-HT$_{1A}$) receptors. Azapirones are partial agonists at the 5-HT$_{1A}$ receptors. Azapirones have no effect on GABA receptors and lack CNS depressant activity.

Pharmacokinetics

Buspirone is the only drug in this class. The onset of action is slow, and maximum therapeutic effects are achieved 3 to 6 weeks after therapy has been initiated. Buspirone is metabolized in the liver and eliminated in urine. The elimination half-life is between 2 and 3 hours. Food increases the drug's bioavailability.

Adverse Reactions

The most common adverse effects associated with buspirone therapy are dizziness, restlessness, headache, nausea, diarrhea, and insomnia. Buspirone produces only minimal sedation.

Precautions

Buspirone should be used with caution in patients with liver or kidney disease.

> ### ● TECH ALERT!
> BusPIRone and buPROPion have look-alike/sound-alike issues.

Miscellaneous Anxiolytic Agents

Hydroxyzine

Hydroxyzine is an antihistamine (see Chapter 24) that is also approved for the treatment of GADs. It is a histamine-1 receptor antagonist. Hydroxyzine may be used in children and adults to reduce anxiety associated with dental and minor medical procedures. It produces a fair bit of sedation but, similar to buspirone, does not produce tolerance or dependence. Other side effects are dizziness, headache, dry mucous membranes, and urinary retention.

Men with prostate disease and lactating women should avoid hydroxyzine, because the antihistamine decreases urine flow and breast milk. Sedation is increased when the drug is taken with other CNS depressants or alcohol (Table 5.3).

> ### ● TECH ALERT!
> HydrOXYzine HCl and hydrOXYzine pamoate have look-alike/sound-alike issues. Verify all prescriptions when the strength and dosage form have been omitted.

> ### ● TECH ALERT!
> HydrOXYzine, hydrALAZINE, and HYDROmorphone have look-alike/ sound-alike issues.

Antidepressants

SSRIs, serotonin-noradrenaline reuptake inhibitors (SNRIs), TCAs, and monoamine oxidase inhibitors (MAOIs) are antidepressants prescribed for the treatment of anxiety disorders (see Chapter 6) (Table 5.4). Fluoxetine and sertraline are SSRIs that are indicated for OCD. Sertraline is also labeled for use in the treatment of panic disorder, social phobia, and PTSD. Venlafaxine is an SNRI and is used in the management of GADs. Clomipramine, a TCA, is indicated for the treatment of OCD.

Treatment of OCD with antidepressants requires higher doses than the treatment of depression, and it takes a longer time for maximum benefits to be achieved. For example, clomipramine may take up to 6 weeks for full effects to be noticed. Maximum benefits of fluoxetine and sertraline are achieved in 1 to 3 weeks.

Mechanism of Action

SSRIs inhibit 5-HT reuptake into the presynaptic neuron, increasing 5-HT availability at postsynaptic receptor sites. SNRIs and TCAs inhibit the reuptake of 5-HT and noradrenaline. MAOI binding increases synaptic availability of 5-HT, noradrenaline, and dopamine.

Adverse Reactions

Some adverse reactions are common to all the antidepressants used in the treatment of anxiety. Others are drug specific. Clomipramine may produce sedation or decreased alertness; fluoxetine, paroxetine, and sertraline may cause insomnia, decreased appetite, dry mouth, dizziness, and agitation or tremor; and paroxetine may also produce headache, nausea, diarrhea, and sexual dysfunction.

No tolerance or dependence is associated with any of the antidepressants. However, some serious side effects are possible. Clomipramine may produce seizures. Serotonin syndrome is a serious condition associated with the use of drugs such as sertraline and fluoxetine. Serotonin syndrome is potentially fatal and produces symptoms of confusion, agitation, diarrhea, tremors, increased blood pressure, and seizures. A detailed description of specific mechanisms of action and pharmacokinetics of these drugs will be discussed in Chapter 6.

> **❶ TECH ALERT!**
>
> ClonazePAM, cloNIDine, and clozapine have look-alike/sound-alike issues.

TABLE 5.3 Miscellaneous Drugs Used in the Treatment of Anxiety

Generic Name	US Brand Name(s) / Canadian Brand(s)	Dosage Forms and Strengths
hydroxyzine HCl[a]	Generics / Atarax	**Capsules**[b]: 10 mg, 25 mg, 50 mg **Injection, solution:** 25 mg/mL, 50 mg/mL **Syrup:** 10 mg/5 mL (2 mg/mL) **Tablets**[c]: 10 mg, 25 mg, 50 mg
hydroxyzine pamoate[a]	Vistaril / Not available	**Capsules**[c]: 25 mg, 50 mg, 100 mg

[a]Generic available.
[b]Available in Canada only.
[c]Available in the United States only.

TABLE 5.4 Antidepressants Used in the Treatment of Anxiety

Generic Name	US Brand Name(s) / Canadian Brand(s)	Dosage Forms and Strengths
clomipramine[a]	Anafranil / Anafranil	**Capsules**[b]: 25 mg, 50 mg, 75 mg **Tablets**[c]: 10 mg, 25 mg, 50 mg
escitalopram[a]	Lexapro / Cipralex, Cipralex Meltz	**Oral solution**[b]: 5 mg/5 mL **Tablets:** 5 mg[b], 10 mg, 20 mg **Tablets (Disintegrating)**[c]: 10 mg, 20 mg
fluoxetine[a]	Prozac, Prozac Weekly, Selfemra, Sarafem / Prozac	**Capsule (Prozac):** 10 mg, 20 mg, 40 mg **Capsule (Prozac Weekly):** 90 mg **Oral solution:** 20 mg/5 mL **Tablets (Prozac, Selfemra):** 10 mg, 15 mg, 20 mg **Tablets, for PMS (Sarafem):** 10 mg, 15 mg, 20 mg
paroxetine[a]	Brisdelle, Paxil, Paxil CR, Pexeva / Paxil, Paxil CR	**Capsule, as mesylate (Brisdelle):** 7.5 mg **Suspension, oral (Paxil)**[b]: 10 mg/5 mL **Tablet, as HCl (Paxil):** 10 mg, 20 mg, 30 mg, 40 mg **Tablets, as mesylate (Pexeva):** 10 mg, 20 mg, 30 mg, 40 mg **Tablets, controlled release (Paxil CR):** 12.5 mg, 25 mg, 37.5 mg
sertraline[a]	Zoloft / Zoloft	**Capsules**[c]: 25 mg, 50 mg, 100 mg **Solution, oral concentrate**[b]: 20 mg/mL **Tablets**[b]: 25 mg, 50 mg, 100 mg
venlafaxine[a]	Effexor XR / Effexor XR	**Capsules, extended release (Effexor XR):** 37.5 mg, 75 mg, 150 mg **Tablets**[b]: 25 mg, 37.5 mg, 50 mg, 75 mg, 100 mg **Tablets, extended release**[b]: 37.5 mg, 75 mg, 150 mg, 225 mg

[a]Generic available.
[b]Available in the United States only.
[c]Available in Canada only.

❶ TECH ALERT!

FLUoxetine, DULoxetine, PARoxetine, and fluvoxaMINE have look-alike/sound-alike issues.

❶ TECH ALERT!

Paxil and Taxol have look-alike/sound-alike issues. Paxil and Plavix also have look-alike/sound-alike issues!

Beta-Adrenergic Antagonists

Rapid heart rate is a common symptom of anxiety. Beta-adrenergic antagonists, also known as beta blockers, are administered to reduce palpitations. Beta-adrenergic antagonists are not approved by the US Food and Drug Administration (FDA) for the treatment of anxiety; however, the beta blockers (e.g., propranolol and nadolol) may be prescribed to control the symptoms that accompany anxiety and to prevent stage fright. Propranolol diminishes sympathetic activity in the brain. Recent studies suggest that propranolol may weaken the formation of stressful memories, making it useful in the treatment of PTSD; however, it is not yet FDA approved for this use.

TECHNICIAN'S CORNER

1. What happens if a patient stops using benzodiazepines abruptly?
2. What is the difference between tolerance and dependence on a drug?

Summary of Drugs Used in the Treatment of Anxiety Disorders

	Generic Name	US Brand Name	Usual Adult Oral Dose and Dosing Schedule	Warning Labels
Benzodiazepines				
	alprazolam	Xanax	**Generalized anxiety disorder:** immediate release 0.25–4 mg daily (in 2–3 divided doses) **Panic disorder:** 1–10 mg/day in 3 divided doses (immediate release); 0.5–6 mg once daily (extended release) **Anxiety associated with depression:** 2.5–3 mg/day in divided doses)	MAY CAUSE DROWSINESS; MAY IMPAIR ABILITY TO DRIVE. AVOID ALCOHOL. MAY BE HABIT FORMING. DO NOT CRUSH, BREAK, OR CHEW (extended release).
	clonazepam	Klonopin	**Panic disorder:** 0.25–1 mg twice a day (maximum, 4 mg/day)	
	clorazepate	Tranxene	**Generalized anxiety disorder:** 7.5–15 mg 2–4 times/day (immediate release); 11.25–22.5 mg once daily (sustained release) **Ethanol withdrawal:** 30 mg dosed 2–4 times/day; increase up to maximum of 90 mg/day (reduce gradually)	
	diazepam	Valium	**Anxiety disorder:** 2–10 mg 2–4 times/day (oral); 2–10 mg every 3–4 hours (IM, IV) **Ethanol withdrawal:** 5–10 mg IV every 3–4 hours as needed	
	lorazepam	Ativan	**Anxiety and sedation:** Oral 1–10 mg daily in 2–3 divided doses **Preprocedure sedation:** 0.05 mg/kg IM (maximum, 4 mg/dose) or 0.044 mg/kg IV (maximum, 2 mg/dose)	
	midazolam	Generic	**Conscious sedation for preoperative procedures:** 0.5–2 mg slow IV every 2–3 min (maximum, 2.5–5 mg)	MAY CAUSE DIZZINESS AND DISORIENTATION. MAY CAUSE PAIN, SWELLING, OR REDNESS AT INJECTION SITE.
	oxazepam	Generic	**Anxiety:** 10–30 mg 3–4 times a day **Ethanol withdrawal:** 15–30 mg 3–4 times a day	MAY CAUSE DROWSINESS; MAY IMPAIR ABILITY TO DRIVE. AVOID ALCOHOL. MAY BE HABIT FORMING. DO NOT CRUSH, BREAK, OR CHEW (extended release).

Summary of Drugs Used in the Treatment of Anxiety Disorders—cont'd

	Generic Name	US Brand Name	Usual Adult Oral Dose and Dosing Schedule	Warning Labels
Azapirones				
	buspirone	generics	7.5–15 mg twice daily (maximum dose, 60 mg/day)	MAY CAUSE DROWSINESS; MAY IMPAIR ABILITY TO DRIVE. TAKE WITH FOOD.
Miscellaneous Anxiolytics				
	hydroxyzine HCl	Atarax	**Anxiety:** 25–100 mg 4 times a day (maximum dose, 400 mg/day) **Ethanol withdrawal:** 50–100 mg IM 4 times a day	MAY CAUSE DROWSINESS; AVOID ALCOHOL MAY INTENSIFY THIS EFFECT.
	hydroxyzine pamoate	Vistaril	**Anxiety:** 50–100 mg IM 4 times a day **Preoperative sedation:** 50–100 mg as a single dose (oral); 25–100 mg (IM)	MAY IMPAIR ABILITY TO DRIVE.
Antidepressants Used in the Treatment of Anxiety Disorders				
	clomipramine	Anafranil	**Obsessive-compulsive disorder:** 25–100 mg/day in divided doses (maximum, 250 mg/day)	MAY CAUSE DIZZINESS OR DROWSINESS; ALCOHOL MAY INTENSIFY THIS EFFECT.
	duloxetine	Cymbalta	**Generalized anxiety disorder:** 60 mg PO once daily	MAY IMPAIR ABILITY TO DRIVE.
	escitalopram	Lexapro, Cipralex[a]	**Generalized anxiety disorder:** 10–20 mg once daily	SWALLOW WHOLE; DO NOT CRUSH OR CHEW (delayed
	fluoxetine	Prozac	**Obsessive-compulsive disorder:** 20–80 mg/day **Panic disorder:** 20 mg/day (maximum, 60 mg/day)	and extended release—Cymbalta, Prozac weekly, Paxil CR, Effexor XR).
	paroxetine	Paxil	**Generalized anxiety disorder:** 20–50 mg/day **Obsessive-compulsive disorder:** 20–60 mg/day **Panic disorder:** 10–60 mg/day (Paxil, Pexeva) or 12.5–75 mg/day (Paxil CR) **Posttraumatic stress disorder:** 12.5–25 mg daily (Paxil CR) 20 mg/day (immediate release) **Social phobias:** 20 mg/day (Paxil) or 12.5–37.5 mg/day (Paxil CR)	DO NOT DISCONTINUE WITHOUT MEDICAL SUPERVISION.
	sertraline	Zoloft	**Obsessive-compulsive disorder:** 50 mg/day (Max 400 mg/day) **Panic disorder, posttraumatic stress disorder, and social phobias:** 50 mg/day (up to 200 mg/day)	
	venlafaxine	Effexor XR	**Generalized anxiety disorder, panic disorder, and social phobias:** 37.5–75 mg once daily (Maximum 225 mg/day); increase by 37.5 mg every 4–7 days	

[a]Available in Canada only. *IM,* Intramuscular.

Key Points

- Anxiety disorders are the leading mental health illness.
- The cause of anxiety disorders may be environmental, biologic, or developmental; associated with socioeconomic conditions; or a combination of several of these individual factors.
- The four major types of anxiety disorders are generalized anxiety disorder, panic disorder, OCD, and PTSD.
- Common physiologic symptoms include increased heart rate, palpitations, shortness of breath, rapid breathing, nausea, sweating, and dry mouth. All of these symptoms are associated with hyperactivity of the autonomic nervous system.

- Generalized anxiety disorder is associated with excessive worry and tension that are experienced daily for longer than 6 months.
- OCD is a condition associated with an inability to control or stop repeated unwanted thoughts or behaviors.
- Panic disorder is a condition associated with repeated sudden onset of feelings of terror.
- A phobia is an irrational fear of things or situations that produce symptoms of intense anxiety.
- Social phobias cause affected individuals to shy away from social situations where they fear embarrassment of humiliation. Fear of public speaking is an example of a social phobia.

- PTSD is a stress disorder that develops in persons who have participated in, witnessed, or been a victim of a terrifying event.
- Anxiety disorder is treated by the administration of anxiolytics and psychotherapy, including cognitive behavioral therapy.
- The mechanism of action for most anxiolytics is to enhance binding of GABA, a neurotransmitter to receptors.
- Benzodiazepines are used in the treatment of anxiety.
- The duration of action for benzodiazepines may be long acting, intermediate acting, or short acting.
- Benzodiazepines can produce a type of amnesia that causes the person receiving the drug to "forget," reducing anxiety associated with future dental or medical procedures.
- All benzodiazepines are capable of producing tolerance and dependence.
- When tolerance develops, increasing doses of a drug are required to achieve the same effects as were achieved previously at lower doses. When drug dependence has developed, the person taking the drug must continue to take the drug to avoid the onset of or psychological withdrawal symptoms (or both).
- All benzodiazepines are scheduled class IV controlled substances in the United States and are targeted substances in Canada.

- Withdrawal symptoms develop soon after discontinuation of benzodiazepines with short half-lives and are delayed after abrupt discontinuation of benzodiazepines that have long half-lives.
- Buspirone is an azapirone that is used to treat anxiety.
- Buspirone does not produce tolerance or dependence. Abrupt discontinuation does not produce withdrawal symptoms.
- Hydroxyzine is an antihistamine that is indicated for the treatment of anxiety. It is used in children and adults to reduce anxiety associated with dental and minor medical procedures.
- TCAs, SSRIs, and MAOIs are antidepressants prescribed for the treatment of anxiety disorders.
- Serotonin syndrome is a potentially life-threatening adverse drug reaction caused by excessive 5-HT that produces symptoms of confusion, agitation, diarrhea, tremors, increased blood pressure, and seizures.
- Beta-adrenergic antagonists are administered to reduce the palpitations associated with anxiety and are also useful for the management of stage fright.

Review Questions

1. Is the following statement true or false? "Women are twice as likely as men to be diagnosed with generalized anxiety disorder."
   a. True
   b. False
2. The_____ treatment of anxiety is associated with increases in drug-receptor binding to the neurotransmitters γ-aminobutyric acid, serotonin, and norepinephrine.
   a. therapeutic
   b. psychological
   c. pharmacologic
   d. physiologic
3. Anxiety disorder is treated by the administration of _____ and psychotherapy.
   a. analgesics
   b. anxiolytics
   c. antiinflammatories
   d. antipsychotics
4. Benzodiazepines are indicated for _____ treatment of anxiety.
   a. short-term
   b. long-term
5. _____ to a drug is said to have developed when the patient must take increasing doses to achieve the same effects as were achieved previously at lower doses.
   a. Dependence
   b. Addiction
   c. Tolerance
   d. none of the above

6. Which of the following benzodiazepines is indicated for the treatment of anxiety disorders, ethanol withdrawal, skeletal muscle relaxation, and seizure disorders?
   a. Alprazolam
   b. Clonazepam
   c. Lorazepam
   d. Diazepam
7. Buspirone is the only drug in this class.
   a. Azapirone
   b. Antihistamine
   c. Amiodarone
   d. a and c
8. _____ is an antihistamine that is indicated for the treatment of anxiety.
   a. Promethazine
   b. Hydroxyzine
   c. Apresoline
   d. none of the above
9. Clomipramine, fluoxetine, and sertraline are antidepressants that are indicated for the treatment of
   a. panic disorders
   b. social phobias
   c. obsessive-compulsive disorder
   d. posttraumatic stress disorder
10. Rapid heart rate is a common symptom of anxiety. Beta-adrenergic antagonists are administered to reduce the palpitations. One example is
    a. Propranolol
    b. Inderal
    c. Nadolol
    d. all of the above

Bibliography

Anxiety Disorders Association of America: Understand the facts Generalized Anxiety Disorder (GAD). Retrieved from https://www.adaa.org/understanding-anxiety/generalized-anxiety-disorder-gad. (Accessed 4 December 2016).

Bourin M: Serotoninergic systems in anxiety, *JSM Anxiety Depress* 1(2):1007, 2016.

Greenberg W, Aronson S: Obsessive-compulsive disorder, *eMedicine* 2016. Retrieved from: http://emedicine.medscape.com/article/1934139-overview. (Accessed 5 December 2016).

Institute for Safe Medication Practices: FDA and ISMP Lists of Look-Alike Drug Names with Recommended Tall Man Letters, 2016.

Lance L, Lacy C, Armstrong L, et al: *Drug information handbook for the allied health professional*, ed 12, Hudson, OH, 2005, APhA Lexi-Comp.

National Institute of Mental Health: Generalized Anxiety Disorders: When worry gets out of control. U.S. Department of Health and Human Services NIH publication no. QF 16-4677, Bethesda, MD, 2016.

National Institute of Mental Health: Panic Disorder: When fear overwhelms. U.S. Department of Health and Human Services NIH publication no. QF 16-4679, Bethesda, MD, National Institute of Mental Health, National Institutes of Health: Anxiety Disorders, 2016. Retrieved from https://www.nimh.nih.gov/health/topics/anxiety-disorders/index.shtml. (Accessed 4 December 2016).

Page C, Curtis M, Sutter M, et al: *Integrated pharmacology*, Philadelphia, 2005, Elsevier Mosby, pp 239–241.

Public Health Agency of Canada: Mood and Anxiety Disorders in Canada, 2014. Retrieved from http://healthycanadians.gc.ca/publications/diseases-conditions-maladies-affections/mental-mood-anxiety-anxieux-humeur/alt/mental-mood-anxiety-anxieux-humeur-eng.pdf. (Accessed 30 November 2016).

Raffa R, Rawls S, Beyzarov E: *Netter's illustrated pharmacology*, Philadelphia, 2005, WB Saunders, pp 65–66.

Ravindran L, Stein MB: The pharmacologic treatment of anxiety disorders: a review of progress, *J Clin Psychiatry* 71(7):839–854, 2010.

Statistics Canada: Section B. Anxiety Disorders, 2015. Retrieved from http://www.statcan.gc.ca/pub/82-619-m/2012004/sections/sectionb-eng.htm. (Accessed 4 December 2016).

6

Treatment of Depression

LEARNING OBJECTIVES

1. Learn the terminology associated with depression and its treatment.
2. List and describe the function of neurotransmitters associated with symptoms of depression.
3. Classify medications used to treat depression.
4. Describe mechanism of action for each class of drugs used to treat depression.
5. Identify significant drug look-alike/sound-alike issues.
6. Identify warning labels and precautionary messages associated with medications used to treat depression.

KEY TERMS

Adjunct drug therapy Initiated to complement the effects of another drug.
Bipolar disorder Mental health illness associated with sudden swings in mood between depression and periods of mania, racing thoughts, distractibility, and increased goal-directed behavior.
Enuresis Bedwetting or uncontrollable urination during sleep.
Major depression Mental health illness associated with persistent feelings of sadness, emptiness, or hopelessness that last for several weeks.

Monoamine oxidase Enzyme found in the liver, intestine, and terminal neuron, responsible for degradation of monoamine neurotransmitters and dietary amines.
Serotonin syndrome Potentially life-threatening adverse drug reaction that produces symptoms of confusion, agitation, diarrhea, tremors, and increased blood pressure and is caused by excessive serotonin.

Overview

It is estimated that more than 15 million Americans experience a major depressive episode annually. At some time in their lives, one in eight Canadians adults will experience a mood disorder such as depression (11.3%) or bipolar disorder (2.6%). Depression affects men, women, and children. Depressive disorder may be precipitated by hormonal changes (premenstrual syndrome, pregnancy, postpartum), substance abuse (alcohol and other drugs), or illness such as Parkinson disease, heart attack, or thyroid dysfunction. Heredity plays a role as well, particularly in bipolar disorder because children born to a parent with bipolar disorder are at increased risk for the illness.

Depressive illness influences most aspects of a person's life and lifestyle. It affects self-esteem, mood, thoughts, eating, and sleeping. Depression reduces the ability to think and concentrate. Feelings of worthlessness or guilt often accompany depressive episodes. As many as 12% of depressed patients contemplate or attempt suicide. Without treatment, symptoms of depression can persist for a few weeks to years.

The three primary types of depressive disorders are major depression, bipolar disorder, and dysthymia. *Major depression* is also called *clinical depression* and is associated with persistent feelings of sadness, emptiness, or hopelessness. These feelings persist for several weeks and are usually accompanied by a lack of interest in activities that were previously thought to be enjoyable, fatigue, irritability, and insomnia or hypersomnia. Sometimes the depression manifests itself in other physical ailments for which no treatments

are able to cure or reduce symptoms. *Bipolar disorder*, formerly called *manic-depressive disorder*, is associated with sudden swings in mood between depression and periods of mania. Mania is associated with hyperactivity, racing thoughts, insomnia, distractibility, and increased goal-directed behavior. Manic periods can last for 1 or more weeks, during which time the person may sleep little and produce a prolific amount of work. Several well-known people such as Vincent Van Gogh are believed to have had bipolar disorder. Dysthymia produces symptoms that are similar to those of major depression; however, the symptoms are less severe. People diagnosed with dysthymia have symptoms that are chronic and, although not typically debilitating, keep the person from functioning well and feeling good.

The causes of depression are not completely known, but a deficiency of certain neurotransmitters is involved. This explains why people with depression cannot "pull themselves together" to get better. Drug treatment is aimed at restoring depleted neurotransmitters to normal levels.

Neurochemistry of Depression

Biogenic Amine Theory

According to the biogenic amine theory, major depression results from a decrease in monoamine neurotransmitters in the brain. This hypothesis was made upon the discovery that patients treated with drugs that deplete monoamine neurotransmitter stores in the

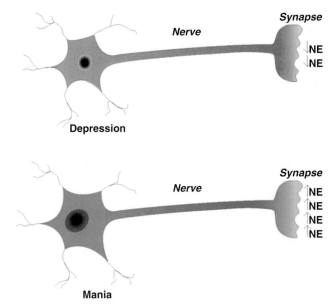

• **Fig. 6.1** Biogenic amine hypothesis. (From Lilley LL, Collins S, Snyder JS: *Pharmacology and the nursing process*, ed 8, St. Louis, 2017, Elsevier.)

neuron develop depression. Neurotransmitter-binding sites are also less sensitive in depressed persons.

If depletion of monoamine neurotransmitters causes depression, what is the effect of excessive levels of these neurotransmitters? Bipolar affective disorder (BPAD), also known as mania, is believed to be associated with increased levels of monoamine neurotransmitters (Fig. 6.1). The complete neurochemistry of BPAD is unclear.

The monoamine neurotransmitters that are thought to be involved in depression and BPAD are norepinephrine (NE), serotonin (5-HT), and dopamine (DA).

Role of Norepinephrine

The neurotransmitter NE plays an important role in the treatment of depression. It is widely distributed in the brain and in the periphery. Decreased levels in the brain are responsible for depression and increased levels in the periphery can cause serious effects such as hypertension.

Role of Serotonin

Serotonin (5-HT) plays an important role in the treatment of depression. 5-HT is an excitatory neurotransmitter. More than nine 5-HT receptors have been identified. 5-HT receptors that have been well studied are 5-HT_{1A}, 5-HT_{2A}, 5-HT_{2C}, and 5-HT_{3}. Drugs that antagonize 5-HT_{2A} and 5-HT_{2C} receptors are used in the treatment of depression and negative-symptom schizophrenia. Drugs that antagonize 5-HT_{3} receptors are used to treat nausea. In addition to improved mood, 5-HT is involved in regulation of the sleep-wake cycle and pain perception.

Role of Dopamine

There are five types of dopamine (DA) receptors. Binding to D2, D3, and D4 receptors is inhibitory, and binding to D1 and D5 is excitatory. DA binding plays less of a role in the treatment and management of depression compared with the neurotransmitters

NE and 5-HT. Drugs that are used in the treatment of Parkinson disease and schizophrenia potentiate the activity of DA (see Chapter 8).

Drugs Used to Treat Depression

Antidepressants are categorized according to the method that they use to potentiate the actions of NE, 5-HT, and DA. Nonspecific antidepressants increase the binding of more than one monoamine neurotransmitter. There are two primary mechanisms of action (MOAs) of marketed antidepressants (Fig. 6.2). One MOA is inhibition of the reuptake of one or more of the monoamine neurotransmitters involved in depression. The other MOA is to block the degradation of monoamine neurotransmitters. The MOAs for drugs used to treat depression may differ, but all antidepressants are equally effective. Selection of one antidepressant over another is based on the patient's ability to tolerate drug side effects. The effects of antidepressants are not immediate and increase over time.

Tricyclic Antidepressants

The tricyclic antidepressants (TCAs) are the oldest class of medication used in the treatment of depression. The effectiveness of newer agents is compared with that of TCAs. The TCAs are used for the treatment and management of several medical conditions in addition to depression. They are also prescribed for *enuresis*, commonly known as bedwetting (imipramine and nortriptyline). They are prescribed for the treatment of obsessive-compulsive disorder (clomipramine) and as *adjunct drug therapy* in the management of chronic pain (amitriptyline, nortriptyline). Doxepin is prescribed for sleep disorders in lower doses than used for depression. Doxepin is also prescribed as a cream for itching.

Mechanism of Action

In depression, sufficient neurotransmitters may be released into the synaptic cleft; however, the neurotransmitters may be returned to the neuron before binding occurs. The TCAs work by producing a nonspecific blockade of the reuptake of monoamine neurotransmitters. The TCAs block the reuptake of NE and 5-HT in the presynaptic neuron and in postsynaptic receptors. When the reuptake of NE and 5-HT back into the neuron is blocked, the neurotransmitters remain in the synaptic cleft longer. The longer the neurotransmitter remains in the synaptic cleft, the greater the opportunity for binding to receptor sites (Fig. 6.3). The TCAs also have some affinity for adrenergic, cholinergic (muscarinic), and histaminic postsynaptic receptors.

Pharmacokinetics

The TCAs are readily absorbed when administered orally. They are lipophilic, so are widely distributed within the central nervous system. The onset of action, duration of action, and half-life ($t\frac{1}{2}$) vary among agents. The $t\frac{1}{2}$ of the TCAs can be as short as 4 hours (imipramine) and as long as 96 hours (nortriptyline). Their long half-lives are associated with their high degree of lipid solubility. The long duration of action of these agents permits once-daily dosing.

The TCAs are metabolized by microsomal enzymes in the liver. Several of the TCAs are metabolized to active metabolites. Amitriptyline is metabolized to nortriptyline, and desipramine is a metabolite of imipramine. They are ultimately eliminated in the urine.

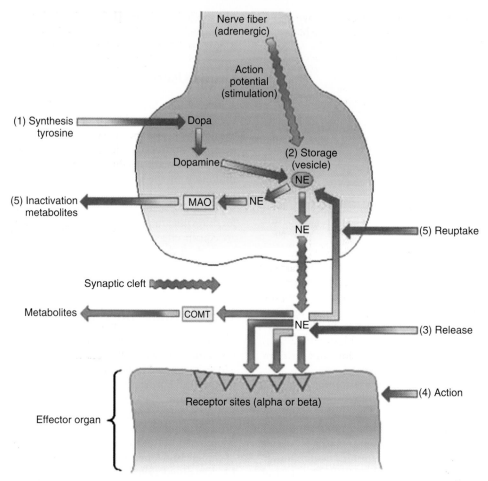

• **Fig. 6.2** Site of neurotransmitter synthesis, storage, release, action, and inactivation. (From Lilley LL, Harrington S, Snyder JS: *Pharmacology and the nursing process*, ed 5, St. Louis, 2007, Mosby.)

• **Fig. 6.3** Mechanism of action for tricyclic antidepressants.

Although the onset of action may be relatively short, maximum antidepressant benefit may take up to 6 weeks to be achieved.

> ● **TECH NOTE!**
> Dry mouth is a side effect of TCAs. It can be relieved by sucking on sugarless candy. TCAs can also increase cravings for sweets!

Adverse Reactions

The TCAs all have a similar structure, so the side effects of the drugs are similar. What varies is the degree to which a particular TCA will produce the side effect. For an example, all TCAs can produce sedation, but some TCAs, such as amitriptyline, have high sedative activity, while other TCAs, such as desipramine, have low sedative activity.

TCA adverse reactions are related to effects produced by increased binding to adrenergic, cholinergic, serotonergic, and histaminic receptors. Increased cardiovascular activity is caused by the rise in NE levels. Hypotension and reflex tachycardia is caused by post-synaptic adrenergic blockade. Sedation, weight gain, and hypotension are produced by histaminic receptor blockade. Blockade of cholinergic (muscarinic) receptors can lead to blurred vision, dry mouth, constipation, urinary retention, confusion, and delirium. The TCAs may also produce photosensitivity.

> ● **TECH NOTE!**
> Prescriptions for small quantities of the TCAs may be written for depressed patients who are believed to be suicidal.

Precautions

Hypotension produced by the TCAs is a problem for elderly adults because they are at increased risk for fainting or falling. The TCAs have a narrow therapeutic index and can produce cardiotoxicity at doses that are six to eight times higher than the therapeutic dose.

> ❶ **TECH ALERT!**
> The TCAs should not be discontinued abruptly; patients should be gradually weaned from the drug.

Selective Serotonin Reuptake Inhibitors

Citalopram (Celexa), escitalopram (Cipralex), fluoxetine (Prozac), fluvoxamine (Luvox), paroxetine (Paxil), sertraline (Zoloft), vilazodone (Viibryd), and vortioxetine (Trintellix) are selective serotonin reuptake inhibitors (SSRIs). The SSRIs are the most widely prescribed antidepressants. They are categorized by their

Tricyclic Antidepressants

Generic Name	US Brand Name(s) / Canadian Brand(s)	Dosage Forms and Strengths
amitriptyline[a]	Generics Elavil, Levate, Novo-Triptyn	**Tablets:** 10 mg, 25 mg, 50 mg, 75 mg, 100 mg[b], 150 mg[b]
desipramine[a]	Norpramin Generic only	**Tablets:** 10 mg, 25 mg, 50 mg, 75 mg, 100 mg, 150 mg[b]
doxepin[a]	Silenor, Zonalon[c] Sinequan Silenor[c]	**Capsules:** 10 mg, 25 mg, 50 mg, 75 mg, 100 mg, 150 mg[d] **Solution, oral concentrate:** 10 mg/mL[b] **Tablet :** 3 mg, 6 mg **Cream**[b]**:** 5% (Zonalon)
imipramine[a]	Tofranil Generics only	**Capsules, as pamoate**[b]**:** 75 mg, 100 mg, 125 mg, 150 mg **Tablets, as HCl:** 10 mg, 25 mg, 50 mg, 75 mg[d]
nortriptyline[a]	Pamelor Aventyl	**Capsules:** 10 mg, 25 mg, 50 mg[b], 75 mg[b] **Solution**[b]**:** 10 mg/5 mL
protriptyline[a]	Vivactil Not available	**Tablets:** 5 mg, 10 mg
trimipramine[a]	Surmontil Generics only	**Capsules:** 12.5 mg[d], 25 mg, 50 mg, 75 mg[d], 100 mg

[a]Generic available.
[b]Available in the United States only.
[c]Zonalon is a cream that is used for the treatment of itching.
[d]Available in Canada only.

MOAs rather than by their chemical structure. The SSRIs are also used in treating obsessive-compulsive disorder, premenstrual dysphoric disorder, and panic disorder. Fluoxetine is also indicated for treatment of anorexia and bulimia.

> **⚠ TECH ALERT!**
>
> The following drugs have look-alike/sound-alike issues:
> clomiPRAMINE and clomiPHENE;
> desipramine and imipramine;
> doxepin and digoxin;
> nortriptyline and amitriptyline;
> trimipramine, imipramine, and triamterene

Mechanism of Action

The SSRIs are potent inhibitors of 5-HT and have little action on the reuptake of NE or DA. They produce a selective blockade of the reuptake of 5-HT at the synaptic cleft. The SSRIs are equally effective as TCAs yet they lack the cardiotoxic effects associated with the TCAs. This makes them the drugs of choice when heart disease is present.

Pharmacokinetics

The SSRIs are well absorbed from the gastrointestinal tract. Some, such as fluoxetine, are metabolized to an active metabolite producing a long duration of action. You may hear about many drug interactions involving SSRIs. This is because they are extensively metabolized via the cytochrome P-450 (CYP450) isoenzyme system in the liver and are highly protein bound. Drug interactions may interfere with the rate of drug clearance of either the SSRI or drug that is administered with it. Therefore the effects and/or side effects of drugs coadministered with SSRIs may be increased.

Adverse Reactions

Insomnia is one of the more common side effects of SSRI administration. Fluoxetine and other SSRIs are dosed once daily in the morning to minimize nighttime sleeplessness. Other side effects include decreased appetite, nausea, agitation or anxiety, and diarrhea. Sexual dysfunction may also occur. The most serious side effects are serotonin syndrome and suicidal ideation. Both conditions are potentially fatal. Suicidal ideation is persistent thoughts of suicide. Symptoms of *serotonin syndrome* are confusion, agitation, diarrhea, tremors, increased blood pressure, and seizures.

> **● TECH NOTE!**
>
> Patients should be advised to suck sugarless candy to control the dry mouth caused by fluvoxamine.

Precautions

The SSRIs are fairly well tolerated, but to avoid adverse reactions, the dose should be increased gradually to desired levels and the dose should be tapered to discontinue the drug. Serotonin syndrome can result from coadministration with monoamine oxidase inhibitors (MAOIs). The SSRIs should be used cautiously in patients with liver disease.

> **● TECH NOTE!**
>
> Doxepin oral concentrate should not be diluted in carbonated beverages.

Monoamine Oxidase Inhibitors

Monoamine Oxidase Inhibitors (MAOIs) are used to treat depression and Parkinson's disease. *Monoamine oxidase* is an enzyme is found in the terminal neuron, liver, intestines, and brain. The enzyme inactivates neurotransmitters that have been released so they do not accumulate when no longer needed. There are two forms of MAO, subtype A (MAOA) and subtype B (MAOB). MOA subtype A is found in the terminal neuron, liver, and intestines. MAO_B is predominantly found in the brain.

> **⚠ TECH ALERT!**
>
> The following drugs have look-alike/sound-alike issues:
> CeleXA, celeBREX and ZyPREXA;
> FLUoxetine and fluvoxaMINE;
> Luvox, Levoxyl, and Lovenox;
> Paxil and Taxol;
> Paxil and Plavix

Mechanism of Action

The MAOIs interfere with the break down of monoamine neurotransmitters and dietary amines (e.g., tyramine) (Fig. 6.4). The MAOIs that are used in the treatment of major depression primarily interfere with the action of MAO_A. Drugs that preferentially interfere with MAO_B are used in the treatment of Parkinson's disease.

Pharmacokinetics

The MAOIs are readily absorbed when taken orally, but elimination is slow. The drugs are categorized as reversible or irreversible inhibitors of MAO according to the time it takes for enzyme levels to return to normal when the drug is discontinued. It takes approximately 3 to 5 days for MAO levels to return to normal on discontinuation of reversible MAOIs. Recovery takes up to 2 weeks when irreversible MAOIs are administered.

Adverse Reactions

The MAOIs were first discovered in the 1950s, but the risk for serious side effects has limited their widespread use. Mild adverse reactions include sedation, dry mouth, urinary retention, constipation, orthostatic hypotension, impotence, and weight gain. The severity of these side effects is equal to or less than that of most TCAs. The most serious adverse reaction is hypertensive crisis.

Hypertensive crisis can be fatal and is caused by drug-drug and drug-food interactions with MAOIs. When MAOIs are administered, their effect on MAO in the liver is to block the break down of dietary amines (e.g., tyramine). As tyramine levels rise in the general circulation the tyramine travels to peripheral sympathetic nerve terminals, where it promotes the release of NE stores. Excess circulating NE causes blood pressure to rise to dangerously high levels and produces excessive stimulation of the heart.

> **● TECH NOTE!**
>
> Symptoms of hypertensive crisis are throbbing headache, neck stiffness, and palpitations.

Selective Serotonin Reuptake Inhibitors

Generic Name	US Brand Name(s) / Canadian Brand(s)	Dosage Forms and Strengths
citalopram[a]	Celexa	**Solution, oral**[b]: 10 mg/5 mL
	Celexa	**Tablet:** 10 mg, 20 mg, 40 mg **Tablet, disintegrating:** 40mg[b]
escitalopram[a]	Lexapro	**Solution, oral:** 1 mg/mL (240 mL)
	Cipralex, Cipralex Meltz	**Tablet:** 5 mg[b], 10 mg, 20 mg
fluoxetine[a]	Prozac, Prozac Weekly, Selfemra, Sarafem	**Capsule:** 10 mg, 20 mg, 40 mg[b] **Capsule, delayed release (Prozac Weekly)**[b]: 90 mg
	Generics	**Solution, oral:** 20 mg/5 mL **Tablet (Sarafem, Selfemra)**[b]: 10 mg, 15 mg, 20 mg
fluoxetine + olanzapine	Symbyax	**Capsules:**
	Not available	fluoxetine 25 mg + olanzapine 3 mg fluoxetine 25 mg + olanzapine 6 mg fluoxetine 25 mg + olanzapine 12 mg fluoxetine 50 mg + olanzapine 6 mg fluoxetine 50 mg + olanzapine 12 mg
fluvoxamine[a]	Luvox	**Capsule, extended release (Luvox CR):** 100 mg, 150 mg
	Luvox	**Tablet:** 25 mg[b], 50 mg, 100 mg
paroxetine[a]	Brisdelle, Paxil, Paxil CR, Pexeva	**Capsule, as mesylate (Brisdelle)**[b]: 7.5 mg **Suspension, oral**[b]: 10 mg/5 mL
	Paxil, Paxil CR	**Tablets, as HCl (Paxil):** 10 mg, 20 mg, 30 mg, 40 mg[b] **Tablets, as controlled release (Paxil CR):** 12.5 mg, 25 mg, 37.5 mg[a] **Tablets, as mesylate (Pexeva)**[b]: 10 mg, 20 mg, 30 mg, 40 mg
sertraline[a]	Zoloft	**Capsules**[c]: 25 mg, 50 mg, 100 mg
	Zoloft	**Solution, oral concentrate:** 20 mg/mL[b] **Tablets**[b]: 5 mg, 50 mg, 100 mg
vilazodone	Viibryd	**Tablets:** 10 mg, 20 mg, 40 mg
	Viibryd	
vortioxetine	Trintellix	Tablet: 5 mg, 10 mg, 20 mg
	Trintellix	

[a]Generic available.
[b]Available in the United States only.
[c]Available in Canada only.

Precautions

To avoid the risk of hypertensive crisis, patients taking MAOIs are advised to avoid eating certain foods and beverages containing high amounts of tyramine (Table 6.1).

Serotonin-Noradrenaline Reuptake Inhibitors

Duloxetine (Cymbalta), desvenlafaxine (Pristiq), levomilnacipran (Fatzima), and venlafaxine (Effexor) are serotonin-noradrenaline reuptake inhibitors (SNRIs). They inhibit the reuptake of 5-HT and NE. Dual inhibition of 5-HT and NE is more effective than inhibition of either 5-HT or NE alone.

Adverse Reactions

Side effects are similar to those of SSRIs, but, unlike the SSRIs, the SNRIs produce anticholinergic side effects, a modest increase in blood pressure, and may cause hepatotoxicity. Common side effects of venlafaxine, desvenlafaxine, and duloxetine are nausea, headache, dry mouth, and dizziness. Sedation is common with venlafaxine and desvenlafaxine. Duloxetine may cause asthenia (weakness).

> **TECH NOTE!**
>
> Patients taking MAOIs should be given a list of tyramine-containing foods and a list of drugs to avoid.

Atypical Antidepressants

Bupropion, mirtazapine, nefazodone, and trazodone, and vortioxetine (Trintellix) are atypical antidepressants. In addition to

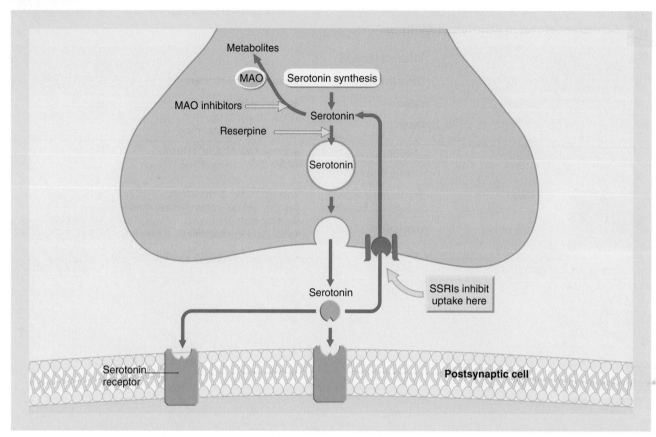

• **Fig. 6.4** Mechanism of action of monoamine oxidase inhibitors. (From Page CP, Hoffman B, Curtis MJ, et al: *Integrated pharmacology*, ed 3, Philadelphia, 2006, Mosby.)

Monoamine Oxidase Inhibitors

Generic Name	US Brand Name(s) Canadian Brand(s)	Dosage Forms and Strengths
moclobemide[ab]	Not available	**Tablets:** 100 mg, 150 mg, 300 mg
	Manerix	
phenelzine[c]	Nardil	**Tablets:** 15 mg
	Nardil	
tranylcypromine[ac]	Parnate	**Tablets:** 10 mg
	Parnate	

[a]Generic available.
[b]Reversible MAOI.
[c]Irreversible MAOI.

TABLE 6.1	**Foods and Beverages to Avoid While Taking Monoamine Oxidase Inhibitors**
Beverages	Chianti, and other red wines, alcohol-free beer, caffeine
Food	Cheeses (especially strong, aged, or processed varieties), sauerkraut, yogurt, raisins, bananas, sour cream, pickled herring, liver (especially chicken liver), dry sausage (including hard salami and pepperoni), canned figs, avocados, turkey, yeast extracts, fava beans, broad bean pods, chocolate
Seasonings	Soy sauce, papaya products (including certain meat tenderizers)

depression, bupropion is used to treat seasonal affective disorder and smoking cessation. Contrave® in a combination drug containing bupropion and naltrexone that is used to treat obesity. Rexulti® (brexpiprazole) is used in the treatment of major depressive disorder and schizophrenia (See chapter 7).

Mechanism of Action

Bupropion is a noradrenaline-DA inhibitor. Mirtazapine affects NE and 5-HT levels. It is metabolized by hepatic microsomal enzymes and is subject to drug interactions involving activation and inhibition of CYP450 isozymes. Trazodone is a weak inhibitor of 5-HT.

> ● **TECH NOTE!**
> Contents of Effexor-XR capsules can be sprinkled onto food.

Adverse Reactions

Although it is well tolerated, doses of bupropion that are greater than 450 mg/day or 150 mg/dose increase the risk for seizures in

Serotonin-Noradrenaline Reuptake Inhibitors

Generic Name	US Brand Name(s) Canadian Brand(s)	Dosage Forms and Strengths
desvenlafaxine[a]	Khedezla, Pristiq	**Tablets, extended release:** 25 mg[b] 50 mg, 100 mg
	Pristiq	
duloxetine[a]	Cymbalta	**Capsules, delayed release:** 20 mg[b], 30 mg, 60 mg
	Cymbalta	
levomilnacipran	Fetzima	**Capsule, extended release:** 20 mg, 40 mg, 80 mg, 120 mg
	Fetzima	
venlafaxine[a]	Effexor-XR	**Capsules, as extended release (Effexor-XR):** 37.5 mg, 75 mg, 150 mg
	Effexor-XR	**Tablets**[b]**:** 25 mg, 37.5 mg, 50 mg, 75 mg, 100 mg
		Tablets, extended release[b]**:** 37.5 mg, 75 mg, 150 mg, 225 mg

[a]Generic available.
[b]Available in the United States only.

Atypical Antidepressants

Generic Name	US Brand Name(s) Canadian Brand(s)	Dosage Forms and Strengths
bupropion[a]	Aplenzin, Forfivo XL, Wellbutrin SR, Wellbutrin XL, Zyban[b]	**Tablets, as HCl:** 75 mg, 100 mg
	Wellbutrin SR, Wellbutrin XL, Zyban	**Tablets, as HCl, extended release 24-hour:** 150 mg, 300 mg (Wellbutrin XL), 450 mg (Forfivo XL)[c]
		Tablets, as hydrobromide, extended release (Aplenzin)[c]**:** 174 mg, 348 mg, 522 mg
		Tablets, as sustained release 12-hour (Wellbutrin SR): 100 mg, 150 mg, 200 mg[c]
bupropion + naltrexone	Contrave	Tablet: 90 mg bupropion + 8 mg naltrexone
	Contrave	
mirtazapine[a]	Remeron, Remeron SolTab	**Tablets:** 15 mg, 30 mg, 45 mg
	Remeron, Remeron RD	**Tablets, orally disintegrating (Remeron SolTab, Remeron RD):** 15 mg, 30 mg, 45 mg
nefazodone	Generics only	**Tablets:** 50 mg, 100 mg, 150 mg, 200 mg, 250 mg
	Not available	
trazodone[a]	Generics only	**Tablets:** 50 mg, 75 mg[d], 100 mg, 150 mg, 300 mg[c]
	Generics only	

[a]Generic available.
[b]Zyban is indicated for smoking cessation.
[c]Available in the United States only.
[d]Available in Canada only.

people with seizure disorders. Mirtazapine may cause drowsiness or dizziness, dry mouth, constipation, blurred vision, diabetes, and suicide ideation. Nefazodone and trazodone produce low to moderate sedation, but they may negatively affect cardiac stimulation. Side effects of trazodone are sedation, hypotension, nausea, and priapism (painful persistent erection). The most common side effect of vortioxetine is nausea (21% to 32%). It may also produce serotonin syndrome (hyperreflexes, nausea/vomiting, sedation, dizziness, sweating, facial flush, restlessness, shivering, and elevated blood pressure).

> ● **TECH NOTE!**
>
> Patients should be advised to avoid discontinuing antidepressants abruptly.

Drugs Used to Treat Bipolar Disorder

Mood stabilizers are used in the treatment of bipolar disorder. Lithium is the oldest of these agents, introduced more than 50 years ago. Medications used in the treatment of seizures have been discovered to effectively treat bipolar disorder.

Lithium is administered to reduce current symptoms of mania and depression, as well as to prevent recurrence of future episodes.

Lithium is rapidly absorbed from the gastrointestinal tract, which accounts for its rapid onset of action. The drug has a long half-life (24 hours), which increases the longer the patient is on lithium therapy. The half-life can double over the course of 1 year's continuous therapy. Lithium is not metabolized and is eliminated unchanged in the urine. Lithium has a narrow therapeutic index. A competitive interaction may occur between lithium and sodium in the kidneys that can result in lithium toxicity. Increased sodium intake can decrease lithium reabsorption. Dehydration can increase lithium reabsorption. Plasma lithium levels and renal function should be monitored regularly to avoid the development of lithium toxicity.

Early-onset side effects associated with lithium carbonate are sedation, nausea, increased urination, dry mouth, difficulty concentrating, and tremor. Adverse reactions associated with long-term use include weight gain, acne, impotence, hypothyroidism, rash, and hair loss. Lithium is contraindicated in pregnancy

and is listed in US Food and Drug Administration pregnancy category D.

Valproic acid, carbamazepine, and lamotrigine are antiseizure drugs with demonstrated efficacy in the treatment of bipolar disorder. They are indicated as an adjunct to lithium therapy or when lithium administration has not produced desired results. Side effects of valproic acid and its salts, divalproex sodium and sodium valproate, include sedation, nausea, ataxia, and liver dysfunction. The side effects of carbamazepine include sedation, dizziness, ataxia, and visual disturbances. Lamotrigine is used in the treatment of bipolar disorder and seizures, and side effects include sedation, nausea, ataxia, blurred vision, double vision, and rash. The use of valproic acid, carbamazepine, and lamotrigine in the treatment of seizure disorder is described in Chapter 9.

> ● **TECH ALERT!**
>
> The following drugs have look-alike/sound-alike issues:
> Wellbutrin SR, and Wellbutrin XL;
> buPROPion and busPIRone;
> Remeron, Remeron SolTab

> ● **TECH ALERT!**
>
> The following drugs have look-alike/sound-alike issues:
>
> Lithium carbonate immediate release and lithium carbonate extended release (both are available in a 300-mg strength)

> ● **TECH NOTE!**
>
> Pharmacy technicians can assist the pharmacist in ensuring optimal drug therapy by alerting the pharmacist when they detect or suspect nonadherence. The pharmacist will determine if intervention is necessary.

TECHNICIAN'S CORNER

1. For patients taking MAOI antidepressants, what kinds of foods can they eat?
2. What is the difference between "feeling blue" and major depression?

Drugs Used in the Treatment of Bipolar Disorder

Generic Name	US Brand Name(s) / Canadian Brand(s)	Dosage Forms and Strengths
lithium carbonate[a] lithium citrate[a]	Lithobid	**Capsules (Carbolith, Lithane):** 150 mg, 300 mg, 600 mg **Syrup, as citrate:** 300 mg/5 mL[b] (8 mmol/5 mL)[c] **Tablets:** 300 mg **Tablets, extended release (Lithobid, Lithmax):** 300 mg, 450 mg[b]
	Carbolith, Lithane, Lithmax	
divalproex sodium[a]	Depakote, Depakote ER	**Capsules, delayed release[b] pellets:** 125 mg **Tablets, enteric coated (Depakote, Epival ECT):** 125 mg, 250 mg, 500 mg **Tablets, extended release (Depakote ER)[b]:** 250 mg, 500 mg
	Epival ECT	

Drugs Used in the Treatment of Bipolar Disorder—cont'd

Generic Name	US Brand Name(s) / Canadian Brand(s)	Dosage Forms and Strengths
carbamazepine[a]	Carbatrol, Carnexiv, Equetro, Epitol, Tegretol, Tegretol Chewable, Tegretol-XR, Teril Tegretol, Tegretol CR, Tegretol Chewtabs	**Capsules, extended release (Carbatrol, Equetro):** 100 mg, 200 mg, 300 mg[b] **Solution, IV infusion (Carnexiv):** 10 mg/mL **Suspension:** 100 mg/5 mL **Tablets, chewable:** 100 mg, 200 mg[c] **Tablets (Tegretol):** 100 mg, 200 mg, 300 mg, 400 mg **Tablets, extended release (Tegretol-XR, Tegretol CR):** 100 mg[b], 200 mg, 400 mg
lamotrigine[a]	Lamictal, Lamictal CD, Lamictal ODT, Lamictal XR Lamictal, Lamictal chewable	**Tablets:** 25 mg, 100 mg, 150 mg, 200 mg[b] **Tablets, as chewable (Lamictal CD):** 2 mg, 5 mg, 25 mg[b] **Tablets, extended release (Lamictal XR)[b]:** 25 mg, 50 mg, 100 mg, 200 mg, 250 mg, 300 mg **Tablets, orally disintegrating (Lamictal ODT)[b]:** 25 mg, 50 mg, 100 mg, 200 mg

[a]Generic available.
[b]Available in the United States only.
[c]Available in Canada only.

Summary of Drugs Used in the Treatment of Depression*

Generic Name	US Brand Name	Usual Adult Oral Dose and Dosing Schedule	Warning Labels
Tricyclic Antidepressants			
amitriptyline	Generic	75–100 mg daily in 1–3 divided doses (maximum 300 mg per day) (oral)	MAY CAUSE DROWSINESS; ALCOHOL MAY INTENSIFY THIS EFFECT. MAY IMPAIR ABILITY TO DRIVE. DO NOT DISCONTINUE WITHOUT MEDICAL SUPERVISION. AVOID PROLONGED EXPOSURE TO SUNLIGHT. MAY DISCOLOR URINE (BLUE-GREEN)—amitriptyline.
desipramine	Norpramin	100–200 mg/day (maximum dose, 300 mg/day in a single or divided doses)	
doxepin	Sinequan	Initiate with 50–150 mg/day and gradually increase to 300 mg/day	
imipramine	Tofranil	Start with 25 mg 3–4 times a day (maximum dose, 300 mg/day)	
nortriptyline	Pamelor	25 mg 3–4 times per day up to 150 mg/day	
protriptyline	Vivactil	15–60 mg daily in 3–4 divided doses	
trimipramine	Surmontil	75–200 mg/day in 1–3 divided doses	
Selective Serotonin Reuptake Inhibitors			
citalopram	Celexa	20–40 mg/day (maximum, 40 mg/day)	MAY IMPAIR ABILITY TO DRIVE. AVOID ALCOHOL. MAY CAUSE DIZZINESS. SWALLOW WHOLE; DO NOT CRUSH OR CHEW (delayed release). DO NOT DISCONTINUE WITHOUT MEDICAL SUPERVISION.
escitalopram	Lexapro	10–20 mg/day	
fluoxetine	Prozac	20–60 mg/day (maximum 80 mg/day) or 90 mg/week (Prozac Weekly)	
fluvoxamine	Generic	100 mg–300 mg daily (divide into 2 doses with larger dose at bedtime)	

Continued

Summary of Drugs Used in the Treatment of Depression*—cont'd

	Generic Name	US Brand Name	Usual Adult Oral Dose and Dosing Schedule	Warning Labels
	paroxetine	Paxil	20 mg/day (Paxil) Maximum dose: 50 mg/day 25 mg once daily (Paxil CR) Maximum dose: 62.5 mg/day	
	sertraline	Zoloft	50–200 mg/day	
	fluoxetine + olanzapine	Symbyax	25 mg fluoxetine/6 mg olanzapine every evening; may increase to 75 mg/18 mg	MAY CAUSE DIZZINESS. MAY IMPAIR ABILITY TO DRIVE. AVOID ALCOHOL.

Monoamine Oxidase Inhibitors

	Generic Name	US Brand Name	Usual Adult Oral Dose and Dosing Schedule	Warning Labels
	moclobemide	Manerix (Canada)	300–600 mg/day divided into two doses per day	TAKE WITH FOOD—moclobemide. AVOID ALCOHOL.
	phenelzine	Nardil	15 mg 3 times a day (maximum 90 mg/day)	MAY CAUSE DIZZINESS OR DROWSINESS.
	tranylcypromine	Parnate	30 mg/day in divided dose (maximum dose, 60 mg/day)	DO NOT DISCONTINUE WITHOUT MEDICAL SUPERVISION.

Serotonin-Noradrenaline Reuptake Inhibitors

	Generic Name	US Brand Name	Usual Adult Oral Dose and Dosing Schedule	Warning Labels
	desvenlafaxine[a]	Khedezla, Pristiq	50 mg once daily	MAY CAUSE DIZZINESS OR DROWSINESS. MAY IMPAIR ABILITY TO DRIVE.
	duloxetine	Cymbalta	40–60 mg/day	AVOID ALCOHOL.
	venlafaxine	Effexor	75–375 mg/day in 2–3 divided doses (immediate release) or 75–225/day (extended release)	TAKE WITH FOOD—venlafaxine. SWALLOW WHOLE; DO NOT CRUSH OR CHEW (extended and sustained release). DO NOT DISCONTINUE WITHOUT MEDICAL SUPERVISION.

Atypical Antidepressants

	Generic Name	US Brand Name	Usual Adult Oral Dose and Dosing Schedule	Warning Labels
	bupropion	Wellbutrin	For depression: 100 mg 2–3 times a day (immediate release); 150 mg twice a day (sustained release); 300 mg once daily (extended release)	MAY CAUSE DIZZINESS OR DROWSINESS. MAY IMPAIR ABILITY TO DRIVE. AVOID ALCOHOL.
	mirtazapine	Remeron	15–45 mg/day (dosed at bedtime)	TAKE WITH FOOD—nefazodone, trazodone
	nefazodone	Generics	200–600 mg/day in two divided doses	
	trazodone	Desyrel	150 mg daily in 2–3 divided doses (maximum dose, 600 mg/day)	
	vortioxetine	Trintellix	10–20 mg once daily	

*Psychiatric drug dosing can vary considerably.
[a]Generic available.

Summary of Drugs Used in the Treatment of Bipolar Affective Disorder*

Generic Name	US Brand Name	Usual Adult Oral Dose and Dosing Schedule	Warning Labels
lithium	Lithonate	900–1800 mg/day in 3–4 divided doses (immediate release) or 900–1200 mg/day in 2 divided doses (sustained release)	MAY CAUSE DIZZINESS OR DROWSINESS; MAY IMPAIR ABILITY TO DRIVE. AVOID ALCOHOL. TAKE WITH FOOD. DRINK PLENTY OF WATER—lithium, Symbyax. SWALLOW WHOLE; DO NOT CRUSH OR CHEW (controlled or slow release). AVOID PREGNANCY—divalproex, carbamazepine, lithium. DO NOT DISCONTINUE WITHOUT MEDICAL SUPERVISION.
divalproex sodium	Depakote	750–1500 mg/day in divided doses	
carbamazepine	Tegretol	400 mg/day in 2 divided doses (maximum, 1600 mg per day)	
lamotrigine	Lamictal	100 mg–200 mg/day	

*Psychiatric drug dosing can vary considerably.

Key Points

- Depressive disorders affect more than 15 million Americans in a given year, and at some time in their lives, 8% Canadians will be affected.
- Depression affects self-esteem, moods, thoughts, eating, sleeping and produces feelings of worthlessness or guilt. It also reduces the ability to think and concentrate.
- Major depression is associated with persistent feelings of sadness, emptiness, or hopelessness.
- Bipolar disorder is associated with sudden swings in mood between depression and periods of mania.
- Dysthymia produces symptoms that are chronic and keep the person from functioning well.
- According to the biogenic amine theory, major depression results from a decrease in monoamine neurotransmitters in the brain.
- Bipolar affective disorder (mania) is believed to be associated with increased levels of monoamine neurotransmitters.
- Monoamine neurotransmitters associated with depression and bipolar disorder are norepinephrine (NE), serotonin (5-HT), and dopamine (DA).
- The mechanisms of action for drugs used to treat depression may differ; however, all antidepressants are equally effective.
- Inhibition of the reuptake of specific monoamine neurotransmitters is one of the ways antidepressants produce their effects. The other mechanism of action is to block the degradation of monoamine neurotransmitters.

- Selection of one antidepressant over another is based on the patient's ability to tolerate drug side effects.
- Tricyclic antidepressants (TCAs) are the oldest class of medication used in the treatment of depression.
- The TCAs are nonspecific reuptake inhibitors of monoamine neurotransmitters.
- The selective serotonin reuptake inhibitors (SSRIs) work by producing selective blockade of the reuptake of 5-HT at the synaptic cleft.
- The SSRIs are equally effective as the TCAs yet lack the cardiotoxic effects associated with TCAs.
- The monoamine oxidase inhibitors (MAOIs) interfere with the degradation of monoamine neurotransmitters and dietary amines (e.g., tyramine).
- Hypertensive crisis is a life-threatening adverse reaction caused by drug-drug and drug-food interactions with MAOIs.
- Lithium is administered to treat bipolar disorder. It reduces current symptoms of mania and depression and prevents recurrence of future episodes.
- Lithium has a narrow therapeutic index.
- Many drugs used to treat seizure disorders (e.g., divalproex sodium and carbamazepine) are also used for the treatment of bipolar disorder.

Review Questions

1. A mental health illness that persists for several weeks and is associated with persistent feelings of sadness, emptiness, or hopelessness that persists for several weeks is _____.
   a. bipolar disorder
   b. obsessive-compulsive disorder
   c. major depression
   d. schizophrenia

2. Wellbutrin is _____.
   a. a noradrenaline-dopamine inhibitor
   b. a monoamine oxidase inhibitor
   c. a selective serotonin reuptake inhibitor
   d. a tricyclic antidepressant

3. Select the antidepressant that is available as an orally disintegrating tablet.
   a. Pristiq
   b. Fetzima
   c. Remeron
   d. Cymbalta

4. The most widely prescribed class of antidepressants is
   a. TCAs
   b. SSRIs
   c. MAOIs
   d. PPIs

5. The brand name for citalopram is
   a. Celexa
   b. Celebrex
   c. Cerebryx
   d. none of the above

6. You receive a prescription for desvenlafaxine 37.5 mg with directions to take one capsule two to three times a day. You consult the pharmacist because
   a. the usual dosing schedule for desvenlafaxine is once daily
   b. desvenlafaxine is not available in 37.5 mg
   c. both a & b
   d. none of the above

7. To avoid the risk of hypertensive crisis, patients taking _____ are advised to avoid eating certain foods containing tyramine.
   a. SSRIs
   b. TCAs
   c. MAOIs
   d. a and b

8. _____ is an example of an atypical antidepressant
   a. fluoxetine
   b. tranylcycpromine
   c. imipramine
   d. mirtazapine

9. Bupropion is indicated for the treatment of depression and smoking cessation.
   a. true
   b. false

10. An example of a 5-HT-noradrenaline reuptake inhibitor is
    a. fluoxetine
    b. sertraline
    c. venlafaxine
    d. nortriptyline

11. Valproic acid, carbamazepine, and lamotrigine are _____ drugs with demonstrated efficacy in the treatment of bipolar disorder.
    a. antiseizure
    b. antidepressant
    c. antimania
    d. antianxiety

12. The oldest drug used to treat bipolar disorder is _____.
    a. fluoxetine
    b. tranylcypromine
    c. lithium
    d. escitalopram

Bibliography

Anxiety and Depression Association of America: 2016. Depression. *Understand the Facts*. Retrieved January 15, 2017 from: https://www.adaa.org/understanding-anxiety/depression.

Kalant H, Grant D, Mitchell J: *Principles of medical pharmacology*, ed 7, Toronto, 2007, Elsevier Canada, A Division of Reed Elsevier Canada, pp 316–333.

Lance L, Lacy C, Armstrong L, et al: *Drug information handbook for the allied health professional*, ed 12, Hudson, OH, 2005, APhA Lexi-Comp.

Neurological protein may hold the key to new treatments for depression-Press release, Toronto, 2010, Centre for Addiction and Mental Health.

Page C, Curtis M, Sutter M, et al: *Integrated pharmacology*, Philadelphia, 2005, Elsevier Mosby, pp 239–241.

Public Health Agency of Canada: What is Depression? 2016. Retrieved Jan 16, 2017 from: http://www.phac-aspc.gc.ca/cd-mc/mi-mm/depression-eng.php.

U.S. Department of Health and Human Services, National Institutes of Health, National Institute of Mental Health: 2015. Depression (NIH Publication No. 15-3561). Bethesda, MD: U.S. Government Printing Office.

7

Treatment of Schizophrenia and Psychoses

LEARNING OBJECTIVES

1. Learn the terminology associated with schizophrenia.
2. Describe the symptoms of schizophrenia.
3. List and describe the function of neurotransmitters associated with the symptoms of schizophrenia and psychoses.
4. Classify medications used to treat schizophrenia and psychoses.
5. Describe the mechanism of action for each class of drugs used to treat schizophrenia and psychoses.
6. Identify warning labels and precautionary messages associated with medications used to treat schizophrenia and psychoses.
7. Identify significant drug look-alike/sound-alike issues.

KEY TERMS

Catatonia Symptom of schizophrenia associated with unresponsiveness and immobility.

Delusion Irrational thoughts or false beliefs that dominate a person's behavior and viewpoint and do not change even when evidence is provided that beliefs are not valid.

Extrapyramidal symptoms Excessive muscle movement (motor activity) associated with use of neuroleptics that includes muscular rigidity, tremor, bradykinesia (slow movement), and difficulty in walking.

Hallucination Visions or voices that exist only in the mind and cannot be seen or heard by others.

Negative symptoms Sign of schizophrenia that is associated with decreased ability to think, plan, or express emotion.

Neuroleptic (antipsychotic) Drug used to treat schizophrenia and psychoses.

Neuroleptic malignant syndrome Potentially fatal reaction to administration of neuroleptic medications. Symptoms include stupor, muscle rigidity, and high temperature.

Positive symptoms Hallucinations, delusions, or other unusual thoughts or perceptions that are symptoms of schizophrenia.

Postural hypotension Drop in blood pressure caused by a change in posture.

Pseudoparkinsonism Adverse reaction to the administration of antipsychotic drugs. Symptoms mimick Parkinson disease.

Psychosis Mental state characterized by disorganized behavior and thought, delusions, hallucinations, and a loss of touch with reality.

Schizophrenia Type of psychosis characterized by delusions of thought, visual or auditory hallucinations (or both), and speech disturbances. Paranoid schizophrenia is characterized by delusions of persecution.

Tardive dyskinesia Inappropriate postures of the neck, trunk, and limbs accompanied by involuntary thrusting of the tongue.

Overview

Schizophrenia is a chronic and major *psychosis* that is characterized by delusions of thought, visual or auditory hallucinations (or both), and speech disturbances. Persons diagnosed with schizophrenia often see visions or hear voices that cannot be seen or heard by others. Paranoid schizophrenia is characterized by delusions of persecution. Paranoid schizophrenia is particularly challenging because the patient may believe that the health care team is prescribing medicines and therapies intended to cause harm.

Schizophrenia affects about more than 21 million people worldwide according to the World Health Organization. The onset typically occurs in the late teens, after puberty begins, to the mid-20s; the onset in men is slightly earlier than in women, who may not develop symptoms until the mid-20s to the early 30s. The onset of symptoms after age 45 years is rare.

Heredity and environmental factors may increase the risk of developing schizophrenia. Schizophrenia runs in families, and 10% of persons diagnosed with schizophrenia have a sibling or relative who has schizophrenia. If the sibling is an identical twin, the risk for schizophrenia increases 40% to 65%. Exposure to viruses, fetal malnutrition, and substance abuse are also thought to influence the development of schizophrenia.

People diagnosed with schizophrenia often exhibit negative symptoms, positive symptoms, and cognitive symptoms. People who exhibit *negative symptoms* may not show visible signs of emotion or facial expressions, or interact socially with others. Speech is monotonous. *Positive symptoms* may appear as bizarre behavior. People with schizophrenia may have delusions. *Delusions* are irrational thoughts or false beliefs that dominate a person's behavior. The person's viewpoint is unlikely to change, even when evidence is provided that the beliefs are not valid. An example of a delusion is the belief that television characters are broadcasting personal messages to the person with schizophrenia. People with schizophrenia may also have visual or auditory *hallucinations*. They respond to visions and voices that only they can see. They may talk to themselves or, when speaking to others, may fail to complete sentences (their thoughts may be finished in their mind). Their thoughts are often disorganized. Schizophrenia may interfere with the performance of routine activities of daily living. Memory loss may impede the person's ability to function on a job. Schizophrenia may also decrease the person's capacity to interpret information and make decisions.

Schizophrenia also produces physical symptoms. The person may be clumsy and appear catatonic or make repetitive movements. People who exhibit symptoms of *catatonia* are unresponsive and immobile.

Neurochemistry of Schizophrenia and Psychoses

Interactions between brain chemicals (e.g., dopamine and serotonin) play a role in schizophrenia. Drugs that block dopamine signals are used in the treatment of schizophrenia. Dopamine pathways project to various emotional areas of the brain involved in cognition and regulation of motivation and emotion. Pathways in the midbrain control muscle movement, and treatments for schizophrenia can produce *pseudoparkinsonism*, Parkinson disease–like symptoms (e.g., tremor and bradykinesia), as a side effect.

Other neurotransmitters that have been identified as playing a role in symptoms of schizophrenia include serotonin, cholecystokinin (CCK), neurotensin, γ-aminobutyric acid (GABA), and glutamate (Fig. 7.1).

Drugs Used to Treat Schizophrenia and Psychosis

Neuroleptics (antipsychotics) are classified by structure and function. Functionally all antipsychotics fall into two classes based on their affinity for dopamine receptors. Dopamine (D_2) is considered the most important neurotransmitter involved the treatment and symptoms of schizophrenia. High-potency neuroleptics have a strong affinity for dopamine receptors. "Atypical" and low-potency antipsychotics have a weaker affinity for dopamine receptors and produce fewer side effects associated with blockade. Dopamine receptor blockade in the nigrostriatal tract produces Parkinson disease–like symptoms (pseudoparkinsonism). Some antipsychotic drugs block serotonin (5-hydroxytryptamine [5-HT]) receptors. They are useful in the treatment of negative symptoms of schizophrenia and protect against long-term motor effects associated with some drugs used to treat psychosis. CCK and neurotensin are peptide neurotransmitters. CCK is thought to be associated with the auditory hallucinations of schizophrenia. psychosis. Drugs that increase neurotensin levels improve negative symptoms of schizophrenia. Abnormalities of the GABA system are believed to be associated with working memory deficits in schizophrenia. Glutamate is an amino acid that acts as an excitatory neurotransmitter in the central nervous system. Drugs that interfere with glutamate signaling in the brain are thought to decrease psychosis.

All antipsychotic agents are equally effective. The selection of agents to treat schizophrenia is based on a balance between the achievement of the desired response and the patient's ability to tolerate drug side effects.

• **Fig. 7.1** The cerebral distribution of dopamine receptors in treated and untreated schizophrenia. (A) Striatal dopamine receptors in untreated schizophrenia. (B) Complete blockade of receptors with typical neuroleptic. (C) Partial blockade of receptors with equally effective dose of clozapine. (From Page CP, Hoffman BB, Curtis MJ, et al: *Integrated pharmacology*, ed 3, Philadelphia, 2006, Mosby.)

First-Generation "Typical" Neuroleptics and Second- and Third-Generation "Atypical" Neuroleptics

Phenothiazines, butyrophenones, and thioxanthenes are categorized as first-generation antipsychotics. They are classified as low, medium, and high potency. The prototype for low-potency antipsychotics is chlorpromazine; medium potency, fluphenazine; and high potency, haloperidol. All other types of antipsychotics are categorized as "atypical." Clozapine (thienobenzodiazepines), risperidone (benzixasoles), and aripiprazole (quinolinones) are examples of atypical antipsychotics.

> **⚠ TECH ALERT!**
>
> The following drugs have look-alike/sound-alike issues: chlorproMAZINE, clomiPRAMINE, and chlorproPAMIDE; fluPHENAZine and fluvoxaMINE; SEROquel and SINEquan

> **● TECH NOTE!**
>
> Phenothiazines are also prescribed for the treatment of nausea and vomiting (chlorpromazine, perphenazine, promethazine).

Mechanism of Action

First-generation antipsychotics block dopamine at postsynaptic receptor sites in the brain. They have a strong alpha-adrenergic blocking action that accounts for the hypotension produced by first-generation antipsychotics (Fig. 7.2). Atypical antipsychotics such as clozapine show strong affinity for serotonin receptors in addition to the dopaminergic receptor blockade.

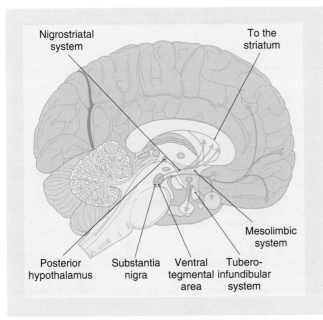

● Fig. 7.2 Dopamine pathways. (From Page CP, Hoffman BB, Curtis MJ, et al: *Integrated pharmacology*, ed 3, Philadelphia, 2006, Mosby.)

> **⚠ TECH ALERT!**
>
> The FDA requires a boxed warning be included in the labeling of all neuroleptics, stating that the treatment of behavioral disorders in elderly patients with dementia with atypical and conventional antipsychotics is associated with increased mortality.

> **⚠ TECH ALERT!**
>
> The FDA requires a boxed warning be included in the labeling of all atypical neuroleptics, stating the agents are associated with hyperglycemia and the onset of diabetes.

Pharmacokinetics

First-generation antipsychotics are well absorbed orally, rectally, and parenterally. They readily cross the blood-brain barrier because of their lipid solubility. They are up to 90% bound to plasma proteins. They are also rapidly metabolized in the liver, and some produce active metabolites. For example, paliperidone is the active metabolite of risperidone. Antipsychotics are eliminated in the urine.

Several antipsychotics are available in slow-release depot formulations for intramuscular injection. The therapeutic effects of slow-release dosage forms (e.g., Invega Sustenna, Haldol deconoate) persist for up to 4 weeks after injection. Atypical antipsychotics are also available in dosage forms designed for rapid action (e.g., Zyprexa Zydis oral disintegrating tablets), extended-release tablets (e.g., Seroquel XR), and every 3 months intramuscular injection (e.g., Invega Trinza).

Adverse Reactions

Up to 80% of the people who are prescribed antipsychotics will experience adverse reactions. Most adverse reactions are predictable and associated with dopaminergic, serotonergic, cholinergic, alpha-adrenergic, or histaminergic blockade (H1). Adverse effects are classified as central nervous system effects and peripheral nervous system effects. Sedation (histamine blockade), confusion, decreased ability to regulate body temperature, weight gain, increased appetite, and increased release of some endocrine hormones are central nervous system effects. Peripheral nervous system adverse effects include blurred vision, dry mouth, and urinary retention (cholinergic blockade). Alpha-adrenergic blockade can cause postural hypotension—a drop in blood pressure caused by a change in posture.

Extrapyramidal effects and tardive dyskinesia are associated with dopaminergic blockade and occur more frequently in elderly patients. *Extrapyramidal symptoms* are exhibited as excessive muscle movement. *Tardive dyskinesia* causes inappropriate postures of the neck, trunk, and limbs, and is accompanied by involuntary thrusting of the tongue and lip smacking. There is no effective prevention or treatment for tardive dyskinesia.

Other adverse effects are hepatotoxicity and jaundice, bone marrow depression, photosensitivity, and failure to ejaculate. Increased release of prolactin can produce pseudopregnancy-type symptoms. Phenothiazines may also increase vitamin B_2 requirements.

> **⚠ TECH ALERT!**
>
> Chlorpromazine oral concentrate and thioridazine oral concentrate are incompatible in enteral formulas (tube feeding).

First Generation Neuroleptics

Phenothiazines

Generic Name	U.S. Brand Name(s)	Dosage Forms and Strengths
	Canadian Brand(s)	
chlorpromazine[a]	Generic only	**Injection, solution:** 25 mg/mL
	Generic only	**Tablets:** 10 mg[b], 25 mg, 50 mg, 100 mg, 200 mg[b]
fluphenazine[a]	Generic only	**Elixir, as hydrochloride**[b]: 2.5 mg/5 mL
	Modecate	**Injection, in oil as deconoate:** 25 mg/mL[b], 100 mg/mL (Modecate)[c]
		Injection, hydrochloride solution[b]: 2.5 mg/mL
		Solution, oral concentrate[b]: 5 mg/mL
		Tablets: 1 mg, 2 mg, 2.5 mg, 5 mg, 10 mg[b]
methotrimeprazine	Not available	**Solution, for injection (Nozinan):** 25 mg/mL
	Nozinan	**Tablet (generics):** 2 mg, 5 mg, 25 mg, 50 mg
perphenazine[a]	Generic only	**Tablets:** 2 mg, 4 mg, 8 mg, 16 mg
	Generic only	
thioridazine[a]	Generic only	**Tablets:** 10 mg, 25 mg, 50 mg, 100 mg
	Not available	

[a]Generic available.
[b]Available in the United States only.
[c]Available in Canada only.

Butyrophenones

Generic Name	U.S. Brand Name(s)	Dosage Forms and Strengths
	Canadian Brand(s)	
haloperidol[a]	Haldol	**Injection, oil, as deconoate:** 50 mg/mL[b]; 100 mg/mL
	Generic only	**Injection, solution, as lactate:** 5 mg/mL
		Solution, oral concentrate: 2 mg/mL
		Tablets: 0.5 mg, 1 mg, 2 mg, 5 mg, 10 mg, 20 mg

[a]Generic available.
[b]Available in the United States only.

Thioxanthenes

Generic Name	U.S. Brand Name(s)	Dosage Forms and Strengths
	Canadian Brand(s)	
thiothixene[a]	Navane	**Capsules:** 1 mg, 2 mg, 5 mg, 10 mg
	Not Available	
zuclopenthixol	Not Available	**Intramuscular injection, as acetate (Clopixol Acuphase):** 50 mg/mL
	Clopixol, Clopixol Acuphase, Clopixol Depot	**Intramuscular injection, as deconoate (Clopixol Depot):** 200 mg/mL
		Tablets: 10 mg, 25 mg

[a]Generic available.

Atypical Neuroleptics

Generic Name	U.S. Brand Name(s) / Canadian Brand(s)	Dosage Forms and Strengths
aripiprazole[a]	Abilify, Abilify Maintena, Abilify Mycite Kit	**Powder for injection (Abilify Maintena):** 300 mg/vial, 400 mg/vial **Tablets:** 2 mg, 5 mg, 10 mg, 15 mg, 20 mg, 30 mg
	Abilify, Abilify Maintena	
asenapine	Saphris	**Tablets, sublingual:** 2.5 mg[b], 5 mg, 10 mg
	Saphris	
brexpiprazole	Rexulti	**Tablet:** 0.25 mg, 0.5 mg, 1 mg, 2 mg, 3 mg, 4 mg
	Rexulti	
cariprazine	Vraylar	**Capsule:** 1.5 mg, 3 mg, 4.5 mg, 6 mg
	Not Available	
clozapine[a]	Clozaril, Fazaclo ODT, Versacloz	**Suspension, oral**[b]**:** 50 mg/mL **Tablets:** 12.5 mg[b], 25 mg, 50 mg, 100 mg, 200 mg **Tablets, oral disintegrating (Fazaclo ODT)**[b]**:** 12.5 mg, 25 mg, 100 mg, 150 mg, 200 mg
	Clozaril	
iloperidone[a]	Fanapt	**Tablets:** 1 mg, 2 mg, 4 mg, 6 mg, 8 mg, 10 mg, 12 mg
	Not available	
loxapine[a]	Adasuve	**Capsules**[b]**:** 5 mg, 10 mg, 25 mg, 50 mg **Injection (Loxapac IM)**[c]**:** 50 mg/mL **Powder, for inhalation (Adasuve)**[b]**:** 10 mg **Tablets**[c]**:** 2.5 mg, 5 mg, 10 mg, 25 mg, 50 mg
	Loxapac IM, Xylac	
lurasidone	Latuda	**Tablets:** 20 mg, 40 mg, 60 mg, 80 mg, 120 mg
	Latuda	
olanzapine[a]	Zyprexa, Zyprexa Relprevv, Zyprexa Zydis	**Injection, powder for reconstitution:** 10 mg **Injection, extended-release powder (Zyprexa Relprevv)**[b]**:** 210 mg, 300 mg, 405 mg **Tablets:** 2.5 mg, 5 mg, 7.5 mg, 10 mg, 15 mg, 20 mg **Tablets, oral disintegrating (Zyprexa Zydis):** 5 mg, 10 mg, 15 mg, 20 mg
	Zyprexa, Zyprexa Zydis	
paliperidon[ab]	Invega, Invega Sustenna	**Suspension, for extended-release injection (Invega Sustenna):** **In United States:** 39 mg/0.25 mL, 78 mg/0.5 mL, 117 mg/0.75 mL, 156 mg/1 mL, 234 mg/1.5 mL **In Canada:** 50 mg/0.5 mL, 75 mg/0.75 mL, 100 mg/1 mL, 150 mg/1.5 mL **Suspension, prefilled syringe (Invega Trinza):** **In United States:** 273 mg/0.875 mL, 410 mg/1.315 mL 546 mg/1.75 mL, 819 mg/2.625 mL **In Canada:** 175 mg/0.875 mL, 350 mg/1.75 m, 525 mg/2.625 mL **Tablet, extended release (Invega):** 1.5 mg[b], 3 mg, 6 mg, 9 mg
	Invega, Invega Sustenna, Invega Trinza	
quetiapine[a]	Seroquel, Seroquel XR	**Tablets:** 25 mg, 50 mg[b], 100 mg, 200 mg, 300 mg, 400 mg[b] **Tablets, extended release (Seroquel XR):** 50 mg, 150 mg, 200 mg, 300 mg, 400 mg
	Seroquel, Seroquel XR	
risperidone[a]	Risperdal, Risperdal Consta	**Injection (Risperdal Consta):** 12.5 mg, 25 mg, 37.5 mg, 50 mg (vials and prefilled syringes) **Solution, oral:** 1 mg/mL **Tablets:** 0.25 mg, 0.5 mg, 1 mg, 2 mg, 3 mg, 4 mg, 5 mg[b] **Tablet, oral disintegrating**[b]**:** 0.5 mg, 1 mg, 2 mg, 3 mg, 4 mg
	Risperdal, Risperdal Consta	
ziprasidone[a]	Geodon	**Capsule:** 20 mg, 40 mg, 60 mg, 80 mg **Injection, powder for reconstitution:**[b] 20 mg
	Zeldox	

[a]Generic available
[b]Available in the United States only.
[c]Available in Canada only.

■ *TECH NOTE!*

Do not mix haloperidol oral concentrate with coffee or tea.

Atypical Neuroleptics

Atypical antipsychotics that are used in the treatment and management of schizophrenia are aripiprazole, asenapine, brexpiprazole, cariprazine, clozapine, iloperidone, lurasidone, olanzapine, paliperidone, quetiapine, risperidone, and ziprasidone. In addition to treating schizophrenia, some antipsychotic drugs are used to treat bipolar disorder. The drugs that are used for bipolar disorder are olanzapine, risperidone, ziprasidone, and quetiapine.

Mechanisms of Action

Atypical antipsychotics act by several mechanisms of action. Some act to stabilize the dopamine system. Some are partial agonists of dopamine (e.g., aripiprazole), and others produce mixed effects on dopamine and serotonin (asenapine). Risperidone, paliperidone, and iloperidone are classified as benzisoxazoles. Loxapine is an atypical antipsychotic drug that is structurally similar to the antidepressant amoxapine. Lurasidone and ziprasidone are classified as benzoisothiazol derivatives. Quetiapine is classified as a dibenzothiazepine.

■ *TECH NOTE!*

Patients, prescribers, and pharmacists must be enrolled in a registry to dispense clozapine.

❗ *TECH ALERT!*

ZyPREXA, CeleXA, and ZyrTEC have look-alike/sound-alike issues.

■ *TECH NOTE!*

Risperidone oral solution should not be diluted with cola or tea.

■ *TECH NOTE!*

Dispense haloperidol, loxapine, risperidone, and aripiprazole oral solutions with the measuring device provided with packaging.

Adverse Reactions

Common side effects of atypical antipsychotics are dizziness, drowsiness, hypotension, headache, confusion, nausea, weight gain, increased urination or urinary retention, thirst, dry mouth, and sexual dysfunction (aripiprazole, asenapine, clozapine, lurasidone and ziprasidone iloperidone, paliperidone, quetiapine and risperidone). Aripiprazole may cause insomnia. Newer atypical antipsychotics

Summary of Drugs Used in the Treatment of Psychosis

	Generic Name	U.S. Brand Name	Usual Adult Oral Dose and Dosing Schedule	Warning Labels
Phenothiazines				
	chlorpromazine	Generics	25–2000 mg/day in 3–4 divided doses (oral) or 300 mg–800 mg/day IM or IV (maintenance dose)	MAY CAUSE DROWSINESS; MAY IMPAIR ABILITY TO DRIVE; AVOID ALCOHOL. MAINTAIN ADEQUATE HYDRATION. AVOID PROLONGED EXPOSURE TO SUNLIGHT. DO NOT DISCONTINUE WITHOUT MEDICAL SUPERVISION. DILUTE ORAL CONCENTRATE BEFORE ADMINISTERING—chlorpromazine, fluphenazine. MAY DISCOLOR URINE (PINK-REDDISH BROWN)—thioridazine. MAY CAUSE DRY MOUTH. CHEWING GUM OR SUCKING SUGARLESS CANDY MAY IMPROVE SYMPTOMS.
	fluphenazine	Generics	**Oral:** 2.5–10 mg/day dosed every 6–8 h (maximum, 20 mg/day) **IM (as HCl):** 2.5 mg–10 mg/day or IM (as deconoate) 12.5 mg every 3 weeks	
	methotrimeprazine	Generics	**Oral:** 50–200 mg/day in 2–3 divided doses **IM:** 75–100 mg given as 3–4 injections/day	
	perphenazine	Generics	4–16 mg 2–4 times a day (maximum, 64 mg/day)	
	thioridazine	Generics	50–100 mg 3 times a day up to 800 mg/day divided in 2–4 doses	
	trifluoperazine	Generics	**Oral:** 2–5 mg twice daily (maximum, 100 mg) **IM:** 1–2 mg every 4–6 h (maximum, 6 mg/24 h)	
Butyrophenones				
	haloperidol	Generics	**Oral:** 0.5–5 mg 2–3 times/day (maximum, 100 mg/day) **IM (lactate):** 2–5 mg every 4–8 h **IM (deconoate):** 10–20 times oral dose (up to 300 mg) once every 4 weeks.	MAY CAUSE DROWSINESS; MAY IMPAIR ABILITY TO DRIVE; AVOID ALCOHOL. DO NOT DISCONTINUE WITHOUT MEDICAL SUPERVISION. DILUTE ORAL CONCENTRATE BEFORE ADMINISTRATION. MAINTAIN ADEQUATE HYDRATION. AVOID PROLONGED EXPOSURE TO SUNLIGHT.

Summary of Drugs Used in the Treatment of Psychosis—cont'd

	Generic Name	U.S. Brand Name	Usual Adult Oral Dose and Dosing Schedule	Warning Labels
Thioxanthenes				
	thiothixene	Navane	2 mg 3 times a day (maximum, 60 mg/day)	MAY CAUSE DROWSINESS; MAY IMPAIR ABILITY TO DRIVE; AVOID ALCOHOL.
	zuclopenthixol	Clopixol	**Injection, as acetate**: 50–150 mg IM every 2–3 days **Injection, as deconoate**: 150–300 mg IM every 2–4 weeks **Tablets**: 10–50 mg/day in 2–3 divided doses	DO NOT DISCONTINUE WITHOUT MEDICAL SUPERVISION. MAINTAIN ADEQUATE HYDRATION. AVOID PROLONGED EXPOSURE TO SUNLIGHT.
Atypical Antipsychotics				
	aripiprazole	Abilify	10–15 mg once daily	MAY CAUSE DIZZINESS OR DROWSINESS—aripiprazole, asenapine, brexpiprazole, clozapine, iloperidone, loxapine, lurasidone, olanzapine, paliperidone, quetiapine, risperidone, ziprasidone MAY IMPAIR ABILITY TO DRIVE—aripiprazole, asenapine, clozapine, loxapine, lurasidone, olanzapine, quetiapine, ziprasidone AVOID ALCOHOL—aripiprazole, asenapine, clozapine, iloperidone, loxapine, lurasidone, olanzapine, quetiapine, ziprasidone MAINTAIN ADEQUATE HYDRATION—asenapine, clozapine, loxapine lurasidone, olanzapine, quetiapine, ziprasidone DO NOT DISCONTINUE WITHOUT MEDICAL SUPERVISION—aripiprazole, asenapine, clozapine, olanzapine, iloperidone, loxapine, lurasidone, quetiapine, ziprasidone ORAL SOLUTION MAY BE MIXED IN MILK, JUICE, WATER, OR COFFEE; AVOID CARBONATED BEVERAGES AND TEA—risperidone. SWALLOW WHOLE; DON'T CRUSH OR CHEW—all extended release
	asenapine	Saphris	Dissolve sublingually 5 mg twice daily	
	brexpiprazole	Rexulti	For depression: Start 0.5–1 mg once daily, increase to 2 mg daily. Max. 3 mg/day	
	clozapine	Clozaril	Begin 12.5 mg 1–2 times a day; increase to 300–450 mg/day (maximum, 900 mg/day)	
	iloperidone	Fanapt	Start 1 mg twice daily; increase to 2 mg twice daily on day 2; then increase by 2 mg twice daily up to 12 mg twice daily (day 7)	
	loxapine	Loxitane	20–100 mg/day divided into 2–4 doses per day	
	lurasidone	Latuda	40–160 mg once daily	
	olanzapine	Zyprexa	5–10 mg/day (maximum, 20 mg/day)	

Continued

Summary of Drugs Used in the Treatment of Psychosis—cont'd

Generic Name	U.S. Brand Name	Usual Adult Oral Dose and Dosing Schedule	Warning Labels
paliperidone	Invega	**Oral:** 6 mg once daily in the morning (maximum, 12 mg/day) **IM, extended release (Invega Sustenna):** Inject 39–234 mg IM once monthly (United States package labeling); 50–150 mg IM once monthly (Canada package labeling) **IM, extended release (Invega Trinza):** 273–819 mg IM once every 3 months (United States package labeling); 175–525 mg IM once every 3 months (Canada package labeling)	
risperidone	Risperdal	2–8 mg/day (oral) or 25 mg every 2 weeks (IM)	
quetiapine	Seroquel, Seroquel XR	Start with 25 mg twice a day; increase to 300–800 mg/day dosed 2–3 times a day **Extended release:** 400–800 mg once daily; start with 50 mg once every evening and increase by 50 mg once daily	
ziprasidone	Geodon	**Oral:** 20 mg twice daily (maximum, 80 mg twice daily) **IM:** 10 mg every 2 h (maximum, 40 mg/day)	

such as ziprasidone and olanzapine have less risk for extrapyramidal symptoms, but they are associated with hyperglycemia and the onset of diabetes. The atypical antipsychotics are also associated with an increased risk for cardiovascular morbidity and mortality. Aripiprazole and asenapine can cause QT interval prolongation, so they should be used cautiously in patients with heart disease.

Precautions

Neuroleptic malignant syndrome is a life-threatening side effect of neuroleptic administration. It produces symptoms of muscle rigidity, increased body temperature (hyperthermia), fluctuating consciousness, and renal failure. Clozapine use is restricted because it can produce a fatal drop in white blood cells (agranulocytosis). Patients on clozapine therapy are required to have white blood cell levels monitored weekly while taking the medication. Antipsychotic agents should be used cautiously in patients with seizure disorders. Low-potency agents and clozapine are most likely to induce seizures. Aripiprazole and asenapine labeling have a boxed warning: Elderly patients with dementia-related psychosis treated with antipsychotic drugs are an increased risk of death. Mortality most commonly occurs due to sudden heart failure, sudden death, or infection. Aripiprazole and asenapine may produce suicidal thoughts.

TECHNICIAN'S CORNER

1. The prevalence of schizophrenia in families in which a sibling or relative has schizophrenia is about 10 times higher than in the general population. What kind of genetic implications does this statement have?
2. Can one live a "normal" life when diagnosed with schizophrenia?

Key Points

- Schizophrenia is a chronic and major psychosis characterized by delusions of thought, visual or auditory hallucinations (or both), and speech disturbances.
- Schizophrenia affects about 1% of the population worldwide.
- The onset typically occurs in the late teens after puberty begins to the mid-20s.
- Symptoms of schizophrenia in women may not develop until the mid-20s to early 30s.

- Neurotransmitters that have been identified as playing a role in schizophrenia are dopamine, serotonin, CCK, neurotensin, GABA, and glutamate.
- Dopamine receptor blockade treats symptoms of schizophrenia but may produce Parkinson disease–like symptoms (pseudoparkinsonism).
- Neuroleptics (antipsychotics) are classified by structure and function.

- Functional classifications for antipsychotics are based on their affinity for dopamine receptors. High-potency antipsychotics have a strong affinity for dopamine receptors. Atypical neuroleptics such as clozapine show strong affinity for serotonin receptors in addition to dopaminergic receptor blockade.
- Atypical neuroleptics are associated with the onset diabetes.
- Atypical neuroleptics are associated with increased mortality in elderly patients with dementia-related psychosis.
- First-generation antipsychotics are well absorbed orally, rectally, and parenterally.

- Typical and atypical neuroleptics are available in slow-release depot formulations for intramuscular injection, and the therapeutic effects persist for up to 4 weeks after injection.
- Up to 80% of the people who are prescribed antipsychotic medications will experience adverse reactions.
- Extrapyramidal effects and tardive dyskinesia are associated with dopaminergic blockade and occur more frequently in elderly patients.
- Neuroleptic malignant syndrome is a life-threatening side effect of antipsychotic drugs.
- Clozapine use is restricted because it can produce a fatal drop in white blood cell levels (agranulocytosis).

Review Questions

1. Schizophrenia runs in families.
   - **a.** true
   - **b.** false
2. Select the drug that is marketed as a oral disintegrating tablet.
   - **a.** Invega
   - **b.** Seroquel
   - **c.** Saphris
   - **d.** Latuda
3. Select the drug that is marketed as a extended release tablet/capsule.
   - **a.** Abilify
   - **b.** Seroquel
   - **c.** Risperdal
   - **d.** Zyprexa
4. Phenothiazines, butyrophenones, and thioxanthines are categorized as _____ neuroleptics.
   - **a.** traditional (typical)
   - **b.** nontraditional (atypical)
5. What causes inappropriate postures of the neck, trunk, and limbs, accompanied by involuntary thrusting of the tongue and lip smacking?
   - **a.** extrapyramidal symptoms
   - **b.** tardive dyskinesia
   - **c.** hyperkinesia
   - **d.** catatonia
6. The use of _____ is restricted because it can produce a fatal drop in white blood cells (agranulocytosis).
   - **a.** quetiapine
   - **b.** clozapine
   - **c.** olanzapine
   - **d.** nifedipine

7. Select the drug that is marketed as an extended duration intramuscular injection
   - **a.** Invega
   - **b.** Mellaril
   - **c.** Clozaril
   - **d.** Seroquel
8. Hallucinations, delusions, or other unusual thoughts or perceptions are _____ symptoms of schizophrenia.
   - **a.** positive
   - **b.** negative
9. Selection of schizophrenia agents is based on a balance between achievement of desired response to the drug and the patient's ability to tolerate drug side effects.
   - **a.** true
   - **b.** false
10. Risperidone is available in which dosage forms?
    - **a.** oral solution
    - **b.** injection
    - **c.** tablet
    - **d.** a, b, and c

Bibliography

FDA. (nd). Drugs@FDA: FDA Approved Drug Products. Retrieved January 28, 2017, from http://www.accessdata.fda.gov/scripts/cder/daf/.

Health Canada. (2017). Drug Product Database. Retrieved January 28, 2017, from https://health-products.canada.ca/dpd-bdpp/index-eng.jsp.

Institute for Safe Medication Practices. (2016). FDA and ISMP Lists of Look-Alike Drug Names with Recommended Tall Man Letters. Retrieved January 31, 2017 from www.ismp.org.

Kalant H, Grant D, Mitchell J: *Principles of medical pharmacology*, ed 7, Toronto, 2007, Elsevier Canada, A Division of Reed Elsevier Canada, pp 303–315.

Keating D, McWilliams S, Schneider I, et al: Pharmacological guidelines for schizophrenia: a systematic review and comparison of recommendations for the first episode, *BMJ Open* 7:e013881, 2017. doi:10.1136/bmjopen-2016-013881.

Lance L, Lacy C, Armstrong L, et al: *Drug information handbook for the allied health professional*, ed 12, Hudson, OH, 2005, APhA Lexi-Comp.

Miyamoto S, Miyake N, Jarskog L, et al: Pharmacological treatment of schizophrenia: a critical review of the pharmacology and clinical effects of current and future therapeutic agents, *Mol Psychiatry* 17:1206–1227, 2012.

National Institutes of Mental Health: *Schizophrenia*. NIH Publication No. 15-3517, Bethesda, 2015, US Department of Health and Human Services. Available at: https://www.nimh.nih.gov/health/publications/schizophrenia-listing.shtml.

Page C, Curtis M, Sutter M, et al: *Integrated pharmacology*, Philadelphia, 2005, Elsevier Mosby, pp 242–247.

8

Treatment of Alzheimer's, Huntington's, and Parkinson's Disease

LEARNING OBJECTIVES

1. Learn the terminology associated with the treatment of Alzheimer's, Huntington's, and Parkinson's disease.
2. Describe the etiology of Alzheimer's, Huntington's, and Parkinson's disease.
3. Classify medications used in the treatment of Alzheimer's, Huntington's, and Parkinson's disease.
4. Describe mechanism of action for each class of drugs used to treat Alzheimer's, Huntington's, and Parkinson's disease.
5. Identify significant drug look-alike/sound-alike issues.
6. Identify warning labels and precautionary messages associated with medications used to treat Alzheimer's, Huntington's, and Parkinson's disease.

KEY TERMS

Acetylcholinesterase Enzyme that degrades the neurotransmitter acetylcholine.

Alzheimer's disease Neurodegenerative disease that causes memory loss and behavioral changes.

ApoE4 allele Defective form of apolipoprotein E that is associated with Alzheimer's disease.

Bradykinesia Slowness in initiating and carrying out voluntary movements.

Cognitive functions The ability to take in information via the senses, process the details, commit the information to memory, and recall it when necessary.

Dementia Condition associated with a loss of memory and cognition.

Huntington's disease Progressive and degenerative disease of neurons that affects muscle movement, cognitive functions, and emotions.

Neurodegeneration Destruction of nerve cells.

Neuroprotective Protects nerve cells from damage.

Parkinson's disease Progressive disorder of the nervous system involving degeneration of dopaminergic neurons and causing impaired muscle movement.

Plaques Substances composed of a protein called beta amyloid that fill the spaces between neurons and interfere with the transmission of signals between neurons.

Pseudoparkinsonism Drug-induced condition that resembles Parkinson's disease.

Tangles Twisted fibers made up of clumps of a protein called tau that interfere with nerve signal transmission.

Alzheimer's Disease

Alzheimer's disease is a neurodegenerative disease that causes memory loss and behavioral changes. According to the National Institutes of Health National Institute on Aging, up to 5.1 million Americans have Alzheimer's disease. More than 500,000 Canadians have Alzheimer's disease or a related dementia. The risk for Alzheimer's disease increases with advancing age. In fact, nearly 5% of the adult population 65 years of age will have Alzheimer's disease. That percentage doubles by age 70 years, and by age 85 years, nearly half of all men and women are estimated to have the disease. Although advancing age is an important risk factor for the development of Alzheimer's disease, *dementia* is not a normal part of the aging process.

Another risk factor for developing Alzheimer's disease is family history. Although less than 5% of the people have familial Alzheimer's disease (FAD), there is a 50% chance of children inheriting the gene that causes Alzheimer's disease. Late-onset Alzheimer's is linked to several nonhereditary genes. Apolipoprotein E (ApoE) helps carry cholesterol in the blood. Approximately 40% of people with Alzheimer's disease have a defective form of ApoE, although not everyone with a defective ApoE4 allele will develop the disease. Only 15% of people with the defective *ApoE4 allele* will develop Alzheimer's disease. Other genes that are associated with the development of Alzheimer's disease are *CLU* (ApoJ/clusterin), *PICALM*, and *CRI* (complement receptor 1). *CLU* and *CRI* play a role in clearing beta amyloid out of the brain. Cell membrane proteins are recycled at the synapse by *PICALM*.

The most commonly reported symptom of Alzheimer's disease is forgetfulness. The person may not recall recent events or names of familiar people or things. This increases as the disease progresses and may interfere with the performance of activities of daily living such as personal hygiene. In the mid to late stages of Alzheimer's disease, the person may have difficulty reading, speaking, writing, and walking. The person may become anxious, angry, and aggressive. In addition, the person may be confused and wander, unable to find his or her way back to where he or she started. Many people confuse the differences between the normal aging process and Alzheimer's disease. Table 8.1 shows some comparisons between the disease and normal aging.

Pathophysiology of Alzheimer's Disease

Alzheimer's disease causes damage to the part of the brain that is involved in memory. The disease causes cholinergic nerve cells in the brain to die. The cerebral cortex shrinks in size, and the ability to think and function diminishes. Abnormal structures, called plaques and tangles, develop in the brain (Fig. 8.1). *Plaques* are dense substances composed of a protein called beta amyloid. The plaques fill the spaces between neurons in the brain and interfere with the transmission of signals between the neurons. *Tangles* look like twisted fibers and are made up of clumps of a protein called tau. Tangles are also thought to block the transmission of messages between neurons. The accumulation of plaques and tangles also produces inflammation, which further damages neurons.

Comorbid conditions such as cerebrovascular disease, high blood pressure, diabetes, sleep apnea, and Parkinson's disease are believed to speed the progression of Alzheimer's disease. Lewy bodies, abnormal clumps of protein, found in people with Alzheimer's disease are also associated with Parkinson's disease. Sleep deprivation can increase beta amyloid deposits. Microvascular infarcts and inflammation, which block blood supply and nourishment to the brain, are common in patients with cerebrovascular disease, diabetes, and Alzheimer's disease.

Role of Neurotransmitters

Several neurotransmitters play a significant role in Alzheimer's disease. The most significant is acetylcholine (ACh). ACh levels gradually decline as the disease progresses producing the symptoms associated with Alzheimer's disease. Glutamate also plays a role in the development of Alzheimer's disease. Glutamate is an excitatory amino acid that is involved in memory formation and learning. There are three classes of glutamatergic receptors. The most important is N-methyl-D-aspartate (NMDA). NMDA is believed to contribute to the process of *neurodegeneration*.

Other neurotransmitters that are believed to play a part in Alzheimer's disease are dopamine, norepinephrine, and serotonin. Reduced nicotinic receptor function is also correlated to impaired memory.

TABLE 8.1	Comparisons Between Alzheimer's Disease and Normal Aging	
Alzheimer's Disease	**Normal Aging**	
Making poor judgments and decisions a lot of the time	Making a bad decision once in a while	
Problems taking care of monthly bills	Missing a monthly payment	
Losing track of the date or time of year	Forgetting which day it is and remembering it later	
Trouble having a conversation	Sometimes forgetting which word to use	
Misplacing things often and being unable to find them	Losing things from time to time	

Courtesy of the National Institute on Aging, Understanding Alzheimer's disease: what you need to know (https://www.nia.nih.gov/alzheimers/publication/understanding-alzheimers-disease/introduction).

• **Fig. 8.1** Disintegrating neurons and tangles. (Courtesy The Alzheimer's Disease Education and Referral Center, National Institute on Aging, Bethesda, MD.)

Drug Treatment for Alzheimer's Disease

Drugs that increase ACh levels at the synapse are used to treat Alzheimer's disease. Drugs that block glutamate activity are also used in the treatment of Alzheimer's disease. Three of the four drugs currently approved for the treatment of Alzheimer's disease are *acetylcholinesterase* (AChE) inhibitors; the other is an NMDA antagonist. AChE is an enzyme that degrades ACh. AChE inhibitors increase levels of ACh. AChE-R appears to protect against the degeneration of cholinergic neurons. *Neuroprotective* agents protect nerve cells from damage.

The AChE inhibitors are typically prescribed for the treatment of mild to moderate disease. The NMDA antagonist is prescribed for moderate to severe disease.

Mechanism of Action and Pharmacokinetics

Donepezil (Aricept), rivastigmine (Exelon), and galantamine (Razadyne, Reminyl) are AChE inhibitors. In addition to AChE inhibition, galantamine slightly increases glutamate activity.

Donepezil is highly protein bound and metabolized by CYP450 isoenzymes and thus subject to drug interactions with drugs that are similarly protein bound and metabolized by enzymes in the liver. Donepezil is available as a swallowable tablet and an oral disintegrating tablet. Its bioavailability is not diminished by food, therefore it may be taken without regard to meals. In contrast, the bioavailability of galantamine is delayed by food; however, the drug is nearly 90% bioavailable, and protein binding and CYP450 metabolism are minimal. Rivastigmine readily crosses the blood-brain barrier, where it is metabolized at central nervous system receptor sites. Cholinesterase inhibition lasts up to 10 hours. Over a 24-hour period, 50% of the drug is released from rivastigmine transdermal patches.

Memantine (Namenda) blocks the actions of glutamate at NMDA receptor sites. This mechanism of action is theorized to protect the neuron from further damage. All dosage forms of memantine exhibit 100% bioavailability. The drug is minimally subject to drug interactions involving CYP450 isozymes; however, alkaline urine can decrease drug clearance by as much as 80%.

Drugs Used in the Treatment of Alzheimer's Disease: Acetylcholinesterase Inhibitors

Generic Name	US Brand Name(s) / Canadian Brand(s)	Dosage Forms and Strengths
donepezil[a]	Aricept, Aricept ODT	**Tablets:** 5 mg, 10 mg, 23 mg[b]
	Aricept, Aricept RDT	**Tablets, oral disintegrating (Aricept ODT, Aricept RDT):** 5 mg, 10 mg
donepezil + memantine[a]	Namzaric	**Capsule, extended release[b]:** 10 mg donepezil + 7 mg memantine; 10 mg donepezil + 14 mg memantine; 10 mg donepezil + 21 mg memantine; 10 mg donepezil + 28 mg memantine;
	Not available	
galantamine[a]	Razadyne, Razadyne ER	**Solution, oral: 4 mg/mL**
	Generics	**Tablets[b]:** 4 mg, 8 mg, 12 mg **Tablets, extended release (Razadyne ER, Reminyl ER):** 8 mg, 16 mg, 24 mg
rivastigmine[a]	Exelon	**Capsules:** 1.5 mg, 3 mg, 4.5 mg, 6 mg
	Exelon, Exelon patch-5, Exelon patch-10, Exelon patch-15,	**Transdermal patch:** 4.6 mg/24 hours, 9.5 mg/24 hours, 13.3 mg/24 hours

[a]Generic available.
[b]Available in the United States only.

Drugs Used in the Treatment of Alzheimer's Disease: *N*-Methyl-D-Aspartate Receptor Inhibitor

Generic Name	US Brand Name(s) / Canadian Brand(s)	Dosage Forms and Strengths
memantine[a,b]	Namenda, Namenda XR	**Solution, oral:** 2 mg/ mL[b]
	Ebixa	**Tablets:** 5 mg, 10 mg **Capsule (Namenda XR)[b]:** 7 mg, 14 mg, 21 mg, 28 mg

[a]Generic available
[b]Available in the United States only.

Summary of Drugs Used in the Treatment of Alzheimer's Disease

Generic Name	US Brand Name	Usual Adult Oral Dose and Dosing Schedule	Warning Labels
donepezil	Aricept	**Tablets/ODT:** 5–23 mg once daily at bedtime	MAY CAUSE DIZZINESS OR DROWSINESS—donepezil, galantamine, rivastigmine, memantine.
donepezil + memantine	Namzaric	**Tablet:** 1 tablet once daily	TAKE WITH FOOD—galantamine, rivastigmine. DISSOLVE IN MOUTH—donepezil ODT.
galantamine	Reminyl	**Tablets:** 4–12 mg twice a day **Extended release Tablets:** 8–24 mg once daily	DO NOT DISCONTINUE WITHOUT MEDICAL SUPERVISION. REMOVE OLD PATCH AND ROTATE SITE OF APPLICATION MAINTAIN ADEQUATE HYDRATION—galantamine.
rivastigmine	Exelon	**Capsules/solution:** 1.5–6 mg twice a day **Transdermal patch:** Apply one patch daily 4.6–13.3 mg once daily	SWALLOW WHOLE; DO NOT CRUSH OR CHEW—donepezil + memantine, galantamine ER, memantine XR. MAY MIX SOLUTION WITH WATER, JUICE OR SODA ONLY—rivastigmine. CAPSULES MAY BE SPRINKLED ON APPLESAUCE—memantine XR.
memantine	Namenda	**Tablets:** 5–10 mg twice a day **Capsules XR:** 7–28 mg once daily	

Food has little effect on absorption, and memantine may be taken without regard to meals.

> **TECH NOTE!**
> In the United States, galantamine was formerly marketed under the brand name Reminyl but is now marketed as Razadyne.

> **TECH NOTE!**
> Rivastimine premixed solution must be consumed within 4 hours of mixing.

Adverse Reactions

Donepezil, galantamine, rivastigmine, and memantine can all produce abdominal pain and cramping, dizziness, diarrhea, nausea, and urinary incontinence. In some patients, donepezil and rivastigmine may increase urinary frequency. Tremor has been reported in all agents except donepezil. Pseudoparkinsonism has been reported with the use of rivastigmine and memantine. Myocardial infarction, erectile dysfunction, and suicide ideation have been reported with memantine.

> **TECH NOTE!**
> Dispense Razadyne solution with manufacturer's calibrated syringe.

Nonpharmacological Measures to Reduce Risks for Alzheimer's Disease

Head injury protection and adoption of a healthy lifestyle that includes reduction in cholesterol, adequate intellectual stimulation, and decreased obesity are modifiable factors that may reduce the risk for Alzheimer's disease. Social interaction keeps the brain stimulated. Some studies have shown that aerobic exercise can reduce risks for obesity, improve cognition, and reduce plaque formation. A diet that includes vegetables, legumes, fruits, cereals, olive oil, decreased saturated fats, dairy products, fish, lean meat, poultry, and antioxidants can reduce vascular disease, a comorbid condition linked to increasing the progression of Alzheimer's disease. Vitamin E, folate, selenium, and other antioxidants are being studied for their possible benefit in preventing Alzheimer's disease.

Parkinson's Disease

Parkinson's disease is a progressive disorder of the nervous system involving degeneration of dopaminergic neurons in the basal ganglia and nigrostriatal pathways in the brain. The basal ganglia are part of the extrapyramidal system that initiates, controls, and modulates movement and posture.

Loss of dopaminergic neurons results in reduction of available dopamine. Symptoms of Parkinson's disease are a result of an imbalance between dopamine and ACh (Fig. 8.2). As the loss of dopaminergic neurons progresses, voluntary muscle movement diminishes.

Approximately 1 million people in the United States have Parkinson's disease (2017). Nearly 100,000 people are living with Parkinson's disease in Canada. The disease disproportionately affects elderly men. The average age at onset of Parkinson's disease is 60 years. The prevalence and incidence (number of new cases) increase with age. The onset of Parkinson's disease in persons under 40 years old is rare and has been associated with ingestion of illicit drugs contaminated with MPTP (1-methyl-4-phenyl-1,2,3,6-tetrahydropyridine).

The etiology of Parkinson's disease is thought to be related to environmental and genetic factors. Recent studies with twins have shown a familial inheritance of the chromosome 4 gene. Environmental causes are associated with pesticide exposure and exposure to drugs that destroy dopaminergic neurons in nigrostriatal pathways. Exposure to pesticides may increase the long-term risk for development of Parkinson's disease from 3% to 5%, according to a cohort study that reviewed surveys of 143,000 participants in the United States, the "Cancer Prevention Study II Nutrition Cohort" begun in 1982. The risks appear to be greater in men than in women. Other environmental toxins that may cause development of Parkinson's disease are carbon monoxide poisoning and heavy metal poisoning (mercury). Infectious diseases such as viral encephalitis are thought to be possible triggers for Parkinson's disease.

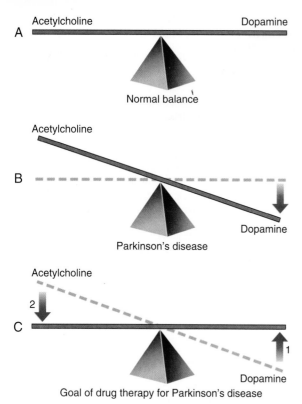

A. Normal balance of acetylcholine and dopamine in the CNS.

B. In Parkinson's disease, a decrease in dopamine results in an imbalance.

C. Drug therapy in Parkinson's disease is aimed at correcting the imbalance between acetylcholine and dopamine. This can be accomplished by either
1. increasing the supply of dopamine or
2. blocking or lowering acetylcholine levels.

• **Fig. 8.2** Balance of acetylcholine and dopamine versus Parkinson's disease. *CNS.* Central nervous system. (From Lilley LL, Harrington S, Snyder JS: *Pharmacology and the nursing process*, ed 5, St. Louis, 2007, Mosby.)

Pseudoparkinsonism is a drug-induced condition that resembles Parkinson's disease. It is caused by administration of drugs that block dopaminergic receptors in the basal ganglia in the brain. Examples of drugs that produce pseudoparkinsonism are neuroleptics (e.g., phenothiazines), administered to treat schizophrenia, and reserpine, a drug that is used to treat hypertension.

Characteristic signs of Parkinson's disease are *bradykinesia* and slowness in initiating and carrying out voluntary movements accompanied by muscle rigidity and tremors. When a person wishes to move her or his arm, the onset of movement is often delayed. When the forward motion begins, movements will be slow, rigid, and tremulous. Tremors are usually present at rest and may reduce the person's ability to perform skilled tasks. Postural and gait abnormalities are also typically present. The person walks with a characteristic shuffle. Other visible signs of Parkinson's disease are a blank facial expression, drooling, and speech impairment.

Cognitive functions may be impaired as well as motor functions. Parkinson's disease can cause memory loss, and affected persons may exhibit signs of dementia. Parkinson's disease can also cause depression.

Parkinson's disease is treated by the administration of pharmaceuticals, exercise, and nutritional support.

Drugs Used to Treat Parkinson's Disease

Mechanism of Action

The strategy for treatment of Parkinson's disease is to restore the balance between dopamine and ACh. This can be accomplished by administering drugs that are synthesized to dopamine, promote the release of existing stores of dopamine, directly stimulate dopamine receptors, or inhibit the degradation of dopamine in the terminal neuron (Fig. 8.3). Dopamine regulates direct and indirect extrapyramidal pathways. The amount of dopamine available for release diminishes as Parkinson's disease progresses because degeneration of dopaminergic neurons increases. This results in unopposed cholinergic excitation and produces the tremors, muscle rigidity, and immobility associated with Parkinson's disease. Stimulation of GABAergic neurons by dopamine (D_2) sends inhibitory feedback to the motor cortex via the indirect pathway. This results in impaired voluntary muscle movement. Anticholinergics may be administered to decrease ACh levels because excessive stimulation of cholinergic neurons causes symptoms of immobility in Parkinson's disease. AChE is the enzyme that degrades ACh.

There is a decrease in the effectiveness of most anti-Parkinson drugs over time because of the disease's progressive neurodegeneration. The efficacy of levodopa and amantadine also declines with long-term therapy because of desensitization of dopamine receptors.

> **TECH NOTE!**
>
> In addition to the treatment of Parkinson's disease, bromocriptine 0.8 mg (Cylcoset) is indicated as adjunct therapy for the treatment of type 2 diabetes mellitus.

> **TECH NOTE!**
>
> Carbidopa/levodopa (Duopa, Duodopa) is also marketed for infusion in an intestinal pump. It is indicated for the treatment of advanced levodopa-responsive Parkinson's disease.

Pharmacokinetics

The absorption, distribution, metabolism, and elimination of drugs used to treat Parkinson's disease vary. Levodopa is a prodrug and a dopamine precursor. It is administered rather than dopamine (which is available for use as a cardiac stimulant), because dopamine does not cross the blood-brain barrier. Although levodopa readily crosses the blood-brain barrier, much of the orally administered drug is metabolized in the gastrointestinal tract and in peripheral tissues (see Fig. 8.3). Only a small percentage actually reaches the neuron to be converted to dopamine. Sustained-release preparations of levodopa can further reduce the bioavailability of levodopa by as much as 30%.

Carbidopa and benserazide are adjuvants that boost the effectiveness of levodopa. Carbidopa and benserazide inhibit the metabolism (decarboxylation) of levodopa in the gastrointestinal tract and peripheral tissues. The bioavailability of levodopa is increased by 75% when combined with carbidopa. Catechol-*O*-methyltransferase (COMT) is the enzyme responsible for peripheral and central metabolism of catecholamines that also metabolizes levodopa. Entacapone and tolcapone are COMT inhibitors that can boost the bioavailability of levodopa by up to 50%.

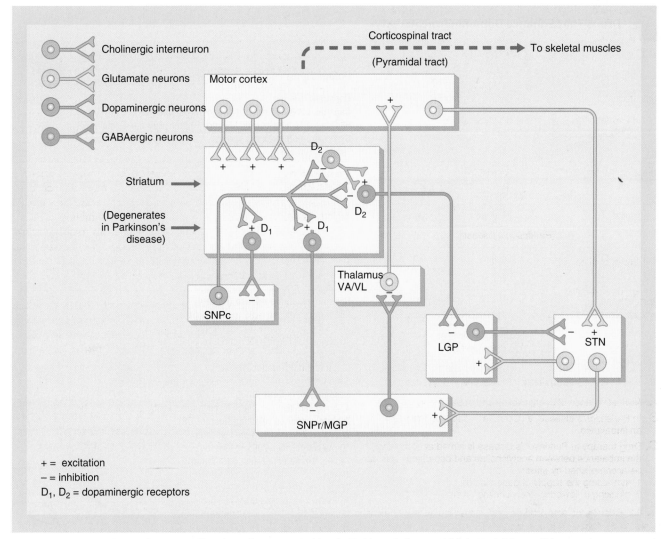

• **Fig. 8.3** Summary of basal ganglia systems involved in Parkinson's disease. *LGP*, Lateral globus pallidus; *SNPc*, substantia nigra pars compacta; *SNPr/MGP*, substantia nigra pars reticula/medial globus pallidus; *STN*, subthalamic nucleus; *VA/VL*, ventroanterior/ventrolateral thalamic nuclei. (From Page C, Curtis M, Sutter M, et al: *Integrated pharmacology*, ed 3, Philadelphia, 2006, Mosby.)

ⓘ TECH ALERT!

The following drugs have look-alike/sound-alike issues:
ReQuip and ReQuip XL
riMANTAdine, and raNITIdine;
Sinemet and Sinemet CR;
selegiline and sertraline;

Common Adverse Reactions

Gastrointestinal distress such as nausea, vomiting, and decreased appetite are common side effects of most of the drugs used to treat Parkinson's disease. Other common side effects are dizziness or lightheadedness, insomnia, and confusion. Hypotension is also associated with most of the drugs used to treat Parkinson's disease. Many of the anti-Parkinson drugs that increase dopamine also produce dry mouth and constipation. Drugs that treat Parkinson's disease can produce auditory and visual hallucinations. People older than the age of 65 years are most susceptible.

▪ TECH NOTE!

High-protein diets and iron supplements may decrease the absorption of Parkinson drugs containing levodopa.

Precautions

Selegiline and rasagiline are monoamine oxidase type B (MAOI$_B$) inhibitors can increase the risk for hypertensive crisis. Patients taking Prolopa (levodopa plus benserazide) may experience sudden drowsiness without warning and should be cautioned about risks for driving accidents. It is recommended that patients with diabetes test their blood glucose levels more frequently when taking Prolopa.

▪ TECH NOTE!

Selegiline and rasagiline are MAOIs. Dispense with list of tyramine-containing foods and beverages to avoid. Dietary restrictions are not required for selegiline patches.

Drugs That Enhance Dopaminergic Activity

Generic Name	US Brand Name(s) Canadian Brand(s)	Dosage Forms and Strengths
amantadine[a]	Gocovri Osmolex ER Generics	**Capsules:** 100 mg **Capsule, extended release (Gocovri, Osmolex ER):** 68.5 mg, 137 mg Gocovri; 129 mg, 193 mg, 258 mg (Osmolex ER) **Syrup, oral:** 50 mg/5 mL **Tablets:** 100 mg[b]
bromocriptine[a]	Parlodel Generics	**Capsules:** 5 mg **Tablets:** 2.5 mg
carbidopa[a]	Lodosyn Not available	**Tablets:** 25 mg
entacapone[a]	Comtan Comtan	**Tablets:** 200 mg
levodopa and carbidopa[a]	Duopa, Rytary, Sinemet, Sinemet CR Duodopa, Sinemet, Sinemet CR	**Capsule, extended release (Rytary):** 23.75 mg carbidopa + 95 mg levodopa; 36.25 mg carbidopa + 145 mg levodopa; 48.75 mg carbidopa + 195 mg levodopa 61.25 mg carbidopa + 245 mg levodopa **Gel, intestinal (Duodopa):** 5 mg carbidopa + 20 mg levodopa per 1 mL **Suspension, enteral (Duopa):** 4.63 mg carbidopa + 20 mg levodopa per 1 mL **Tablets, extended release (Sinemet CR):** 25 mg carbidopa + 100 mg levodopa, 50 mg carbidopa + 200 mg levodopa **Tablets, immediate release (Sinemet):** 10 mg carbidopa + 100 mg levodopa, 25 mg carbidopa + 100 mg levodopa, 25 mg carbidopa + 250 mg levodopa **Tablets, immediate oral disintegrating:** 10 mg carbidopa + 100 mg levodopa, 25 mg carbidopa + 100 mg levodopa, 25 mg carbidopa + 250 mg levodopa
levodopa and benserazide	Not available Prolopa	**Capsules:** 50 mg levodopa + 12.5 mg benserazide 100 mg levodopa + 25 mg benserazide 200 mg levodopa + 50 mg benserazide
levodopa, carbidopa, and entacapone	Stalevo Stalevo	**Tablets:** carbidopa 12.5 mg + levodopa 50 mg + entacapone 200 mg carbidopa 18.75 mg + levodopa 75 mg + entacapone 200 mg carbidopa 25 mg + levodopa 100 mg + entacapone 200 mg carbidopa 31.5 mg + levodopa 125 mg + entacapone 200 mg carbidopa 37.5 mg + levodopa 150 mg + entacapone 200 mg carbidopa 50 mg + levodopa 200 mg + entacapone 200 mg
pramipexole[a]	Mirapex, Mirapex ER Mirapex	**Tablets:** 0.125 mg, 0.25 mg, 0.5 mg, 0.75 mg[b], 1 mg, 1.25 mg, 1.5 mg **Tablets, extended release (Mirapex ER)[b]:** 0.375 mg, 0.75 mg, 1.5 mg, 2.25 mg, 3 mg, 3.75 mg, 4.5 mg
rasagiline[a]	Azilect Azilect	**Tablets:** 0.5 mg, 1 mg
ropinirole[a]	ReQuip, ReQuip XL Generics	**Tablets:** 0.25 mg, 0.5 mg[b], 1 mg, 2 mg, 3 mg[b], 4 mg[b], 5 mg **Tablets, extended release[b]:** 2 mg, 4 mg, 6 mg, 8 mg, 12 mg

Drugs That Enhance Dopaminergic Activity—cont'd

Generic Name	US Brand Name(s) Canadian Brand(s)	Dosage Forms and Strengths
selegiline[a] (L-deprenyl)	Eldepryl, Zelapar Emsam Generics	**Capsules (Eldepryl):** 5 mg **Tablets:** 5 mg **Tablets, oral disintegrating (Zelapar)**[b]**:** 1.25 mg **Transdermal Patch (Emsam)**[b]**:** 6 mg/24 hr, 9 mg/24 hr, 12 mg/24 hr
tolcapone[a]	Tasmar Not available	**Tablets:** 100 mg

[a]Generic available.
[b]Available in the United States only.

Drugs That Reduce Cholinergic Activity

Generic Name	US Brand Name(s) Canadian Brand(s)	Dosage Forms and Strengths
benztropine[a]	Cogentin Generics	**Injection:** 1 mg/mL **Tablets:** 0.5 mg[b], 1 mg, 2 mg
trihexyphenidyl[a]	Generic only Generic only	**Elixir:** 2 mg/5 mL **Tablets:** 2 mg, 5 mg

[a]Generic available.
[b]Available in the United States only

Summary of Drugs Used in the Treatment of Parkinson's Disease

Generic Name	US Brand Name	Usual Adult Oral Dose and Dosing Schedule	Warning Labels
Drugs That Increase Dopamine Levels			
amantadine	Generics	100 mg twice a day up to 300–400 mg/day	MAY CAUSE DIZZINESS; MAY IMPAIR ABILITY TO DRIVE. AVOID ALCOHOL. DO NOT DISCONTINUE WITHOUT MEDICAL SUPERVISION. AVOID IRON SUPPLEMENTS WITHIN 2 HOURS OF DOSE—levodopa/carbidopa, levodopa, carbidopa and entacapone, levodopa and benserazide. MAY CAUSE SUDDEN, EXCESSIVE DROWSINESS—Prolopa. SWALLOW WHOLE; DO NOT CRUSH OR CHEW (sustained release, Prolopa).
bromocriptine	Parlodel	Start 1.25 mg twice/day; increase to 40–100 mg/day	
entacapone	Comtan	200 mg up to 8 times a day (Only effective in combination with levodopa/carbidopa)	
levodopa and carbidopa	Sinemet	**Immediate release:** carbidopa 25 mg/levodopa 100 mg 3–4 times a day (maximum, carbidopa 200 mg/levodopa 2000 mg) **Sustained release:** carbidopa 50 mg/levodopa 200 mg 2 times a day (maximum, carbidopa 400 mg/levodopa 1600 mg)	
levodopa and benserazide	Prolopa	Initiate 1 capsules Prolopa (100–25 mg) 1–2 times a day; increase to 4–8 capsules daily in 4–6 divided doses	
levodopa, carbidopa and entacapone	Stalevo	Individualized (maximum, 1600 mg/day)	

Continued

Summary of Drugs Used in the Treatment of Parkinson's Disease—cont'd

Generic Name	US Brand Name	Usual Adult Oral Dose and Dosing Schedule	Warning Labels
pramipexole	Mirapex	Start 0.125 mg/day in 3 divided doses; increase to 1.5–4.5 mg/day	TAKE WITH FOOD—bromocriptine, Prolopa. AVOID FOODS HIGH IN TYRAMINE—rasagiline, selegiline. MAY DISCOLOR URINE—Stavelo, tolcapone, entacapone, Sinemet. SWALLOW WHOLE; DO NOT CRUSH OR CHEW—ReQuip XL, Mirapex ER.
rasagiline	Azilect	0.5–1 mg once daily	
ropinerole	ReQuip	Start 0.25 mg 3 times/day; increase weekly to a maximum 24 mg/day	
selegiline	Eldepryl	5 mg twice a day or 10 mg once daily	
tolcapone	Tasmar	100 mg 3 times a day	
Anticholinergics			
benztropine	Cogentin	0.5–6 mg/day (usual dose 1–2 mg at bedtime)	MAY CAUSE DROWSINESS; MAY IMPAIR ABILITY TO DRIVE. AVOID ALCOHOL. MAINTAIN ADEQUATE HYDRATION. DO NOT DISCONTINUE WITHOUT MEDICAL SUPERVISION.
trihexyphenidyl	Generics	5–15 mg/day in 3–4 divided doses	

Drugs That Deplete Stores of Dopamine

Generic Name	US Brand Name(s) Canadian Brand(s)	Dosage Forms and Strengths
tetrabenazine[a]	Xenazine	**Tablets:** 12.5 mg[b], 25 mg
	Nitoman	

[a]Generic available.
[b]Strength available in the United States only.

Drugs That Reduce Cholinergic Activity

Anticholinergics are administered as adjunctive treatment of Parkinson's disease and to lessen drug-induced extrapyramidal symptoms. Side effects are dizziness, sedation, confusion, dry mouth, blurred vision, constipation, urinary retention, heat intolerance, hypotension, and hallucinations.

Huntington's Disease

Huntington's disease is another progressive and degenerative disease of neurons that affects muscle movement, cognitive functions, and emotions. Huntington's disease is similar to Parkinson's disease in that it is associated with defects in the basal ganglia. Unlike Parkinson's disease, it produces excessive, abnormal muscle movement rather than immobility.

Huntington's disease is a hereditary disorder. It affects approximately one person in every 10,000. Children born to a parent who has Huntington's disease have a 50% chance of inheriting the gene for the disease. If the gene is inherited, the child will develop Huntington's disease at some point. The onset of Huntington's disease typically occurs in middle age (30 to 50 years); symptoms rarely occur after age 55. Juvenile onset is associated with rapid progression of symptoms and shorter life expectancy. Patients may live with the illness for 10 to 30 years.

Characteristic symptoms of Huntington's disease are tremors, rhythmic oscillations or circular movements around the ankles or wrists, and sudden abnormal movements. Movements are typically repetitive. Choreiform movements, unpredictable, irregular, and jerking motions, are also signs of the disease. The person may also have speech impairment and difficulty swallowing and may exhibit facial grimaces.

Huntington's disease also causes emotional and intellectual changes. The person has difficulty concentrating, which worsens as the disease progresses. Irritability, mood swings, and depression are other symptoms of the disease. Cognitive impairment may appear as fixation on an idea, slowed thinking and responses, memory problems, and difficulty sequencing activities.

Neurochemistry of Huntington's Disease

Huntington's disease causes defects in the basal ganglia that result in increased concentrations of dopamine and decreased activity of the enzymes that synthesize GABA and ACh. Deficient levels of ACh and GABA lead to hyperactivity of dopaminergic neurons in nigrostriatal pathways. The balance between GABA, ACh, and dopamine is upset, and this produces the excessive muscle movement associated with Huntington's disease.

Summary of Drugs Used in the Treatment of Huntington's Disease

Generic Name	US Brand Name	Usual Adult Oral Dose and Dosing Schedule	Warning Labels
Drugs That Decrease Dopamine Levels			
tetrabenazine	Xenazine, Nitoman (Canada)	25–37.5 mg 2–3 times/day (maximum, 50 mg/day)	MAY CAUSE DROWSINESS; MAY IMPAIR ABILITY TO DRIVE; LIMIT ALCOHOL. DO NOT DISCONTINUE WITH MEDICAL SUPERVISION. DILUTE ORAL CONCENTRATE BEFORE ADMINISTRATION—haloperidol. MAINTAIN ADEQUATE HYDRATION—haloperidol. AVOID PROLONGED EXPOSURE TO SUNLIGHT—haloperidol.

Drugs Used to Treat Huntington's Disease

Tetrabenzine (Xenazine) is the only drug approved by the US Food and Drug Administration for the treatment of Huntington's disease.

Mechanism of Action

Tetrabenzine decreases excessive dopaminergic activity. This is accomplished by depleting stores of dopamine in the neuron. Drugs that block dopamine receptors may also be administered.

Common Side Effects

Side effects of tetrabenazine are hypotension, sedation, constipation, dizziness, depression, and pseudoparkinsonism.

Drugs That Block Dopamine Receptors

Neuroleptics (e.g., haloperidol, fluphenazine, risperidone and olanzapine) have been administered to control choreiform movements but are not approved by the FDA for this purpose. Side effects include sedation, confusion, weight gain, increased appetite, blurred vision, dry mouth, urinary retention, constipation, postural hypotension, pseudoparkinsonism, extrapyramidal symptoms, tardive dyskinesia, photosensitivity, and sexual dysfunction.

TECHNICIAN'S CORNER

1. According to the most current research, a brain-healthy diet is one that reduces the risk of heart disease and diabetes, encourages good blood flow to the brain, and is low in fat and cholesterol. What sort of physical, mental, and social activities can be added to daily living to delay the onset of Alzheimer's disease?
2. What are public health strategies to reduce the risk of Parkinson's disease in young person's 1) exposed to street drugs or 2) environmental toxins?

Key Points

- Cognitive impairment and memory loss are symptoms of Alzheimer's, Huntington's, and Parkinson's disease.
- Risk factors for Alzheimer's disease are age and heredity.
- Abnormal structures called plaques and tangles form and interfere with the transmission of messages between neurons.
- Alzheimer's disease causes cholinergic nerve cells in the brain to die.
- Alzheimer's disease is treated with drugs that increase acetylcholine levels or drugs that block glutamate activity.
- AChE is an enzyme that degrades ACh. AChE inhibitors increase levels of ACh.
- Three of the drugs approved for the treatment of Alzheimer's disease are AChE inhibitors. They are donepezil (Aricept), rivastigmine (Exelon), and galantamine (Reminyl).
- Memantine (Namenda) blocks the actions of glutamate at the NMDA receptor.
- Parkinson's disease is a progressive disorder of the nervous system involving degeneration of dopaminergic neurons in the basal ganglia of the brain.
- Symptoms of Parkinson's disease are caused by an imbalance between dopamine and acetylcholine.
- The average age at onset of Parkinson's disease is 60 years. Men are more often affected than women.
- Environmental factors (e.g., exposure to pesticides, carbon monoxide poisoning) and infectious diseases (e.g., viral encephalitis and syphilis) can increase the risk for Parkinson's disease.
- Antipsychotic drugs can cause pseudoparkinsonism, a drug-induced condition that resembles Parkinson's disease.
- Physical signs of Parkinson's disease are bradykinesia, muscle rigidity, tremors, postural and gait abnormalities, and walking with a characteristic shuffle. Other visible signs of Parkinson's disease are blank facial expression, drooling, and speech impairment.
- Levodopa is a prodrug and is a dopamine precursor.
- Benserazide, carbidopa, and tolcapone are combined with levodopa to inhibit levodopa's metabolism and increase its effects.
- Dizziness, hypotension, confusion, and gastrointestinal distress are common side effects of most of the drugs used to treat Parkinson's disease. People older than the age of 65 years are most susceptible to side effects of anti-Parkinson drugs.
- Side effects of anticholinergic drugs are dry mouth, blurred vision, constipation, and urinary retention.
- The effectiveness of anti-Parkinson drugs decline over time due to the progressive nature of the disease. The efficacy of levodopa and amantadine also declines with long-term therapy because of desensitization of dopamine receptors.
- Selegiline and rasagiline are MAOI$_B$ and are associated with a risk for hypertensive crisis.
- Huntington's disease is a progressive and degenerative disease of neurons that affects muscle movement, cognitive functions, and emotions.
- Huntington's disease is a hereditary disorder.

- Characteristic symptoms of Huntington's disease are choreiform movements (e.g., unpredictable, irregular, and jerking tremors), rhythmic oscillations or circular movements around the ankles or wrists, and sudden abnormal movements.

- In Huntington's disease, the balance between GABA, acetylcholine, and dopamine is upset, which produces the excessive muscle movement associated with Huntington's disease.
- Huntington's disease is primarily treated with drugs that decrease excessive dopaminergic activity.

Review Questions

1. Parkinson's disease is a progressive disorder of the nervous system that is associated with an imbalance between _____ and _____.
   a. epinephrine, dopamine
   b. dopamine, serotonin
   c. acetylcholine, norepinephrine
   d. dopamine, acetylcholine
2. The most commonly reported symptom of Alzheimer's disease is _____.
   a. pain
   b. forgetfulness
   c. heart problems
   d. incontinence
3. Drugs that increase _____ levels at the synapse are used to treat Alzheimer's disease.
   a. dopamine
   b. acetylcholine
   c. serotonin
   d. glutamate
4. Which drug is marketed in blister packaging to protect it from moisture?
   a. ReQuip XL
   b. Mirapex ER
   c. Sinemet CR
   d. Aricept ODT/Aricept RDT
   e. Duopa/Duodopa
5. The warning label MAY CAUSE DIZZINESS should be placed on prescriptions dispensed for Aricept and Namenda.
   a. true
   b. false

6. _____ is a prodrug and is a dopamine precursor.
   a. Levodopa
   b. Carbidopa
   c. Cogentin
   d. ReQuip
7. The effects of levodopa are increased by combining the drug with all of the following EXCEPT:
   a. tolcapone
   b. carbidopa
   c. selegiline
   d. benserazide
8. _____ is a common side effect of most of the drugs used to treat Parkinson's disease.
   a. Headache
   b. Gastrointestinal distress
   c. Muscle spasms
   d. Flulike symptoms
9. You receive a prescription for ReQuip XL 2 mg take one tablet three times a day for Parkinson's disease. You consult the pharmacist because _____.
   a. ReQuip XL is not available in 2 mg
   b. the usual dosing schedule for ReQuip XL is once daily
   c. ReQuip XL is not used for the treatment of Parkinson's disease
   d. none of the above
10. Huntington's disease is treated with drugs that _____ excessive dopaminergic activity.
   a. increase
   b. decrease

Bibliography

Ascherio A, Chen H, Weisskopf MG, et al: Pesticide exposure and risk for Parkinson's disease, *Ann Neurol* 60:197–203, 2006. Wiley-Liss, Inc., A Wiley Company.

Bourne C, Clayton C, Murch A, et al: Cognitive impairment and behavioural difficulties in patients with Huntington's disease, *Nurs Stand* 20:41–44, 2006.

FDA. (nd). Drugs@FDA: FDA Approved Drug Products, nd. Retrieved July 28, 2018, from http://www.accessdata.fda.gov/scripts/cder/daf/.

Geerts H: Pharmacology of acetylcholinesterase inhibitors and N-methyl-D-aspartate receptors for the combination therapy in the treatment of Alzheimer's disease, *J Clin Pharmacol* 46:8S–16S, 2006.

Health Canada: Drug Product Database, 2017. Retrieved July 28, 2018, from, https://health-products.canada.ca/dpd-bdpp/index-eng.jsp.

Institute for Safe Medication Practices: FDA and ISMP Lists of Look-Alike Drug Names with Recommended Tall Man Letters, 2016. Retrieved January 31, 2017 from www.ismp.org.

Nance MA, Paulsen JS, Rosenblatt A, et al: A Physician's Guide to the Management of Huntington Disease, 2013. M. Meijer & C. M. Forsyth (Eds).

Retrieved January 31, 2017 from: http://www.huntingtonsociety.ca/wp-content/uploads/2013/10/PhysGuide2013_WebsiteCopy_Reduced1.pdf.

National Institute on Aging: Alzheimer's Disease Medications Fact Sheet NIH Publication No. 16-AG-3431 (Vol. Alzheimer's Disease Education and Referral Center), 2016. Retrieved January 31, 2017 from https://www.nia.nih.gov/alzheimers/publication.

National Institute on Aging: 2014-2015 Alzheimer's Disease Progress Report Advancing Research Toward a Cure: U.S. Department of Health and Human Services, 2015. Retrieved January 31, 2017 from www.nia.nih.gov/alzheimers.

National Institute on Aging: Understanding Alzheimer's Disease: What You Need to Know, June 2011, Department of Health and Human Services, National Institutes of Health NIH Publication No. 11-5441. Available at https://www.nia.nih.gov/alzheimers/publication/understanding-alzheimers-disease/introduction.

National Institute of Neurological Disorders and Stroke National Institutes of Health: Parkinson's Disease—Challenges, Progress and Promise, 2015. Bethesda: US Department of Health and Human Services. Retrieved at: https://catalog.ninds.nih.gov/ninds/product/Parkinson-s-Disease-Challenges-Progress-and-Promise/15-5595.

National Institute of Neurological Disorders and Stroke National Institutes of Health: Parkinson's Disease—Hope through research, 2015. Bethesda, MD: US Department of Health and Human Services. NINDS, Publication date December 2014. NIH Publication No. 15-139.

Nordberg A: Mechanisms behind the neuroprotective actions of cholinesterase inhibitors in Alzheimer's disease, *Alzheimer Dis Assoc Disord* 20(Suppl 1):S12–S18, 2006.

Parkinson Society Canada: Fact Sheet, 2012. Retrieved from www.parkinson.ca.

Page C, Curtis M, Sutter M, et al: *Integrated pharmacology*, Philadelphia, 2005, Mosby, pp 242–247, 261–262.

Raffa R, Rawls S, Beyzarov E: *Netter's illustrated pharmacology*, Philadelphia, 2005, WB Saunders, pp 77–78, 80–82.

Smetanin P, Kobak P, Briante C, et al: *Rising Tide: the impact of dementia on Canadian society*, Toronto, ON, 2010, Alzheimer's Society of Canada.

Tarsy D: Patient Education: Parkinson disease treatment options- education, support, and therapy (Beyond the Basics), 2016. UptoDate, Inc., Wolters Kluwer.

USP Center for Advancement of Patient Safety: Use caution–avoid confusion, USP Quality Review No. 79, Rockville, MD, April 2004, USP Center for Advancement of Patient Safety.

9

Treatment of Seizure Disorders

LEARNING OBJECTIVES

1. Learn the terminology associated with seizures.
2. Describe the etiology of seizure disorders.
3. Compare and contrast the function of neurotransmitters associated with symptoms of seizure disorders.
4. Classify medications used in the treatment of seizure disorders.
5. Identify significant drug look-alike/sound-alike issues.

6. Describe mechanism of action for each class of drugs used to treat seizure disorders.
7. Identify significant drug interactions.
8. Identify warning labels and precautionary messages associated with medications used to treat seizure disorders.

KEY TERMS

Absence seizure A seizure in which the person experiences a brief period of unconsciousness and stares vacantly into space.

Anoxia Lack of oxygen to the brain.

Aura Unusual sensation, auditory, visual, or olfactory hallucination that is experienced just before the onset of a seizure.

Complex focal seizures Seizure disorder that produces a blank stare, disorientation, repetitive actions, and memory loss.

Convulsions Sudden contraction of muscles that is caused by seizures.

Eclampsia A life-threatening condition that can develop in pregnant women that causes high blood pressure and seizures.

Epilepsy A recurrent seizure disorder characterized by a sudden, excessive, disorderly discharge of cerebral neurons.

Febrile seizure A seizure associated with a sudden spike in body temperature.

Generalized seizure A seizure that spreads across both cerebral hemispheres. Includes tonic-clonic, myoclonic, and absence seizures.

Generalized tonic-clonic seizure A seizure that causes stiffening of the limbs, difficulty breathing, and jerking movements and is followed by disorientation and limbs that become limp.

Gingival hyperplasia Excess growth of gum tissue that may overgrow the teeth.

Hirsutism Excessive growth of body hair (especially in women).

Myoclonic seizure A seizure that is characterized by jerking muscle movements and is caused by contraction of major muscle groups.

Seizure threshold A person's susceptibility to seizures.

Simple focal seizure A seizure that affects only one part of the brain and causes the person to experience unusual sensations or feelings.

Status epilepticus Medical emergency that is characterized by repeated generalized seizures that can deprive the brain of oxygen.

Overview

Epilepsy is one of the oldest known brain disorders and was described as early as 3000 years ago in ancient Babylon. The word *epilepsy* is derived from the Greek word for "attack" because the ancient Greeks believed a person having a seizure was being attacked by demons. The World Health Organization estimates that 50 million people worldwide have epilepsy. Approximately 8 per 1000 people in the United States (approximately 2.2 million people) and 5 per 1000 people in Canada are diagnosed with epilepsy. The seizure risk increases with age. By 75 years, 3% of the population will have had a seizure caused by age-related cerebrovascular disease that deprives the brain of oxygen. Epilepsy is a type of seizure disorder that is associated with having experienced two or more seizures. Seizures are characterized by a sudden, excessive, disorderly discharge of cerebral neurons. Seizures may also be caused by conditions that range from injury to illness. Half of all seizures have no known cause. When the cause is known, the origin may

be birth defects, infection (meningitis, acquired immunodeficiency syndrome [AIDS]), perinatal injury, malignant tumors, lead poisoning, head trauma, or *eclampsia* (a life-threatening condition that can develop in pregnant women). Wearing seat belts, motorcycle helmets, and bike helmets can reduce the risk for seizures that are caused by head injury. The onset of a seizure may be preceded by an aura. An *aura* is an unusual sensation, auditory, visual, or olfactory hallucination that is experienced just before the onset of a seizure. In other words, the person may hear, see, or smell something distinctive immediately before the seizure activity begins. These signs of an upcoming seizure are important because they indicate the location of abnormal neuronal firing in the cerebrum.

> **● TECH NOTE!**
> Flashing or strobe lights such as those used in fire alarms systems can trigger seizures in individuals with epilepsy.

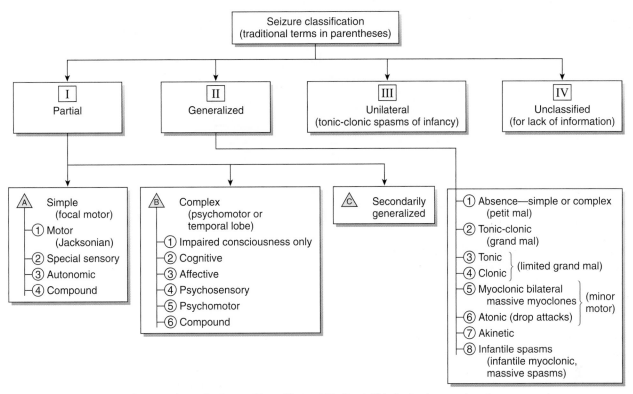

• **Fig. 9.1** Classifications of seizures. (From Clayton BD, Stock YN: *Basic pharmacology for nurses*, ed 12, St. Louis, 1997, Mosby.)

Febrile seizures in children are associated with an infection causing a sudden spike in temperature; aggressive treatment with fever reducers is indicated to prevent more seizures. Most children who have febrile seizures will not develop epilepsy.

External causes of seizures include metabolic disturbance, hypoglycemia, electrolyte imbalance, drug and alcohol withdrawal, and use of drugs that lower the *seizure threshold*. Stroke and heart attack can cause seizures because the brain becomes deprived of oxygen (*anoxia*).

Seizure Classifications

There are two major seizure classifications (Fig. 9.1): generalized seizures and focal or partial seizures. *Generalized seizures* spread across both of the cerebral hemispheres, while partial seizures are confined to a single hemisphere. Tonic-clonic (Fig. 9.2), myoclonic, and absence seizures are generalized seizures. *Tonic-clonic* and *myoclonic seizures* start with a stiffening of the limbs and difficulty breathing; are followed by jerking movements and loss of bladder and bowel control; and on conclusion (postictal phase), the limbs become limp and the person may be disoriented. The jerking muscle movement associated with *generalized tonic-clonic* seizures is sometimes referred to as a *convulsion*.

Petit mal seizures are also called absence seizures. This type of seizure is associated with a characteristic vacant or absent stare during the seizure. Absence seizures occur more commonly in children. They are barely noticeable to onlookers because no major muscle twitching is exhibited. *Status epilepticus* is a medical emergency that is characterized by repeated, generalized seizures that deprive the brain of oxygen. Antiseizure medicines must be administered intravenously to persons with status epilepticus.

Approximately 60% of people with epilepsy have focal seizures. Focal (partial) seizures involve only one cerebral hemisphere. Focal seizures are classified as simple or complex. *Simple focal seizures* may cause the arms, face, or legs to twitch, and visual, olfactory, or auditory hallucinations may occur. *Complex focal seizures* often begin with a blank stare. The person becomes disoriented and engages in repetitive actions during the seizure. When the seizure is over, the person does not have any memory of the seizure. Psychomotor and temporal lobe seizures are complex partial seizures.

Neurochemistry of Seizures

When there is an abnormality in nerve signaling by neurotransmitters, seizures result. People with epilepsy have an abnormally high level of excitatory neurotransmitters coupled with a low level of inhibitory neurotransmitters. This accounts for the excess neuronal firing that occurs with seizure disorders. γ-Aminobutyric acid (GABA) is an inhibitory neurotransmitter that plays an important role in epilepsy. An excitatory neurotransmitter that plays a role in epilepsy is the amino acid glutamate. Some seizures are linked to a defect in the genes that control the ion channels that open and close to regulate the influx of chloride, sodium, and calcium into the neuron.

Drugs Used to Treat Seizure Disorders

The goal of treatment of epilepsy and other seizure disorders is to reduce the incidence of seizures by suppressing seizure activity. Successful achievement of this therapeutic goal is dependent on correctly classifying the seizure type and selecting an appropriate drug for seizure type, with optimal drug administration and serum monitoring. Monodrug therapy is preferred to lower the incidence

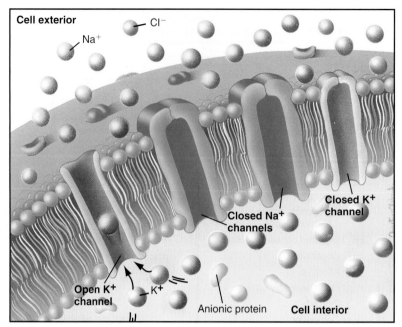

• **Fig. 9.2** Role of ion channels. (From Patton KT, Thibodeau GA: *Anatomy and physiology*, ed 9, St. Louis, 2016, Elsevier.)

of adverse effects, reduce the incidence of drug interactions, improve adherence to drug therapy, and lower medication costs.

Drugs That Modulate Ion Channels

The aim of pharmaceutical treatment of seizure is to suppress seizure activity. This is accomplished by control of ion channels. Neuronal firing is inhibited by drugs that delay the inflow of sodium, potassium, and calcium ions. Drugs that act on ion channels are phenytoin, carbamazepine, oxcarbazepine, eslicarbazine, lamotrigine, gabapentin, pregablin, levetiracetam, zonisamide, lacosamide, and ethosuximide. Gabapentin and pregabalin are structurally similar to GABA; however, they do not produce their effects by binding to GABA$_A$ receptors. Instead, they both act on ion channels. Gabapentin acts on sodium channels and pregabalin acts on calcium channels. They are effective in treating partial and generalized seizures. Fosphenytoin is used to treat status epilepticus and seizures occurring during neurosurgery. Carbamazepine and oxcarbazepine are used to treat generalized and complex focal seizures. Ethosuximide and methsuximide are two of only a few drugs that target absence seizures. Carbamazepine and gabapentin are also used in the management of neuropathic pain (see Chapter 10) and bipolar disorder (see Chapter 6).

Pharmacokinetics

The absorption of phenytoin and carbamazepine is variable and is influenced by particle size as well as by inactive ingredients in manufacturers' formulations. This influences bioavailability. Erratic serum blood levels can lead to poor seizure control, therefore switching between different manufacturers' formulations should be avoided, if possible. Ninety percent of phenytoin is protein bound, so drug interactions involving protein binding are common. Patients taking phenytoin must periodically have their blood levels monitored. Phenytoin can alter the rate of metabolism of other coadministered drugs that use the same metabolic system. For example, phenytoin can reduce the effectiveness of oral contraceptives as well as other antiseizure drugs.

Fosphenytoin is converted to phenytoin by enzymes in the blood (phosphatases). It has a short half-life of approximately 8 minutes. Unlike phenytoin, which can be administered orally or parenterally, fosphenytoin is only available for parenteral use and is administered intravenously or intramuscularly. It is 100% bioavailable.

Lamotrigine and levetiracetam are rapidly absorbed orally. Oral absorption of zonisamide is slow to moderate. All three drugs have greater than 95% bioavailability. Protein binding is less than 50% so there are fewer drug interactions than with some of the other antiseizure medications. Lower doses of lamotrigine are required when taken with valproic acid. Higher doses are required when taken with enzyme-inducing drugs.

Common Adverse Reactions

Sedation, dizziness, ataxia, and nausea are common side effects of all of the drugs. Several agents have drug-specific side effects. Phenytoin and fosphenytoin may cause *hirsutism* (excessive growth of body hair, especially in women) and *gingival hyperplasia* (excessive growth of gum tissue). Infants born to women who take phenytoin during pregnancy may be born with cleft palate. Phenytoin may also decrease folic acid, calcium, and vitamin D absorption; vitamin supplements may be recommended. Carbamazepine and oxcarbazepine may cause double vision (diplopia), bruising, and jaundice. Zonisamide may produce kidney stones.

Precautions

Phenytoin and fosphenytoin are known teratogens, and prenatal exposure may increase risk for congenital malformations. Carbamazepine should be protected from light and moisture. Moisture can decrease the potency by as much as 30%.

• TECH NOTE!

Therapeutic blood levels for phenytoin are best maintained by dispensing the same manufacturer's formulation every time a prescription is filled. Avoid switching if possible.

Drugs That Inhibit Ion Channels

Generic Name	US Brand Name(s) / Canadian Brand(s)	Dosage Forms and Strengths
carbamazepine[a]	Carbatrol, Carnexiv, Equetro, Epitol, Tegretol, Tegretol-XR, Teril Tegretol, Tegretol CR	**Capsules, extended release (Carbatrol, Equetro)[b]:** 100 mg, 200 mg, 300 mg **Infusion, IV (Carnexiv)[b]:** 10 mg/mL **Suspension (Tegretol, Teril):** 100 mg/5 mL **Tablets, chewable:** 100 mg, 200 mg **Tablets (Epitol, Tegretol):** 200 mg **Tablets, extended release (Tegretol-XR):** 100 mg[b], 200 mg, 400 mg
eslicarbazepine	Aptiom Aptiom	**Tablets:** 200 mg, 400 mg, 600 mg, 800 mg
ethosuximide[a]	Zarontin Zarontin	**Capsules (Zarontin):** 250 mg **Syrup (Zarontin):** 250 mg/5 mL
fosphenytoin[a]	Cerebyx Cerebyx	**Injection, solution:** 50 mg/mL phenytoin sodium equivalents (PE)
gabapentin[a]	Gralise, Horizant, Neurontin Neurontin	**Capsules:** 100 mg, 300 mg, 400 mg **Solution, oral[b]:** 250 mg/5 mL **Tablets:** 300 mg[b], 600 mg, 800 mg **Tablets, extended release (Horizant)[b]:** 300 mg, 600 mg
lacosamide	Vimpat Vimpat	**Injection, solution:** 10 mg/mL **Solution, oral[b]:** 10 mg/mL **Tablets, oral:** 50 mg, 100 mg, 150 mg, 200 mg
lamotrigine[a]	Lamictal, Lamictal CD, Lamictal ODT kit, Lamictal XR Lamictal	**Tablets (Lamictal):** 25 mg, 100 mg, 150 mg, 200 mg[b] **Tablets, as chewable (Lamictal CD):** 2 mg, 5 mg, 25 mg[b] **Tablets, extended release (Lamictal XR)[b]:** 25 mg, 50 mg, 100 mg, 200 mg, 250 mg, 300 mg **Tablets, oral disintegrating (Lamictal ODT)[b]:** 25 mg, 50 mg, 100 mg, 200 mg
levetiracetam[a]	Keppra, Keppra XR, Roweepra, Spritam Keppra	**Injection, solution[b]:** 5 mg/mL, 10 mg/mL, 15 mg/mL, 100 mg/1 mL **Solution, oral[b]:** 100 mg/mL **Tablet, for oral suspension (Spritam)[b]:** 250 mg, 500 mg, 750 mg, 1000 mg **Tablets:** 250 mg, 500 mg, 750 mg, 1000 mg[b] **Tablets, extended release (Keppra XR)[b]:** 500 mg, 750 mg
methsuximide	Celontin Not Available	**Capsules:** 150 mg, 300 mg
oxcarbazepine	Oxtellar XR, Trileptal Trileptal	**Suspension:** 60 mg/mL **Tablets:** 150 mg, 300 mg, 600 mg **Tablets, Extended Releases[b]:** 150 mg, 300 mg, 600 mg
phenytoin[a]	Dilantin, Phenytek Dilantin, Dilantin Infatab	**Capsule, extended release:** 30 mg[c], 100 mg, 200 mg[b], 300 mg[b] **Injection, solution:** 50 mg/mL **Suspension:** 30 mg/5 mL[c], 125 mg/5 mL **Tablets, chewable (Dilantin Infatab):** 50 mg
pregabalin[a]	Lyrica, Lyrica CR Lyrica	**Solution, oral:** 20 mg/mL **Tablet, extended release (Lyrica CR):** 82.5 mg, 165 mg, 330 mg **Capsules:** 25 mg, 50 mg, 75 mg, 100 mg[b], 150 mg, 200 mg[b], 225 mg, 300 mg
rufinamide	Banzel Banzel	**Suspension, oral[b]:** Lyrica CR 40 mg/mL **Tablets:** 100mg[c], 200 mg, 400 mg
zonisamide[a]	Zonegran Not available	**Capsules:** 25 mg, 50 mg, 100 mg

[a]Generic available.
[b]Available in the United States only.
[c]Available in Canada only.

> **● TECH NOTE!**
>
> Dilantin is compatible in normal saline. Intravenous solution is stable for 14 hours at room temperature when diluted to 2 mg/mL. Dilantin chewable tablets should be followed by a glass of water.

> **! TECH ALERT!**
>
> The following drugs have look-alike/sound-alike issues:
> TEGretol XR, TEGretol, and TRENtal;
> OXcarbazepine and carBAMazepine;
> LaMICtal and LamISIL;
> lamoTRIgine and lamiVUDine

> **● TECH NOTE!**
>
> Pregabalin (Lyrica) is a C-V controlled substance in the United States.

Drugs That Potentiate GABA

GABA is an inhibitory neurotransmitter. The GABA receptor regulates the movement of chloride ion into the neuron. Chloride ions are negatively charged. The influx of chloride ions inhibits formation of action potentials suppressing neuronal hyperactivity and seizures.

Valproates, barbiturates (e.g., phenobarbital), and benzodiazepines (e.g., clonazepam) are classifications of drugs that potentiate GABA. Other drugs that produce this effect are ritagabine, tiagabine, topiramate, felbamate. Phenobarbital was the first drug used to treat seizures. It is indicated in the treatment of generalized tonic-clonic seizures and partial seizures and is administered to children to control febrile seizures. Valproates are described as "broad-spectrum" antiseizure drugs because they are effective in treating all types of seizures. They are one of the few antiseizure drugs indicated for the treatment of absence seizures. Benzodiazepines are indicated for the treatment of status epilepticus (intravenous diazepam), absence seizures and myoclonic seizures (clonazepam), and partial seizures (clorazepate). The mechanism of action and pharmacokinetics of benzodiazepines are discussed in detail in Chapter 5.

Mechanism of Action

One of the mechanisms of action for valproates and their derivatives is to enhance the inhibitory actions of GABA. Other mechanisms of action may be involved, including actions on potassium channels that result in membrane stabilization. Tiagabine blocks the reuptake of GABA in the synapse and vigabatrin enhances GABA activity by binding to GABA transaminase (GABA-T), the enzyme that inactivates GABA.

Pharmacokinetics

The effectiveness of all valproic acid derivatives is expressed as valproic acid activity. All valproates are rapidly absorbed when administered orally and have 100% bioavailability. Up to 10% of the drug is passed in breast milk, limiting the use of valproates during lactation. Valproates are up to 95% protein bound, so drug interactions involving protein binding must be considered when dispensing other drugs with them, including other antiseizure medicines such as phenobarbital and phenytoin. The oral absorption of tiagabine is rapid. It is nearly 95% protein bound (i.e., making it susceptible to drug interactions involving protein binding). Vigabatrin has a short half-life, but its effects persist even after blood levels of the drug declines. Antacids decrease the absorption of gabapentin by 20%. The absorption of tiagabine is reduced by foods that have a high fat content. Primidone is a barbiturate used to treat seizures. Primidone is metabolized to phenobarbital. Phenobarbital is capable of self-inducing the enzymes that metabolize it and many other drugs such as phenytoin and valproic acid. It is implicated in many drug interactions involving enzyme induction. The absorption of phenobarbital is moderately slow; however, the drug is readily distributed throughout the central nervous system because of its high degree of lipid solubility. Bioavailability is 100%.

Common Adverse Reactions

Common adverse reactions of divalproex, phenobarbital, primidone, and tiagabine are dizziness, confusion, drowsiness, unsteadiness, and nausea. Phenobarbital may produce hyperactivity, rather than sedation, in children. Divalproex may cause diplopia (double vision), and vigabatrin can cause irreversible tunnel vision. Other adverse effects for divalproex are bruising or weight gain, hair loss, tremor, irregular menstruation. Phenobarbital, diazepam, and clonazepam may cause tolerance and dependence. Respiratory depression is a serious side effect of phenobarbital and intravenous diazepam. Diazepam and clonazepam may impair learning.

> **! TECH ALERT!**
>
> The following drugs have look-alike/sound-alike issues:
> Cerebyx, CeleBREX, and CeleXA;
> DepaKOTE, DepaKENE, and Depakote ER

> **! TECH ALERT!**
>
> Phenobarbital is a controlled drug (C2) in Canada. Diazepam, clobazam, and clonazepam are controlled substances (C-IV) in the United States and targeted substances in Canada.

> **● TECH NOTE!**
>
> Depakote sprinkles may be mixed into soft foods.

> **! TECH ALERT!**
>
> Prescriptions for phenobarbital may be written using the grain strength. Pharmacy technicians must know how to convert grain strength to milligram strength. Check manufacturer label to see whether 60 or 65 mg is used for the gr 1 conversion.

> **● TECH NOTE!**
>
> Diazepam for injection is stable for 24 hours at room temperature in concentrations of 0.1 mg or less with normal saline, D_5W, or lactated Ringer solution in glass containers.

> **● TECH NOTE!**
>
> Rectal diazepam should not be used more than five times per month or one episode every 5 days.

Drugs That Inhibit Glutamate

Perampenal is a glutamate antagonist that is used to treat partial-onset seizures with or without secondary generalized seizures. It

Drugs That Potentiate GABA

Generic Name	US Brand Name(s) Canadian Brand(s)	Dosage Forms and Strengths
clobazam[a]	Onfi	**Suspension, oral**[b]: 2.5 mg/mL **Tablets:** 10 mg, 20 mg[b]
	Frisium	
clonazepam[a]	Klonopin	**Tablets (Klonopin, Rivotril):** 0.25 mg[c], 0.5 mg, 1 mg, 2 mg
	Rivotril	
diazepam[a]	Diastat, Diastat AcuDial, Valium	**Injection, solution:** 5 mg/mL **Solution, oral:** 1 mg/mL, 5 mg/mL[b] **Rectal gel (Diastat):** 5 mg/mL (2.5 mg, 5 mg[c], 10 mg, 15 mg[c] and 20 mg pre-filled syringes) **Tablets:** 2 mg, 5 mg, 10 mg
	Diastat, Valium	
divalproex sodium[a] valproic acid[a]	Depacon, Depakene, Depakote Delayed Release, Depakote ER	**Capsules, as valproic acid (Depakene):** 250 mg **Capsules, delayed releasepellets (Depakote):** 125 mg **Injection, solution (Depacon):** 100 mg/mL **Syrup, as valproic acid (Depakene):** 250 mg/5 mL **Tablets, as divalproex sodium delayed release (Depakote, Epival):** 125 mg, 250 mg, 500 mg **Tablets, as divalproex sodium extended release (Depakote ER):** 250 mg, 500 mg
	Depakene Epival	
felbamate[a]	Felbatol	**Suspension, oral:** 600 mg/5 mL **Tablets:** 400 mg, 600 mg
	Not available	
phenobarbital[a]	Not Available	**Elixir:** 5 mg/mL **Injection, solution:** 30 mg/mL, 120 mg/mL **Tablets:** 15 mg, 30 mg, 60 mg, 100 mg
	Generics	
primidone[a]	Mysoline	**Tablets:** 50 mg[b], 125 mg[c], 250 mg
	Generics	
tiagabine[a]	Gabatril	**Tablets:** 2 mg, 4 mg, 12 mg, 16 mg
	Not available	
topiramate[a]	Qudexy XR, Topamax, Trokendi XR	**Capsules, sprinkle:** 15 mg, 25 mg **Capsules, extended release (Qudexy XR, Trokendi XR)**[b]: 25 mg, 50 mg, 100 mg, 150 mg, 200 mg **Tablets:** 25 mg, 50 mg[b], 100 mg, 200 mg
	Topamax	
vigabatrin[a,b]	Sabril Viagdrone	**Powder for oral suspension:** 500 mg packets **Tablets:** 500 mg
	Sabril	

[a]Generic available.
[b]Available in the United States only.
[c]Available in Canada only.

is the only drug in its class. Perampenal inhibits glutamate, the primary excitatory neurotransmitter in the central nervous system. This reduces the generation and spread of seizures.

Pharmacokinetics

Perampenal is rapidly absorbed when taken orally. The rate of absorption is reduced if it is taken with food but the extent of absorption is not affected.

Common Adverse Reactions

Dizziness (36%), somnolence (16%), fatigue (10%), irritability (9%), falls (7%), nausea (7%), ataxia (5%), balance disorder (4%), gait disturbance (4%), vertigo (4%), and weight gain (4%) are the most common side effects. Less common side effects are serious or life-threatening psychiatric and behavioral changes such as aggression, hostility, or homicidal thoughts. The FDA requires a box warning in the product label.

Miscellaneous

The precise mechanism of action for brivaracetam (Briviact, Brivlera) is unknown. The drug is used to treat partial-onset seizures. The most common side effects are drowsiness, dizziness, and nausea or vomiting.

TECHNICIAN'S CORNER

1. If you see someone experiencing a seizure, what would you do?
2. What would be the best advice you can give a patient with epilepsy about his or her medication?

> **TECH NOTE!**
>
> Briviact (brivaracetam) is a C–V controlled substance in the United States.

Glutamate Receptor Antagonist

Generic Name	US Brand Name(s) / Canadian Brand(s)	Dosage Forms and Strengths
perampanel	Fycompa / Fycompa	**Suspension, oral:** 0.5 mg/mL **Tablet:** 2 mg, 4 mg, 6 mg, 8 mg 10 mg 12 mg

Miscellaneous

Generic Name	US Brand Name(s) / Canadian Brand(s)	Dosage Forms and Strengths
brivaracetam	Briviact / Brivlera	**Solution, intravenous[a]:** 10 mg/mL **Solution, oral[a]:** 10 mg/mL **Tablet:** 10 mg, 25 mg, 50 mg, 75 mg, 100 mg

[a]Available in the United States only.

Summary of Drugs Used for the Treatment of Seizures*

	Generic Name	Brand Name	Usual Adult Oral Dose and Dosing Schedule	Warning Labels
Drugs That Inhibit Ion Channels				
	carbamazepine[a]	Tegretol	800–1200 mg/day in 2 divided doses (XR) or 3–4 divided doses other formulations	MAY CAUSE DROWSINESS; MAY IMPAIR ABILITY TO DRIVE—all AVOID ALCOHOL—all DO NOT DISCONTINUE WITHOUT MEDICAL SUPERVISION—all SWALLOW WHOLE; DO NOT CRUSH OR CHEW—extended release TAKE WITH FOOD—carbamazepine, ethosuximide, gabapentin, methsuximide, oxcarbazepine, phenytoin, pregabalin, rufinamide AVOID ANTACIDS—gabapentin, phenytoin SHAKE WELL—suspension TAKE WITH A FULL GLASS OF WATER—chewable tablets
	eslicarbazepine	Aptiom	800–1600 mg once daily	
	ethosuximide[a]	Zarontin	Start 250 mg twice a day; increase up to 1500 mg/day	
	fosphenytoin[a]	Cerebyx	**Status epilepticus:** IV loading dose: 15–20 mg/kg (PE) administered at rate of 100–150 mg/min **Nonemergent maintenance dose:** 10–20 mg/kg (PE)/day administered IM or IV	
	gabapentin[a]	Neurontin	300–600 mg 3 times/day	

Summary of Drugs Used for the Treatment of Seizures—cont'd

	Generic Name	Brand Name	Usual Adult Oral Dose and Dosing Schedule	Warning Labels
	lacosamide[a]	Vimpat	Start 50 mg twice daily; increase up to 400 mg/day in 2 divided doses	MAY BE HABIT FORMING—pregabalin STORE AT ROOM TEMPERATURE; DISCARD UNUSED
	lamotrigine[a]	Lamictal	100–500 mg/day in 1–2 divided doses	PORTION 7 WEEKS AFTER OPENING— lacosamide oral solution
	levetiracetam[a]	Keppra	1000–3000 mg/day in 2 divided doses	
	methsuximide	Celontin	300–1200 mg/day in 1–2 divided doses	
	oxcarbazepine	Trileptal	600–2400 mg/day in 2 divided doses	
	phenytoin	Dilantin	100 mg 3–4 times a day	
	pregabalin[a]	Lyrica	150–600 mg dosed 2–3 times a day	
	rufinamide	Banzel	400–3200 mg/day in 2 divided doses	
	zonisamide	Zonegran	100–600 mg/day in 1 or 2 divided doses	
Drugs That Potentiate GABA				
	clobazam[a]	Onfi (Frisium)	5–15 mg/day (up to 80 mg as necessary) in 1–2 divided doses	MAY CAUSE DROWSINESS; MAY IMPAIR ABILITY TO DRIVE—clobazam, clonazepam, diazepam, divalproex Na+, phenobarbital, tiagabine, topiramate, vigabatrin
	clonazepam[a]	Klonopin (Rivatril)	1.5–20 mg/day in 3 divided doses	AVOID ALCOHOL—clobazam, clonazepam, diazepam, divalproex Na+, phenobarbital, tiagabine, topiramate, vigabatrin
	diazepam[a]	Valium	**Oral:** 2–10 mg/day in 2–4 divided doses **Rectal gel:** 0.2–0.5 mg/kg/day	DO NOT DISCONTINUE WITHOUT MEDICAL SUPERVISION—all SWALLOW WHOLE; DO NOT CRUSH OR CHEW—extended release
	divalproex sodium[a] valproic acid[a]	Depakote	10–60 mg/kg/day in 2–3 divided doses (delayed release) or once daily (extended release)	TAKE WITH FOOD—divalproex Na+, tiagabine, vigabatrin SHAKE WELL—suspension (vigabatrin) TAKE WITH A FULL GLASS OF
	felbamate	Felbatol	1200–3600 mg/day in 3–4 divided doses	WATER—chewable tablets MAY BE HABIT FORMING—
	phenobarbital[a]	Generics	50–100 mg 2–3 times a day	phenobarbital, clonazepam, diazepam
	primidone[a]	Mysoline	Start 100–125 mg at bedtime; increase to 250 mg 3–4 times/day	
	tiagabine[a]	Gabatril	Start 4 mg once daily; increase up to 56 mg/day in 2–4 divided doses	
	topiramate[a]	Topamax	200–400 mg/day in 2 divided doses (maximum 1600 mg/day) (Extended release tablets dosed once daily)	
	vigabatrin	Sabril	500–1500 mg twice per day	
Drugs That Inhibit Glutamate				
	perampanel	Fycompa	Start 2 mg; maintenance 8–12 mg once daily	MAY CAUSE DROWSINESS; MAY IMPAIR ABILITY TO DRIVE. AVOID ALCOHOL. DON'T DISCONTINUE WITHOUT MEDICAL SUPERVISION
Miscellaneous				
	brivaracetam	Briviact, Brivlera	25–100 mg twice daily	MAY CAUSE DIZZINESS OR DROWSINESS; DON'T DRIVE STORE ORAL SOLUTION AT ROOM TEMPERATURE

*Doses of medications used to treat seizures can vary considerably from patient to patient and depending on the specific condition being treated.
[a]Generic available.

Key Points

- Epilepsy is a type of seizure disorder that is characterized by a sudden, excessive, disorderly discharge of cerebral neurons.
- People with epilepsy have an abnormally high level of excitatory neurotransmitters, coupled with a low level of inhibitory neurotransmitters.
- Half of all seizures have no known cause.
- Known causes of seizures include birth defects, infection (meningitis, AIDS), tumors, head trauma, high fevers, hypoglycemia, drug and alcohol withdrawal, and cerebrovascular disease.
- Wearing seat belts, motorcycle helmets, and bike helmets can reduce head injury and injury-related seizures.
- Status epilepticus is a medical emergency that is characterized by repeated generalized seizures that deprive the brain of oxygen.
- Status epilepticus is treated with intravenous medications.
- Seizures are treated with drugs that modulate ion channels, potentiate GABA, and/or inhibit glutamate.
- The goal of treatment of epilepsy and other seizure disorders is to reduce the incidence of seizures by suppressing seizure activity.
- Therapeutic blood levels for phenytoin are best maintained by dispensing the same manufacturer's formulation each time a prescription is filled.
- Carbamazepine should be protected from light and moisture. Moisture can decrease the potency by as much as 30%.
- Antacids decrease the absorption of gabapentin by 20%. The absorption of tiagabine is reduced by foods that have a high fat content.
- Phenobarbital is a controlled substance in Canada.
- Benzodiazepines used in the treatment of seizures are controlled substances in the United States and targeted substances in Canada.
- Drug therapy with antiepileptic drugs increases the risk for suicide ideation and behavior.

Review Questions

1. All of the following drugs are controlled or targeted substances in Canada and/or the United States EXCEPT _____
   a. clonazepam.
   b. diazepam.
   c. phenytoin.
   d. pregabalin.
2. Febrile seizures in children are associated with an _____, causing a sudden spike in temperature.
   a. injury
   b. injection
   c. infection
   d. a, b, and c
3. The only major seizure classification is generalized seizures.
   a. true
   b. false
4. A medical emergency that is characterized by repeated generalized seizures and deprives the brain of oxygen is called
   a. status epilepticus.
   b. myoclonic epilepticus.
   c. absence epilepticus.
   d. tonic-clonic status.
5. The goal of treatment of epilepsy and other seizure disorders is to reduce the incidence of seizures by _____ seizure activity.
   a. stopping
   b. sedating
   c. suppressing
   d. shocking
6. _____ is administered IV in the management of status epilepticus and seizures after neurosurgery.
   a. Tiagabine
   b. Carbamazepine
   c. Valproic acid
   d. Fosphenytoin
7. You receive a prescription for Topimax 100 mg 1 tablets QID. You consult with the pharmacist because Topimax is _____
   a. not prescribed 100 mg per dose.
   b. QID.
   c. Not marketed as 100 mg tablets.
   d. a capsule.
8. You receive a prescription for gabapentin 500 mg 1 tablet TID. You consult with the pharmacist because gabapentin is _____
   a. not prescribed in a dose greater than 100 mg.
   b. not prescribed TID.
   c. not marketed as 500 mg tablets.
   d. Not prescribed for seizures.
9. Phenytoin was the first drug that was used to treat seizures.
   a. true
   b. false
10. An unusual sensation or, auditory, visual, or olfactory hallucination that is experienced just before the onset of a seizure is called a(n)
   a. halo.
   b. aura.
   c. vision.
   d. hallucination.

Bibliography

FDA: Drugs@FDA: FDA Approved Drug Products, nd. Available from: http://www.accessdata.fda.gov/scripts/cder/daf/. (Retrieved 28 June 2018).

Glauser T, Shinnar S, Gloss D, et al: Evidence-based guideline: Treatment of convulsive status epilepticus in children and adults: Report of the Guideline Committee of the American Epilepsy Society, *Epilepsy Curr* 16(1):48–61, 2016.

Health Canada: Drug Product Database. 2018, from https://health-products.canada.ca/dpd-bdpp/index-eng.jsp. (Retrieved 28 June 2018).

Institute for Safe Medication Practices: FDA and ISMP lists of look-alike drug names with recommended tall man letters. 2016.

Kalant H, Grant D, Mitchell J: *Principles of medical pharmacology*, ed 7, Toronto, 2007, Elsevier Canada, A Division of Reed Elsevier Canada, pp 223–235.

National Institute of Neurological Disorders and Stroke National Institutes of Health: *Hope through research: the epilepsies and seizures*, NIH Publication No. 15-156. Bethesda, 2015, National Institutes of Health.

Page C, Curtis M, Sutter M, et al: *Integrated pharmacology*, Philadelphia, 2005, Elsevier Mosby, pp 257–259.

Patsalos PN: The clinical pharmacology profile of the new antiepileptic drug perampanel: A novel noncompetitive AMPA receptor antagonist, *Epilepsia* 56:12–27, 2015. doi:10.1111/epi.12865.

Raffa RB, Rawls SM, Beyzarov EP: *Netter's illustrated pharmacology*, Philadelphia, 2005, WB Saunders, pp 67–70.

Schmidt D, Schachter SC: Drug treatment of epilepsy in adults, *BMJ* 348:g2546, 2014.

USP Center for Advancement of Patient Safety: *Use caution: avoid confusion*, USP Quality Review No. 79. Rockville, MD, 2004, USP Center for Advancement of Patient Safety.

10

Treatment of Pain and Migraine Headache

LEARNING OBJECTIVES

1. Learn the terminology associated with the treatment of pain and migraine headache.
2. Describe the etiology of pain and migraine headache.
3. Compare and contrast the treatment of nociceptive pain and neuropathic pain.
4. Compare and contrast the function of neurotransmitters associated with pain and migraine headache symptoms.
5. Classify medications used in the treatment of pain and migraine headache.
6. Describe mechanisms of action for each class of drugs used to treat pain and migraine headache.
7. Identify significant drug look-alike/sound-alike issues.
8. Identify warning labels and precautionary messages associated with medications used to treat pain and migraine headache.
9. Identify significant drug interactions.

KEY TERMS

Acute pain Sudden pain that results from injury or inflammation and is usually self-limiting.

Acupuncture Nonpharmacologic treatment for pain that involves the application of needles to precise points on the body.

Analgesic Drug that reduces pain.

Arthritis Condition that is associated with joint pain.

Biofeedback Nonpharmacologic treatment for pain that involves relaxation techniques and gaining self-control over muscle tension, heart rate, and skin temperature.

Breakthrough pain Pain that occurs in between scheduled doses of analgesics.

Cephalgia Head pain.

Chronic pain Pain that persists for a long period of time that is worsened by psychological factors and is resistant to many medical treatments.

Cluster headache Intensely painful vascular headache that occurs in groups and produces pain on one side of the head.

Diabetic neuropathy Peripheral nerve disorder caused by diabetes that produces numbness, pain, or tingling in the feet or legs.

Dysphoria Feeling of emotional or mental discomfort, restlessness, and depression; the opposite of euphoria.

Endorphins, enkephalins, and dynorphin Substances released by the body in response to painful stimuli that act as natural painkillers.

Euphoria State of intense happiness or well-being; the opposite of dysphoria.

Hyperalgesia Heightened sensitivity to pain that can result from treatment of chronic pain with high-dose opioids.

Inflammation A response to tissue irritation or injury that is marked by signs of redness, swelling, heat, and pain.

Migraine Vascular headache that is often accompanied by nausea and visual disturbances.

Neuropathic pain Type of pain associated with nerve injury caused by trauma, infection, or chronic diseases such as diabetes.

Nociceptors Thin nerve fibers in skin, muscle, and other body tissues that carry pain signals.

NSAID Nonsteroidal antiinflammatory drug.

Opiate naïve No current exposure to opioids.

Opioid Naturally occurring or synthetically derived analgesic with properties similar to those of morphine.

Shingles Reoccurring and painful skin rash caused by the herpes zoster virus.

Substance P Peptide that is involved in the production of pain sensations and controls pain perception.

Trigeminal neuralgia Painful condition that produces intense, stabbing pain in areas of the face innervated by branches of the trigeminal nerve.

Overview

Most people will experience some type of physical pain in their lifetime. *Acute pain* is triggered by an injury, burn, infection, or some other stimuli and is self-limiting. *Chronic pain* may persist for years and is often inadequately controlled by pharmaceuticals or other pain management therapies. There is a strong psychological component to pain that is frequently underestimated. Psychological factors can influence a person's tolerance for pain and can determine whether the outcome of treatment is successful. To reduce anxieties associated with pain and the need for higher doses of pain medications, hospitalized patients may be permitted to control the frequency of administration of their doses of pain medications. Patient-controlled analgesia (PCA) is done using a device that is connected to the patient's intravenous line. The patient pushes a button to deliver a measured dose of pain medication.

Pain is often categorized by its origin. *Neuropathic pain* is associated with a nerve injury caused by trauma, infection, or chronic disease such as diabetes. Chronic pain is often of neuropathic origin. Nociceptive pain is caused by stimulation of nociceptors in viscera (lungs, gastrointestinal [GI], heart) or skin, muscle, soft tissue, or bone (somatic). *Nociceptors* are thin nerve fibers located in the skin, muscle, and other body tissues that carry pain signals. The division of pain into distinct categories is somewhat simplistic because multiple pathophysiologic mechanisms are probably involved. A multimodal approach to pain management is recommended because untreated pain can affect all body systems. It may produce increased heart rate, anxiety, and muscle spasms and/or decreased immune response and intestinal motility.

Conditions That Produce Pain

Inflammation

Inflammation is an important source of pain. *Inflammation* is a response to tissue irritation or injury that is marked by signs of redness, swelling, heat, and pain. Sport injuries, *arthritis*, trauma caused by motor vehicle, workplace, or home accidents, sprains, fractures, burns, cuts, and bruises may all produce inflammation. Infection can also produce painful inflammation.

Low Back Pain

Nearly one-third of adults will experience low back pain in any given year, making it one of the most common types of pain. Despite its high prevalence, only 20% of people experiencing low back pain seek medical attention.

Acute low back pain produces symptoms that last less than 6 weeks. Chronic low back pain can persist indefinitely and may produce leg pain or widespread body pain or restrict spinal movement.

Burns

Severe burns can produce excruciating pain. Third-degree burns are the most severe because the skin has been destroyed. First-degree burns are less severe than second- or third-degree burns.

Diabetic Neuropathy

Uncontrolled diabetes can lead to damage to peripheral nerves. Nerve damage results in numbness, pain, or tingling of the feet or legs. Symptoms of *diabetic neuropathy* become more severe as the disease progresses.

Phantom Limb

Pain may be referred. This means that the place where pain symptoms are most strongly felt may be different than the actual origin of the painful stimuli. Patients who have had a limb amputated may describe pain in the area where the limb was removed. It is believed that although the limb is no longer present, the nerves that innervated the limb are remapped or rewired, permitting nerve messages to continue to be received. The ability of the brain to restructure itself and adapt to injury is called plasticity.

Shingles

Shingles produces a reoccurring and painful skin rash and is caused by the herpes zoster virus. The herpes zoster virus, which causes chicken pox, lays dormant in nerve endings until activated. Shingles cannot be cured.

Trigeminal Neuralgia

Trigeminal neuralgia produces headache and intense stabbing pain in areas of the face innervated by branches of the trigeminal nerve (lips, eyes, nose, scalp, forehead, upper jaw, and lower jaw). Approximately 1% to 2% of persons with multiple sclerosis develop trigeminal neuralgia.

Pain Signal Transmission

The pain message begins with stimulation of nociceptors in peripheral tissues. The signal is converted to an electrical impulse (transduction) that then travels to the dorsal horn of the spinal cord (transmission), where it is augmented or diminished by the release of neurotransmitters, amino acids, and neuropeptides (modulation) and then carried to the brain where the pain message is interpreted (perception) (Fig. 10.1).

When an injury occurs, proteins (cytokines) are released that produce painful inflammation. Prostaglandins, important mediators of pain, are also synthesized. Histamine, bradykinin, and serotonin (5-hydroxytryptamine [5-HT]) are also released in response to tissue injury and are part of the immune system response. They produce inflammation, vasodilation, and pain. Glutamate is an amino acid neurotransmitter that enhances the response to painful stimuli. *Substance P* and neurokinin A are peptides that are involved in the modulation of pain sensations that are transmitted to the brain and control how pain is perceived. *Endorphins, enkephalins, and dynorphins* are opioid peptides that bind to opioid receptors in the brain and spinal cord and block or dull the pain sensations by inhibiting the release of substance P and glutamate. They act like natural painkillers (Fig. 10.2).

Drugs Used to Treat Pain

Opioids

Opiates are naturally occurring substances that are derived from the opium poppy and have been used for more than 2000 years to induce sleep and *euphoria* and to relieve diarrhea. Morphine and heroin are examples of opiates. *Opioid* is a term used to describe a drug that acts like morphine, whether naturally occurring or synthetically derived. Opiates and opioid drugs produce analgesia. *Analgesics* are drugs that reduce pain sensations and alter pain perception. Opioid analgesics are less effective in treating neuropathic pain.

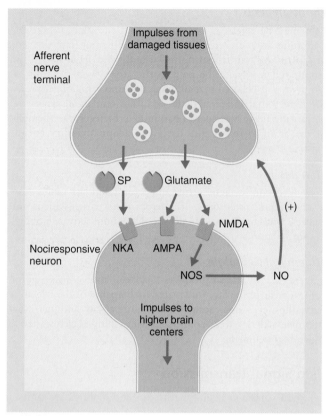

SP = substance P
NO = nitric oxide
NKA = neurokinin A

• **Fig. 10.1** Mechanism of pain perception. (From Page C, Curtis M, Sutter M, et al: *Integrated pharmacology*, ed 3, Philadelphia, 2006, Mosby.)

Some opioid analgesics are also used to treat opioid dependence. When detoxification is achieved, a maintenance dose is continued. Methadone and buprenorphine are examples of opioid agonists that are administered for management of drug dependence. Opioid antagonists such as naltrexone are also used to treat drug and alcohol dependence.

Mechanism of Action

Opioids bind to opioid receptors located in the dorsal route of the spinal cord, brainstem, thalamus, hypothalamus, and limbic system to decrease painful sensations and raise the pain threshold.

There are several types of opioid receptors. The effects and adverse reactions produced by opioid drugs are related to the receptors that are stimulated by the drugs. Mu (μ) receptor stimulation produces analgesia, euphoria, respiratory depression, pupillary constriction, decreased GI motility, and physical dependence. Kappa (κ) receptor binding produces analgesia, sedation, pupillary constriction, *dysphoria,* and hallucinations. Delta (δ) receptor stimulation produces analgesia and decreases contractions of smooth muscle.

Classification of Opioids

Agonists

Opioids are categorized according to their action at the opioid receptor. Opioid agonists (e.g., codeine, morphine, and oxycodone) produce analgesia and other adverse effects associated with stimulation of the specific opioid receptor. Partial agonists produce incomplete activation of the opioid receptor, producing less than maximum response.

Antagonists

Antagonists (e.g., naloxone) bind to the opioid receptor but do not activate it. They interfere with agonist binding. Antagonists

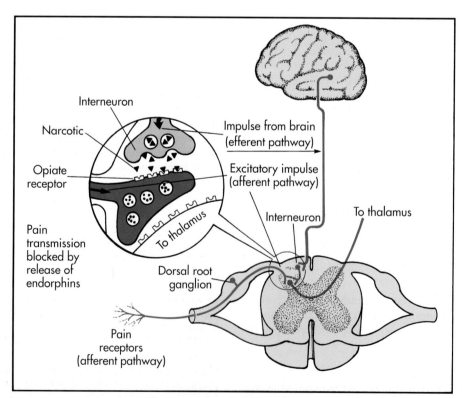

• **Fig. 10.2** Descending pathway and endorphin response. The biologic receptors of the enkephalins and endorphins are located close to known pain receptors in the periphery and ascending and descending pain pathways. (From McCance KL, Huether SE: *Pathophysiology,* ed 7, St. Louis, 2014, Elsevier.)

are administered when reversal of the action of an opioid agonist is desired.

Mixed Agonist/Antagonists

The response produced by some opioids is mixed. Sometimes the opioid behaves like an agonist, and sometimes it behaves like an antagonist (e.g., buprenorphine, butorphanol, and nalbuphine). Agonist activity is exhibited if the patient has had no recent exposure to an opioid agonist *(opiate naïve)*. If the patient is currently taking an opioid agonist, the mixed agonist/antagonist exhibits antagonist activity.

Pharmacokinetics

The analgesic effect produced by opioid agonists is often compared with morphine. When switching between agents or dosage forms, the equivalent analgesic dose must be calculated to achieve the same level of pain relief. Oral absorption of opioid agonists, partial agonists, and mixed agonist/antagonist is varied. Many orally administered opioids exhibit significant first-pass metabolism. The average onset of action of orally administered opioids is approximately 30 minutes after administration. The onset of action of most parenterally administered opioids occurs within 10 to 15 minutes. A few opioids (meperidine, pentazocine, and butorphanol) begin working in less than 5 minutes. Peak effects are achieved between 30 minutes and 2 hours. The duration of action for immediate-release opioids ranges between 2 and 6 hours. The duration of action for controlled-release opioid analgesics may last for up to 72 hours (e.g., fentanyl patches). Patients who have been prescribed long-acting opioid dosage forms (e.g., Kadian, Exalgo) may also be prescribed short-acting opioids to control *breakthrough pain* that may occur between scheduled doses of the long-acting analgesic.

> ● **TECH NOTE!**
>
> Butorphanol is often prescribed for migraine headache pain.

> ● **TECH NOTE!**
>
> Immediate-release opioids are used to manage breakthrough pain.

Adverse Reactions

Adverse effects of opioid agonists, partial agonists, and mixed agonist/antagonists are determined by the extent to which they bind to specific opioid receptors. Common side effects caused by acute use are sedation, constipation, and GI upset (Table 10.1). Opioid agonists and partial agonists may produce tolerance and dependence. Tolerance requires increasing doses to produce the same effects. Dependence causes users to continue taking opioids to avoid withdrawal symptoms. Dependence may be physical or psychological. Overdose may lead to respiratory depression and death. Chronic use may additionally produce *hyperalgesia* (a heightened sensitivity to pain that can result from treatment of chronic pain with high-dose opioids), sexual dysfunction, and decreased immune response.

Precautions

Access to opioid agonists, partial agonists, and most mixed agonist/antagonists is restricted in the United States (schedule C-I through C-V) and Canada (straight and verbal narcotics) because they produce tolerance and dependence.

TABLE 10.1	Opioid-Induced Side Effects and Adverse Effects by Body System
Body System	**Side Effect or Adverse Effect**
Central nervous system	Sedation, disorientation, euphoria, lightheadedness, dysphoria, lowered seizure threshold, and tremors
Cardiovascular system	Hypotension, palpitations, and flushing
Respiratory tract	Respiratory depression and aggravation of asthma
Gastrointestinal tract	Nausea, vomiting, constipation, and biliary tract spasm
Genitourinary tract	Urinary retention
Other	Itching, rash, and wheal information

From Lilley LL, Harrington S, Snyder JS: *Pharmacology and the nursing process,* ed 5, St. Louis, 2007, Mosby.

> ● **TECH ALERT!**
>
> The following drugs have look-alike/sound-alike issues:
> oxyCODONE and oxyCONTIN
> HYDROcodone, HYDROmorphone, and oxyCODONE
> morphine and oxyMORphone;
> AVINza and INVanz

> ● **TECH NOTE!**
>
> Duragesic patches are worn for 72 hours and should be dispensed with instructions on proper storage and disposal to prevent accidental overdose or poisoning.

Opioid Antagonists

Opioid antagonists are indicated for the reversal of respiratory depression caused by opioid use. Respiratory depression may be produced by drugs administered during surgery for general anesthesia, may occur in infants born to opioid-dependent women, and occur in opioid overdose. The opioid antagonist naltrexone is indicated for the treatment of opioid overdose and the management of drug and alcohol dependence. Naltrexone may produce drowsiness. The warning labels MAY CAUSE DROWSINESS, MAY IMPAIR ABILITY TO DRIVE, and AVOID ALCOHOL should be applied to prescription vials. Both naltrexone and naloxone can precipitate withdrawal symptoms in patients who are opioid dependent.

> ● **TECH ALERT!**
>
> Naloxone and naltrexone have look-alike/sound-alike issues.

> ● **TECH NOTE!**
>
> Buprenorphine tablets may only be prescribed for the treatment of opioid dependency. Valid prescriptions are written by prescribers who have a Drug Enforcement Administration (DEA) No. specifically for buprenorphine.

> ● **TECH NOTE!**
>
> US Pharmacies must be enrolled in the Transmucosal Immediate Release Fentanyl Risk Evaluation and Mitigation Strategy (TIRF REMS) Access Program to dispense or distribute transmucosal immediate release fentanyl products (e.g., ABSTRAL, ACTIQ, FENTORA, Lazanda, and SUBSYS).

Text continued on p. 107

Opioid Agonists

Generic Name	US Brand Name(s) / Canadian Brand Name(s)	Dosage Forms and Strengths	Controlled Substance Schedule
codeine[a]	Generics Codeine Contin	**Injection:** 30 mg/mL[b] **Syrup, oral:** 5 mg/mL[b] **Tablets, controlled release (Codeine Contin)[b]:** 50 mg, 100 mg, 150 mg, 200 mg **Tablets, as phosphate[b]:** 15 mg, 30 mg, 60 mg **Tablets, as sulfate[c]:** 15 mg, 30 mg, 60 mg	**C-II** (US) **Straight narcotic** (Canada)
codeine and acetaminophen (APAP)[a]	Tylenol with Codeine No. 3, Tylenol with Codeine No. 4 ratio-LENOLTEC No. 1, ratio-LENOLTEC No. 2, ratio-LENOLTEC No. 3, ratio-LENOLTEC No. 4 Tylenol with Codeine No. 2, Tylenol with Codeine No. 3, Tylenol with Codeine No. 4	**Elixir/Suspension:** 120 mg APAP + 12 mg codeine **Tablets:** 300 mg APAP + 8 mg codeine + 15 mg caffeine[b] **Tablets (Tylenol with Codeine No. 2):** 300 mg APAP + 15 mg codeine + 15 mg caffeine[b] **Tablets (Tylenol with Codeine No. 3):** 300 mg APAP + 30 mg codeine (in Canada Tylenol #3 also contains 15 mg caffeine) **Tablets (Tylenol with Codeine No. 4):** APAP 300 mg and codeine 60 mg	**In the US:** APAP + codeine Elixir (**C-V**), tablets (**C-III**) **In Canada:** APAP + caffeine + codeine 8 mg (**Schedule II, exempt narcotic**), tablets containing APAP, caffeine + 15 mg or 30 mg codeine (**Verbal narcotic**); tablets containing APAP + codeine 60 mg (**Straight narcotic**)
fentanyl[a]	ABSTRAL, Actiq, Duragesic, FENTORA, Ionsys, Lazanda, Sublimaze, SUBSYS ABSTRAL, Duragesic, FENTORA	**Injection, solution (Sublimaze):** 50 mcg/mL **Lozenge (ACTIQ)[c]:** 200 mcg, 400 mcg, 600 mcg, 800 mcg, 1200 mcg, 1600 mcg **Nasal Spray (Lazanda)[c]:** 100 mcg, 300 mcg, 400 mcg **Sublingual Spray (SUBSYS):** 100 mcg, 200 mcg, 400 mcg, 600 mcg, 800 mcg, 1200 mcg, 1600 mcg **Tablets, buccal (FENTORA):** 100 mcg, 200 mcg, 400 mcg, 600 mcg, 800 mcg **Tablets, sublingual (ABSTRAL):** 100 mcg, 200 mcg, 300 mcg, 400 mcg, 600 mcg, 800 mcg **Transdermal (Duragesic, Ionsys):** 12 mcg, 25 mcg, 37.5 mcg[c], 40 mcg[c], 50 mcg, 62.5 mcg[c], 75 mcg, 87.5 mcg[c], 100 mcg	**C-II** (All dosage forms in the US) **Straight narcotic** (All dosage forms in Canada)
hydrocodone[a]	Hysingla, Zohydro ER Generics	**Capsule, extended release (Zohydro ER):** 10 mg, 15 mg, 20 mg, 30 mg, 40 mg, 50 mg **Syrup[b]:** 1 mg/mL **Tablet, extended release:** 20 mg, 30 mg, 40 mg, 60 mg, 80 mg, 100 mg, 120 mg (Hysingla)	**C-II** (All dosage forms in the US) **Straight Narcotic** (All dosage forms in Canada)
hydrocodone and acetaminophen[a]	Anexsia 5/325, Anexsia 7.5/325, Norco Not available	**Solution:** 7.5 mg hydrocodone and 325 mg APAP/15 mL **Tablets:** 2.5 mg hydrocodone + 325 mg APAP; 5 mg hydrocodone + 325 mg APAP; 7.5 mg hydrocodone + 325 mg APAP; 10 mg hydrocodone + 325 mg APAP	**C-II** (All dosage forms in the US):

Opioid Agonists—cont'd

Generic Name	US Brand Name(s) Canadian Brand Name(s)	Dosage Forms and Strengths	Controlled Substance Schedule
hydrocodone and ibuprofen[a]	Represain Not available	**Tablets:** 2.5 mg/200 mg, 5 mg/200 mg, 7.5 mg/200 mg, 10 mg/200 mg	**C-III**
hydromorphone[a]	Dilaudid, Dilaudid-HP, Exalgo Dilaudid, Dilaudid-HP, Dilaudid-HP Plus, Hydromorph Contin, Jurnista	**Capsules, controlled release (Hydromorph Contin):** 3 mg, 4.5 mg, 6 mg, 9 mg, 12 mg, 18 mg, 24 mg, 30 mg **Injection, powder for reconstitution (Dilaudid):** 250 mg per vial **Injection, solution:** 1 mg/mL, 2 mg/mL, 4 mg/mL, 10 mg/mL (Dilaudid-HP); 20 mg/mL, 50 mg/mL, 100 mg/mL **Liquid, oral (Dilaudid):** 1 mg/mL **Tablets, extended release (Exalgo, Jurnista):** 4 mg[b], 8 mg, 12 mg, 16 mg, 32 mg **Tablets, immediate release (Dilaudid,):** 1 mg[b], 2 mg, 4 mg, 8 mg **Suppository**[b]**:** 3 mg	**C-II** (US) **Straight narcotic** (Canada)
levorphanol[a]	Generics Not available	**Tablets:** 1 mg, 2 mg, 3 mg	**C-II** (US)
meperidine[a]	Demerol Demerol	**Injection, solution (vials and prefilled syringe):** 10 mg/mL, 25 mg/mL[c], 50 mg/mL, 75 mg/mL[c], 100 mg/mL[c] **Solution, oral**[c]**:** 50 mg/5 mL **Tablets:** 50 mg, 100 mg[c]	**C-II** (US) **Straight narcotic** (Canada)
methadone[a]	Dolophine, Methadose Metadol, Metadol-D Methadose	**Injection, solution:** 10 mg/mL **Solution, oral:** 5 mg/5 mL, 10 mg/5 mL **Solution, oral concentrate (Methadose, Metadol):** 10 mg/mL **Tablets (Dolophine, Metadol):** 1 mg[b], 5 mg, 10 mg, 25 mg[b] **Tablets, dispersible For oral solution (Methadose):** 40 mg	**C-II** (US) **Straight narcotic** (Canada)
morphine[a]	Arymo ER, Astramorph/PF, Duramorph, Infumorph, Kadian, MS Contin, Oramorph SR Doloral, Kadian, M-Eslon, MS Contin, MS IR, Statex	**Capsules, extended release:** **(M-Eslon):** 10 mg, 15 mg, 30 mg, 60 mg, 100 mg, 200 mg **Capsules, sustained release (Kadian):** 10 mg, 20 mg, 30 mg[c], 40 mg[c], 50 mg, 60 mg[c], 70 mg[c], 80 mg[c], 100 mg, 130 mg[c], 150 mg[c], 200 mg[c] **Injection, extended release for epidural:** 10 mg/mL **Injection, epidural, intrathecal (Astramorph/PF, Duramorph):** 0.5 mg/mL, 1 mg/mL **Injection, solution:** 2 mg/mL, 4 mg/mL[c], 5 mg/mL, 8 mg/mL[c], 10 mg/mL, 15 mg/mL, 25 mg/mL, 50 mg/mL[b] **Solution, oral (Doloral):** 20 mg/mL, 1 mg/mL[b], 5 mg/mL[b], 10 mg/mL[b], 10 mg/5 mL[c], 20 mg/5 mL[c], 100 mg/5 mL[c]	**C-II** (US) **Straight narcotic** (Canada)

Continued

Opioid Agonists—cont'd

Generic Name	US Brand Name(s) / Canadian Brand Name(s)	Dosage Forms and Strengths	Controlled Substance Schedule
		Solution, oral drops (Statex): 20 mg/mL, 50 mg/mL Syrup: 1 mg/mL, 5 mg/mL, 10 mg/mL Suppositories: 5 mg, 10 mg, 20 mg, 30 mg Tablets, controlled release (MS Contin): 15 mg, 30 mg, 60 mg, 100 mg, 200 mg Tablets, immediate release (MS IR): 5 mg, 10 mg, 20 mg, 30 mg Tablets, sustained release (Oramorph SR): 15 mg, 30 mg, 60 mg, 100 mg	
morphine + naltrexone	Embeda Not available	Capsules, extended release: 20 mg morphine + 0.8 mg naltrexone 30 mg morphine + 1.2 mg naltrexone 50 mg morphine + 2 mg naltrexone 60 mg morphine + 2.4 mg naltrexone 80 mg morphine + 3.2 mg naltrexone 100 mg morphine + 4 mg naltrexone	C-II
oxycodone[a]	Oxaydo, OxyContin, Roxicodone, Xtampza ER OxyNEO, Oxy IR, Supeudol	Capsule, extended release (Xtampza ER)[c]: 9 mg, 13.5 mg, 18 mg, 27 mg, 36 mg Capsules, immediate release: 5 mg Solution, oral: 5 mg/5 mL Solution, oral concentrate: 20 mg/mL Tablets, immediate release (Oxy IR, Oxaydo, Supeudol): 5 mg, 7.5 mg, 10 mg, 15 mg[c], 20 mg, 30 mg[c] Tablets, extended release (OxyContin, OxyNEO): 5 mg[b], 10 mg, 15 mg, 20 mg, 30 mg, 40 mg, 60 mg, 80 mg	C-II Straight narcotic (Canada)
oxycodone and acetaminophen[a]	Percocet, Roxicet Generics	Tablets (Percocet): 2.5 mg/325 mg, 5 mg/325 mg, 7.5 mg/325 mg, 10 mg/325 mg	C-II (US) Straight narcotic (Canada)
oxycodone and aspirin	Percodan Generics	Tablets: 5 mg oxycodone/325 mg aspirin	C-II (US) Straight narcotic (Canada)
oxymorphone[a]	Opana Not available	Tablets: 5 mg, 10 mg Tablets, extended release: 5 mg, 7.5 mg, 10 mg, 15 mg, 20 mg, 30 mg, 40 mg	C-II

[a]Generic available.
[b]Available in Canada only.
[c]Available in the United States only.

Mixed Agonist/Antagonists

Generic Name	US Brand Name(s) / Canadian Brand(s)	Dosage Forms and Strengths	Controlled Substance Schedule (C-I, C-II, C-III, C-IV, C-V)
buprenorphine	Belbuca Buprenex, Butrans, Probuphine, Sublocade Butrans	Film, buccal (Belbuca): 0.075 mg, 0.15 mg, 0.3 mg, 0.45 mg, 0.6 mg[c], 0.75 mg[c], 0.9 mg[c] Implant (Probuphine): 80 mg base/implant Injection, solution (Buprenex): 0.3 mg/mL Solution, extended release for injection (Sublocade): 100 mg/0.5 mL, 300 mg/1.5 mL Tablets, sublingual (Subutex): 2 mg, 8 mg Transdermal, weekly patch (Butrans): 7.5 mg/hr[c], 15 mg/hr, 5 mcg/hr, 10 mcg/hr, 20 mcg/hr	C-III (US) Straight narcotic (Canada)

Mixed Agonist/Antagonists—cont'd

Generic Name	US Brand Name(s) / Canadian Brand(s)	Dosage Forms and Strengths	Controlled Substance Schedule (C-I, C-II, C-III, C-IV, C-V)
buprenorphine and naloxone[a]	Bunavail, Suboxone, Zubsolv / Suboxone	**Film, buccal: (Bunavail):** 2.1 mg burprenorphine and 0.3 mg naloxone, 4.2 mg burprenorphine and 0.7 mg naloxone, 6.3 mg burprenorphine and 1 mg naloxone **Tablets, sublingual (Zubsolv):** 0.7 mg burprenorphine and 0.18 mg naloxone, 1.4 mg burprenorphine and 0.36 mg naloxone, 2.9 mg burprenorphine and 0.71 mg naloxone, 5.7 mg burprenorphine and 1.4 mg naloxone, 8.6 mg burprenorphine and 2.1 mg naloxone, 11.4 mg burprenorphine and 2.9 mg naloxone **Tablets, sublingual (Suboxone):** 2 mg buprenorphine and 0.5 mg naloxone, 8 mg buprenorphine and 2 mg naloxone, 4 mg buprenorphine and 1 mg naloxone (United States only), 12 mg buprenorphine and 3 mg naloxone, 16 mg buprenorphine and 4 mg naloxone (Canada only)	**C-III** (US) **Straight narcotic** (Canada)
butorphanol[a]	Generics / Generics	**Injection:** 1 mg/mL, 2 mg/mL[b] **Intranasal solution:** 10 mg/mL (1 mg/spray)	**C-IV** (US) **Straight narcotic** (Canada)
morphine and naltrexone	Embeda / Not available	**Capsule, extended release:** 20 mg morphine and 0.8 mg naltrexone, 40 mg morphine and 1.2 mg naltrexone, 50 mg morphine and 2 mg naltrexone, 60 mg morphine and 2.4 mg naltrexone, 80 mg morphine and 3.2 mg naltrexone, 100 mg morphine and 4 mg naltrexone	
nalbuphine[a]	Generics / Generics	**Injection, solution:** 10 mg/mL, 20 mg/mL[b]	**Schedule G Controlled (Canada)**
oxycodone and naloxone	Not available / Targin	**Tablets:** 5 mg oxycodone and 2.5 mg naloxone, 10 mg oxycodone and 5 mg naloxone, 20 mg oxycodone and 10 mg naloxone, 40 mg oxycodone and 20 mg naloxone	**Straight narcotic (Canada)**
pentazocine	Talwin / Talwin	**Injection, solution:** 30 mg/mL **Tablets:** 50 mg[c]	Straight narcotic (Canada)
pentazocine and naloxone	Generics / Not available	**Tablets:** 50 mg pentazocine + 0.5 mg naloxone	C-IV

[a]Generic available.
[b]Strength available in the United States only.
[c]Strength available in Canada only.

Opioid Overdose: A Public Health Issue

Opioid use and opioid overdose is epidemic in the United States and Canada. Approximately 115 Americans die each day from an opioid overdose, according the the U.S. Centers for Disease Control and Prevention. In Canada, 2458 people died of an opioid overdose in 2016, according to Health Canada. Naloxone is an opioid antagonist that available for emergency use to reduce death due to opioid overdose. Forty-six states have laws that address access to naloxone for opioid overdose. As many as 40 states allow pharmacists to dispense naloxone to the general public without a physician prescription. In Canada and in the United States, pharmacists may dispense intranasal and injectable kits of naloxone. The kits are publically funded in Canada and may be dispensed free of charge. Naloxone is marketed as a nasal spray (2 mg and 4 mg per spray) and an injectable kit for use by the general public.

TECH NOTE!

Evzio® is a prefilled auto-injector containing naloxone that is injected into the thigh. After administration it is necessary to monitor the breathing of the patient and administer a second dose within 2 to 3 minutes if they don't awaken. The nasal spray is administered while the patient is lying on their back. Place the nozzle inside one nostril and press the plunger to release the dose. After administration, turn the patient onto their side.

Opioid Antagonists

Generic Name	US Brand Name(s) / Canadian Brand(s)	Dosage Forms and Strengths	Usual Adult Dose
naloxone[a]	Evzio, Narcan / Generics	**Injection, solution:** 0.4 mg/mL, 1 mg/mL, 2 mg/0.4 mL **Nasal Spray:** 4 mg/spray	0.4–2 mg IV every 2–3 min; repeat every 20–60 min Auto-injector (Evzio): inject 1 dose into the thigh. Repeat if necessary Nasal Spray: 1 spray in one nostril, repeat in 2–3 minutes as necessary
methylnaltrexone	Relistor / Relistor	**Solution, for injection:** 8 mg/0.4 mL, 12 mg/0.6 mL **Tablet:** 150 mg	450 mg orally or 12 mg subcutaneously once daily for opioid induced constipation
naltrexone[a]	Vivitrol / ReVia	**Powder, for injection (Vivitrol):** 380 mg per vial **Tablets (ReVia):** 50 mg	Tablets: Start 25 mg; 50 mg/day or 100–150 mg 3 times a week (up to 800 mg/day) Injection: 380 mg IM every 4 weeks (Vivitrol)

[a]Generic available.

Summary of Drugs Used to Manage Drug Dependence or Reverse Effects of Opioids

Generic Name	Dose	Onset[a] (min)	Duration[a] (min/h)	Route
buprenorphine	Opioid dependence	30–60 PO	12 h (2 mg) up to 72 h (>16 mg)	IV, PO
buprenorphine and naloxone	Opioid dependence			
methadone	Opioid dependence	30	24–36 h	PO
naloxone	Reverse opioid-induced respiratory depression of overdose	2	30 min	IM, IV, subcutaneous, nasal spray
naltrexone	Alcohol dependence	15–30	50 mg (24 h) 100 mg (48 h) 150 mg (72 h)	PO

[a]Varies according to dose and route of administration.

Summary of Opioid Analgesics

	Generic Name	US Brand Name	Usual Adult Oral Dose and Dosing Schedule	Warning Labels
Opioid Agonists				
	codeine	Generics	**Immediate release, IM and subcut injection:** 15–60 mg every 4–6 h (up to 360 mg/day) **Controlled release:** 50–300 mg every 12 h	MAY CAUSE DROWSINESS; MAY IMPAIR ABILITY TO DRIVE. AVOID ALCOHOL. TAKE WITH FOOD. MAY BE HABIT FORMING. TAKE EACH DOSE WITH A FULL GLASS OF WATER. SWALLOW WHOLE; DO NOT CRUSH OR CHEW—controlled release and delayed release. ROTATE SITE OF APPLICATION—transdermal. TAKE ON AN EMPTY STOMACH—Opana
	codeine and acetaminophen	Tylenol with Codeine #3	1–2 tablets every 4 h (maximum, 4 g daily)	

Summary of Opioid Analgesics—cont'd

Generic Name	US Brand Name	Usual Adult Oral Dose and Dosing Schedule	Warning Labels
fentanyl	Duragesic, Subsys SL	**For pain (opiate naïve):** Apply one 25–100 mcg/h (up to 300 mcg for severe chronic pain) transdermal system every 72 h **Breakthrough cancer pain in opioid-tolerant patients:** Spray a 100–1600 mcg dose under the tongue; may repeat once after 30 minutes (Subsys®). Separate treatments by at least 4 hours.	
hydrocodone and acetaminophen	Anexsia	1–2 tablets every 4–6 h (maximum dose, hydrocodone 60 mg and APAP 4 g/day)	
hydrocodone and ibuprofen	Repraxain	1 tablets every 4–6 h	
hydromorphone	Dilaudid, Exalgo	**For pain (opiate naïve):** **IM/Subcut:** 1–2 mg every 2–3 h prn **IV:** 0.2–1 mg every 2–3 h **PCA:** 0.2 mg/mL (range, 0.05 to 0.4 mg) **Capsule, controlled release (Hydromorph Contin):** 3–30 mg every 12 h **Tablet, controlled release (Exalgo):** 8–32 mg once daily **Rectal:** Insert 3–6 mg rectally every up to every 3 to 4 hours **Oral (immediate release):** 2–8 mg every 3–4 h	
levorphanol	Generics	**For pain (opiate naïve):** 2–4 mg every 6–8 h (maximum 12 mg daily)	
meperidine	Demerol	**For pain (opiate naïve):** **Oral, IM, and subcut:** 50–150 mg every 3–4 h	
methadone	Methadose	**For pain (opiate naïve):** **Oral:** 2.5–10 mg every 8–12 h **IV, IM, subcut:** 2.5–10 mg every 8–12 h **Detoxification (oral):** 20–40 mg/day; maintenance dose 80–120 mg/day	
morphine	MS Contin, Kadian	**For pain (opiate naïve):** **Oral (prompt release):** 10–30 mg every 3–4 h **Oral (extended release and sustained release capsules e.g., Kadian, M-Eslon):** Individualized 1–2 times daily **Controlled release (tablet e.g., Arymo ER, Morphabond ER, MS Contin):** Individualized every 8–12 h **PCA:** 0.5–2.5 mg, lock out interval: 5–10 min **IM, subcut:** 5–20 mg every 4 h as needed **Rectal:** 10–20 mg rectally every 4 hours	
oxycodone	OxyContin, OxyNeo	**For pain (opiate naïve):** **Immediate release (e.g., Oxy IR, Oxaydo):** 5–10 mg every 6 h **Controlled release (capsule e.g., Xtampza ER):** Individualized; initiate 9 mg every 12 hours **Controlled release (tablet e.g., OxyContin, OxyNeo):** 10–40 mg every 12 h	
oxycodone and acetaminophen	Percocet	1–2 tablets every 4–6 h (maximum, 4 g APAP daily)	
oxymorphone	Opana	**Oral tablet (immediate release):** 10–20 mg every 4–6 hours **Oral tablet (extended release):** 5–10 mg every 12 hours	

Continued

Summary of Opioid Analgesics—cont'd

	Generic Name	US Brand Name	Usual Adult Oral Dose and Dosing Schedule	Warning Labels
Mixed Agonist/Antagonists				
	buprenorphine	Buprenex, Butrans	**Buprenex (opiate naïve): IM, IV:** 0.3 mg every 6–8 h **Butrans:** Apply 1 patch every 7 days	MAY CAUSE DROWSINESS; MAY IMPAIR ABILITY TO DRIVE. AVOID ALCOHOL. MAY BE HABIT FORMING.
	buprenorphine and naloxone	Suboxone	**Opioid dependence:** 4–24 mg/day titrated according to avoid withdrawal symptoms	
	butorphanol	Stadol	**Acute pain (IM, IV):** 1–4 mg every 3–4 h **Labor pain:** 1–2 mg within 4 h of anticipated delivery	

❗ TECH ALERT!

Fentanyl SL spray (Subsys®) is not bioequivalent to other fentanyl dosage forms so is not substituted on a mcg-per-mcg basis.

❗ TECH ALERT!

Product selection errors are common because of many strength combinations for hydrocodone and acetaminophen.

Nonopioid Analgesics

Nonsteroidal Antiinflammatory Drugs, Salicylates, and Acetaminophen

Nonsteroidal antiinflammatory drugs *(NSAIDs)*, salicylates (aspirin), and acetaminophen are widely used in the treatment of pain with or without inflammation. NSAIDs and aspirin have analgesic, antiinflammatory, and antipyretic properties. An antipyretic is a drug that is capable of reducing fever. NSAIDs action and effectiveness are similar to those of aspirin (ASA).

Mechanism of Action

Similar to aspirin, NSAIDs decrease prostaglandin synthesis by inhibiting the action of cyclooxygenase-1 (COX-1) and cyclooxygenase-2 (COX-2). Most NSAIDs are not selective. COX-1 is expressed continuously and is found throughout the body. It is important for regulation of platelet aggregation and the biosynthesis of prostaglandins that protect the gastric mucosa. COX-2 is formed in selected cells as part of the immune response. COX-2 is involved in the biosynthesis of prostaglandins responsible for pain and inflammation. The analgesic effect of acetaminophen is thought to additionally be caused by inhibition of COX-3 in the brain.

Pharmacokinetics

Aspirin and NSAIDs are well absorbed orally. Aspirin is a weak acid (acetylsalicylic acid), and the rate of absorption varies according to the pH of stomach, small intestine, and urine. Enteric-coated aspirin is released in the pH of the intestine rather than in the stomach. Aspirin is eliminated in the urine. Acidification of the urine with vitamin C can increase rate of reabsorption, and sodium bicarbonate enhances elimination (see Chapter 2).

NSAIDs are structurally dissimilar; however, they are biologically similar. Oral absorption is good and bioavailability ranges between 80% and 99%. They are all highly protein bound, more than 97%, and they all are primarily eliminated in the urine.

▪ TECH NOTE!

Ofirmev is a parenteral dosage form of acetaminophen approved by the US Food and Drug Administration (FDA) in 2010.

Adverse Reactions

All of the NSAIDs and aspirin can produce nausea, GI bleeding, and ulceration. NSAIDs can cause fluid retention, leading to increased blood pressure. Some NSAIDs can produce dizziness. Serious side effects include salicylism (aspirin), hepatotoxicity (ketorolac), and agranulocytosis (indomethacin, flurbiprofen). Celecoxib (Celebrex) remains the only selective COX-2 inhibitor currently in use. Acetaminophen can cause hepatotoxicity.

❗ TECH ALERT!

The maximum daily adult dose for acetaminophen and aspirin is 4 g.

❗ TECH ALERT!

Acetaminophen doses for children are calculated based on body weight. Consumers should dispense the dose using the calibrated measuring device that is supplied with the product.

Drug Treatment for Neuropathic Pain

Neuropathic pain is associated with nerve injury caused by trauma, infection, or chronic diseases such as uncontrolled diabetes and is often treated with different drugs than are used to treat pain of nociceptive origin. Neuropathic pain is unique because pain sensations are felt even after the injury is healed. When nerves are damaged, the body may make adaptations to compensate for the nerve damage. These changes can lead to persistent nerve pain. Nerve injury can lead to sensitization of nerve terminals. This lowers the threshold for neuron firing (action potential) and increases the response to stimuli. Nerve damage can result in a reorganization of nerves. The rewiring sometimes goes haywire, causing painful sensations even after limbs have been amputated. Another cause of neuropathic pain is changes in the sodium and calcium ion channels that result in increasing or decreasing levels of ions involved in neuronal firing. Nerve injuries can also cause a loss of inhibitory

Commonly Used Nonopioid Analgesics

	Generic Name	Brand Name	Usual Adult Dose	Side Effects	Warning Labels
Salicylates					
	aspirin	Ecotrin, Bayer, Anacin	325–650 mg every 4–6 h (maximum, 4 g/day)	GI upset, bleeding, tinnitus, salicylism	TAKE WITH FOOD.
	diflunisal	Dolobid	250–500 mg twice a day	GI upset, rash, drowsiness, jaundice	TAKE WITH FOOD. MAY CAUSE DIZZINESS OR DROWSINESS. AVOID ASPIRIN AND RELATED DRUGS.
p-Aminophenol					
	acetaminophen	Tylenol	325–650 mg every 4–6 h (maximum, 4 g/day)	Skin, liver toxicity, kidney toxicity	
Indoles					
	indomethacin	Indocin	25–50 mg 2–3 times a day	GI upset, headache, dizziness (drowsiness— sulindac), tinnitus, agranulocytosis (fatigue, apnea— indomethacin)	TAKE WITH FOOD. MAY CAUSE DIZZINESS OR DROWSINESS. AVOID ASPIRIN AND RELATED DRUGS.
	sulindac	Generics	150–200 mg twice a day maximum, 400 mg per day		
	etodolac	Generics	200–400 mg every 6–8 h		
Phenylpropionic Acid					
	flurbiprofen	Generics	200–300 mg/day in 2-4 divided doses	GI upset, headache, tinnitus, dizziness, kidney toxicity (ibuprofen)	TAKE WITH FOOD. MAY CAUSE DIZZINESS OR DROWSINESS. AVOID ASPIRIN AND RELATED DRUGS.
	ibuprofen	Motrin	200–800 mg every 4–8 h (maximum, 3200 mg/day)		
	ketoprofen	Generics	50–75 mg 3–4 times a day		
		Generics (extended release)	200 mg once a day		
	oxaprozin	Daypro	1200 mg once a day		
Naphthylpropionic Acids					
	naproxen	Naprosyn Naprosyn DS Napralen	**Immediate release:** Start 500 mg (Naproxen[a])-550 mg (Anaprox); then 250–275 mg every 6–12 h	GI upset, headache, tinnitus, rash, dizziness	TAKE WITH FOOD. MAY CAUSE DIZZINESS OR DROWSINESS. AVOID ASPIRIN AND RELATED DRUGS.
	naproxen sodium	Anaprox Anaprox DS	**Delayed release** (EC Naprosyn): 375–500 mg twice daily **Controlled release** (Napralen): 750–1500 mg once daily (maximum 1500 mg/day)		
Naphthyalkanones					
	nabumetone	Generics	1000–2000 mg/day dosed 1–2 times/day	GI upset, dizziness, agranulocytosis	TAKE WITH FOOD. MAY CAUSE DIZZINESS OR DROWSINESS. AVOID ASPIRIN AND RELATED DRUGS.
Anthranilic Acids					
	meclofenamate	Generics	50–100 mg every 4–6 h (maximum, 400 mg/day)	GI upset, headache, dizziness, increased urination	TAKE WITH FOOD. MAY CAUSE DIZZINESS OR DROWSINESS. AVOID ASPIRIN AND RELATED DRUGS.

Continued

Commonly Used Nonopioid Analgesics—cont'd

	Generic Name	Brand Name	Usual Adult Dose	Side Effects	Warning Labels
Pyrroleacetic Acid					
	tolmetin	Generics	200–600 mg 3 times a day		TAKE WITH FOOD.
	ketorolac	Toradol, Sprix	**Nasal Spray:** Inhale 1 spray in each nostril every 6–8 hours **PO:** 10 mg every 4–6 h (maximum, 40 mg/day) **IM:** Inject 10–30 mg IM every 4–6 h	GI upset, headache, dizziness, rash, liver toxicity (ketorolac), palpitations (tolmetin)	MAY CAUSE DIZZINESS OR DROWSINESS. AVOID ASPIRIN AND RELATED DRUGS. DISCARD CONTENTS OF NASAL SPRAY 24 HOURS AFTER OPENING
Phenylacetic Acid					
	diclofenac	Cambia, Flector, Zorvolex, Voltaren, Voltaren XR, Voltaren Rapide (Canada)	**Capsule:** 18–35 mg 3 times a day **Powder, for suspension (Cambia):** Mix 1 packet in 1–2 ounces of water and drink **Transdermal Patch:** apply 1 patch twice daily **Immediate release:** 50 mg 2–4 times a day (oral) **Controlled release:** 100 mg once daily (maximum, 200 mg/day)	GI upset, pain, nausea and vomiting, ulceration	TAKE WITH FOOD. MAY CAUSE DIZZINESS OR DROWSINESS. AVOID ASPIRIN AND RELATED DRUGS. SHAKE WELL—Cambia SWALLOW WHOLE; DO NOT CRUSH OR CHEW. —extended release
	diclofenac + misoprostol	Arthrotec-50, Arthrotec-75	100–150 mg diclofenac tablet 2–3 times per day		
Oxicams					
	meloxicam	Mobic	7.5–15 mg once a day	GI upset, constipation or diarrhea, gas, dizziness, edema, GI bleeding, hypertension	TAKE WITH FOOD. MAY CAUSE DIZZINESS OR DROWSINESS. AVOID ASPIRIN AND RELATED DRUGS. SWALLOW WHOLE; DO NOT CRUSH OR CHEW.
	piroxicam	Feldene	20 mg once a day		
COX-2 Inhibitors					
	celecoxib	Celebrex	100–200 mg twice a day	GI upset, GI ulceration, heart attack, stroke	TAKE WITH FOOD. MAY CAUSE DIZZINESS OR DROWSINESS. AVOID ASPIRIN AND RELATED DRUGS.

[a]550 mg naproxen Na = (500 mg naproxen base).

pathways such as the γ-aminobutyric acid (GABA) pathways (described in Chapter 8).

Drugs used in the treatment of neuropathic pain include antidepressants (amitriptyline, duloxetine), antiseizure drugs (gabapentin, lamotrigine), local anesthetics (lidocaine, mexiletine), and capsaicin. The tricyclic antidepressants are often used as first-line agents for the treatment of neuropathic pain. They inhibit the reuptake of neurotransmitters (e.g., norepinephrine and 5-HT) at receptor sites in the spinal cord that are responsible for modulating pain sensation. Duloxetine is a 5-HT–noradrenaline reuptake inhibitor that has been shown to be effective in reducing pain caused by fibromyalgia and diabetic neuropathy. There is little evidence to support the use of selective 5-HT reuptake inhibitors for the management of neuropathic pain.

Gabapentin, pregabalin, and carbamazepine are antiseizure drugs that are used for the treatment of diabetic neuropathy, nerve pain caused by herpes virus infection, and trigeminal neuralgia. Topiramate enhances inhibitory effects of GABA in addition to its action on voltage-dependent sodium channels. These drugs are discussed in detail in Chapter 9.

Lidocaine is a local anesthetic used in the treatment of neuropathic pain. Lidocaine blocks sodium channels and may be administered intravenously or topically. Lidocaine patches are indicated for the treatment of nerve pain caused by herpes infection (shingles). Capsaicin is derived from chili peppers. It is applied topically and it depletes substance P from nerve terminals. It is indicated for the treatment of diabetic neuropathy and shingles.

● TECH NOTE!

Pregabalin (Lyrica) is a class V (C-V) controlled substance.

Nondrug Treatment of Pain

The treatment of pain, especially chronic pain, requires a multi-modal approach that includes drug therapy and nondrug therapy. Nondrug therapies that may be supportive are education, physical therapy, occupational therapy, *biofeedback*, cognitive behavioral therapy (counseling), *acupuncture*, chiropractic medicine, and transcutaneous electrical stimulation (TENS) (Fig. 10.3). The TENS device delivers electrical impulses through the skin that causes contraction and numbness. This blocks the transmission of pain messages to the spinal cord by peripheral nerves. Cryotherapy (cold packs) and heat packs can reduce swelling, which can also decrease pain.

● **Fig. 10.3** Transcutaneous nerve stimulation unit. (From Proctor D, Niedzwiecki B, et al: *Kinn's the medical assistant*, ed 13, St. Louis, 2017, Elsevier.)

Commonly Used to Treat Neuropathic Pain

	Generic Name	Brand Name	Usual Adult Dose	Side Effects	Warning Labels
Antidepressants	amitriptyline	Elavil	25–100 mg at bedtime	Sedation, dry mouth, urinary retention, nausea, blurred vision, photosensitivity	MAY CAUSE DROWSINESS; ALCOHOL MAY INTENSIFY THIS EFFECT. MAY IMPAIR ABILITY TO DRIVE. DO NOT DISCONTINUE WITHOUT MEDICAL SUPERVISION. MAY DISCOLOR URINE (BLUE-GREEN). AVOID PROLONGED EXPOSURE TO SUNLIGHT.
	desipramine	Norpramin	25–150 mg/day in 1–2 doses		
	imipramine	Tofranil	25–150 mg daily in 1–2 divided doses		
Antiseizure Drugs	gabapentin	Neurontin Gralise	1200–3600 mg in 3 divided doses	Dizziness, confusion, fatigue, ataxia and nausea, double vision, blurred vision, dry mouth, and constipation	MAY CAUSE DROWSINESS; MAY IMPAIR ABILITY TO DRIVE. AVOID ALCOHOL. TAKE WITH FOOD. DO NOT DISCONTINUE WITHOUT MEDICAL SUPERVISION. SHAKE WELL. SWALLOW WHOLE; DO NOT CRUSH OR CHEW—controlled release. AVOID ANTACIDS WITHIN 2 H OF DOSE—gabapentin, phenytoin. AVOID PREGNANCY—phenytoin.
	pregabalin	Lyrica, Lyrica CR	50–100 mg 3 times a day Extended release: Initial, 165 mg orally once daily after an evening meal; Increase to 330 mg once daily within 1 week.		
	carbamazepine	Tegretol	400–800 mg twice a day (maximum 1200 mg/day)	Nausea, vomiting, sedation, dizziness, ataxia, bruising, jaundice, and visual disturbances	

Continued

Commonly Used to Treat Neuropathic Pain—cont'd

	Generic Name	Brand Name	Usual Adult Dose	Side Effects	Warning Labels
Topicals					
	lidocaine	Lidoderm	1–3 patches up to 12 h/day	Numbness, local irritation	ROTATE SITE OF APPLICATION—Lidoderm, Qutenza.
	capsaicin	Zostrix, Qutenza (patch)	Apply 3–4 times a day Patch: 1 to 4 patches once every 3 months	Burning, stinging	WASH HANDS AFTER USE—capsaicin. REMOVE PATCH AFTER 60 MINUTES

ªNot FDA approved.

Headache

International Headache Society (IHS) classifications for primary headaches include migraine headache, tension-type headache, cluster headache, and trigeminal *cephalgia*. Tension headache is the most common of the primary headaches. It produces bilateral pain, affecting both sides of the head, is mild to moderate in intensity, and is described as having a pressing or tightening quality. Left untreated, tension headaches may last for 30 minutes to up to 7 days. A *cluster headache* is a frequently reoccurring headache that produces severe pain on one side of the head. Cluster headaches may last 15 to 90 minutes and occur more frequently in men.

Migraine Headache

In the United States, up to 18.2% of women and 6.5% of men experience migraine headaches annually. Up to 24% of Canadians will experience a migraine headache in their lifetime. Migraine headache occurs infrequently in children younger than 10 years of age; the onset is typically between 10 and 29 years old. The prevalence is greatest between 30 and 39 years old and tapers after 60 years old. The probability of developing migraines may be as high as 70% if both parents get migraine headaches.

Once thought to be a vascular headache, it is now believed that migraine pain occurs as a result of biochemical and hormonal changes involving serotonergic and adrenergic pain modulating systems. 5-HT is most commonly implicated; however, prostaglandins, catecholamines, histamine, substance P, and neuroexcitatory amino acids are also thought to play a role.

Migraine headaches are typically unilateral, affecting only one side of the head; however, the headache can spread to the opposite side. IHS classifications include migraine with aura, migraine without aura, menstrual migraine, and chronic migraine. Chronic migraine can occur from overuse of medicines used in the treatment of migraine. An aura is an unusual sensation that is experienced just before the onset of the migraine headache. An aura may present as a temporary flashing light, blind spots, double vision, a smell, paresthesia, weakness, or aphagia (loss of language).

Severe throbbing pain is characteristic of migraines, as are nausea, photophobia (eyes are sensitive to the light), and phonophobia (sensitivity to noise). Resting in a quiet area with the lights off can sometimes improve migraine symptoms. Physical activity worsens migraine symptoms. Acute migraine attacks can last between 4 and 72 hours; the average is 29 hours. Migraine headaches occur more frequently in women than in men.

Pathophysiology of Migraine Headaches

Migraine headaches are triggered by numerous events, including stress, insufficient sleep, red wine, caffeine, strong odors, smoke, changes in the weather, and exposure to bright or flashing lights. The trigger sets off a series of events that starts with the release of vasoactive neuropeptides that cause blood vessels in the brain to first constrict and then dilate. The trigger produces vasospasms, which reduce blood flow to the brain. Platelets in the blood clump together and cause the release of 5-HT, which further constricts blood vessels. This triggers afferent signals via the trigeminal nerve to release prostaglandins and other neurochemicals that dilate blood vessels, produce inflammation, and stimulate nociceptors. This causes the throbbing head pain characteristic of migraine headaches.

Drug Treatment for Migraine Headache

Treatment of migraines is aimed at stopping the current migraine attack (abortive therapy) and preventing future migraines. Simple analgesics, combination analgesics, 5-HT agonists, ergot alkaloids, antidepressants (tricyclic antidepressants, selective 5-HT reuptake inhibitors, and monoamine oxidase inhibitors), beta blockers, and antiseizure drugs are used in the treatment and prevention of migraine headaches. The overall goal of therapy is to treat attacks rapidly and consistently with minimal adverse effects; decrease the frequency, intensity, and duration of headaches; restore the patient's ability to function; and minimize the use of rescue and backup medications (Table 10.2).

> ● **TECH NOTE!**
>
> *Triptan* is a common ending for drugs used in the treatment of migraine headache.

Treatment of Acute Migraine Headache

Simple Analgesics and Combination Analgesics

Simple analgesics (aspirin, acetaminophen, ibuprofen, and naproxen) are often effective in stopping mild to moderate migraine headaches if taken early and in high doses. The effective dose of aspirin or acetaminophen used to treat migraine headache (up to 1000 mg per dose) is higher than the usual dose recommended for the treatment of mild to moderate tension headache (325–650 mg per dose). Codeine, caffeine, and butalbital may be added to aspirin and acetaminophen to form combination analgesics. Simple analgesics and combined analgesics (aspirin and NSAIDs) reduce pain and decrease inflammation associated with migraine headache.

Triptans

The triptans are the most widely prescribed drugs for the treatment of migraine headaches. They are administered during an acute attack to lessen symptoms and to stop the headache from progressing to more severe migraine symptoms. They are administered at the first sign of an impending migraine (aura).

TABLE 10.2 Quality of Evidence for Drugs Used in the Acute Treatment of Migraine Headache

Drug Category	Drug	Quality of Evidence of Effectiveness[a]
Simple analgesics	acetaminophen	B
	aspirin	A
	ibuprofen	A
	naproxen Na+	A
Combination analgesics	aspirin + acetaminophen + caffeine	A
	aspirin + butalbital + caffeine	C
Ergotamine and ergotamine combinations	ergotamine	B
	ergotamine + caffeine	B
	dihydroergotamine nasal spray	A
	dihydroergotamine subcut, IM, IV	B
Triptans	almotriptan, eletriptan, frovatriptan, naratriptan, rizatriptan, sumatriptan, zolmitriptan	A
Opioid analgesics	butorphanol nasal spray	A
	codeine + acetaminophen	A
	meperidine IM, IV	B

[a]Quality of the evidence (grade A, B, or C [A, multiple well-designed randomized, clinical trials directly relevant to the recommendation; B, some evidence from randomized clinical trials, but the scientific support was not optimal; and C, the US Headache Consortium achieved consensus on the recommendation in the absence of relevant randomized, controlled trials.])

TECH ALERT!

The following drugs have look-alike/sound-alike issues:
Axert and Antivert;
Amerge and Amaryl;
sumatriptan and zolmitriptan;
Maxalt and Maxair

Mechanism of Action
The triptans are selective 5-HT receptor agonists. They have a high affinity for 5-HT$_{1B}$ and 5-HT$_{1D}$ receptors, which stimulate vasoconstriction (Fig. 10.4).

Pharmacokinetics
The triptans are available for administration via mouth, in the nose, and by injection. Subcutaneous injection produces the most rapid response and is the most effective route of administration; however, intranasal administration is also rapid and has fewer adverse reactions. Oral formulations have slower onsets of action. The half-life of the triptans range between 2 hours and 25 hours. Triptans that have a long half-life, such as frovatriptan (24 hours) and naratriptan (8 hours), are more effective in reducing headache reoccurrence.

Adverse Reactions
The vasoconstriction caused by triptans is responsible for their therapeutic effects but can result in serious cardiac side effects, including arrhythmia, angina, coronary vasospasm, and myocardial infarction (heart attack). Vasoconstriction can also cause high blood pressure and stroke. Less serious and more common side effects are pain, tightness, and burning at the site of injection; dizziness; nausea; hot flashes; dry mouth; and fatigue.

Precautions
Overuse of triptans should be avoided. Nearly all triptans are restricted to two doses per 24 hours. Frovatriptan is restricted to three doses per 24 hours. The safety of treating more than four migraines per month has not been established for most of the triptans.

TECH NOTE!

Maxalt-MLT contains phenylalanine.

TECH NOTE!

Review sumatriptan nasal directions carefully—only one spray in one nostril is indicated.

Comparison of Triptans

Generic Name (Brand Name)	Onset (min)	Repeat Time (h)	Route	Headache[a] Effectiveness (%)	Dose (mg)[b]
almotriptan (Axert)	30	2	PO, tablet	57–68	25
eletriptan (Relpax)	30	2	PO, tablet	54–65 / 68–77	40 / 80
frovatriptan (Frova)	30	2	PO, tablet	40	2.5
naratriptan (Amerge)	30	4	PO, tablet	48	2.5

Continued

Comparison of Triptans—cont'd

Generic Name (Brand Name)	Onset (min)	Repeat Time (h)	Route	Headache[a] Effectiveness (%)	Dose (mg)[b]
rizatriptan (Maxalt, Maxalt-MLT)	30	2	PO, tablet	73	10
		2	Wafer		
sumatriptan (Imitrex)	10–15	1	subcut	80–85	6
	15	2	Nasal	60–86	20
	30	2	PO, tablet	51–61	50
zolmitriptan (Zomig)	30	2	PO, tablet	59–69	2.5
		2	Wafer		
	10–15		Nasal	24–61	5

[a]Percentage patients reporting pain relief at 2 hours after dosing.
[b]Dose associated with headache effectiveness (%).

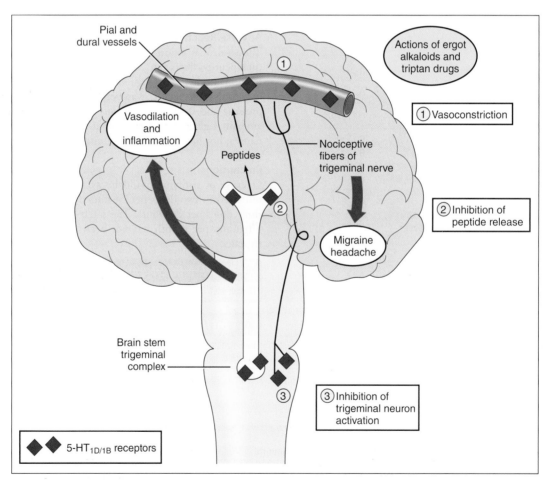

• **Fig. 10.4** Mechanism of action for triptan drugs. (From Brenner GM, Stevens CW: *Brenner and Stevens' pharmacology*, ed 5, Philadelphia, 2018, Elsevier.)

Drugs Used in the Acute Treatment of Migraine Headache: Triptans Dosage Forms and Strength

Generic Name	US Brand Name(s) Canadian Brand(s)	Dosage Forms and Strengths
almotriptan[a]	Axert	**Tablets:** 6.25 mg, 12.5 mg
	Axert	
eletriptan[a]	Relpax	**Tablets:** 20 mg, 40 mg
	Relpax	
frovatriptan[a]	Frova	**Tablets:** 2.5 mg
	Frova	
naratriptan[a]	Amerge	**Tablets:** 1 mg, 2.5 mg
	Amerge	
rizatriptan[a]	Maxalt, Maxalt-MLT	**Tablets (Maxalt):** 5 mg, 10 mg
	Maxalt, Maxalt-RPD	**Tablets, disintegrating (Maxalt-MLT):** 5 mg, 10 mg **Wafer (Maxalt-RPD):** 5 mg, 10 mg
sumatriptan[a]	Imitrex, Onzetra Xsail, Zembrace Symtouch	Capsule, for nasal inhalation (Onzetra Xsail): 11 mg **Injection, as solution:** 3 mg/0.5 mL[a], 4 mg/0.5 mL[a], 6 mg/0.5 mL
	Imitrex	**Intranasal solution:** 5 mg, 20 mg (100 µL unit dose spray device) **Powder, for nasal inhalation (Onzetra Xsail)[b]:** 11 mg **Tablets:** 25 mg, 50 mg, 100 mg
zolmitriptan[a]	Zomig, Zomig-ZMT	**Nasal solution:** 2.5 mg/spray, 5 mg/spray
	Zomig, Zomig-Rapimelt	**Tablets:** 2.5 mg, 5 mg[b] **Tablets, disintegrating (Zomig-ZMT, Zomig-Rapimelt):** 2.5 mg, 5 mg[b]
sumatriptan + naproxen Na[+a]	Treximet	**Tablets:** 60 mg naproxen Na[+] + 10 mg sumatriptan, 500 mg naproxen Na[+] + 85 mg sumatriptan
	Not available in Canada	

[a]Generic Available.
[b]Available in the United States only.

Summary of Triptans Used in the Treatment of Migraine Headaches

Generic Name	US Brand Name	Usual Adult Oral Dose and Dosing Schedule	Warning Labels
almotriptan	Axert	**Oral:** 6.25–12.5 mg as a single dose; repeat dose in 2 h if needed (maximum, 25 mg in 24 h)	DO NOT EXCEED RECOMMENDED DOSAGE. IF NO IMPROVEMENT AFTER FIRST DOSE, DO NOT TAKE A SECOND DOSE.
eletriptan	Relpax	**Oral:** 20–40 mg as a single dose; repeat dose in 2 h if needed (maximum, 80 mg in 24 h)	
frovatriptan	Frova	**Oral:** 2.5 mg as a single dose; repeat dose in 2 h if needed (maximum, 7.5 mg in 24 h)	
naratriptan	Amerge	**Oral:** 1–2.5 mg as a single dose; repeat dose in 4 h if needed (maximum, 5 mg in 24 h)	
rizatriptan	Maxalt	**Oral:** 5–10 mg as a single dose; repeat dose in 2 h if needed (maximum, is 30 mg [15 mg if also receiving propranolol] in 24 h)	
sumatriptan	Imitrex	**Oral:** 25 mg, 50 mg, or 100 mg as a single dose; repeat dose in 2 h if needed (maximum, 200 mg in 24 h) **Nasal powder:** Inhale 22 mg (2 nose pieces) in one nostril; repeat dose in 2 h if needed (maximum, 44 mg in 24 h) **Nasal spray:** 1–2 sprays (5 mg, 10 mg), or 1 spray (20 mg) in one nostril; repeat dose in 2 h if needed (maximum, 40 mg in 24 h) **Subcut injection:** 6 mg as a single injection; repeat dose in 1 h if needed	DO NOT INJECT MORE THAN 2 DOSES (6 MG) IN 24 H. USE SPRAY IN ONE NOSTRIL ONLY. IF NO IMPROVEMENT AFTER FIRST DOSE, DO NOT TAKE A SECOND DOSE.

Continued

Summary of Triptans Used in the Treatment of Migraine Headaches—cont'd

Generic Name	US Brand Name	Usual Adult Oral Dose and Dosing Schedule	Warning Labels
zolmitriptan	Zomig	**Oral:** 2.5–5 mg as a single dose; repeat dose in 2 h if needed (maximum, 10 mg in 24 h) **Nasal solution:** 1 spray as a single dose; repeat dose in 2 h if needed	IF NO IMPROVEMENT AFTER FIRST DOSE, DO NOT TAKE A SECOND DOSE.
sumatriptan + naproxen sodium	Treximet	Take 1 tablet for migraine; may repeat dose in 2 h if needed	DO NOT EXCEED 2 DOSES PER 24 H. MAY CAUSE DIZZINESS OR DROWSINESS. SWALLOW WHOLE; DO NOT CUT, CRUSH, OR CHEW. TAKE WITH A FULL GLASS OF WATER.

Summary of Nontriptan Drugs Used to Treat Migraine Headaches

Generic Name	Brand Name	Usual Adult Dose	Side Effects	Warning Labels
dihydroergotamine mesylate	D.H.E. 45 Migranal	1 mg IM IV or SC; repeat in 1 h if needed (maximum, 6 mg/week) 1 spray in each nostril; repeat after 15 min if needed (maximum, 8 sprays/week)	Numbness	DO NOT EXCEED RECOMMENDED DOSAGE. DO NOT ASSEMBLE SPRAYER UNTIL READY TO USE.
ergotamine tartrate	Ergomar	2 mg every 30 min until relief (maximum, 6 mg/day or 10 mg/week)	Nausea, vomiting, numbness, chest pain, abdominal pain	DO NOT EXCEED RECOMMENDED DOSAGE.
butorphanol	Generics	1 spray in one nostril, may repeat in 60–90 min if needed (maximum, 4 doses/day)	Drowsiness, dizziness, nausea, constipation, dry mouth	MAY CAUSE DROWSINESS; MAY IMPAIR ABILITY TO DRIVE. AVOID ALCOHOL. TAKE WITH FOOD. MAY BE HABIT FORMING.
codeine 30 mg + acetaminophen	Tylenol #3	1–2 tablets every 4 h (maximum, 4 g daily)	Drowsiness, dizziness, nausea, constipation	

IM, intramuscularly; *IV,* intravenously; *SC,* subcutaneously.

Drugs Used for the Prevention of Migraine Headaches

	Generic Name	US Brand Name(s) Canadian Brand(s)	Dosage Forms and Strengths
Beta Blockers			
	propranolol[a]	Inderal LA Inderal LA	**Tablets:** 10 mg, 20 mg, 40 mg, 60 mg, 80 mg **Tablets, extended release (Inderal LA):** 60 mg, 80 mg, 120 mg, 160 mg
Antiepileptic Drugs			
	divalproex sodium	Depakote	**Tablets:** 250 mg, 500 mg
	topiramate	Topamax, Qudexy XR, Trokendi XR Topamax	**Tablets:** 25 mg, 50 mg, 100 mg, 200 mg, 300 mg, 400 mg **Capsule, extended release (Qudexy XR, Trokendi XR):** 25 mg, 50 mg, 100 mg, 150 mg, 200 mg
Tricyclic Antidepressants			
	amitriptyline	Generics Elavil	**Tablets:** 10 mg, 20 mg, 50 mg, 75 mg, 100 mg[b], 150 mg[b]
Neuromuscular Blockers			
	onabotulinumtoxinA	Botox Botox	**Powder for injection:** 50 unit[b], 100 units, 200 units[b]

Drugs Used for the Prevention of Migraine Headaches—cont'd

Generic Name	US Brand Name(s) Canadian Brand(s)	Dosage Forms and Strengths
Miscellaneous		
Flunarizine	Not Available Generics	**Capsule:** 5 mg

[a]Generic available.
[b]Strength available in the United States only.

Summary of Drugs Used for the Prevention of Migraine Headaches

	Generic Name	Brand Name	Usual Adult Dose	Side Effects	Warning Labels
Beta Blockers					
	propranolol	Inderal Inderal-LA	80–240 mg/day every 6–8 h or 80–240 mg/day (long acting)	Hypotension, lethargy	MAY CAUSE DIZZINESS OR DROWSINESS AND IMPAIR ABILITY TO DRIVE.
Antiepileptic Drugs					
	topiramate	Topamax, Qudexy XR, Trokendi XR	100 mg/day in 1–2 divided doses		
	divalproex Na$^+$	Depakote	250 mg twice daily up to 1000 mg/day	Sedation, nausea, Ataxia, and liver dysfunction	MAY CAUSE DROWSINESS AND IMPAIR ABILITY TO DRIVE. AVOID ALCOHOL. TAKE WITH FOOD.
Tricyclic Antidepressants					
	amitriptyline	generics Elavil	10–150 mg/day (start at 25 mg/day, inc by 25 mg/week)		MAY CAUSE DROWSINESS AND IMPAIR ABILITY TO DRIVE. AVOID ALCOHOL. TAKE WITH FOOD.
Neuromuscular Blockers					
	onabotulinumtoxinA	Botox	155 Units administered IM as 5 Units/injection divided across 31 injection sites within 7 specific head and neck muscle areas	Neck pain, stiffness, myasthenia, myalgia, muscle pain, pain at inj. site, botulism, blepharedema	
Miscellaneous					
	flunarizine	Generics	10 mg at bedtime		MAY CAUSE DROWSINESS

Other Acute Treatments for Acute Migraine Headaches

Ergot alkaloids and 5-HT agonists are also prescribed as migraine abortive therapy. Information about these agents is found in the **Summary of Nontriptan Drugs Used to Treat Migraine Headaches** table.

Migraine Preventive Agents

Migraine preventive therapy is offered to persons who use abortive medication more than twice per week or when acute-acting agents are contraindicated or have failed to relieve the headache. They are also offered to people who experience six or more migraine headaches per month. They may be offered to people experiencing only three to four migraines if the migraine produces moderate to severe impairment (requires bed rest). Beta blockers (see Chapter 22), tricyclic antidepressants (see Chapter 6), onabotulinumtoxinA (a neuromuscular blocker), neuromuscular blocking agents (see Chapter 13), and antiseizure drugs (see Chapter 9) are all prescribed for prophylaxis (prevention) of migraine headaches.

TECHNICIAN'S CORNER

1. Describe the difference between neuropathic and muscular pain. Can they be intertwined?
2. A patient who has suffered for years with chronic pain asks, "Is there anything else I can do besides take pain medicines for my pain?" What can you tell the patient?

Key Points

- Acute pain may be triggered by an injury, burn, infection, or some other stimuli and be self-limiting.
- Chronic pain may persist for years and is often inadequately controlled by pharmaceuticals.
- Psychological factors can influence a person's tolerance for pain and can determine whether the outcome of treatment is successful.
- Patient-controlled analgesia (PCA) permits patients to control the frequency of administration of their dose of pain medications.
- Neuropathic pain is associated with nerve injury caused by trauma, infection, or chronic diseases such as uncontrolled diabetes and is often treated with different drugs than other types of pain.
- Osteoarthritis, gout, burns, trauma, and low back pain are examples of pain with a nociceptor origin.
- Painful stimuli trigger the release of neurotransmitters, amino acids, and peptides that carry signals to increase sensitivity to the pain or to dull the painful sensations.
- Histamine, bradykinins, serotonin, prostaglandins, glutamate, and substance P are involved in the transmission of signals for pain sensation and pain perception.
- Endorphans, enkephalin, and dynorphin are the body's natural painkillers and bind to opioid receptors.
- Opioids are naturally occurring or synthetically derived drugs that act like morphine and are used to treat pain.
- Opioid receptors are mu (μ), kappa (κ), and delta (δ), and stimulation produces analgesia. The euphoria, dysphoria, respiratory depression, pupillary constriction, decreased GI motility, and physical dependence associated with opioid use are linked to specific receptors.
- Opioid agonists activate μ, κ, or δ receptors.
- Antagonists bind to the opioid receptor but do not activate it.
- Mixed agonist/antagonists behave like an agonist when the patient has had no recent exposure to an opioid agonist (opiate naïve).
- Equianalgesic doses of opioids produce equivalent pain relief regardless of dosage form.
- Opioid agonists, partial agonists, and most mixed agonist/antagonists are restricted substances because they produce tolerance and dependence.
- Opioid antagonists and some mixed agonist/antagonists are used to treat drug dependence and opioid-induced respiratory depression.

- Nonsteroidal antiinflammatory drugs (NSAIDs), acetaminophen, and aspirin are widely used in the treatment of pain with or without inflammation.
- NSAIDs and aspirin have analgesic, antiinflammatory, and antipyretic properties.
- Acetaminophen does not reduce inflammation.
- Aspirin and NSAIDs decrease prostaglandin synthesis by inhibiting the action of cyclooxygenase (COX), an enzyme involved in the biosynthesis of prostaglandins. Prostaglandins are important mediators of pain.
- All of the NSAIDs and aspirin can produce nausea, GI bleeding, and GI ulceration.
- Enteric-coated aspirin is released in the pH of the intestine rather than in the stomach.
- Migraine headaches are triggered by numerous events, including stress, consumption of certain foods, red wine, caffeinated beverages, and exposure to bright or flashing lights.
- During a migraine, blood vessels in the brain dilate, produce inflammation, and stimulate nociceptors, causing the throbbing head pain characteristic of migraine headaches.
- Treatment of migraines is aimed at stopping the current migraine attack and preventing future migraines.
- Simple and combined analgesics, serotonin agonists, and ergot alkaloids are used in the treatment of acute migraine headache.
- Tricyclic antidepressants, selective serotonin reuptake inhibitors, monoamine oxidase inhibitors, beta blockers, and neuromuscular blocking agents antiseizure drugs can be used in the prevention of migraine headaches.
- Triptans are selective serotonin receptor agonists and are the most widely prescribed drugs for the treatment of acute migraine headaches.
- Triptans that have long half-lives, frovatriptan and naratriptan, are more effective in preventing headache reoccurrence.
- The use of triptans is restricted to a maximum of two or three doses per 24 hours. The safety of treating more than four migraines per month has not been established for most of the triptans.
- The vasoconstriction caused by triptans is partially responsible for their therapeutic effects but can result in serious effects, including arrhythmia, angina, myocardial infarction, and stroke.

Review Questions

1. _____ pain may be triggered by an injury, burn, infection, or some other stimuli and be self-limiting.
   a. Chronic
   b. Dull
   c. Acute
   d. Nerve
2. The most common of all arthritic conditions is _____.
   a. gout
   b. osteoarthritis
   c. rheumatoid arthritis
   d. ankylosis

3. _____ are hormones that trigger pain response from peripheral nociceptors.
   a. Histamines
   b. Serotonins
   c. Prostaglandins
   d. Norepinephrines
4. *Opiate* is a term used to describe _____ derived drugs that act like morphine.
   a. naturally
   b. synthetically
   c. both a and b
   d. none of the above

5. What US controlled substance schedule does oxycodone fall into?
   a. C-II
   b. C-III
   c. C-IV
   d. C-V
6. Naloxone (Narcan), which is indicated for reversal of respiratory depression caused by opioid use and opioid overdose, is an example of an
   a. agonist
   b. antagonist
7. NSAIDs have analgesic, antiinflammatory, and antipyretic properties.
   a. true
   b. false
8. The only COX-2 inhibitor that remains currently in use is
   a. rofecoxib, Vioxx
   b. valdecoxib, Bextra
   c. acetaminophen, Tylenol
   d. celecoxib, Celebrex

9. Migraine headaches are triggered by numerous events, including _____.
   a. stress or consumption of certain foods
   b. red wine or caffeinated beverages
   c. exposure to bright or flashing lights
   d. all of the above
10. _____ are the most widely prescribed drugs for the treatment of migraine headaches.
    a. Ergot alkaloids
    b. Antiseizures
    c. Antidepressants
    d. Triptans

Bibliography

Adelman J, Lewit E: Comparative aspects of triptans in treating migraine, *Clin Cornerstone* 4:1–19, 2001.

Bennett M, Smith S, Torrance N, et al: Can pain be more or less neuropathic? Comparison of symptom assessment tools with ratings of certainty by clinicians, International Association for the Study of Pain, *Pain* 122:289–294, 2006.

BMJ: 2016. Migraine headache in adults, from: http://bestpractice.bmj.com/info/. (Retrieved 24 April 2017).

DeMaagd G: The pharmacological management of migraine, part 1 overview and abortive therapy, *P T* 33(7):2008.

Gawel M, Aschoff J, May A, et al: Zolmitriptan 5 mg nasal spray: efficacy and onset of action in the acute treatment of migraine—Results from Phase I of the REALIZE study, *Headache* 7–16, 2005.

Kalant H, Grant D, Mitchell J: *Principles of medical pharmacology*, ed 7, Toronto, Elsevier Canada, A Division of Reed Elsevier Canada, pp 236–251.

Kampman K, et al: National practice guideline for the use of medications in the treatment of addiction involving opioid use: American Society of Addiction Medicine, *J Addict Med* 9(5):358–367, 2015.

Kelmann L: *Pain characteristics of acute migraine attack, headache*, Ames, IA, 2006, Blackwell Publishing.

Kidd B: Osteoarthritis and joint pain: topical review, International Association for the Study of Pain, *Pain* 123:6–9, 2006.

Lipton RB, Bigal ME, Diamond M, et al: Migraine prevalence, disease burden, and the need for preventive therapy, *Neurology* 68:343–349, 2007.

Macfarlane G, Jones G, Hannaford P: Managing low back pain presenting in primary care: where do we go from here? International Association for the Study of Pain, *Pain*, 122 219–222, 2006.

Marcus D: Treatment of nonmalignant chronic pain, *Am Fam Physician* 61:1–8, 2000.

Matcher B, Young WB, Rosenberg JH, et al: Evidence-Based Guidelines for Migraine Headache in the Primary Care Setting: Pharmacological Management of Acute Attacks, US Headache Consortium, (nd). Available online at: http://tools.aan.com/professionals/practice/pdfs/gl0087.pdf.

National Institute of Neurological Disorders and Stroke (2014). Chronic Pain: Hope through research, Bethesda, MD, NINDS, National Institutes of Health, U.S. Department of Health and Human Services, NIH Publication No. 14-2406.

Page C, Curtis M, Sutter M, et al: *Integrated pharmacology*, Philadelphia, 2005, Elsevier Mosby, pp 272–274.

Raffa RB, Rawls SM, Beyzarov EP: *Netter's illustrated pharmacology*, Philadelphia, 2005, Saunders, p 85.

Silberstein SD, Holland S, Freitag F, et al: Evidence-based guideline update: pharmacologic treatment for episodic migraine prevention in adults: report of the Quality Standards Subcommittee of the American Academy of Neurology and the American Headache Society, *Neurology* 78:1337–1345, 2012.

Sun-Edelstein C, Rapoport AM: Update on the pharmacological treatment of chronic migraine, *Curr Pain Headache Rep* 20(6):2016. doi:10.1007/s11916-015-0533-9.

Teng J, Mekhail N: Neuropathic pain: mechanisms and treatment options, World Institute of Pain, *Pain Pract* 3:8–21, 2003.

USP Center for Advancement of Patient Safety: *Use caution: avoid confusion. USP Quality Review No. 79*, Rockville, MD, 2004, USP Center for Advancement of Patient Safety.

11

Treatment of Sleep Disorders and Attention-Deficit Hyperactivity Disorder

LEARNING OBJECTIVES

1. Learn the terminology associated with sleep disorders and attention-deficit hyperactivity disorder (ADHD).
2. Discuss the reasons why sleep is necessary.
3. Describe the phases of a normal sleep cycle.
4. Describe symptoms associated with sleep deprivation.
5. Describe the types of sleep disorders.
6. Describe the function of neurotransmitters associated with symptoms of sleep.
7. Classify medications used in the treatment of sleep disorders.
8. Describe mechanism of action for each class of drugs used to treat sleep disorders.
9. Identify warning labels and precautionary messages associated with medications used to treat sleep disorders.
10. Describe the etiology of ADHD.
11. Classify medications used in the treatment of ADHD.
12. Describe mechanism of action for each class of drugs used to treat ADHD.
13. Identify warning labels and precautionary messages associated with medications used to treat ADHD.
14. Identify significant drug look-alike/sound-alike issues.

KEY TERMS

Hypnotic Drug that induces sleep.
Insomnia Condition characterized by difficulty falling asleep, staying asleep, or both.
Melatonin Hormone that is released by the pineal gland that makes a person feel drowsy.
Non-REM sleep Stages 1 through 4 of the sleep cycle.
Rapid eye movement (REM) sleep The stage of sleep when dreaming occurs.

Rebound hypersomnia Condition associated with excessive sleep that follows long-term insomnia or the use of drugs that depress REM and non-REM sleep.
Sedative Drug that causes relaxation and promotes drowsiness.
Stimulant Drug that increases activity in the brain and is used to treat ADHD and narcolepsy.

Overview

Sleep is a necessary biological function for the growth and maintenance of a healthy body. Sleep is needed for a healthy immune system and nervous system. Our physical and mental agility, memory, emotional and social functioning are also improved when we get sufficient sleep.

The body's sleep cycle is influenced by circadian rhythms. Circadian rhythms are biological changes that occur according to time cycles. The human body operates on a 24-hour clock; however, this clock can be manipulated by external time cues. Sunlight is the primary external time cue. Changes in sunlight and darkness are picked up by the retina in the back of the eye. The retina sends signals to the pineal gland in the brain. The pineal gland controls the release of *melatonin*, a hormone that makes people feel drowsy in addition to regulating body temperature and hormone secretion. The fact that our normal sleep–wake cycle is linked to sunlight

explains why people who work the night shift may feel uncontrollably drowsy in the middle of the night, and it explains why workplace accidents occur more frequently in the middle of the night than during the day.

The amount of time a person needs to sleep ranges between 5 and 16 hours per day. The amount of sleep needed can vary according to age. Infants may sleep up to 16 hours per day, teenagers require as much as 9 hours, and adults need as little as 5 to 8 hours. The patterns of sleep change as people age. Elderly adults often sleep for shorter time spans, sleep more lightly, and dream less than they did as young adults, although their overall sleep requirement may not change.

The normal sleep pattern involves five stages of sleep (Fig. 11.1). In *Stage 1,* the person sleeps lightly and can be awakened easily. Sudden muscle contractions of the limbs may occur similar to when a person is startled while awake, and the eyes move slowly back and forth. In *stage 2,* sleep eye movements stop, and brain

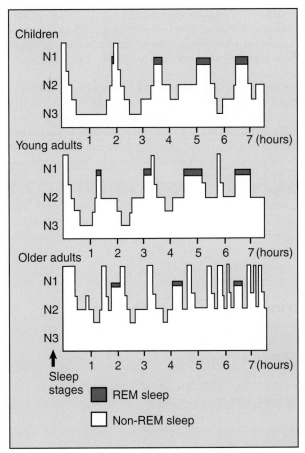

• **Fig. 11.1** Normal sleep cycle. *REM*, Rapid eye movement. (From McCance KL, Huether SE: *Pathophysiology*, ed 7, St. Louis, 2014, Elsevier.)

activity decreases. *Stage 3* and *stage 4* sleep are deep sleep. Brain activity slows (delta waves). It is difficult to wake someone from stage 3 or stage 4 sleep; if awakened, the person feels disoriented. The final stage of sleep is known as *rapid eye movement (REM) sleep* because of the characteristic eye movements that occur. This is the sleep cycle where dreaming occurs, and it lasts between 90 minutes and 110 minutes. REM sleep is crucial to normal emotional and physical functioning. Approximately 2 hours per night is spent in REM sleep. The thalamus and cerebral cortex actively communicate with each other during REM sleep. The cortex is the region of the brain involved in learning and interpretation of information.

Signs of sleep deprivation are a drowsy feeling during the day with or without micro-sleeps and falling asleep within 5 minutes of lying down. Insufficient sleep can interfere with concentration, affecting work and school. Studies attribute as many as 100,000 motor vehicle accidents in the United States each year to sleep deprivation. The rate for sleep deprivation–related motor vehicle accidents is similar to driving under the influence of alcohol. Sleep deprivation can also trigger seizures, paranoia, and hallucinations.

Factors that contribute to the inability to get adequate sleep are numerous and include sleep apnea, restless legs syndrome, consumption of caffeinated beverages and foods near bedtime, use of prescription and nonprescription drugs, psychiatric disorders, substance abuse, and chronic illness. Chronic illnesses that can interfere with sleep are gastroesophageal reflux disorder, cardiovascular disease, diabetes, and chronic pain, among others.

Sleep Disorders

Nearly one in three adults in the United States and Canada report that they get insufficient sleep. *Insomnia* is a sleep disorder that affects nearly 60 million Americans each year and up to one-third of the world population. It is categorized according to the length of time the symptoms persist. Acute insomnia typically has a sudden onset and lasts less than 3 months. Patients may have difficulty initiating sleep, maintaining sleep, poor sleep quality, and/or a short duration of sleep. Chronic insomnia lasts longer than 3 months for at least 3 nights per week. It is may be associated with a psychiatric or medical condition such as pain.

As many as 12% of the people who say they have insomnia complain about periodic leg movements. Restless legs syndrome is reported in up to 12 million Americans and is more common in elderly adults. Diabetes, pregnancy, and anemia can also cause restless leg syndrome. Sleep apnea is a sleep disorder that affects up to 25 million people in the United States. Approximately 1 in 5 Canadian adults have mild sleep apnea and 1 in 15 Canadians are at high risk for developing sleep apnea. The condition is associated with an interruption in the supply of oxygen during sleep, which causes the person to awaken. Sleep apnea can increase the risk for cardiovascular disorders such as hypertension, myocardial infarction, and stroke. People with sleep apnea also have an increased risk for arrhythmias, heart failure, diabetes, and obesity. Rarely, sleep apnea is fatal. Sudden death occurs from respiratory arrest during sleep.

Narcolepsy is the least common of the sleep disorders. It affects approximately 1 in 2000 people. It is characterized by falling asleep suddenly and without warning. Attacks may last between a few seconds and 30 minutes. In most cases the cause is unknown; however, some patients with narcolepsy have low levels of the brain chemical that controls wakefulness and arousal (hypocretin). The disorder is not usually hereditary, although it may run in some families.

Treatment of Sleep Disorders

Insomnia

Pharmacological treatments for insomnia are recommended only for short-term use. Prescription drugs, nonprescription drugs, and natural remedies are commercially available, and all produce drowsiness that enables the person to drift off to sleep (improve sleep latency) and stay asleep (improve sleep maintenance). Drugs that are used to treat insomnia are benzodiazepines, benzodiazepine receptor agonists, and melatonin. It is important to note that drugs that promote sleep do not result in a normal pattern of sleep. They alter *non-REM* and REM sleep. This can result in *rebound hypersomnia* and increased dreaming once the drugs are discontinued. Guidelines recommend prescribing the lowest effective dose and close monitoring of *sedative-hypnotics* (drugs that induce relaxation drowsiness) and sleep because most of the prescription drugs used to treat insomnia are habit forming (e.g., benzodiazepines).

Benzodiazepines and Benzodiazepine Receptor Agonists

Benzodiazepines (e.g., temazepam) and benzodiazepine-receptor agonists (e.g., zopiclone, zaleplon and zolpidem) are prescribed for the short-term treatment of insomnia.

Mechanism of Action and Pharmacokinetic. Benzodiazepines decrease neuronal excitability by opening Cl⁻ channels. The mechanism of action, pharmacokinetics, and adverse reactions of benzodiazepines were discussed in detail in Chapter 5.

The mechanism of action of benzodiazepine receptor agonists is similar to the benzodiazepines. Zaleplon, zolpidem, eszopiclone, and zopiclone act on benzodiazepine receptors subtype v-1. They modulate the GABA-A receptor chloride channel to reduce neuronal excitability. Zolpidem is available as an immediate-release tablet, controlled-release tablet, lingual spray, and sublingual tablet. Peak effects vary according to dosage form administered (≈50 minutes for the oral spray to 90 minutes for the oral tablet). Zolpidem is a biphasic controlled release formulation. Food reduces absorption, so zolpidem should be taken on an empty stomach.

Adverse Drug Effects. Nearly all of the benzodiazepine and benzodiazepine receptor agonists are controlled substances and can produce tolerance and dependence. Sedation and dizziness are other side effects common to all. Zaleplon may also produce photosensitivity, and eszopiclone and zopiclone can produce a bitter or metallic taste. Driving, preparing food and engaging in other activities while asleep, with no recollection of the behaviors, has been reported with zolpidem.

Miscellaneous Drugs Used for the Treatment of Insomnia

Doxepin (Silenor) is an antidepressant (see Chapter 6) that is marketed as a low dose (3 mg and 6 mg) for sleep disorders. Ramelteon (Rozerem) is a selective melatonin receptor agonist. Melatonin is a hormone that regulates the circadian rhythm sleep–wake cycle. Ramelteon is indicated for insomnia caused by difficulty falling asleep.

Adverse Drug Effects. Ramelteon may cause headache, dizziness, and gastrointestinal (GI) upset. It may also cause temporary memory loss and sleep walking. Doxepin may increase drowsiness and it may produce nausea.

Benzodiazepines and Benzodiazepine Receptor Agonists Used in the Treatment of Insomnia

Generic Name	US Brand Name(s) / Canadian Brand(s)	Dosage Forms and Strengths
Benzodiazepines		
estazolam[a]	Generics	**Tablets:** 1 mg, 2 mg
	Not available	
flurazepam[a]	Generics only	**Capsules:** 15 mg, 30 mg
	Generics only	
quazepam	Doral	**Tablets:** 15 mg
	Not available	
temazepam[a]	Restoril	**Capsules:** 7.5 mg[b], 15 mg, 22.5 mg[b], 30 mg
	Restoril	
triazolam[a]	Halcion	**Tablet:** 0.125 mg[b], 0.25 mg
	Generics only	
Benzodiazepine Receptor Agonists		
eszopiclone[a]	Lunesta	**Tablets:** 1 mg, 2 mg, 3 mg
	Not available	
zaleplon[a]	Sonata	**Capsules:** 5 mg, 10 mg
	Not available	
zolpidem[a]	Ambien, Ambien CR, Edluar, Intermezzo, Zolpimist	**Oromucosal spray (Zolpimist)[b]:** 5 mg **Tablets (Ambien)[b]:** 5 mg, 10 mg **Tablets, controlled release (Ambien CR)[b]:** 6.25 mg, 12.5 mg
	Sublinox	**Tablets, sublingual (Edluar, Intermezzo)[b]:** 1.75 mg, 3.5 mg, 5 mg, 10 mg **Tablet, ODT (Sublinox)[c]:** 5 mg, 10 mg
zopiclone[a]	Not available	**Tablets:** 5 mg, 7.5 mg
	Imovane	

[a]Generic available.
[b]Available in the United States only.
[c]Available in Canada only.

Miscellaneous Drugs Used for the Treatment of Insomnia

Generic Name	US Brand Name(s) Canadian Brand(s)	Dosage Forms and Strengths
doxepin[a]	Silenor	**Tablets:** 3 mg, 6 mg
	Silenor	
ramelteon[a]	Rozerem	**Tablets:** 8 mg
	Not available	

[a]Generic available.

Over-the-Counter Medications and Herbals Used in the Treatment of Insomnia

Generic Name	US Brand Name(s) Canadian Brand(s)	Dosage Forms and Strengths
diphenhydramine[a]	Nytol Quickcaps, Simply Sleep, Sleep-Eze 3, Unisom SleepMelts, Unisom SleepGels, Sleepinal, Sominex	**Capsules:** 25 mg, 50 mg **Solution, oral:** 6.25 mg/5 mL[b], 12.5 mg/5 mL, 25 mg/5 mL **Tablets:** 25 mg, 50 mg **Tablets, ODT (Unisom SleepMelts):** 25 mg
	Extra Strength Nytol Quickgels, Extra Strength Nytol tabs, Jack & Jill Bedtime, Simply Sleep, Sleep-Eze	
doxylamine[a]	Aldex AN, Doxytex, Unisom SleepTabs	**Solution, oral:** 2.5 mg/2.5 mL **Suspension, oral:** 2.5 mg/2.5 mL **Tablets:** 25 mg **Tablets, chewable:** 5 mg
	Unisom	
melatonin[a]	Generics	**Capsules:** 2.5 mg **Capsules, extended release:** 10 mg **Tablet:** 1 mg, 3 mg, 5 mg
	Generics	
valerian[a]	Generics	**Capsule:** 400 mg, 500 mg, 530 mg **Extract:** 50 mg, 250 mg
	Generics	

[a]Generic available.
[b]Available in Canada only.

OTC and Natural Remedies for Insomnia

Several natural remedies have proven effectiveness for promoting sleep; they are melatonin and valerian root. Melatonin is a hormone that is produced by the pineal gland; it is sensitive to light changes and tells the body it is time to sleep. Doses of 3 mg to 5 mg have been used for treatment of short-term insomnia and enhancement of sleep. The greatest evidence for efficacy of melatonin is in prevention of jet lag. The use of valerian root dates back more than 2000 years. Galen recommended it for the treatment of insomnia. A dose of 600 mg aqueous extract, taken 1 hour before bedtime, has been shown to be effective. Diphenhydramine and doxylamine are other (OTC) drugs that are used for short-term relief of insomnia.

Adverse Drug Effects. Diphenhydramine and doxylamine should be avoided in men who have benign prostatic hypertrophy because they cause urinary retention. The antihistamines may also reduce the milk supply of breastfeeding women.

Nonpharmacological Treatments

It is best to avoid the things that can cause sleeplessness when possible. Insomnia prevention tips include the following:

- Avoid stimulants close to bedtime. Caffeinated beverage such as colas, tea, chocolate, fortified water, OTC decongestants, and ephedra containing herbals are **stimulants** and can cause insomnia if consumed near bedtime.
- Adopt a regular sleeping schedule. A routine sleep schedule provides a cue that sleep time is approaching.
- Avoid daytime naps. Naps disrupt the normal sleep cycle.
- Create a safe, comfortable sleeping environment, if possible. Fears about safety and extremes in temperature can prevent sleep.
- Do not go to bed hungry, if possible. Hunger can prevent sleep.
- Exercise 20 to 30 minutes each day (not at bedtime). Maximum benefits are achieved if exercise is performed 5 to 6 hours before bedtime. Exercise before bedtime can interfere with sleep.
- Avoid ambient lighting produced by electronic devices such as cell phones, tablets, laptops and televisions. Turn off devices before bedtime.
- Do not lie in bed awake. If you do not fall asleep, get up and engage in a nonstimulating activity such as reading. Try to go to sleep again in about 10 minutes.

Summary of Drugs Used in the Treatment of Insomnia

	Generic Name	US Brand Name	Usual Adult Oral Dose and Dosing Schedule	Controlled Substance Schedule (United States)	NAPRA[a] Schedule (Canada)	Warning Labels
Benzodiazepine and Benzodiazepine Receptor Agonists						
	eszopiclone	Lunesta	1–3 mg at bedtime	C-IV		MAY CAUSE DROWSINESS; MAY IMPAIR THE ABILITY TO DRIVE. AVOID ALCOHOL. MAY BE HABIT FORMING. TAKE 30 MIN BEFORE BEDTIME.
	estazolam	Generics	1–2 mg at bedtime	C-IV		
	flurazepam	Dalmane	15–30 mg at bedtime	C-IV	TS[b]	
	quazepam	Doral	7.5–15 mg at bedtime	C-IV		
	temazepam	Restoril	7.5–30 mg at bedtime	C-IV	TS	
	triazolam	Halcion	0.125–0.25 mg at bedtime	C-IV	TS	
	zaleplon	Sonata	5–20 mg at bedtime	C-IV		
	zolpidem	Ambien	Dissolve 1 tab (5–10 mg) under tongue each night (Intermezzo SL, Edular SL) 6.25–12 mg immediately before bed (extended release)	C-IV		
	zopiclone	Imovane	3.75–7.5 mg at bedtime			
Miscellaneous						
	doxepin	Silenor	3–6 mg 30 min before bedtime			MAY CAUSE DROWSINESS; MAY IMPAIR THE ABILITY TO DRIVE—all. AOID TAKING AFTER EATING A HIGH FAT MEAL—ramelteon. AVOID ALCOHOL—all. SWALLOW WHOLE; DO NOT CRUSH OR CHEW—extended release. DISSOLVE SUBLINGUALLY—Edluar, Sublinox. MAY BE HABIT FORMING—all targeted and controlled substances.
	ramelteon	Rozerem	8 mg at bedtime			

[a]NAPRA, National Association of Pharmacy Regulatory Authorities.
[b]TS, Targeted substance.

Narcolepsy

Narcolepsy is a relatively rare condition in which a person suddenly falls asleep, often in response to an emotional stimulus such as laughter or fear. The primary treatment for narcolepsy is the administration of stimulants. Stimulants used in the treatment of narcolepsy include amphetamine, methylphenidate, modafinil, and armodafinil. Modafinil and armodafinil are nonamphetamine stimulants. The drugs' mechanisms of action are not fully known, but it is believed they stimulate alpha$_1$-adrenergic receptor sites. Modafinil and armodafinil are also prescribed for the treatment of sleep apnea. Amphetamine and methylphenidate are stimulants that are classified as sympathomimetics. A sympathomimetic is a drug that mimics the effects produced by stimulation of the sympathetic nervous system. A detailed discussion of amphetamine and methylphenidate is described in the section on treatment for attention-deficit hyperactivity disorder (ADHD).

Side Effects and Precautions

The most common adverse effects produced by armodafinil and modafinil are headache, nausea, insomnia, and dizziness. The drugs may produce tolerance and dependence and are C-IV controlled substances in the United States. Stevens-Johnson syndrome, a fatal drug rash, has been linked to modafinil use. Armodafinil and modafinil may decrease the effect of oral contraceptives.

● *TECH NOTE!*

Warning labels that should be affixed to prescription vials for modafinil are:
AVOID ALCOHOL.
MAY DECREASE THE EFFECT OF ORAL CONTRACEPTIVES.
MAY BE HABIT FORMING.

● *TECH NOTE!*

Modafinil should be taken in the morning to avoid insomnia.

Attention-Deficit Hyperactivity Disorder

Attention-Deficit Hyperactivity Disorder (ADHD) is the most commonly diagnosed childhood behavioral disorder. In the United States, more than 10% of school-age children (5 to 17 years) have ADHD. In Canada, the percentage ranges between 5% and 12%. Although most statistics are gathered about children, ADHD affects adolescents and adults, too.

Symptoms of ADHD are also commonly observed in children without ADHD, making diagnosis challenging (Fig. 11.2). These symptoms are hyperactivity, restlessness, an inability to sit still when required, impulsiveness, inattention, distractibility, forgetfulness, and an inability to complete tasks. All children sometimes exhibit these behaviors. A diagnosis of ADHD should only be made when these behaviors occur more frequently than would be expected for the child's age and if the behavior interferes with two or more areas of the child's life. These areas are defined as school, playground, home, community, and social relationships.

There are three subtypes of ADHD: they are predominantly hyperactive-impulsive, predominantly inattentive, and combined type. It is important to note that children who are diagnosed with predominantly inattentive type (attention-deficit disorder [ADD]) rarely exhibit hyperactivity and impulsiveness. Learning disorders such as dyslexia occur in approximately 20% to 30% of children with ADHD.

There is no single cause for ADHD. Genetics is most strongly linked to ADHD. Up to 25% of children who have a parent, sibling, or other close family relative with ADHD also have ADHD. The rate is only 5% in the general population.

Exposure to environmental agents such as cigarette smoke and alcohol during pregnancy has shown to increase the risk for ADHD. Exposure to high levels of lead-based paint also increases the risk. This is an important risk factor for children who live in older urban cities and attend school in old buildings that were painted with lead-based paint before it was banned. There is also an increased risk of ADHD in children who live in developing countries that still use leaded gasoline.

Some people believe that consumption of food additives and sugar can make ADHD worse. When placed on a diet that restricted these food additives, approximately 5% of children with ADHD showed improvement in symptoms.

Treatments for Attention-Deficit Hyperactivity Disorder

A variety of drug treatments are available for treating patients with ADHD however, medications cannot cure ADHD. They only control symptoms. The most effective therapy for ADHD involves drug treatment in addition to behavioral therapy. The goal of behavioral therapy is to decrease anxiety and improve relationships and social skills.

Look for signs of ADHD.

Put a check mark next to each one that sounds like your child. ☑

My child often…
☐ is moving something—fingers, hands, arms, feet, or legs.
☐ walks, runs, or climbs around when others are seated.
☐ has trouble waiting in line or taking turns.
☐ doesn't finish things.
☐ gets bored after just a short while.
☐ daydreams or seems to be in another world.
☐ talks when other people are talking.
☐ gets frustrated with schoolwork or homework.
☐ acts quickly without thinking first.
☐ is sidetracked by what is going on around him or her.

● **Fig. 11.2** Checklist for signs of attention-deficit hyperactivity disorder (ADHD). (Courtesy National Institute of Mental Health, Bethesda, MD.)

Drugs Used for the Treatment of Narcolepsy

Generic Name	US Brand Name(s) / Canadian Brand(s)	Dosage Forms and Strengths	Usual Adult Dose	US Controlled Substance Schedule
armodafinil[a]	Nuvigil / Not available	**Tablets:** 50 mg, 150 mg, 200 mg, 250 mg	150–250 mg every morning	C-IV
modafinil[a]	Provigil / Alertec	**Tablets:** 100 mg, 200 mg[b]	200–400 mg daily once daily.	C-IV

[a]Generic available.
[b]Available in the United States only.

Pharmaceutical treatment of ADHD is achieved with the administration of amphetamines and nonamphetamine stimulants. Amphetamines behave differently in people who have ADHD than they do in people without ADHD. They decrease hyperactivity and improve focus, rather than producing hyperactivity and a lack of focused behavior.

> **⊘ TECH ALERT!**
>
> The following drugs have look-alike/sound-alike issues:
> Ritalin, Ritalin SR, and Ritalin LA

Mechanism of Action and Pharmacokinetics

Amphetamines are sympathomimetics structurally similar to norepinephrine. They work via three primary mechanisms: they stimulate the release of norepinephrine, block monoamine oxidase (further increasing catecholamine levels), and stimulate the release of dopamine. Increased stimulation of adrenergic receptors by norepinephrine is responsible for the increased alertness, responsiveness, wakefulness, and reduced awareness of fatigue.

Amphetamines are well absorbed from the GI tract, and their lipid solubility enables them to cross the blood-brain barrier. They are metabolized in the liver and eliminated in the urine. Lisdexamfetamine is a prodrug that is metabolized to dextroamphetamine. Amphetamines are manufactured in immediate-release, sustained-release, and extended-release dosage forms. The duration of action varies according to the dosage form administered. Atomoxetine is a nonamphetamine stimulant. It inhibits the reuptake of norepinephrine.

> **● TECH NOTE!**
>
> Stimulants should be taken in the morning to avoid insomnia.

> **● TECH NOTE!**
>
> Metadate CD and Ritalin LA capsules may be opened and the contents sprinkled on cold applesauce.

Adverse Reactions

The most common side effects produced by amphetamines are decreased appetite, nausea, stomachache, anxiety, and irritability. They can also cause insomnia. Insomnia can be minimized if the last dose is taken before 6 PM. Sympathetic nervous system stimulation produced by amphetamines is responsible for these drugs' cardiovascular effects. Amphetamines can cause increased heart rate, palpitations, and arrhythmia. Other side effects produced by amphetamines are dizziness and tremor. Doses greater than therapeutic doses can produce amphetamine syndrome, a type of drug-induced psychosis.

> **● TECH NOTE!**
>
> The following warning labels should be affixed to prescription vials for amphetamines:
> TAKE WITH FOOD.
> MAY BE HABIT FORMING.
> SWALLOW WHOLE; DO NOT CRUSH OR CHEW (sustained-release and extended-release).
> ROTATE SITE OF APPLICATION (Daytrana patch).

Precautions

Amphetamines have a high abuse potential. They are all Schedule C-II controlled substances in the United States. They are also controlled in Canada (National Association of Pharmacy Regulatory Authorities schedule C1). Atomoxetine is not a controlled substance.

> **● TECH NOTE!**
>
> The methylphenidate transdermal patch (Daytrana) should be worn for only 9 hours each day and then removed.

> **TECHNICIAN'S CORNER**
>
> 1. Does diet and lack of exercise or lack of attention have anything to do with the number of children diagnosed with ADHD?
> 2. What would you recommend to someone with a sleep disorder who does not want to take any sleep aids?

Drugs Used for the Treatment of Attention-Deficit Hyperactivity Disorder

Generic Name	US Brand Name(s) Canadian Brand(s)	Dosage Forms and Strengths
amphetamine	Adzenys XR-ODT, Dynanavel XR, Evekeo	**Suspension, oral:** 1.25 mg/mL, 2.5 mg/mL **Tablet:** 5 mg, 10 mg **Tablets, extended release, disintegrating:(Adzenys XR-ODT):** 3.1 mg, 6.3 mg, 9.4 mg, 12.5 mg, 15.7 mg, 18.8 mg
	Not available	
amphetamine + dextroamphetamine[a]	Adderall XR	**Capsules, extended release (Adderall XR):** 5 mg, 10 mg, 15 mg, 20 mg, 25 mg, 30 mg
	Adderall XR	
dextroamphetamine[a]	Dexedrine,	**Capsules, extended release (Dexedrine spansule):** 5 mg[b], 10 mg, 15 mg
	Dexedrine, Dexedrine Spansule	**Tablets: immediate release (Dexedrine):** 5 mg
dexmethylphenidate[a]	Focalin, Focalin XR	**Capsule, extended release:** 5 mg, 10 mg, 15 mg, 20 mg, 25 mg, 30 mg, 35 mg, 40 mg
	Not available	**Tablets:** 2.5 mg, 5 mg, 10 mg

Drugs Used for the Treatment of Attention-Deficit Hyperactivity Disorder—cont'd

Generic Name	US Brand Name(s) / Canadian Brand(s)	Dosage Forms and Strengths
lisdexamfetamine	Vyvanse Vyvanse	**Capsules:** 10 mg, 20 mg, 30 mg, 40 mg, 50 mg, 60 mg, 70 mg **Tablet, chewable:** 10 mg, 20 mg, 30 mg, 40 mg, 50 mg, 60 mg
methylphenidate[a]	Aptensio XR, Cotempla XR-ODT, Concerta, Daytrana, Metadate CD, Metadate ER, Methylin, Quillichew, Ritalin, Ritalin LA, Ritalin SR Biphentin, Concerta, Foquest, Ritalin, Ritalin SR	**Capsules, biphasic extended release (Aptensio XR, Biphentin, Metadate CD, Ritalin LA):** 10 mg, 20 mg, 30 mg, 40 mg, 50 mg, 60 mg, 15 mg (Aptensio XR, Biphentin) and 80 mg (Biphentin only) **Capsule, controlled release (Foquest)[c]:** 25 mg, 35 mg, 45 mg, 55 mg, 70 mg, 85 mg, 100 mg **Capsule, for suspension (Qullivant XR):** 5 mg/mL **Solution, oral (Methylin):** 2 mg/mL, 1 mg/mL **Tablets, chewable:** 2.5 mg, 5 mg, 10 mg **Tablets, chewable extended release (Quillichew):** 20 mg, 30 mg, 40 mg **Tablets, extended release (Concerta):** 18 mg, 27 mg, 36 mg, 54 mg **Tablets, extended release (Metadate ER):** 10 mg, 20 mg **Tablets, immediate release (Ritalin):** 5 mg[b], 10 mg, 20 mg **Tablet, oral disintegrating (Cotempla XR-ODT):** 8.6 mg, 17.3 mg, 25.9 mg **Tablets, sustained release (Ritalin SR):** 20 mg **Transdermal patch (Daytrana):** 10 mg/9 hr, 15 mg/9 hr, 20 mg/9 hr, 30 mg/9 hr
atomoxetine[a]	Strattera Strattera	**Capsules:** 10 mg, 18 mg, 25 mg, 40 mg, 60 mg, 80 mg, 100 mg

[a]Generic available.
[b]Available in the United States only.
[c]Available in Canada only.

Summary of Drugs Used in the Treatment of Attention-Deficit Hyperactivity Disorder

Generic Name	Brand Name	Usual Child Dosage	Controlled Substance Schedule (Canada)
Amphetamines			
amphetamine + dextroamphetamine (Immediate release)	Adderall	2.5–40 mg/day (1–2 doses/day)	C-II (CDSA I)
amphetamine + dextroamphetamine (Extended release)	Adderall XR	5–30 mg every morning	C-II (CDSA I)
dextroamphetamine (Immediate release)	Dexedrine, Dextrostat	2.5–40 mg 1–2 doses per day	C-II (CDSA I)
dexmethylphenidate	Focalin	2.5–20 mg/day given as 2 doses/day	C-II (CDSA III)
lisdexamfetamine	Vyvanse	30–70 mg once daily	C-II (CDSA III)
methylphenidate (Immediate release)	Ritalin	10–20 mg twice a day up to 60 mg/day	C-II (CDSA III)

Continued

Summary of Drugs Used in the Treatment of Attention-Deficit Hyperactivity Disorder—cont'd

	Generic Name	Brand Name	Usual Child Dosage	Controlled Substance Schedule (Canada)
	methylphenidate (Extended release)	Concerta	18–72 mg once daily	C-II (CDSA III)
		Ritalin LA	20 mg once a day up to 60 mg/day	C-II (CDSA III)
		Metadate CD	20 mg once a day up to 60 mg/day	C-II (CDSA III)
		Cotempla XR-ODT	17.3-51.8 mg/day	C-II
		Metadate ER	May replace methylphenidate immediate release (IR) when 8-hr dosage of methylphenidate ER corresponds to the titrated 8-hour dosage of methylphenidate IR (maximum 60 mg/day)	C-II (CDSA III)
	methylphenidate (Sustained release)	Ritalin SR	20–30 mg daily (May replace of immediate release tablets when 8-hr dosage of methylphenidate SR corresponds to the titrated 8-hour dosage of methylphenidate IR; not to exceed 60 mg/day)	C-II (CDSA III)
	methylphenidate (Transdermal patch)	Daytrana	1 patch worn for 9 h per day	C-II (CDSA III)
Nonamphetamine	atomoxetine	Strattera	40–80 mg/day in 1–2 divided doses (Maximum 100 mg per day)	Not Controlled

Key Points

- Sleep is needed for a healthy immune system and nervous system, healthy emotional and social functioning, as well as physical and mental agility.
- The pineal gland controls the release of melatonin, a hormone that makes people feel drowsy.
- Infants may sleep up to 16 hours per day, teenagers require as much as 9 hours, and adults need as little as 5 to 8 hours. Patterns of sleep change as people age.
- There are five stages of sleep (four non–REM stages and REM).
- Dreaming occurs during REM sleep and is crucial to normal emotional and physical functioning.
- Sleep apnea can increase the risk for hypertension, myocardial infarction, and stroke, and is linked to arrhythmias, heart failure, diabetes, and obesity.
- Sleep apnea, restless legs syndrome, consumption of caffeinated beverages and foods, use of prescription and nonprescription drugs, and chronic illness can cause insomnia.
- Pharmacological treatment for insomnia is recommended for short-term use.
- Prescription drugs, nonprescription drugs, and herbal remedies are commercially available, and all produce drowsiness that enables the person to drift off to sleep and stay asleep.
- Prescription drugs used to treat insomnia are benzodiazepines and nonbenzodiazepine sedative-hypnotics.
- Drugs that promote sleep do not result in a normal pattern of sleep. They alter non-REM and REM sleep.
- Rebound hypersomnia and increased dreaming occur after the drugs are discontinued.

- The mechanism of action for zaleplon, zolpidem, eszopiclone, and zopiclone is similar to that of benzodiazepines.
- Melatonin and valerian root are herbal remedies that have proven effectiveness for promoting sleep.
- Insomnia prevention tips include (1) avoid stimulants close to bedtime; (2) adopt a regular sleeping schedule; (3) avoid daytime naps; (4) create a safe comfortable sleeping environment, if possible; (5) do not go to bed hungry, if possible; (6) exercise; and (7) do not lie in bed awake.
- Stimulants are administered for the treatment of narcolepsy.
- ADHD is the most commonly diagnosed childhood behavioral disorder.
- Symptoms of ADHD are hyperactivity, restlessness, an inability to sit still when required, impulsiveness, inattention, distractibility, forgetfulness, and an inability to complete tasks.
- The most effective therapy for ADHD involves a combination of drug treatments and behavioral therapy.
- Pharmaceutical treatment of ADHD is achieved with the administration of amphetamines and nonamphetamine stimulants.
- The most common side effects produced by amphetamines are decreased appetite, nausea, stomachache, anxiety, insomnia, and irritability.
- Amphetamines have a high abuse potential and are controlled substances in the United States and Canada.
- The methylphenidate patch (Daytrana) should be applied to the hip area. It should not be worn for more than 9 hours per day.

Review Questions

1. Not getting enough sleep does not affect the immune system, nervous system, or emotional and social functioning of the body.
   a. True
   b. False
2. Circadian rhythms are biological changes that occur according to _____ cycles.
   a. growth
   b. age
   c. time
   d. health
3. The pineal gland controls the release of _____, a hormone that makes people feel drowsy in addition to regulating body temperature and hormone secretion.
   a. serotonin
   b. melatonin
   c. dopamine
   d. acetylcholine
4. Select the drug that is NOT a controlled or targeted substance in the United States and Canada.
   a. Adderall
   b. Ritalin
   c. Restoril
   d. Strattera
5. Pharmacological treatment for insomnia is recommended for long-term use.
   a. True
   b. False
6. You receive a prescription for Concerta 10 mg 1 tablet once daily. You consult with the pharmacist because_____
   a. methylphenidate is not marketed as 10 mg.
   b. Concerta is not available in a 10 mg tablet.
   c. Ritalin is not dosed once daily.
   d. the dose is too low.
7. Zaleplon and zolpidem are benzodiazepines.
   a. True
   b. False
8. The primary treatment for ADHD is administration of stimulants.
   a. True
   b. False
9. Pharmaceutical treatment of insomnia is achieved with the administration of all of the following EXCEPT _____.
   a. methylphenidate
   b. zolpidem
   c. temazepam
   d. doxepin
10. Amphetamines have a high abuse potential and are classified as Schedule _____ controlled substances in the United States.
    a. C-I
    b. C-II
    c. C-IV
    d. C-III

Bibliography

American Academy of Sleep Medicine. "Rising prevalence of sleep apnea in U.S. threatens public health." ScienceDaily. ScienceDaily, 29 September 2014. www.sciencedaily.com/releases/2014/09/140929105443.htm.

Centers for Disease Control. 1 in 3 Adults Don't Get Enough Sleep. Retrieved March 2, 2017, from https://www.cdc.gov/media/releases/2016/p0215-enough-sleep.html.

Centers for Disease Control. (2015). Attention Deficit Hyperactivity Disorder- Fast Stats. Retrieved March 2, 2017, from https://www.cdc.gov/nchs/fastats/adhd.htm.

Ford ES, Wheaton AG, Cunningham TJ, et al: Trends in outpatient visits for insomnia, sleep apnea, and prescriptions for sleep medications among US adults: findings from the National Ambulatory Medical Care Survey, 1999-2010, Sleep 37:1283–1293, 2014.

FDA. (nd). Drugs@FDA: FDA Approved Drug Products. Retrieved July 10, 2018, from http://www.accessdata.fda.gov/scripts/cder/daf/.

Health Canada. (2017). Drug Product Database. Retrieved July 10, 2018, from https://health-products.canada.ca/dpd-bdpp/index-eng.jsp.

Institute for Safe Medication Practices. (2015). List of Confused Drugs. Retrieved September 9, 2017, from https://www.ismp.org/tools/confuseddrugnames.pdf.

Institute for Safe Medication Practices. (2016). FDA and ISMP Lists of Look-Alike Drug Names with Recommended Tall Man Letters.

Kalant H, Grant D, Mitchell J: Principles of medical pharmacology, ed 7, Toronto, 2007, Elsevier Canada, A Division of Reed Elsevier Canada, pp 339–342.

National Institute of Mental Health: Attention deficit hyperactivity disorder, Bethesda (MD), 2016, National Institute of Mental Health, National Institutes of Health, US Department of Health and Human Services. https://www.nimh.nih.gov/health/topics/attention-deficit-hyperactivity-disorder-adhd/index.shtml.

National Institute of Neurological Disorders and Stroke, National Institute of Health, U.S. Department of Health and Humans Services: Brain basics: understanding sleep, Bethesda, 2017, National Institute of Neurological disorders and stroke. NIH publication No. 17-3440-c.

Public Health Agency of Canada: Fast Facts from the 2009 Canadian Community Health Survey—Sleep Apnea Rapid Response, 2010. Retrieved March 5, 2011, from http://www.phac-aspc.gc.ca/cd-mc/sleepapnea-apneesommeil/pdf/sleep-apnea.pdf.

Ramar K, Olson EJ: Management of Common Sleep Disorders, American Academy of Family Physicians 88(4):2013. http://www.aafp.org/afp.

Raffa R, Rawls S, Beyzarov E: Netter's illustrated pharmacology, Philadelphia, 2005, WB Saunders, pp 80–82.

Toward Optimized Practice. (2015). Assessment to Management of Adult Insomnia Clinical Practice Guideline. Retrieved March 2, 2017, from www.topalbertadoctors.org.

UNIT III

Drugs Affecting the Musculoskeletal System

The proper functioning of the joints of musculoskeletal system is crucial for purposeful movement because it provides form, support, stability, and movement to the body. A number of body systems support the function of muscle tissues and the proper functioning of the joints of the skeleton. Overexertion or trauma may cause muscle strain, muscle pain (myalgia), muscle bruising (contusion), or sprains. Muscle tension in the head and neck can cause tension headaches. Diseases of the musculature may be caused by autoimmune disorders (e.g., multiple sclerosis and rheumatoid arthritis); infection by bacteria, viruses, or parasites that can produce myositis, *tetanus*, or poliomyelitis; and genetics (e.g., muscular dystrophy). Inflammatory disorders (e.g., bursitis and arthritis) affect large weight-bearing joints (e.g., hip, knees) and are characterized by morning stiffness, limited joint motion, and deep achy pain on movement.

In Unit III, pharmacotherapy for muscle spasms, conditions requiring neuromuscular blockade, gout, rheumatoid arthritis, osteoarthritis, osteoporosis, and Paget disease are described. A brief description of each disorder is provided, followed by a description of the drugs indicated for treatment that includes mechanisms of action, adverse reactions, strength(s), and dosage forms. Musculoskeletal disorders such as inflammation and pain are treated with nonsteroidal anti-inflammatory drugs (NSAIDS), locally acting corticosteroids, and skeletal muscle relaxants. Biological response modifiers (e.g. Humira®) are used in the treatment of autoimmune disorders such as rheumatoid arthritis. Non-pharmacological therapy to prevent injury and wear and tear of the skeletal and muscular systems (e.g., daily exercise) is also discussed.

12

Neuromuscular Blockade and Muscle Spasms

KEY TERMS

Acetylcholinesterase Enzyme that degrades acetylcholine and reverses acetylcholine-induced depolarization.

Amyotrophic lateral sclerosis (ALS) Degenerative disease that causes muscle wasting and muscle weakness. ALS is also known as Lou Gehrig disease.

Anaphylactic shock Acute, life-threatening allergic reaction that produces peripheral vasodilation, bronchospasm, laryngeal edema, and airway obstruction.

Botulinum toxin Toxin produced by the bacterium *Clostridium botulinum* that causes muscle paralysis.

Central-acting muscle relaxants Drugs that produce relaxation of muscles by blocking nerve transmission between the spinal cord and muscles.

Cerebral palsy Neurologic disorder that affects muscle movement and coordination.

Clonus Involuntary rhythmic muscle contraction that causes the feet and wrists to involuntarily flex and relax.

Depolarizing neuromuscular blockers Drugs that act as agonists at acetylcholine receptor sites and produce sustained depolarization whereby the receptors to convert to an inactive state.

Endotracheal intubation Process of inserting a tube into the trachea or windpipe to facilitate mechanical ventilation.

End plate Projection extending off the end of a motor neuron where the neurotransmitter acetylcholine is released.

Multiple sclerosis Autoimmune disease that causes progressive damage to nerves resulting in spasticity, pain, mood changes, and other physical symptoms.

Neuromuscular junction Space between motor neuron end plate and the muscle sole plate that neurotransmitters must cross.

Nondepolarizing competitive blockers Drugs that compete with acetylcholine for binding sites. When acetylcholine binding is inhibited, muscle contraction is blocked.

Peripheral-acting muscle relaxants Drugs that block nerve transmission between the motor end plate and skeletal muscle receptors.

Sarcomere Contracting unit of muscle fibers.

Sole plate Portion of the membrane of muscle cells that receives messages transmitted by motor neurons.

Spasticity Motor disorder that causes increased muscle tone, exaggerated tendon jerks, and hyperexcitable muscles.

Tetanus Potentially fatal condition characterized by continuous muscle spasm that is caused by exposure to the nerve toxin produced by the bacterium *Clostridium tetani*. It is also known as "lockjaw."

Overview

Skeletal muscles contract as a response to messages transmitted between peripheral nerves and muscles by neurotransmitters. Acetylcholine (ACh) is the primary neurotransmitter that sends messages between nerve cells and muscle cells. The process begins with the release of ACh from vesicles located in the motor neuron end plate. The *end plate* is a projection extending off the end of one of the branches of the motor neuron. The end of the motor neuron may be divided into as many as 200 branches. The *sole plate* is the portion of the membrane of muscle cells that receives messages transmitted by motor neurons.

Drugs that block nerve transmission between the motor end plate and skeletal muscle receptors are classified as *peripheral-acting muscle relaxants*. Peripheral-acting drugs are further classified according to their mechanism of action. They are classified as *nondepolarizing competitive blockers* and depolarizing blockers. *Central-acting muscle relaxants* are direct-acting agents that bind to and block calcium channels. Skeletal muscle relaxants that work by CNS depression (i.e., block nerve transmission between the spinal cord and muscles) are examples of central-acting muscle relaxants.

The release of ACh produces skeletal muscle contraction. Calcium increases ACh release. Drugs that decrease the release ACh or deplete ACh levels in the neuron also cause skeletal muscle relaxation. *Botulinum toxin* and magnesium are examples of drugs that decrease the release of ACh. Black widow spider venom causes a massive release of ACh from vesicles that is independent of calcium. The venom causes muscle contractions and cramping. If untreated, depletion of ACh causes paralysis. The effect of ethanol on ACh is dose dependent.

> ### ● TECH NOTE!
>
> The US Food and Drug Administration (FDA) has issued a warning that onabotulinumtoxin type A (Botox) and botulinum toxin rimabotulinumtoxin type B (Myobloc) injections may spread beyond the injection site and the toxins' effects may produce respiratory failure and death (2010).

Indication

Neuromuscular blocking agents have been used historically by Indigenous peoples of South America. They were first used in surgery in 1942 and continue to be used currently to induce a controlled, temporary state of paralysis. They are most commonly used in general anesthesia for endotracheal intubation to facilitate mechanical ventilation. *Endotracheal intubation* is the process of inserting a tube into the trachea or windpipe. Onabotulinum-toxinA, commonly known as Botox, is a neuromuscular blocking drug that is used in an outpatient setting. Its use is becoming widespread, and it has been FDA approved for a variety of conditions, including temporary removal of wrinkles, treatment of excessive sweating, spasticity, uncontrollable blinking, and chronic migraine (headache more than 15 days per month).

Care must be taken when transcribing and filling orders for neuromuscular blocking drugs because they can cause severe injury or death. To prevent possible injury or death, the United States Pharmacopoeia (USP) Interdisciplinary Safe Medication Use Expert Committee has compiled a list of recommendations for the safe use of neuromuscular blocking agents. The recommendations listed in Box 12.1 are modified for pharmacy-specific application.

> ### ❶ TECH ALERT!
>
> Institute for Safe Medication Practices (ISMP) Canada recommends adoption of the USP standards for drug vials containing neuromuscular blocking agents. The lids of the vials are clearly marked "Paralyzing Agent" or "Warning: Paralyzing Agent" (Fig. 12.1).

Mechanism of Action

Depolarizing neuromuscular blockers are agonists at nicotinic receptors. They bind to ACh receptors, where they produce

> ### •BOX 12.1 Safe Management of Neuromuscular Blocking Agents: Recommendations for Pharmacy Practice
>
> **Product Selection**
> - Procurement managers should select products that have distinctive names and packaging to avoid sound-alike/look-alike issues.
>
> **Product Storage**
> - Neuromuscular blocking drugs should be stored apart from other drugs.
> - Storage of neuromuscular blocking drugs should be confined to primary care areas and pharmacy areas that care for mechanically ventilated patients.
> - Storage conditions for undiluted and diluted solutions should be clearly marked.
>
> **Limit Access**
> - Neuromuscular blocking drugs should be kept in sealed "intubation kits" or "anesthesia kits" until use is needed.
> - Opened vials should be immediately discarded or returned to the seal kit after use.
> - Neuromuscular blocking drugs should NOT be dispensed in unit dose carts or delivered to general nursing units unless in a sealed kit.
> - Neuromuscular blocking drugs should be stored in a single access drawer when stored in drug storage devices such as Pyxis and AccuDose-Rx.
> - Neuromuscular blocking drugs requiring refrigeration should be stored in a separate area away from other refrigerated drugs.
>
> **Auxiliary Labels or Warning Labels**
> - Neuromuscular blocking drugs should always be dispensed with the auxiliary label "WARNING: Paralyzing agent. (Use requires mechanical ventilatory assistance.)"
> - Overwraps should be considered for individual vials of neuromuscular blocking drugs stored outside of pharmacy and anesthesiology areas, especially drugs stored in the refrigerator.
> - Affix preprinted syringe labels to syringes filled with neuromuscular blocking drugs at the time the drug is drawn up to avoid risks associated with unlabeled syringes.
>
> **Ordering Practices and Dispensing**
> - Contact prescriber for complete directions when medication orders for neuromuscular blocking agents are written with 'as needed' (PRN) directions.
> - Verify patient identity and drug identity with barcode readers when available.
>
> *Adapted from United States Pharmacopoeia Interdisciplinary Safe Medication Use Expert Committee recommendations.*

sustained depolarization. Prolonged depolarization causes receptors to convert to their inactive state. Depolarization is the process whereby the cell undergoes a shift in electric charge. Positive ions enter the cell (e.g., calcium). When the endplate potential exceeds 15 mV, an action potential is produced (Fig. 12.2). The receptors become desensitized, and contractions are prevented until the receptors return to their preactivated state.

Succinylcholine is the only depolarizing neuromuscular blocker currently available. Similar to ACh, it is rapidly inactivated by cholinesterase enzymes. Cholinesterase enzymes are synthesized in the liver and are responsible for the breakdown of succinylcholine.

Nondepolarizing Neuromuscular Blockers

Most nondepolarizing neuromuscular blockers are competitive antagonists at prejunctional and postjunctional receptors. At low doses, they produce no effects of their own when they bind to receptor sites; instead, they compete with ACh for binding sites. At high doses, nondepolarizing drugs weaken neuromuscular transmission and reduce the action of *acetylcholinesterase*, the enzyme that reverses ACh-induced depolarization.

> **TECH NOTE!**
>
> "-curonium" and "-curium" are common endings for nondepolarizing neuromuscular blockers.

Pharmacokinetics

Most neuromuscular blocking drugs are poorly absorbed from the gastrointestinal tract, so they are administered parenterally. They have low lipid solubility, and they do not easily cross the blood-brain barrier. They are highly water soluble and are primarily eliminated in the urine. Vecuronium is also metabolized in the liver, and its rate of elimination may be decreased if the patient has liver disease. The onset of action is rapid (1 to 4 minutes), and duration of action is short (10 to 90 minutes). This requires a continuous infusion to be administered. An exception is the duration of action for the botulinum toxins, which may last up to 12 weeks. Nondepolarizing neuromuscular blocking drugs have a longer onset and longer duration of action than depolarizing neuromuscular blocking drugs because they are not broken down by the enzyme acetylcholinesterase.

> **TECH NOTE!**
>
> Botox injections are made from a substance derived from the toxin that causes botulism (botulinum toxin).

• **Fig. 12.1** Examples of lids for vials containing neuromuscular blocking agents. (Reprinted with permission from ISMP Canada.)

Adverse Reactions

Common side effects are muscle pain, itching, or burning at the injection site. Hypotension, flushing (vasodilation), tachycardia, or bradycardia may also occur. Allergic actions that occur may be life threatening. They may appear as rash and redness on the face and neck or may be serious enough to produce bronchospasm, laryngospasm, and anaphylactic shock. Other life-threatening adverse reactions are respiratory depression and cardiac arrest and pulmonary edema. Depolarizing neuromuscular blockers (e.g., succinylcholine) cause potassium channels to remain open, producing hyperkalemia. Excess potassium may produce cardiac arrest. OnabotulinumtoxinA injections may produce muscle weakness in the injected muscles. This may cause droopy eyelid muscles *(blepharoptosis),* headache, nausea, flulike syndrome, redness, and muscle weakness.

> **TECH NOTE!**
>
> **Anaphylactic shock** is an acute, life-threatening allergic reaction that produces peripheral vasodilation, bronchospasm, laryngeal edema, and airway obstruction.

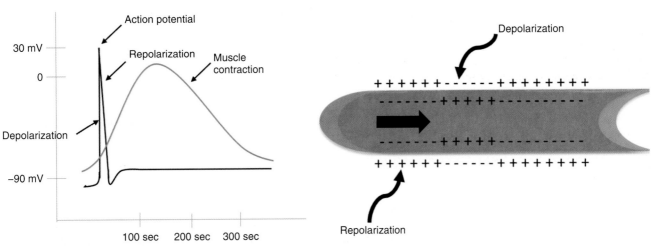

• **Fig. 12.2** Depolarization process.

Neuromuscular Blockers

Generic Name	US Brand Name(s) / Canadian Brand(s)	Dosage Forms and Strengths
Depolarizing Neuromuscular Blocking Drugs		
succinylcholine[a][b]	Anectine, Quelicin	Injection, solution: 20 mg/mL, 100 mg/mL[b]
	Quelicin	
Nondepolarizing Neuromuscular Blocking Drugs		
atracurium[a]	Generic	Injection, solution: 10 mg/mL
	Generic	
abobotulinumtoxinA	Dysport	Powder for injection: 300 units/vial, 500 units/vial
	Dysport	
onabotulinumtoxinA	Botox, Botox Cosmetic	Powder for injection: 50 units/vial[c], 100 units/vial, 200 units/vial[c]
	Botox, Botox Cosmetic	
rimabotulinumtoxinB (botulinum toxin type B)	Myobloc	Injection, solution: 5000 units/vial
	Not available	
incobotulinumtoxinA	Xeomin	Powder for injection: 50 units/vial, 100 units/vial
	Xeomin, Xeomin Cosmetic	
cisatracurium[a]	Nimbex	Injection, solution: 2 mg/mL, 10 mg/mL[c]
	Generics	
pancuronium[a]	Generics	Injection, solution: 1 mg/mL, 2 mg/mL
	Not available	
rocuronium[a]	Generics	Injection, solution: 10 mg/mL
	Generics	
vecuronium[a]	Generics	Powder for injection: 10 mg/vial, 20 mg/vial
	Not available	

[a]Generic available.
[b]Available in Canada only.
[c]Available in the United States only.

Reversal of Neuromuscular Blockade

Drugs that reverse the effects of neuromuscular blockade must always be readily available any time the drugs are administered. Anticholinesterase drugs inhibit the degradation of ACh by the enzyme acetylcholinesterase at the *neuromuscular junction*. This causes ACh to accumulate. Increasing ACh produces skeletal muscle contraction. Anticholinesterase drugs are most effective after the process of spontaneous recovery from neuromuscular blocking drugs has begun.

> **▌ TECH NOTE!**
>
> Tubocurarine, formerly used in anesthesia, is the synthetic version of curare, a natural paralytic drug used by South American Indian hunters to immobilize prey.

Adverse Reactions

Edrophonium and neostigmine may produce salivation, muscle twitching, muscle weakness, abdominal cramping, nausea, increased bronchial secretions, and difficulty breathing.

Strategies for Safe Use of Neuromuscular Blocking Agents

Neuromuscular blocking drugs are classified "high alert" by the Interdisciplinary Safe Medication Use Expert Committee of the USP because improper use can result in permanent injury, respiratory arrest, and death. Problems associated with neuromuscular blocking drugs have been attributed to improper product selection, improper storage conditions, inappropriate dosing, improper labeling, and inadequate patient monitoring. Improper product selection is caused by similar product packaging and sound-alike drug names. Drug names that sound alike pose problems in dispensing regardless of the type of drug. Look-alike packaging is a problem that can be attributed to drug manufacturers, as well as pharmacies dispensing drugs (see **Chapter 4**). Neuromuscular blocking drugs may be repackaged for unit of use in institutional care settings. Infusion bags and syringes that have been prepared by the pharmacy look alike. Neuromuscular blocking drugs have been administered in the place of vaccines, intravenous flush solutions, and antibiotics by mistake. A pharmacy that fails to securely affix the label onto the infusion bag or syringe of a neuromuscular blocking drug has created a potentially life-threatening situation for a patient. Additional medicine errors occur from inaccurate sterile compounding, dispensing of incorrect drug concentrations, and placing incorrect doses in automated dispensing machines.

> **❶ TECH ALERT!**
>
> Zemuron and remeron have look-alike/sound-alike issues.

Summary of Drugs Used to Reverse the Effects of Neuromuscular Blocking Drugs

Generic Name	US Brand Name	Warnings and Storage Conditions
edrophonium	Enlon	STABLE AT ROOM TEMPERATURE.
neostigmine	Bloxiverz	STABLE AT ROOM TEMPERATURE. PROTECT FROM LIGHT (injection solution).
pyridostigmine	Mestinon	SWALLOW WHOLE; DON'T CRUSH OR CHEW—SR tab PROTECT FROM MOISTURE

> **▌ TECH NOTE!**
>
> Discard solutions of doxacuronium that are discolored or have particles.

Drugs That Reverse the Effects of Neuromuscular Blockade

Generic Name	US Brand Name(s) Canadian Brand(s)	Dosage Forms and Strengths
edrophonium	Enlon	**Injection, solution:** 10 mg/mL
	Not available	
neostigmine[a]	Bloxiverz	**Injection, solution:** 0.5 mg/mL, 1 mg/mL, 2.5 mg/mL[b]
	Generics	**Tablets:** 15 mg[b]
pyridostigmine[a]	Mestinon, Regonol	**Injection, solution (Regonol):** 5 mg/mL[c]
	Mestinon, Mestinon SR	**Syrup:** 60 mg/5 mL[c]
		Tablets: 60 mg
		Tablets, sustained release (Mestinon SR, Mestinon Timespan): 180 mg

[a]Generic available.
[b]Available in Canada only
[c]Available in the United States only.

Summary of Neuromuscular Blocking Drugs

Generic Name	US Brand Name	Warnings and Storage Conditions
succinylcholine	Quelicin	PARALYZING AGENT KEEP REFRIGERATED (2°–8°C). PROTECT FROM LIGHT Multidose vials stable at room temperature for 14 days.
atracurium	Generics	PARALYZING AGENT KEEP REFRIGERATED (2–8°C). PROTECT FROM LIGHT Stable at room temperature for 14 days. Infusion solutions should be used within 24 h of preparation.
abobotulinumtoxinA	Dysport	PARALYZING AGENT KEEP REFRIGERATED (2–8°C). PROTECT FROM LIGHT After dilution: Refrigerated solutions should be used within 24 h of preparation.
onabotulinumtoxinA	Botox	PARALYZING AGENT KEEP REFRIGERATED (2–8°C). After dilution: Refrigerated solutions should be used within 24 h of preparation.
incobotulinumtoxinA	Xeomin	PARALYZING AGENT KEEP REFRIGERATED (2–8°C). After dilution: Refrigerate and use within 24 h; discard unused portion.
rimabotulinumtoxinB	Myobloc	PARALYZING AGENT KEEP REFRIGERATED; DO NOT FREEZE. After dilution: Use within 4 h and discard unused portion. PROTECT FROM LIGHT.
cisatracurium	Nimbex	PARALYZING AGENT KEEP REFRIGERATED; DO NOT FREEZE (2–8°C). PROTECT FROM LIGHT. Once warmed to room temperature: Use within 21 days.
pancuronium	Generics	PARALYZING AGENT KEEP REFRIGERATED (2–8°C). DO NOT STORE IN PLASTIC SYRINGE. Stable for 6 months if stored at room temperature. If mixed, use within 48 hours.

Continued

Summary of Neuromuscular Blocking Drugs—cont'd

Generic Name	US Brand Name	Warnings and Storage Conditions
rocuronium	Generics	PARALYZING AGENT KEEP REFRIGERATED. If unopened, use within 60 days after removal from refrigerator. Once opened use within 30 days. If mixed, use within 24 h and discard unused portion.
vecuronium	Generics	PARALYZING AGENT KEEP REFRIGERATED. PROTECT FROM LIGHT. Before dilution: May store at room temperature. After dilution: Refrigerate and use within 24 h if reconstituted with sterile water or use within 5 days if reconstituted with bacteriostatic water.

TREATMENT OF MUSCLE SPASMS

Overview

Spasticity is a debilitating motor disorder that affects up to 12 million people worldwide. Symptoms of spasticity are increased muscle tone, exaggerated tendon jerks, and hyperexcitability of the stretch reflex. Spasticity can also cause muscle weakness, decreased endurance, and reduction in the capacity to make voluntary muscle movements. It may be accompanied by pain.

Spasticity may interfere with the normal performance of self-care and activities of daily living, inhibit effective walking, cause fatigue and stiffness, and disturb sleep.

Stroke, spinal cord injury, cerebral palsy, muscle trauma (e.g., whiplash), multiple sclerosis, head injury, and metabolic diseases such as *amyotrophic lateral sclerosis* (ALS; Lou Gehrig disease) can all cause spasticity. In fact, 65%–78% of people with spinal cord injuries and 65% of people who have had a stroke will develop spasticity.

Spasticity can be aggravated by a variety of factors. Fatigue, pain, stress, fever, cold, constipation, immobility, and hormonal changes can all worsen symptoms of spasticity.

Pathophysiology of Spasticity

Any condition that can damage the brain or spinal cord can cause spasticity. Regardless of the cause, the progression to spasticity follows a specific pattern, and the degree of spasticity is related to the duration since the original injury. The four phases are (1) decreased muscle contractility; (2) excessive muscle tone and increased reflex activity lasting from days to years; (3) decreased reflex excitability; and (4) stiff, contracted muscles.

Conditions That Produce Spasticity

Spinal Cord Injury

Spinal cord injury may produce muscle paralysis and loss of tendon reflexes in the region below the level of spinal cord injury immediately after the injury. Within a few weeks, this period of spinal shock ends and is followed by a period of increased muscle tone, exaggerated tendon jerks, and involuntary muscle spasms. It is believed that spasticity develops because the neurons that branch out from the spinal cord to the muscles and tissues of the body (lower motor neurons) grow new synapses that increase response to stretching of the muscle. Normal inhibitory control of sustained neuron firing is lost during the recovery period after spinal cord injury. What follows are unopposed motor neuron excitability. As muscle fibers atrophy, the number of sarcomeres decreases, and connective tissue increases. *Sarcomeres* are units within muscle fibers responsible for muscle contraction.

Spinal cord injury also results in *clonus*, involuntary rhythmic muscle contraction that produces involuntarily flexing and relaxation of the feet and wrists.

Stroke

Stroke can cause a lesion to form in the brain or spinal cord, which results in unopposed motor neuron excitability by normal inhibitory mechanisms.

Cerebral Palsy

Spasticity caused by *cerebral palsy* follows the same pathophysiologic pathway as stroke and spinal cord injury. Treatment is complicated because spasticity impairs effective muscle movement in some people with cerebral palsy and helps maintain posture, making walking easier in other people.

Amyotrophic Lateral Sclerosis

In people who have ALS, upper motor neurons (which carry messages from the brain down to the spinal cord) are damaged. Changes in the presynaptic membrane result in the release of ACh from its storage vesicle. This ultimately causes desensitization of motor nerves, muscle weakness, and cell death.

> **TECH NOTE!**
> The myelin sheath around neurons acts as an electrical insulator and increases the velocity of impulse transmission.

Multiple Sclerosis

Multiple sclerosis is an autoimmune disease that causes damage to myelinated nerves. Lesions damage nerves in the CNS and cause spasticity, pain, fatigue, dysfunction of the bladder and bowel, impotence, cognitive dysfunction, and changes in mood or depression. Nerve damage and symptoms get progressively worse over time.

Muscle Strain

Muscle strain, sprains, fibromyalgia, tension headache, low back pain, and neck pain can cause muscle spasm, stiffness, and pain.

When spasms are present, it is typically related to local injury or irritation of a specific muscle group.

Neurotransmitters Involved in Spasticity

Spasticity is a symptom of upper motor neuron syndrome. The cause may be excess activity of neurotransmitters that carry excitatory messages, such as ACh and glutamate, or decreased activity or a deficiency of inhibitory transmitters, such as γ-aminobutyric acid (GABA) and glycine. Defective glycine receptors are associated with a rare disease that causes an exaggerated startle reflex called hyperekplexia. This produces intense muscle contractions known as hypertonia. The excitatory actions of glutamate are described in more detail in **Chapter 8**. The inhibitory action of GABA is described in **Chapter 5**.

Drugs Used to Treat Spasticity

To manage spasticity, a variety of nonpharmaceutical treatments have been tried. Electrical stimulation, cold packs (cryotherapy), biofeedback, splinting, positioning, and physical therapy have all been proposed. These nondrug therapies may support pharmacologic treatments.

Drugs used in the treatment of spasticity are grouped according to the site of action and are classified as central acting and peripheral acting. Peripheral-acting drugs act directly on contractile mechanisms in the muscle. Central-acting drugs may be further categorized according to their mechanism of action. Some drugs are GABAergic. They act on GABA receptors in the CNS. Another group of drugs act at alpha$_2$-adrenergic receptor sites.

Peripheral-Acting Drugs

Botulinum Toxins

Botulinum toxins type A and B are used for the treatment of cervical dystonia. Cervical dystonia is a painful condition in which the neck muscles contract involuntarily. The toxins have also been studied in the treatment of poststroke spasticity and cerebral palsy. Only botulinum toxins type A are indicated for the treatment of blepharospasms. The toxin is injected locally to inhibit presynaptic release of ACh at the neuromuscular junction. This causes temporary paralysis in the muscle(s) that have received the injections. The onset of effect begins 3 to 7 days after injections are administered and lasts 3 to 6 months. Resistance develops with repeated use and injections, and the frequency of injection should be limited to no sooner than every 3 months.

Dantrolene

Dantrolene is indicated for the treatment of spasticity associated with spinal cord injury, stroke, cerebral palsy, multiple sclerosis, and malignant hyperthermia. Malignant hyperthermia causes severe muscle contractions and fever. Dantrolene reduces spasticity by weakening hyperexcited muscles. It acts directly on contractile mechanisms in skeletal muscle. Dantrolene inhibits calcium-dependent excitation-contraction. The use of dantrolene in the treatment of some spastic conditions is limited because the drug produces muscle weakness. Muscle weakness is undesirable when treating spasticity associated with spinal cord injury or ALS. Other adverse effects produced by dantrolene include sedation, fatigue, diarrhea, and hepatotoxicity. Dalfampridine (Ampyra) is a potassium channel blocker that is used to improve walking in patients with multiple sclerosis. The most common side effects are urinary tract infections, insomnia, headache, dizziness, nausea, and weakness.

Peripheral-Acting Drugs Used for the Treatment of Spasticity

Generic Name	US Brand Name(s) / Canadian Brand(s)	Dosage Forms and Strengths
dalfampridine	Ampyra	**Tablet, extended release:** 10 mg
	Not available	
dantrolene[a]	Dantrium, Revonto Ryanodex	**Capsules:** 25 mg, 50 mg[b], 100 mg
	Dantrium	**Injection, powder for reconstitution:** 20 mg/vial, 250 mg/vial

[a]Generic available.
[b]Available in the United States only.

Central-Acting Drugs

Central-acting skeletal muscle relaxants reduce spasticity by binding to receptor sites that control motor movement in the brain and spinal cord. The mechanism of action of these drugs is to enhance the actions of GABA, an inhibitory neurotransmitter, or to stimulate alpha$_2$-adrenergic receptors.

GABAergic Drugs

Drugs That Bind Directly to GABA Receptors

Baclofen is indicated for the treatment of spasticity associated with spinal cord injury and multiple sclerosis. Baclofen is structurally similar to the neurotransmitter GABA and is particularly useful in treatment of spasticity associated with spinal cord injury.

Mechanism of Action and Pharmacokinetic. The site of action for baclofen is the spinal cord, where it acts as an agonist at GABA$_B$ receptor sites. It reduces pain linked to spasticity by inhibiting the release of substance P (**Chapter 10**). The ability of baclofen to cross the blood-brain barrier is limited, so its effectiveness is augmented by administering the drug intrathecally. Intrathecal solutions are injected directly into the cerebrospinal fluid (CSF). Surgery is required to implant the intrathecal delivery system. The pump needs to be refilled every 1 to 6 months and must be replaced every 5 to 7 years.

Adverse Reactions. Adverse reactions include dizziness, drowsiness, headache, nausea, orthostatic hypotension, confusion, and weakness. Sudden discontinuation can cause withdrawal symptoms. Rebound spasticity, hallucinations, itching, hyperthermia, and seizures are signs and symptoms of withdrawal syndrome.

Central-Acting Drugs Used for the Treatment of Spasticity (Bind to GABA Receptors)

Generic Name	US Brand Name(s) / Canadian Brand(s)	Dosage Forms and Strengths
baclofen[a]	Gablofen, Lioresal	**Solution, intrathecal injection:** 0.05 mg/mL, 0.5 mg/mL, 1 mg/mL[b], 2 mg/mL
	Lioresal	**Tablets:** 10 mg, 20 mg

[a]Generic available.
[b]Available in the United States only.

Drugs That Enhance Gamma-Aminobutyric Acid Binding

Diazepam is classified as a central-acting agent because its site of action the brainstem and the spinal cord. It is the most commonly used benzodiazepine for the treatment of spasticity, and it is effective in treating hyperactive reflexes and painful muscle spasms. It improves range of motion and decreases anxiety and sleeplessness—both conditions can aggravate spasticity. Diazepam is a C-IV controlled substance in the United States and a targeted substance in Canada. A detailed discussion of the pharmacokinetics and adverse reactions of the benzodiazepines is found in **Chapters 5** and **9**.

> ! TECH ALERT!
>
> diazePAM and dilTIAZem have look-alike/sound-alike issues.

Alpha₂-Adrenergic Drugs

Alpha$_2$-adrenergic agonists (e.g., tizanidine) act like naturally occurring neurotransmitters to screen out unnecessary sensory messages that cause spasticity. They reduce muscle tone and the frequency of muscle spasms in people who have had spinal cord injuries, cerebral palsy, and stroke.

Mechanism of Action and Pharmacokinetics. Spasticity is reduced when drugs like tizanidine are administered because they prevent the release of excitatory neurotransmitters in the spinal cord and increase the actions of the inhibitory neurotransmitter glycine. Painful muscle spasms are diminished because the drugs interfere with the release of substance P, the neurotransmitter involved in the production of pain sensations and pain perception (see **Chapter 10**).

Adverse Reactions. Tizanidine produces sedation, hypotension, and dizziness.

> ● TECH NOTE!
>
> Skeletal muscle relaxants should not be combined with alcohol. Alcohol increases the CNS depression produced by the skeletal muscle relaxants, causing excessive drowsiness and decreased alertness.

> ! TECH ALERT!
>
> Carisoprodol is a C-IV controlled substance in the United States. When carisoprodol is combined with codeine, it is a schedule C-III controlled substance in the United States.

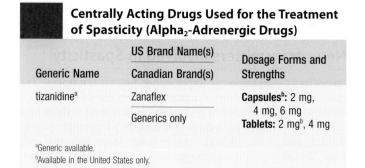

Centrally Acting Drugs Used for the Treatment of Spasticity (Alpha₂-Adrenergic Drugs)

Generic Name	US Brand Name(s) / Canadian Brand(s)	Dosage Forms and Strengths
tizanidine[a]	Zanaflex Generics only	**Capsules**[b]: 2 mg, 4 mg, 6 mg **Tablets:** 2 mg[b], 4 mg

[a]Generic available.
[b]Available in the United States only.

> ! TECH ALERT!
>
> tiZANidine and tiaGABine have look-alike/sound-alike issues.

Miscellaneous

Cyproheptadine is an antihistamine that is used in the treatment of spasticity associated with spinal cord injury, as well as to treat baclofen withdrawal symptoms however, this use is not approved by the FDA. Its mechanism of action appears to be linked to its effects on the neurotransmitters serotonin, histamine, and ACh.

Drugs Used to Treat Muscle Strain

Skeletal muscle relaxants are used to treat muscle stiffness, pain, and spasms associated with muscle tension, strain, sprains, or injury. Drugs in this category include carisoprodol, chlorzoxazone, cyclobenzaprine, metaxalone, methocarbamol, and orphenadrine. These skeletal muscle relaxants are central acting; however, the mechanism of action is unknown. It is believed their actions may be related to their sedative effects on the CNS.

Common adverse effects are dizziness, drowsiness, and blurred vision. Additional adverse effects are discoloration of urine—chlorzoxazone (orange to reddish purple) and methocarbamol (black, brown, or green).

Skeletal muscle relaxants should be used along with nonpharmaceutical therapies such as rest, exercise, cryotherapy, heat, and physical therapy.

Central-Acting Drugs Used for the Treatment of Spasticity (Enhance GABA Binding)

	Generic Name	US Brand Name(s) / Canadian Brand(s)	Dosage Forms and Strengths
	diazepam[a]	Diastat, Diazepam Intensol, Valium Diastat, Valium	**Rectal gel (Diastat):** 5 mg/mL as 2.5 mg, 10 mg and 20 mg prefilled syringes **Solution, for injection**[b]: 5 mg/mL **Oral, solution:** 1 mg/mL **Oral concentrate (Diazepam Intensol):** 5 mg/mL **Tablets (Valium):** 2 mg, 5 mg, 10 mg

[a]Generic available.
[a]Available in Canada only.

Central-Acting Drugs Used for the Treatment of Muscle Strain

	Generic Name	US Brand Name(s) Canadian Brand(s)	Dosage Forms and Strengths
	carisoprodol[a]	Soma Not available	**Tablets:** 250 mg, 350 mg
	chlorzoxazone[a]	Generics Not available	**Tablets:** 250 mg, 375 mg, 500 mg, 750 mg
	cyclobenzaprine[a]	Amrix Generics	**Capsules, extended release (Amrix):** 15 mg, 30 mg **Tablets:** 5 mg[b], 7.5 mg[b],10 mg
	metaxalone[a]	Skelaxin Not available	**Tablets:** 400 mg, 800 mg
	methocarbamol[a]	Robaxin Robaxin	**Tablets:** 500 mg, 750 mg **Solution, for injection:** 100 mg/mL
	orphenadrine[a]	Generics Orphenace	**Solution, for injection:** 30 mg/mL (2 mL) **Tablets, extended release:** 100 mg
Combination Products			
	carisoprodol + aspirin[a]	Generics Not available	**Tablets:** 200 mg carisoprodol + 325 mg aspirin
	carisoprodol + aspirin + codeine[a]	Generics Not available	**Tablets:** 200 mg carisoprodol + 325 mg aspirin + 16 mg codeine
	chlorzoxazone + acetaminophen	Not available Acetazone Forte, Back Aid Forte[c]	**Tablets:** 250 mg chlorzoxazone + 300 mg acetaminophen
	chlorzoxazone + acetaminophen + codeine	Not available Acetazone Forte C8	**Tablets:** 250 mg chlorzoxazone + 300 mg acetaminophen + 8 mg codeine
	methocarbamol + aspirin	Generic Extra Strength Muscle and Backache Relief with ASA, Methoxisal Extra Strength[c], Robaxisal Extra Strength	**Tablets:** 400 mg methocarbamol + 325 mg aspirin[b]; 400 mg methocarbamol + 500 mg aspirin[c]
	methocarbamol + aspirin + codeine	Not available Methoxisal C[1/8], Robaxisal C ¼, Robaxisal C ½	**Tablets:** 400 mg methocarbamol + 500 mg aspirin + 8 mg codeine; 400 mg methocarbamol + 500 mg aspirin + 16.2 mg codeine; 400 mg methocarbamol + 500 mg aspirin + 32.4 mg codeine
	methocarbamol + acetaminophen	Not available Extra Strength Tylenol Back Pain, Extra Strength Body Pain Night, Robaxacet, Robaxacet Extra Strength	**Tablets:** 400 mg methocarbamol + 325 mg acetaminophen; 400 mg methocarbamol + 500 mg acetaminophen
	methocarbamol + acetaminophen + codeine	Not available Robaxacet-8	400 mg methocarbamol + 325 mg acetaminophen + 8 mg codeine

Continued

Central-Acting Drugs Used for the Treatment of Muscle Strain—cont'd

Generic Name	US Brand Name(s) Canadian Brand(s)	Dosage Forms and Strengths
methocarbamol + ibuprofen	Not available	**Tablets:** 500 mg methocarbamol + 200 mg ibuprofen
	Axum, Motrin Platinum Muscle and Body, Robax Platinum	
orphenadrine + caffeine + aspirin	Generic	**Tablets:** 25 mg orphenadrine + 30 mg caffeine + 385 mg aspirin; 50 mg orphenadrine + 60 mg caffeine + 770 mg aspirin
	Not available	

aGeneric available.
bAvailable in the United States only.
cOver the counter in Canada.

Summary of Drugs Used in the Treatment of Spasticity

Generic Name	US Brand Name	Usual Adult Oral Dose and Dosing Schedule	Warning Labels
Central-Acting Skeletal Muscle Relaxants			
baclofen	Lioresal	**Oral:** 5 mg 3 times a day (maximum, 80 mg/day)	MAY CAUSE DIZZINESS OR DROWSINESS. MAY IMPAIR ABILITY TO DRIVE. AVOID ALCOHOL. TAKE WITH FOOD—baclofen. MAY DISCOLOR URINE—chlorzoxazone, methocarbamol. MAY BE HABIT FORMING—diazepam. SWALLOW WHOLE; DO NOT CRUSH OR CHEW—cyclobenzaprine, orphenadrine extended release.
carisoprodol	Soma	250–350 mg 4 times a day	
chlorzoxazone	Generics	250–350 mg 3 times a day and at bedtime	
cyclobenzaprine	Generics	5–10 mg 3 times a day (immediate release); 15–30 mg once daily (extended release)	
diazepam	Valium	**Oral:** 2–10 mg 3–4 times a day **IM or IV:** 5–10 mg every 3–4 hours if needed	
metaxolone	Skelaxin	800 mg 3–4 times a day	
methocarbamol	Robaxin	**Oral:** 1.5 g 4 times a day (up to 8 g/day) for 48 hrs then 750 mg orally every 4 hours, 1.5 g 3 times a day, or 1g 4 times a day	
orphenadrine	Generics	**Oral:** 100 mg twice a day	
tizanidine	Zanaflex	2–4 mg 1–4 times a day (maximum, 36 mg/day)	
Direct-Acting Skeletal Muscle Relaxants			
dantrolene	Dantrium	25–100 mg 3 times a day	MAY CAUSE DIZZINESS OR DROWSINESS. MAY IMPAIR ABILITY TO DRIVE. AVOID ALCOHOL. PROTECT FROM LIGHT AND MOISTURE.

TECHNICIAN'S CORNER

1. Why does the blood-brain barrier prevent some drugs from entering the brain?
2. You are in charge of inventory in the pharmacy and need to alert everyone about the potential of medication errors that can occur with neuromuscular blocking drugs. What would be the best way to alert everyone?

Key Points

- Skeletal muscles contract as a response to messages transmitted between peripheral nerves and muscles by neurotransmitters.
- Acetylcholine (ACh) is the primary neurotransmitter that sends messages between nerve cells and muscle cells.
- The release of ACh produces skeletal muscle contraction. Calcium increases ACh release. Drugs that block nerve transmission between the motor end plate and skeletal muscle receptors are classified as *peripheral-acting muscle relaxants*.
- Skeletal muscle relaxants that work by central nervous system depression (i.e., block nerve transmission between the spinal cord and muscles) are called *central-acting muscle relaxants*.
- Drugs that decrease the release ACh or deplete ACh levels in the neuron cause skeletal muscle relaxation.
- Care must be taken when transcribing and filling orders for neuromuscular blocking drugs because they can cause severe injury or death.
- The vial lids of the neuromuscular blocking drug must be clearly marked "Paralyzing Agent" or "Warning: Paralyzing Agent."
- The actions of neuromuscular blocking drugs are reversed by administering anticholinesterase drugs (e.g., neostigmine). They inhibit the degradation of ACh by the enzyme acetylcholinesterase.
- Neuromuscular blocking drugs are classified "high alert" by the Interdisciplinary Safe Medication Use Expert Committee of the United States Pharmacopoeia, because improper use can result in permanent injury, respiratory arrest, and death.

- Problems associated with neuromuscular blocking drugs can be avoided by proper product selection, storage conditions, and labeling; appropriate dosing; and patient monitoring.
- Spasticity is a debilitating motor disorder that affects up to 12 million people worldwide. It interferes with the normal performance of activities of daily living.
- Stroke, spinal cord injury, cerebral palsy, muscle trauma, multiple sclerosis, head injury, and amyotrophic lateral sclerosis can cause spasticity.
- There are four phases to the development of spasticity: (1) decreased muscle contractility; (2) excessive muscle tone and increased reflex activity lasting from days to years; (3) decreased reflex excitability; and (4) stiff, contracted muscles.
- Nonpharmaceutical treatments of spasticity are electrical stimulation, cold packs (cryotherapy), biofeedback, splinting, positioning, and physical therapy.
- Skeletal muscle relaxants are used to treat muscle stiffness, pain, and spasms associated with muscle tension, strain, sprains, or injury.
- Drugs used in the treatment of spasticity are grouped according to the site of action and are classified as central acting and peripheral acting.
- Peripheral-acting drugs act at the neuromuscular junction or directly on contractile mechanisms in the muscle.
- Dantrolene is a peripheral-acting drug that acts directly on contractile mechanisms in skeletal muscle.
- Baclofen is a central-acting drug that looks and acts like GABA, a naturally occurring neurotransmitter.

Review Questions

1. The neurotransmitter that is primarily responsible for transmitting messages between nerve cells and muscle cells is _____.
   a. dopamine
   b. epinephrine
   c. acetylcholine
   d. GABA
2. You prepare a solution of BOTOX. The solution should be _____.
   a. Stored at room temperature until use
   b. Stored in the refrigerator until use
   c. Discarded if not used within 24 hours
   d. Stored in the freezer
3. Botox has not been FDA approved for cosmetic use.
   a. true
   b. false

4. Most neuromuscular blocking drugs are poorly absorbed from the gastrointestinal tract so they are administered _____.
   a. topically
   b. enterally
   c. parenterally
   d. transdermally
5. _____ is the most commonly used benzodiazepine for the treatment of spasticity, and it is effective in treating hyperactive reflexes and painful muscle spasms.
   a. Alprazolam
   b. Diazepam
   c. Clonazepam
   d. Lorazepam

6. Neuromuscular blocking drugs are classified "_____" by the Interdisciplinary Safe Medication Use Expert Committee of the USP.
   a. dangerous
   b. high alert
   c. low alert
   d. use with caution

7. Where should most neuromuscular blocking drugs be stored?
   a. in alphabetical order on the shelf
   b. with the oral solutions
   c. with the fast movers
   d. apart from other drugs

8. Neuromuscular blocking drugs should always be dispensed with what auxiliary label?
   a. WARNING: Paralyzing agent. (Use requires mechanical ventilatory assistance.)
   b. WARNING: Allergic reactions possible.
   c. KEEP IN REFRIGERATOR UNTIL READY TO USE.
   d. FOR ONE TIME USE ONLY.

9. The effect of botulinum toxins in reducing spasticity lasts up to _____.
   a. 2 weeks
   b. 4 weeks
   c. 8 weeks
   d. 12 weeks

10. Medication errors can easily happen with nondepolarizing neuromuscular blocking drugs because _____.
   a. all packages look the same
   b. some drugs have look-alike/sound-alike names
   c. doses are all the same.
   d. all are made by same manufacturer

Bibliography

Adams MM, Hicks AL: Spasticity after spinal cord injury, *Spinal Cord* 43:577–586, 2005.

FDA. Drugs@FDA: FDA Approved Drug Products: U.S. Department Health and Human Services; nd Retrieved July 16, 2018 from: http://www.accessdata.fda.gov/scripts/cder/daf/.

Gallichio J: Pharmacologic management of spasticity following stroke, *Phys Ther* 84:973–981, 2004.

Health Canada. Drug Product Database 2017 Retrieved July 16, 2018 from: https://health-products.canada.ca/dpd-bdpp/index-eng.jsp.

Honda M, Sekiguchi Y, Sato N, et al: Involvement of imidazoline receptors in the centrally acting muscle-relaxant effects of tizanidine, *Eur J Pharmacol* 445:187–193, 2002.

ISMP: Neuromuscular Blocking Agents: Sustaining Packaging Improvements over Time, *ISMP Canada Safety Bullletin* 14(7):2014.

Kalant H, Grant D, Mitchell J: *Principles of medical pharmacology*, ed 7, Toronto, 2007, Elsevier Canada, A Division of Reed Elsevier Canada, pp 176–180.

Lewis C: Botox cosmetic: a look at looking good, U.S. Food and Drug Administration, FDA Consumer Magazine. Retrieved from https://permanent.access.gpo.gov/lps1609/www.fda.gov/fdac/features/2002/402_botox.html.

Matthey P, Wang P, Finegan B, et al: Rocuronium anaphylaxis and multiple neuromuscular blocking drug sensitivities, *CJA* 47(9):890–893, 2000.

Mehta S, Burry L, Fischer S, et al: Canadian survey of the use of sedatives, analgesics, and neuromuscular blocking agents in critically ill patients, *Crit Care Med* 34:374–380, 2006.

Ozcakir S, Sivrioglu K: Botulinum toxin in poststroke spasticity, *Clin Med Res* 5(2):132–138, 2007.

Patel D, Soyode O: Pharmacologic interventions for reducing spasticity in cerebral palsy, *Indian J Pediatr* 72:869–872, 2005.

Phillips M, Williams R: Improving the safety of neuromuscular blocking agents: a statement from the USP Safe Medication Use Expert Committee, *Am J Health Syst Pharm* 63:139–142, 2006.

USP Center for Advancement of Patient Safety: Use caution–avoid confusion, USP Quality Review No. 79, Rockville, MD, April 2004, USP Center for Advancement of Patient Safety.

Zafonte R, Lombard L, Elovic E: Antispasticity medications: uses and limitations of enteral therapy, *Am J Phys Med Rehabil* 83(Suppl):S50–S58, 2004.

13

Treatment of Gout, Osteoarthritis, and Rheumatoid Arthritis

LEARNING OBJECTIVES

1. Learn the terminology associated with drugs used in the treatment of gout, osteoarthritis, and rheumatoid arthritis.
2. Describe the signs and symptoms of gout, osteoarthritis, and rheumatoid arthritis.
3. List and classify medications used in the treatment of gout, osteoarthritis, and rheumatoid arthritis.
4. Describe the mechanism of action for each class of drugs used in the treatment of gout, osteoarthritis, and rheumatoid arthritis.
5. Identify warning labels and precautionary messages associated with medications used in the treatment of gout, osteoarthritis, and rheumatoid arthritis.

KEY TERMS

Arthritis An inflammatory condition that produces joint pain.
Autoantibody Abnormal antibody that attacks healthy cells and tissue.
Autoimmune disease Disease that occurs when the immune system turns against the parts of the body it is designed to protect.
Gout Disease characterized by deposits of urate crystals in the joints that produces inflammation. It is caused by hyperuricemia.
Hyperuricemia Condition in which urate levels build up in the blood.

Rheumatoid arthritis Chronic disease characterized by inflammation and remodeling of the joints.
Rheumatoid factor Immunoglobulin (antibody) that is present in many people who have rheumatoid arthritis.
Synovium Thin layer of tissue that lines the joint space.
Tumor necrosis factor Inflammatory cytokine released as part of the immune response and found in synovial fluid of people with rheumatoid arthritis.
Urates Product of purine metabolism. Urate crystals may accumulate in joints and produce inflammation and pain.
Uricosuric Drug that increases the renal clearance of urates.

Overview

Gout, also called gouty arthritis, is a disease that is associated with hyperuricemia. *Hyperuricemia* is a condition in which urate levels build up in the blood serum. *Urates* are the product of the metabolism of purines. Population studies show that the prevalence of hyperuricemia in men is greater than in women until menopause, when the rates equalize. Before puberty, boys and girls both have low serum urate levels.

In the United States and Canada, approximately 6% men and 2% women have gout. Hyperuricemia and gout are also associated with cardiovascular disease, hyperlipidemia, and hypertension. It is likely that the relationship between hypertension and hyperuricemia is attributable to decreased renal clearance resulting in accumulation of urate. Hyperuricemia increases the risk of coronary heart disease and stroke partly because of its role in producing hyperlipidemia. Hyperlipidemia causes atherosclerosis, a buildup of lipids in arteries that leads to clogged arteries. Hyperuricemia worsens heart failure.

Hyperuricemia is a risk factor for diabetes and is associated with increased insulin resistance. Obesity increases the risk for gout. Weight loss reduces hyperuricemia and insulin resistance. Hyperuricemia can cause kidney disease and make preexisting kidney disease worse. Exposure to lead in the environment can also increase the risk for development of gout.

Pathophysiology of Gout

Gout is characterized by a build up of urate crystals in joints; there they produce inflammation and pain. Deposits of uric acid are called *tophi* (singular, tophus) and look like lumps under the skin around the joints and at the rim of the ear (Fig. 13.1).

The joints most commonly affected are the big toe, foot, ankle, knee, wrist, finger, and elbow. Consumption of foods or beverages high in dietary purines can produce a flare-up of gout symptoms. For example, beer consumption increases the risk of an acute attack, perhaps because beer contains high levels of purine (Box 13.1).

Some people with gout will experience sharp needlelike painful symptoms, but some people will have no symptoms at all. Acute gout attacks usually resolve spontaneously in 7 to 10 days without treatment; however, people with symptoms may benefit from treatment. Chronic gout is a condition in which there is persistent

• **Fig. 13.1** Gouty arthritis. (From Swartz MH: *Textbook of physical diagnosis*, ed 7, Philadelphia, 2014, Elsevier.)

• **BOX 13.1** **Purine Content of Foods**

Foods considered high in purine content include:
• Alcoholic beverages
• Fish, seafood, and shellfish, including anchovies, sardines, herring, mussels, codfish, scallops, trout, and haddock
• Meats, such as bacon, turkey, veal, and venison, and organ meats such as liver and sweetbreads

Foods considered moderate in purine content include:
• Meats such as beef, chicken, duck, pork, and ham
• Crab, lobster, oysters, and shrimp
• Vegetables and beans such as asparagus, cauliflower, kidney beans, lentils, lima beans, peas, mushrooms, and spinach
• Grains: oatmeal, whole wheat bread, and cereal

Foods considered low in purine content include:
• Dairy products: skim milk and cheese
• Eggs
• Fruit and most vegetables (except those listed above)
• Grains: enriched bread and cereal

---

presence of uric acid crystals in and around the joint. The uric acid crystals may form disfiguring tophi (clumps of uric acid crystals) around the joint. Chronic gout that develops over a period of years may cause permanent joint or kidney damage.

Drugs Used to Treat Gout

Drugs prescribed for the treatment of gout include antiinflammatories, uricosurics, and inhibitors of uric acid synthesis. Colchicine is one of the oldest agents used to treat gout. It is extracted from the autumn crocus plant. It may be used treat or prevent symptoms. Colchicine penetrates inflammatory cells and inhibits their ability to respond to irritation. Colchine is most effective if taken at the first signs of an acute gout attack. Common adverse reactions associated with the use of colchicine include nausea, vomiting, and diarrhea. Rare serious adverse reactions are bone marrow suppression and renal failure.

Uricosurics

A *uricosuric* is a drug the increases the renal clearance of urates. Urate-lowering drugs are indicated for patients who experience frequent attacks of gout (more than 2–3 attacks per year) in order to prevent further gout attacks. Probenecid is a uricosuric that

Anitinflammatories Used in the Treatment of Gout

Generic Name	US Brand Name(s) / Canadian Brand(s)	Dosage Forms and Strengths
colchicine[a]	Colcrys, Mitigare / Generics	**Capsule (Mitigare):** 0.6 mg **Tablets:** 0.6 mg

[a]Generic available.

inhibits the reabsorption of uric acid in the renal tubules and thereby promotes the elimination of urates. Nausea, vomiting, and worsening of preexisting kidney stones are adverse reactions to probenecid.

Uricosurics Used in the Treatment of Gout

Generic Name	US Brand Name(s) / Canadian Brand(s)	Dosage Forms and Strengths
probenecid[a]	Generics / Not Available	**Tablets:** 500 mg
Combination probenecid + colchine[a]	Generics / Not available	**Tablets:** 500 mg probenecid + 0.5 mg colchicine

[a]Generic available.

> **TECH NOTE!**
> Thiazide diuretics (e.g., hydrochlorothiazide) and low-dose aspirin are known to increase urate levels.

Inhibitors of Uric Acid Synthesis

Xanthine Oxidase Inhibitors

Xanthine oxidase inhibitors block the final enzymatic step in the synthesis of uric acid. Allopurinol and febuxostat are xanthine oxidase inhibitors. Allopurinol is readily absorbed when administered orally and is easily eliminated in the urine. Nausea, drowsiness, headache, diarrhea, and an itchy skin rash are adverse reactions linked to allopurinol use. Febuxostat (Uloric) is more selective than allopurinol. Gout flare-ups have been reported when febuxostat therapy is initiated. Common adverse reactions are nausea, vomiting headache, diarrhea, and changes in appetite. Serious adverse events that have been reported with febuxostat include myocardial infarction, stroke, atrial fibrillation. Patients are advised to report muscle pain, an early sign of rhabdomyolysis—a breakdown of muscle tissue that can lead to acute renal failure.

Metabolism of Uric Acid

Recombinant Urate Oxidase Enzymes

Recombinant urate oxidase enzymes lower uric acid levels by metabolizing uric acid to the water-soluble benign purine metabolite allantoin, which is excreted in the urine. Pegloticase (Krystexxa)

Inhibitors of Uric Acid Synthesis

Generic Name	US Brand Name(s) Canadian Brand(s)	Dosage Forms and Strengths
allopurinol[a]	Aloprim, Zyloprim Zyloprim	**Injection, powder for reconstitution (Aloprim)**[b]: 500 mg **Tablet (Zyloprim):** 100 mg, 200 mg[c], 300 mg
febuxostat	Uloric Uloric	**Tablets:** 40 mg[b], 80 mg

[a]Generic available.
[b]Available in the United States only.
[c]Available in Canada only.

is US Food and Drug Administration (FDA) approved for patients with chronic gout. Rasburicase (Elitek, Fasturtek) is indicated for the treatment of hyperuricemia in patients receiving chemotherapy that has elevated uric acid. Pegloticase and rasburicase are administered intravenously. Patients may experience infusion reactions such as rash, itching, redness, and anaphylaxis. Additional adverse reactions of pegloticase include nausea and vomiting, constipation or diarrhea, fatigue, arthralgia, upper respiratory infection, fever, heart failure, and hypotension.

Recombinant Urate Oxidase Inhibitors

Generic Name	US Brand Name(s) Canadian Brand(s)	Dosage Forms and Strengths
pegloticase	Krystexxa Not available	**Solution, for IV infusion:** 8 mg/mL
rasburicase	Elitek Fasturtek	**Powder, for injection:** 1.5 mg/vial

IV, intravenous.

Nonpharmacologic Therapy for Gout

Prevention tips include weight loss and consumption of a low purine diet. The purine content of selected food is shown in Box 13.1. Foods high in purines are meat (especially liver), fish (anchovies), dried beans, peas, and gravy. Beer and spirits are also known to increase purine levels. Low-fat dairy products have low purine levels.

Osteoarthritis

Arthritis is a condition that produces joint pain. Inflammation of the fluid that surrounds the joint (synovial fluid) contributes to the pain associated with osteoarthritis. Osteoarthritis is the most common of all arthritic conditions. It is the leading cause of musculoskeletal pain. Symptoms of osteoarthritis are joint pain, stiffness, swelling, and crepitus (creaking joints). Pain may occur after activity or at rest. Risk factors for osteoarthritis are previous joint injury or surgery, obesity, increasing age, muscle weakness, and occupations that involve excessive joint use.

Acetaminophen, aspirin, and nonsteroidal antiinflammatory drugs (NSAIDs) are used to control pain.

Nonsteroidal Antiinflammatory Drugs

The principal antiinflammatories used for the treatment of acute gout and osteoarthritis are NSAIDs and corticosteroids. The most commonly prescribed NSAID for gout is indomethacin; however, ibuprofen, ketoprofen, and naproxen are also administered. The cyclooxygenase-2 (COX-2) inhibitor celecoxib may also be prescribed for the treatment of acute gout. Celecoxib remains the only COX-2 inhibitor available for sale in the United States and Canada. As per FDA requirements, manufacturers of all NSAIDs must print a boxed warning in the package insert describing the risk for cardiovascular toxicity and GI ulceration. The mechanism of action, pharmacokinetics, and additional adverse reactions for NSAIDS are discussed in Chapter 10.

> **❶ TECH ALERT!**
>
> The following drugs have look-alike/sound-alike issues:
> CeleBREX, CeleXA, and Cerebyx;

Rheumatoid Arthritis

Rheumatoid arthritis (RA) is an *autoimmune disease* that is characterized by inflammation of the lining of the joints. An autoimmune disease occurs when the immune system turns against the parts of the body it is designed to protect. The body attacks its own cells, thinking they are germs or a harmful foreign substance. No one knows exactly why autoimmunity develops. It is believed that several factors may be involved. The trigger may be exposure to a virus, environmental toxins, the sun, genetics, hormonal changes, drugs, pregnancy, or some combination of any of these things. What is known is that autoimmunity can affect any organ of the body.

In addition to chronic inflammation, RA produces pain, joint damage, and disability. According to the National Institutes of Health (2016), 1.5 million Americans have RA. Nearly one in every 100 Canadians is living with RA, according to the Canadian

Usual Dosage and Warnings for Drugs Used in the Treatment of Gout

	Generic Name	US Brand Name	Usual Adult Oral Dose and Dosing Schedule	Warning Labels
Antiinflammatories				
	colchine	Generics	**Oral, prevention:** 0.6 mg 1–2 times/day; may decrease to 0.6 mg 3 times a week **Oral, acute attack:** 1.2 mg at first sign of flare followed by 0.6 mg in 1 hour. MAX 1.8 mg over 1 hour	AVOID ALCOHOL. TAKE WITH A LOT OF WATER.
Uricosuric				
	probenecid	Generics	250 mg twice daily for 1 week, followed by 500 mg twice daily (Maximum 2000 mg/day)	TAKE WITH FOOD. TAKE WITH A LOT OF WATER. AVOID ASPIRIN.
Inhibitors of Uric Acid Synthesis				
	allopurinol[a]	Zyloprim	**Gout:** 200–600 mg/day orally; (Start 100 mg/day; increase weekly)	TAKE WITH FOOD. AVOID ALCOHOL. MAY CAUSE DIZZINESS OR DROWSINESS. TAKE WITH A LOT OF WATER (10–12 GLASSES/DAY).
	febuxostat	Uloric	**Hyperuricemia-gout:** 40–80 mg/day	TAKE WITH A GLASS OF WATER.
Recombinant Urate Oxidase Enzyme				
	pegloticase	Krystexxa	**Chronic gout:** 8 mg IV over 2 h every 2 weeks	MIX BY GENTLY INVERTING IV BAG; DO NOT SHAKE. REFRIGERATE DILUTED SOLUTION. USE WITHIN 4 H OF RECONSTITUTION—pegloticase.
	rasburicase	Elitek, Fasturtek	**Hyperuricemia (with malignancy):** 0.2 mg/kg as a 30-min infusion once daily for up to 5 days	

[a]Top 200 Drugs From Kane SP. ClinCalc DrugStats Database, Version 18.0. ClinCalc: http://clincalc.com/DrugStats. Updated February 3, 2018. Accessed July 24, 2018.
IV, Intravenous.

Nonsteroidal Antiinflammatory Drugs

Generic Name	US Brand Name Canadian Brands	Dosage Forms and Strengths
celecoxib[a]	Celebrex	**Capsule:** 50 mg[b], 100 mg, 200 mg, 400 mg[b]
	Celebrex	
indomethacin[a]	Indocin, Tivorbex	**Capsule:** 25 mg, 50 mg, 20 mg and 40 mg (Tivorbex)[b] **Powder for injection:** 1 mg base/vial **Suppository:** 50 mg, 100 mg[c] **Suspension, oral use:** 25 mg/5 mL
	Generics	
ibuprofen[a]	Advil, Motrin	**Capsule:** 200 mg[d] **Suspension, oral:**[d] 100 mg/5 mL **Tablets:** 200 mg[d], 300 mg[e], 400 mg[e], 600 mg[e]
	Advil, Motrin	
ketoprofen[a]	Generics	**Capsule:** 25 mg[b], 50 mg, 75 mg[b] **Capsule, extended release**[b]: 200 mg **Suppository:** 100 mg[c] **Tablet, enteric coated**[c]: 50 mg, 100 mg **Tablet, extended release**[c]: 200 mg
	Generics	
naproxen[a]	Naprosyn, EC-Naprosyn	**Tablet:** 125 mg[c], 250 mg, 375 mg, 500 mg **Tablet, extended release:**[c] 750 mg **Tablet, delayed release (EC-Naprosyn):** 375 mg, 500 mg
	Naprosyn	

Nonsteroidal Antiinflammatory Drugs—cont'd

Generic Name	US Brand Name / Canadian Brands	Dosage Forms and Strengths
naproxen Na[+a]	Aleve, Anaprox, Anaprox DS, Naprelen	**Tablet**: 200 mg[db], 220 mg[dc], 275 mg, 550 mg (Anaprox DS),
	Aleve, Anaprox, Anaprox DS	**Tablet, extended release (Naprelen)**: 375 mg, 500 mg, 750 mg

[a]Generic available.
[b]Available in the United States only.
[c]Available in Canada only.
[d]Over-the-counter.
[e]Over-the-counter in Canada only.

Arthritis Society (2011). RA is 2 to 3 times more common in women than in men. Although children have been diagnosed with juvenile RA, the onset of the disease is usually between 30 and 50 years.

Most people who have RA have high levels of *rheumatoid factor* (RF), an immunoglobulin (antibody) that regulates other antibodies made by the body. RF is not specific to RA, so its presence is part of the diagnosis for RA but is not a definitive diagnostic tool.

There are three distinct phases of the disease. In phase 1, the joint lining *(synovium)* or synovial membrane becomes inflamed, causing swelling, pain, and stiffness (Fig. 13.2). In phase 2, rapid cell growth causes the synovium to thicken. In phase 3, inflamed cells in the synovium release enzymes that digest bone and cartilage. This results in more pain and disability. The damaging, chronic cycle of inflammation is stimulated by proinflammatory cytokines (Fig. 13.3) such as interleukins (ILs) and *tumor necrosis factor* (TNF-α). Rheumatoid arthritis causes more than joint problems. Other symptoms of RA are fatigue, weakness, flulike symptoms, nodules that form under the skin, muscle pain, decreased appetite, depression, and dry mouth.

RA and other autoimmune diseases that affect the musculoskeletal system are treated using pharmacologic and nonpharmacologic therapies. Drug therapy is aimed at suppressing inflammation, pain, and immune system response. Drugs that are used to suppress inflammation and reduce joint swelling and pain include glucocorticosteroids (e.g., dexamethasone and prednisone), NSAIDs (e.g., celecoxib and naproxen), and salicylates (aspirin).

Disease-modifying antirheumatic drugs (DMARDs) are an important group of drugs that slow the progression of RA. Azathioprine and methotrexate (immunosuppressive drugs), hydroxychloroquine (an antimalarial), sulfasalazine, and leflunomide are examples of DMARDS. Another class of DMARDS, called biologic response modifiers, includes TNF inhibitors (e.g., adalimumab, certolizumab etanercept, and golimumab infliximab), IL antagonists (e.g., anakinra), the antimalarial hydroxychloroquine, and gold salts.

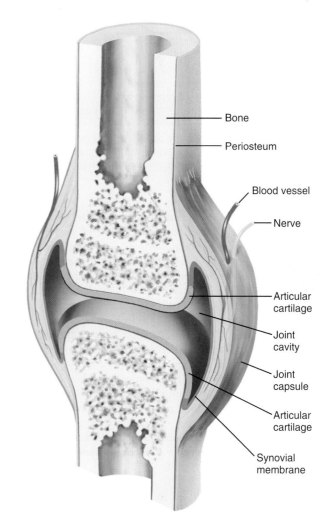

• **Fig. 13.2** Synovial joint. (From Vidic B, Suarez FR: *Photographic atlas of the human body*, St. Louis, 1984, Mosby.)

Labels: Bone, Periosteum, Blood vessel, Nerve, Articular cartilage, Joint cavity, Joint capsule, Articular cartilage, Synovial membrane

❶ TECH ALERT!

The following drugs have look-alike/sound-alike issues:
hydrocortisone, cortisone, and hydrocodone;
Medrol and Mebaral;
methylprednisolone and medroxyprogesterone;
prednisone, prednisolone, Pramosone, and primodone

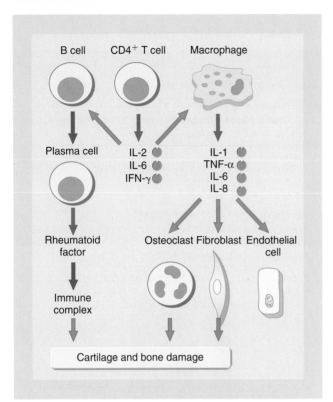

• **Fig. 13.3** Cytokine network in the pathogenesis of rheumatoid arthritis. (From Page C, Curtis M, Sutter M, et al: *Integrated pharmacology*, ed 3, Philadelphia, 2006, Mosby.)

Glucocorticosteroids

Glucocorticosteroids are prescribed to suppress inflammation, reduce flare-ups, and treat pain associated with RA. Oral prednisone and intraarticular injections of corticosteroids may sometimes be given when only one or two joints are involved. Glucocorticosteroids have immunosuppressive actions, and they inhibit the synthesis of antibodies that are responsible for attacking the body's healthy cells. They decrease the accumulation of cells that mobilize to fight when the body believes it is under attack, such as leukocytes and T cells. They interfere with the binding of antibodies to receptor sites on the cell surface. Glucocorticosteroids are potent antiinflammatory drugs too. They decrease the synthesis of proinflammatory substances—prostaglandins (see Chapter 10), leukotrienes, cytokines, arachidonic acid, and macrophages—that are released as part of the inflammatory response and cause swelling, pain, irritation, and other effects. Glucocorticosteroids may also be prescribed for the treatment of ulcerative colitis, allergic reactions, cerebral edema, and septic shock or used as a diagnostic agent for endocrine disorders.

Pharmacokinetics

The absorption, distribution, metabolism, and elimination of glucocorticosteroids vary according to the dosage form administered. In general, oral dosage forms are well absorbed in the GI tract and are readily distributed. Metabolism occurs in the liver. Glucocorticosteroids are eliminated in urine.

Adverse Reactions

The adverse effects produced by glucocorticosteroids are numerous and affect all body systems. In the CNS, they cause insomnia and euphoria. In the cardiovascular system, they produce edema and hypertension. In the endocrine system, they may produce hyperglycemia, leading to diabetes. Short-term use of glucocorticosteroids can also cause nausea and weight gain. Other adverse drug effects are osteoporosis, acne, cataracts, poor wound healing, increased risk of infection, and ulceration in the GI tract.

Precautions

Glucocorticosteroids may initially produce muscle weakness. This is a serious problem for people with myasthenia gravis, given that muscle weakness is a symptom of the disease. Glucocorticoid immunosuppressive effects are important to their therapeutic action; however, immunosuppression increases the risk for infections and lead to poor wound healing. Alternate-day therapy can minimize some adverse effects caused by glucocorticosteroids. Long-term use of glucocorticosteroids may increase the need for potassium; vitamins A, B_6, C, and D; folate; calcium; zinc; and phosphorous supplementation.

Disease-Modifying Antirheumatic Drugs

Disease-modifying antirheumatic drugs (DMARDs) slow the disease progression of RA rather than provide symptomatic relief. DMARDs described in this chapter include selected immunosuppressives, TNF inhibitors, IL antagonists, antimalarials, lefluonomide, gold salts, penicillamine, and sulfasalazine.

Immunosuppressives

Immunosuppressive drugs interfere with the formation of immune cells by damaging RNA and DNA needed for cell replication. They may also block immune system response to autoantibodies. An *autoantibody* is an abnormal antibody that attacks healthy cells and tissue.

Azathioprine, cyclophosphamide, cyclosporine, and methotrexate are immunosuppressive drugs used to treat RA. Methotrexate was one of the first drugs used for the treatment of RA, and it continues to be used as monotherapy or along with other DMARDs. It works by inhibiting the formation of folates that are needed for purine synthesis; thus folic acid supplementation is prescribed with methotrexate. Methotrexate also decreases cytokine and immunoglobulin production and COX-2 activity, reducing both inflammation and immune system activity. In addition to RA, methotrexate is prescribed for the treatment of leukemias; neoplasms; psoriasis; breast, lung, and head and neck cancer; GI tract and testes cancers; and osteosarcoma.

Azathioprine blocks purine synthesis to cause DNA damage and suppresses T cell–mediated immune system responses. Cyclophosphamide interferes with DNA synthesis and cell replication. It inhibits B-cell antibody production and T-cell activity, suppresses cytokine and immunoglobulin production, and suppresses the antigen-induced response to T cells. Because of toxicity, cyclophosphamide is reserved for severe, active disease. Cyclophosphamide is also prescribed for the treatment of other cancers, such as leukemia, breast, ovarian, endometrial, and testicular cancer, and to prevent rejection of bone marrow transplants. Cyclosporine is used with azathioprine or glucocorticosteroids to treat severe RA. It selectively interferes with T-cell proliferation and IL production. The result is a decreased immune system response to autoantibodies. Cyclosporine is also prescribed for the prevention of organ transplant rejection and severe psoriasis.

> ⓘ *TECH ALERT!*
>
> The following drugs have look-alike/sound-alike issues: cycloSPORINE, cycloSERINE, and cyclophosphamide;

Glucocorticoids Used in the Treatment of Rheumatoid Arthritis

Generic Name	US Brand Name(s) / Canadian Brand(s)	Dosage Forms and Strengths
dexamethasone[a]	Generics Generics	**Elixir:** 0.5 mg/5 mL **Oral concentrate:**[b] 1 mg/mL **Solution, injection:** 4 mg/mL, 10 mg/mL **Tablet:** 0.5 mg, 0.75 mg, 1 mg[b], 1.5 mg[b], 2 mg, 4 mg, 6 mg[b]
hydrocortisone[a]	Cortef, Solu-Cortef Cortef, Solu-Cortef	**Injection, powder for reconstitution (Solu-Cortef):** 100 mg, 250 mg, 500 mg, 1000 mg **Tablets:** 5 mg[b], 10 mg, 20 mg
methylprednisolone[a]	A-Methapred, Depo-Medrol, Medrol, Solu-Medrol Depo-Medrol, Medrol, Solu-Medrol	**Suspension, injection:** 20 mg/mL, 40 mg/mL, 80 mg/mL **Powder, for injection:** 40 mg/vial, 125 mg/vial, 500 mg/vial, 1 g/vial, 2 g/vial[b] **Tablet:** 2 mg[b], 4 mg, 8 mg[b], 16 mg, 32 mg[b]
prednisone[a]	Prednisone Intensol, Rayos Winpred	**Solution, for oral use (Prednisone Intensol):** 5 mg/ml **Tablet, delayed release (Rayos):** 1 mg, 2 mg, 5 mg **Tablet:** 1 mg, 2.5 mg[b], 5 mg, 10 mg[b], 20 mg[b], 50 mg
prednisolone[a]	Orapred ODT, Pediapred, Prelone Pediapred	**Solution, oral (Pediapred):** 5 mg/5 mL **Syrup (Prelone):** 15 mg/5 mL[b] **Tablet[b]:** 5 mg **Tablet, disintegrating[b]:** 10 mg, 15 mg, 30 mg
triamcinolone[a]	Aristospan, Kenalog-10, Kenalog-40, Zilretta Kenalog-10, Kenalog-40	**Suspension, extended release; intra-articular injection:**[b] 32 mg/vial **Suspension, injectable:** 5 mg/mL[b], 10 mg/mL, 20 mg/mL[b], 40 mg/mL

[a]Generic available.
[b]Available in the United States only.

Precautions and Adverse Reactions

Adverse reactions to azathioprine include nausea, vomiting, infections, hepatotoxicity, cytopenias, and myelosuppression. Cyclophosphamide may produce alopecia, nausea, infertility, infections, hemorrhagic cystitis, bladder cancer, hypoglycemia, and bone marrow depression. Adverse reactions to cyclosporine include kidney toxicity, infections, nausea, abdominal pain, mouth sores, gingival hyperplasia, headache, hirsutism, weight gain, hepatotoxicity, and hypertension. Methotrexate's side effects include nausea, vomiting, diarrhea, GI ulceration, rash, photosensitivity, hair loss, bone marrow depression, hepatotoxicity, renal toxicity, and stomach pain.

> **● TECH NOTE!**
> Reconstituted solution of azathioprine must be mixed by gently swirling, not shaking.

> **● TECH NOTE!**
> Cyclosporine oral solution must be dispensed in a glass container. Dispense the same manufacturer's product each time (bioavailability issues).

> **● TECH NOTE!**
> For cyclosporine solution for injection:
> - DO NOT REFRIGERATE.
> - PROTECT FROM LIGHT.
> - DILUTE SOLUTION AND USE IMMEDIATELY. Stable for 6 h in plastic IV bags or 24 h in glass.

Antimalarials

Antimalarials have antiinflammatory and analgesic properties that are useful in the management of RA. Although the exact mechanism of action is unknown, antimalarials are known to accumulate inside cell structures, where they raise the pH and interfere with processes that are normally stimulated when the body thinks its own cells are harmful antigens. An antigen is a substance that stimulates an immune response.

Precautions and Adverse Reactions

The most common adverse reaction is GI irritation; however, hydroxychloroquine can cause permanent damage to the retina, resulting in blindness. This adverse reaction is associated with long-term chronic use (greater than 5 years) at doses greater than 6.5 mg/kg per day. Additional adverse reactions include nausea, stomach pain, visual disturbances, and tinnitus.

Miscellaneous Disease-Modifying Antirheumatic Drugs

Leflunomide is a DMARD that is approved for the treatment of RA and selectively blocks the replication of lymphocytes by interfering with pyrimidine synthesis. Sulfasalazine was developed by combining an anti-infective agent (sulfapyridine) with an aspirin-like antiinflammatory agent (5-aminosalicylic acid). Sulfasalazine slows the progression of RA. Sulfasalazine takes approximately 2 to 3 months to produce maximum effects. Gold compounds are used in the treatment of RA; however, their use is limited because of side effects, cost, and lack of sustained effectiveness. Gold compounds are believed to affect the function of B cells and macrophages, part of the immune system response. They decrease the release of

Immunosuppressives Used in the Treatment of Rheumatoid Arthritis

Generic Name	US Brand Name(s) Canadian Brand(s)	Dosage Forms and Strengths
azathioprine[a]	Azasan, Imuran	**Injection, powder for reconstitution:** 50 mg vial[b], 100 mg vial[c]
	Imuran	**Tablets:** 25 mg[c], 50 mg, 75 mg[c], and 100 mg[c]
cyclophosphamide[a]	Generics	**Capsule:**[c] 25 mg, 50 mg
	Procytox	**Injection, powder for reconstitution:** 200 mg[b], 500 mg, 1 g, 2 g **Tablets:**[b] 25 mg, 50 mg
cyclosporine[a]	Gengraf, Neoral, Sandimmune	**Capsules, modified (Gengraf, Neoral):** 10 mg[b], 25 mg, 50 mg[b], 100 mg
	Neoral, Sandimmune	**Capsules, nonmodified (Sandimmune):**[c] 25 mg, 50 mg, 100 mg **Solution, for injection, (Sandimmune):** 50 mg/mL **Solution, oral:** 100 mg/mL
methotrexate[a]	Otrexup, Otrexup PFS, Rasuvo, Rheumatrex, Trexall, Xatmep	**Injection, powder for reconstitution:** 1000 mg[c] **Injection, solution:** 2.5 mg/mL, 10 mg/mL, 20 mg/mL, 25 mg/mL, 50 mg/mL, **Solution, oral (Xatmep):** 2.5 mg/mL (2 mg base) **Solution, for subcutaneous injection (Otrexup):** 7.5 mg/0.4 mL, 10 mg/0.4 mL, 12.5 mg/0.4 mL, 15 mg/0.4 mL, 17.5 mg/0.4 mL, 20 mg/0.4 mL, 22.5 mg/0.4 mL, 25 mg/0.4 mL
	Methotrexate, Metoject Subcutaneous	**Solution, for subcutaneous injection (Metoject Subcutaneous, Rasuvo):** 7.5 mg/0.15 mL[c], 10 mg/0.20 mL[c], 12.5 mg/0.25 mL[c], 15 mg/0.30 mL[c], 17.5 mg/0.35 mL, 20 mg/0.4 mL, 22.5 mg/0.45 mL, 25 mg/0.5 mL, 30 mg/0.6 mL **Solution, for injection (prefilled syringe):**[c] 7.5 mg/0.3 mL, 7.5 mg/0.75 mL, 10 mg/0.4 mL, 10 mg/mL, 15 mg/0.6 mL, 15 mg/0.15 mL, 20 mg/0.8 mL **Tablets:** 2.5 mg, 5 mg[c], 7.5 mg[c], 10 mg, 15 mg[c]

[a]Generic available.
[b]Available in Canada only.
[c]Available in the United States only.

Antimalarials Used in the Treatment of Rheumatoid Arthritis

Generic Name	US Brand Name(s) Canadian Brand(s)	Dosage Forms and Strengths
hydroxychloroquine[a]	Plaquenil	**Tablets:** 200 mg
	Plaquenil	

[a]Generic available.

antibodies and cytokines and inhibit the action of collagenase. Gold compounds may be delivered by mouth or intramuscular injection. The onset of action is slow, and it can take 4 to 6 months before maximum effectiveness is achieved. Gold compounds can produce temporary remission in approximately 50% of the people who respond favorably to the drug. Penicillamine has antiinflammatory actions and alters the immune system response. This makes it useful in the treatment of RA. It inhibits T-cell function and blocks collagen cross-linking. Tofacitinib is a jak kinase (JAK) inhibitor. It fights inflammation from inside the cell.

Precautions and Adverse Reactions

Common side effects of sulfasalazine are GI upset, increased sensitivity to sunlight, allergy, crystalluria, impaired folic acid absorption, and damage to white blood cells (cytopenias). Leflunomide adverse reactions include nausea, diarrhea, rash, hair loss, liver dysfunction, and fetal toxicity. Adverse reactions to auranofin and gold sodium thiomalate include itching rash, metallic taste, sore mouth, photosensitivity, cytopenias, interstitial pneumonia, and proteinuria. Penicillamine adverse reactions include rash, GI upset, and nephrotoxicity.

> **⚠ TECH ALERT!**
>
> The following drugs have look-alike/sound-alike issues:
> sulfaSALAzine and sulfADIAZINE;
> Ridura and Cardura;
> penicillAMINE and penicillin

Biologic Response Modifiers

Many DMARDs are biologic response modifiers. They interfere with the inflammatory process by reducing mediators of the inflammatory response. They inhibit the release of cells that mobilize to fight what the body believes is a harmful invasion and inhibit

Miscellaneous Disease-Modifying Antirheumatic Drugs

Generic Name	US Brand Name(s) / Canadian Brand(s)	Dosage Forms and Strengths
auranofin	Ridaura	**Capsules:** 3 mg
	Ridaura	
leflunomide[a]	Arava	**Tablets:** 10 mg, 20 mg, 100 mg
	Arava	
gold sodium thiomalate	Not available	**Injection, solution:** 10 mg/mL, 25 mg/mL, 50 mg/mL
	Myochrysine	
penicillamine[a]	Cupramine, Depen	**Capsules (Cupramine):** 250 mg
	Cupramine	**Tablets (Depen):** 250 mg
sulfasalazine[a]	Azulfidine, Azulfidine EN-tabs	**Tablets (Azulfidine):** 500 mg
	Salazopyrin, Salazopyrin EN-tabs	**Tablets, enteric coated (Azulfidine EN-tab, Salazopyrin EN-tabs):** 500 mg
tofacitinib	Xeljanz, Xeljanz XR	**Tablets:** 5 mg, 10 mg[b]
	Xejanz	**Tablet, extended release (Xeljanz XR):** 11 mg

[a]Generic available.
[b]Available in the United States only.

the release of substances that produce inflammation. Chronic inflammation can cause degeneration of nerves, bones, and muscles.

Biologic response modifiers interfere with the activity of immune system mediators such as cytokines, leukocytes, B cells, and T cells. TNF is a cytokine that is released by specialized cells to fight what the body believes is a harmful invasion. High levels of TNF are found in the synovial fluid of people with RA, and the factor is responsible for joint-damaging inflammation. TNF-α inhibitors are genetically engineered drugs that block the inflammatory process triggered by high concentrations of TNF. They prevent cell lysis (destruction) and release of the substances that cause inflammation.

Adalimumab, certolizumab, golimumab, and infliximab are monoclonal antibodies that bind to TNF-α to reduce mediators of the inflammatory response. Etanercept is a fusion protein that inhibits TNF-α. Abatacept is a fusion protein. Unlike the TNF-α inhibitor etanercept, abatacept blocks T-cell activation. Rituximab works by depleting circulating B cells. Anakinra is a genetically engineered interleukin (IL) receptor antagonist. Anakinra interferes with the binding of the ILs that promote inflammatory responses. Drug-receptor binding results in fewer lymphocytes and macrophages in synovial fluid. Tocilizumab inhibits IL-6 and may be administered with methotrexate or given as monotherapy.

> ### TECH NOTE!
> Cytotoxic waste (e.g., cyclophosphamide methotrexate and azathioprine), including bags, sets, tubing, drug vials and gloves, must be properly disposed of in the cytotoxic waste containers.

Precautions and Adverse Reactions

Monoclonal antibodies (e.g., adalimumab, infliximab), abatacept, and etanercept increase the risk for opportunistic infections. The most commonly reported opportunistic infections are tuberculosis and fungal infections. In addition to opportunistic infections, other adverse reactions common to "-mabs" are rash, pruritus, nausea, headache, and injection site redness and itchiness. Redness, itching, and swelling at the injection site are the most common side effects of etanercept. The most common side effects of abatacept are headache, dizziness, nausea, and hypertension. Adverse reactions to anakinra include redness or irritation at the injection site, infections, and bone or muscle weakness. In rare cases the body recognizes the "mabs" as nonhuman proteins and produces antibodies to the drugs, resulting in allergic and immune system reactions such as anaphylactic shock. Abatacept and etanercept may also produce anaphylactic shock. TNF-α inhibitors are associated with the development of secondary cancers. Fatal infusion reactions can occur with rituximab and tocilizumab that may be fatal.

> ### TECH NOTE!
> "-mab" is the common ending for monoclonal antibody drugs (e.g., TNF-α inhibitors and IL inhibitors).

Biologic Response Modifiers Used in the Treatment of Rheumatoid Arthritis

Generic Name	US Brand Name(s) / Canadian Brand(s)	Dosage Forms and Strengths
abatacept	Orencia	**Powder, for injection:** 250 mg/vial
	Orencia	**Solution, for injection[a]:** 125 mg/mL
adalimumab	Amjevita, Cyltezo Humira	**Injection, solution (Single use vial and pre-filled syringe):** 40 mg/0.8 mL, 40 mg/0.4 mL[a], 20 mg/0.4 mL[b] (Amjevita)
	Humira	
anakinra	Kineret	**Injection, solution:** 100 mg/0.67 mL (150 mg/mL pre-filled syringe)
	Kineret	

Continued

Biologic Response Modifiers Used in the Treatment of Rheumatoid Arthritis—cont'd

Generic Name	US Brand Name(s) Canadian Brand(s)	Dosage Forms and Strengths
certolizumab pegol	Cimzia	**Powder, for injection solution:** 200 mg/mL
	Cimzia	**Solution, for subcutaneous injection:** 200 mg/mL (Single use vial and prefilled syringe)
etanercept	Enbrel, Erelzi	**Injection, powder for reconstitution (Enbrel):** 25 mg/vial
	Brenzys, Enbrel	**Injection, solution** (prefilled syringe): 25 mg/0.5 mL(Erelzi), 50 mg/mL (Brenzys, Enbrel)
golimumab	Simponi, Simponi Aria	**Solution for injection (prefilled syringe):** 50 mg/0.5 mL, 100 mg/1 mL
	Simponi, Simponi IV	**Solution for IV:** 50 mg/4 mL
infliximab	Inflectra, Ixifi, Remicade, Renflexis	**Injection, powder for reconstitution:** 100 mg vial
	Inflectra, Remicade, Remsima	
rituximab	Rituxan, Rituxan Hycela	**Solution, for injection:** 10 mg/mL vial
	Rituxan, Rituxan SC	**Subcutaneous injection (Rituxan SC, Rituxan Hycela):** 1400 mg/11.7 mL, 1600 mg/13.4 mL
tocilizumab	Actemra	**Solution, for injection:** 80 mg/4 mL, 200 mg/10 mL, 400 mg/20 mL
	Actemra	**Subcutaneous injection:** 162 mg/0.9 mL

[a]Generic available.
[b]Available in the United States only.

Dosage and Warnings for Drugs Used in the Treatment of Rheumatoid Arthritis

Generic Name	US Brand Name	Usual Adult Oral Dose and Dosing Schedule	Warning Labels
dexamethasone	Generics	0.75–9 mg/day given in 2–4 divided doses	TAKE WITH FOOD. DO NOT DISCONTINUE ABRUPTLY. TAKE AT THE SAME TIME EACH DAY. TAKE WITH A FULL GLASS OF WATER.
hydrocortisone	Cortef	20–240 mg once daily or on alternate days 100–500 mg IV; May repeat IM/IV every 2, 4, or 6 hrs until stable (up to 48–72 hrs)	
methylprednisolone[a]	Medrol	4–48 mg PO daily in 4 divided doses or 10–40 mg IM or IV infused over several minutes	
prednisone	Generics	**Acute:** 5–60 mg PO once daily (May administer twice the daily dose every other day)	
NSAIDS			
celecoxib[a]	Celebrex	**Gout, acute:** 800 mg immediately, then 400 mg every 12 hours for 7 days **Osteoarthritis:** 200 mg/day in 1–2 divided doses **RA:** 100–200 mg twice a day	TAKE WITH FOOD. AVOID ASPIRIN AND RELATED PRODUCTS. MAY CAUSE DIZZINESS OR DROWSINESS. SWALLOW WHOLE; DO NOT CRUSH OR CHEW—EC-Naprosyn.
ibuprofen[a]	Motrin	400–800 mg 3–4 times a day (maximum, 3200 mg/day)	
naproxen[a]	Anaprox, Naprosyn	**Gout:** 750 mg, followed by 250 mg every 8 hrs until attack over **Osteoarthritis/RA:** 500–1000 mg/day in 2 divided doses	

Dosage and Warnings for Drugs Used in the Treatment of Rheumatoid Arthritis—cont'd

Generic Name	US Brand Name	Usual Adult Oral Dose and Dosing Schedule	Warning Labels
Antimalarials			
hydroxychloroquine[a]	Plaquenil	**RA:** 400–600 mg/day; when optimal response is reached (4–12 weeks), reduce dose to 200–400 mg/day	AVOID ANTACIDS (and kaolin products) WITHIN 2 H OF DOSE. TAKE WITH FOOD. AVOID PROLONGED EXPOSURE TO SUNLIGHT.
Immunosuppressives			
azathioprine	Imuran	**RA:** 1 mg/kg/day for 6–8 weeks; increase every 4 weeks up to 2.5 mg/kg/day	TAKE WITH FOOD. AVOID PREGNANCY.
cyclosporine	Neoral, Sandimmune	**RA:** 2.5–5 mg/kg/day in 2 divided doses	AVOID ALCOHOL AVOID GRAPEFRUIT JUICE AVOID PREGNANCY.
methotrexate	Rheumatrex	**RA:** 7.5 mg PO or SC once a week or 2.5 mg PO every 12 h for 3 doses/week (maximum, 20 mg/wk)	TAKE WITH A FULL GLASS OF WATER. AVOID ALCOHOL. AVOID ASPIRIN and NSAIDs. AVOID PROLONGED EXPOSURE TO SUNLIGHT. AVOID PREGNANCY.
Biologic Response Modifiers			
adalimumab[a]	Humira	40 mg SC every other week (if not taking methotrexate may increase to 40 mg/week)	PROTECT FROM LIGHT. REFRIGERATE; DO NOT FREEZE.
certolizumab	Cimzia	400 mg SC, given as two 200-mg subcut injections at weeks 0, 2, and 4; then 200 mg SC every other week OR 400 mg once every 4 weeks	REFRIGERATE; DO NOT FREEZE. ROTATE SITE OF INJECTION. PROTECT FROM LIGHT
golimumab	Simponi Aria, Simponi	2 mg/kg IV infusion over 30 minutes at weeks 0 and 4, then every 8 weeks (Simponi Aria); 50 mg SC once monthly (in combination with methotrexate)	ROTATE SITE OF INJECTION. REFRIGERATE; DON'T FREEZE PROTECT FROM LIGHT DO NOT SHAKE.
infliximab	Remicade	3 mg/kg IV infusion at 2 and 6 weeks after first dose; repeat in 8 weeks; maintenance, 3–10 mg/kg at 4- or 8-week intervals (in combination with methotrexate)	REFRIGERATE; DO NOT FREEZE. GENTLY SWIRL RECONSTITUTED PRODUCT; DO NOT SHAKE AFTER MIXING, DISCARD ANY UNUSED PORTION.
rituximab	Rituxan	500–1000 mg IV on days 1 and 15; repeat every 16–24 weeks based on clinical evaluation	REFRIGERATE DO NOT FREEZE. GENTLY INVERT IV BAG TO MIX TO AVOID FOAMING. AFTER MIXING, DISCARD ANY UNUSED PORTION.
tocilizumab	Actemra	**RA:** 4 mg/kg IV every 4 weeks; maximum, 8 mg/kg 162 mg SC every other week or weekly depending on response and weight	REFRIGERATE DO NOT FREEZE. GENTLY INVERT IV BAG TO MIX TO AVOID FOAMING. AFTER MIXING, DISCARD ANY UNUSED PORTION.
Other Biologic Response Modifiers			
abatacept	Orencia	**Psoriatic arthritis/RA:** 500–1000 mg IV infusion; repeat doses at 2 and 4 weeks after first infusion and every 4 weeks thereafter. **RA/Psoriatic arthritis:** 125 mg SC weekly	REFRIGERATE; DO NOT FREEZE. PROTECT FROM LIGHT. USE WITHIN 24 H OF MIXING; DISCARD UNUSED PORTION.
anakinra	Kineret	100 mg SC once daily	ROTATE SITE OF INJECTION. GENTLY SWIRL TO DISSOLVE. REFRIGERATE. PROTECT FROM LIGHT.
etanercept	Enbrel	**Psoriatic arthritis/RA:** 50 mg once weekly	ROTATE SITE OF INJECTION. DO NOT SHAKE. REFRIGERATE. PROTECT FROM LIGHT.

Continued

Dosage and Warnings for Drugs Used in the Treatment of Rheumatoid Arthritis—cont'd

Generic Name	US Brand Name	Usual Adult Oral Dose and Dosing Schedule	Warning Labels
DMARDs			
leflunomide	Arava	Start 100 mg/day for 3 days; decrease to 10–20 mg/day	AVOID PROLONGED EXPOSURE TO SUNLIGHT—auranofin, sulfasalazine.
sulfasalazine	Azulfidine	Start 500–1000 mg/day; increase to 2000–3000 mg/day in 2 divided doses (enteric-coated tablets)	MAINTAIN ADEQUATE HYDRATION—sulfasalazine. MAY DISCOLOR URINE (or skin)—orange-yellow, sulfasalazine.
auranofin	Ridura	6 mg/day in 1–2 divided doses (maximum, 9 mg/day)	
gold sodium thiomalate	Aurolate	Start 10 mg/week (IM); increase to 25–50 mg/wk for 20 weeks or toxicity occurs; if effective, continue 25–50 mg every 2–4 weeks indefinitely	DISCARD IF DARKENED (solution should be clear or pale yellow).
penicillamine	Cupramine	125–250 mg/day (may increase dose every 1–3 months to maximum, 1500 mg/day)	TAKE ON AN EMPTY STOMACH.
tofacitinib	Xeljanz	5 mg twice a day or 11 mg extended release tablet once daily	SWALLOW WHOLE (Xeljanz XR)

ᵃTop 200 Drugs From Kane SP. ClinCalc DrugStats Database, Version 18.0. ClinCalc: http://clincalc.com/DrugStats. Updated February 3, 2018. Accessed July 24, 2018.
PO, orally; *SC,* subcutaneously

TECHNICIAN'S CORNER

1. Celebrex is the only prescriptive COX-2 inhibitor left on the market. Discuss the FDA's or Health Canada's role in identifying postmarket drug safety issues.
2. Diets that are low in purine have been recommended to prevent gout attacks. What foods might be recommended to patients with gout?

Key Points

- Gout is the primary disease associated with hyperuricemia, a condition in which urate levels build up in the blood serum.
- The joints most commonly affected by gout are the big toe, foot, ankle, knee, wrist, finger, and elbow. Urate crystals build-up in joints and cause inflammation and pain.
- Urate-lowering drugs are prescribed for the treatment of gout.
- Urate-lowering drugs reduce inflammation, dissolve urate crystals, and/or increase urinary elimination of urates.
- A uricosuric is a drug the increases the renal clearance (elimination) of urate crystals.
- Colchicine is the oldest drug used for the treatment of acute gouty arthritis pain.
- Probenecid is a uricosuric used in the treatment of gout.
- Allopurinol, a xanthine oxidase inhibitor, blocks the final enzymatic step in the synthesis of uric acid.
- A low purine diet is recommended to prevent gout attacks.
- Certain meats, fish, and beer increase the risks of an acute gout attack, perhaps because they contain high levels of purines.
- Pegloticase and rasburicase are recombinant urate oxidase enzymes that convert uric acid to a water-soluble purine that is excreted in the urine.
- Nonsteroidal antiinflammatory drugs (NSAIDs) and aspirin (ASA) are widely used in the treatment of pain and inflammation caused by gout and arthritis.

- Rheumatoid arthritis is an autoimmune disease in which the immune system attacks its own cells. It is characterized by inflammation of the lining of the joints.
- Drug therapy for rheumatoid arthritis is aimed at suppressing inflammation, pain, and immune system response to minimize further joint destruction, preservation of body functions, and prevention of disability.
- Glucocorticosteroids have immunosuppressive actions and are prescribed to suppress inflammation, reduce flare-ups, and treat pain.
- Antimalarials have antiinflammatory and analgesic properties that are useful in the management of rheumatoid arthritis.
- Biologic response modifiers act to inhibit the release of cells that mobilize to fight what the body believes is a harmful invasion and inhibit the release of substances that produce inflammation.
- Immunosuppressive drugs interfere with the formation of immune cells by damaging RNA and DNA needed for cell replication.
- Tumor necrosis factor-α (TNF-α) inhibitors are genetically engineered drugs that block the inflammatory process triggered by high concentrations of TNF.
- Methotrexate blocks purine synthesis needed for lymphocyte cell proliferation, reducing inflammation, and immune system activity.

- Leflunomide interferes with pyrimidine synthesis, and when used along with methotrexate, both pathways in the cell division process for lymphocytes are blocked.
- Sulfasalazine is a combination of an antiinfective agent and an aspirin-like antiinflammatory agent, and it is used to treat RA.
- Gold compounds are used in the treatment of RA and work by decreasing the release of antibodies and cytokines and inhibiting the action of collagenase, actions that are part of the immune response.
- Penicillamine is used in the treatment of RA because it has antiinflammatory actions and alters immune system response.

Review Questions

1. _____is the primary disease associated with hyperuricemia.
   a. Arthritis
   b. Gout
   c. Osteoporosis
   d. Kidney stones
2. All of the listed drugs are prescribed for the treatment of gout EXCEPT _____.
   a. colchicine
   b. clozapine
   c. allopurinol
   d. indomethacin
3. You receive a prescription for rasburicase (Elitek, Fasturtek) 1 mg IM. You consult with the pharmacist about the prescription because _____.
   a. rasburicase is a tablet
   b. rasburicase is an oral solution
   c. rasburicase in administered by IV infusion
   d. is an investigational drug in the United States or Canada
4. You receive a prescription for Uloric 8 mg QID. You consult with the pharmacist because _____.
   a. Uloric is not marketed as 8 mg
   b. Uloric is typically prescribed once daily
   c. Uloric is administered IV
   d. Uloric is an injectable drug
5. Diets _____ in purine have been recommended to prevent gout attacks.
   a. high
   b. low
6. The brand name for allopurinol is _____.
   a. Zyban
   b. Zomig
   c. Zyloprim
   d. Zyrtec
7. A uricosuric is a drug that decreases the renal clearance of urates.
   a. true
   b. false
8. A disease that occurs when the immune system turns against the parts of the body it is designed to protect is called a(n) _____.
   a. autoimmune disease
   b. viral disease
   c. immune disease
   d. bacterial disease
9. Which of the following drugs is indicated for the treatment of active rheumatoid arthritis, ankylosing spondylitis, and chronic plaque psoriasis?
   a. Enbrel
   b. Remicade
   c. Humira
   d. Kineret
10. _____ are prescribed commonly to suppress inflammation, reduce flare-ups, and treat pain associated with multiple sclerosis, myasthenia gravis, systemic erythematosus, myositis, and rheumatoid arthritis.
   a. Mineralocorticoids
   b. Glucocorticosteroids
   c. Anabolic steroids
   d. All of the above

Bibliography

Becker M, Jolly M: Hyperuricemia and associated diseases, *Rheum Dis Clin North Am* 32:275–293, 2006.

FDA: Drugs@FDA: FDA Approved Drug Products, nd. Retrieved May 22, 2017, from http://www.accessdata.fda.gov/scripts/cder/daf/.

Health Canada: Drug Product Database, 2017. Retrieved May 22, 2017, from https://health-products.canada.ca/dpd-bdpp/index-eng.jsp.

Kalant H, Grant D, Mitchell J: *Principles of medical pharmacology*, ed 7, Toronto, 2007, Elsevier Canada, A Division of Reed Elsevier Canada, p 381.

Institute for Safe Medication Practices: FDA and ISMP Lists of Look-Alike Drug Names with Recommended Tall Man Letters, 2016.

National Institute of Arthritis and Musculoskeletal and Skin Dieases: Gout, 2016. Retrieved February 22, 2017, from https://www.niams.nih.gov/Health_Info/Gout/default.asp.

National Institute of Arthritis and Musculoskeletal and Skin Diseases: Rheumatoid Arthritis, Bethesda, MD, 2017, NIAMS, National Institutes of Health, U.S. Department of Health and Human Services. NIH Publication No. 17–4179. Retrieved from https://www.niams.nih.gov/health-topics/rheumatoid-arthritis#tab-treatment.

Page C, Curtis M, Sutter M, et al: *Integrated pharmacology*, Philadelphia, 2005, Mosby, pp 450–451.

Pohar S, Murphy G: *Febuxostat for prevention of gout attacks* [Issues in emerging health technologies issue 87], Ottawa, 2006, Canadian Agency for Drugs and Technologies in Health.

Rai SK, Avina-Zubieta JA, McCormick N, et al: Rising incidence and prevalence of gout in the canadian general population [abstract], *Arthritis Rheumatol* 67(Suppl 10):2015. http://acrabstracts.org/abstract/rising-incidence-and-prevalence-of-gout-in-the-canadian-general-population/. (Accessed 25 February 2017).

Robinson PC, Dalbeth N: Advances in pharmacotherapy for the treatment of gout, *Expert Opin Pharmacother* 16(4):533–546, 2015. doi:10.151 7/14656566.2015.997213.

The Arthitis Society: Gout—Causes, Symptoms and Treatment, 2016. http://arthritis.ca/manage-arthritis/educational-resources-tools/printed-publications.

Underwood M: Diagnosis and management of gout, *BMJ* 332:1315–1319, 2006.

USP Center for Advancement of Patient Safety: Use caution—avoid confusion, USP Quality Review No. 79, Rockville, MD, April 2004, USP Center for Advancement of Patient Safety.

14

Treatment of Osteoporosis and Paget's Disease of the Bone

LEARNING OBJECTIVES

1. Learn the terminology associated with osteoporosis and Paget's disease of the bone.
2. Describe the signs and symptoms of osteoporosis.
3. List causes of osteoporosis.
4. Describe the signs and symptoms of Paget's disease of the bone.
5. List and classify medications used in the treatment of osteoporosis and Paget's disease of the bone.
6. Describe the mechanism of action for each class of drug used in the treatment of osteoporosis and Paget's disease of the bone.
7. Identify significant drug look-alike and sound-alike issues.
8. Identify warning labels and precautionary messages associated with medications used to treat osteoporosis and Paget's disease of the bone.

KEY TERMS

Bone mineral density Test measurement that is taken to determine the degree of bone loss.
Bone resorption Process during which bone is broken down into mineral ions (e.g., calcium).
Osteoblasts Cells responsible for bone formation, deposit, and mineralization of the collagen matrix of bone.

Osteoclasts Cells responsible for bone resorption.
Osteoporosis Chronic, progressive disease of bone characterized by loss of bone density and bone strength and resulting in increased risk for fractures.
Remodeling Process of continual turnover of bone.

Osteoporosis

An estimated 10.2 million men and women in the United States and 1.4 million people in Canada have osteoporosis. It is the most common disease of bone and affects women more often than men. *Osteoporosis* is a chronic, progressive disease characterized by loss of bone density and bone strength. It increases the risk for fractures (Fig. 14.1). The risk for osteoporosis increases with age, increasing from 4% of women ages 50 to 59 years up to 52% by age 80 years. The risk is increased in people with low bone mass (decreased *bone mineral density* [BMD]). Fifty-four percent of adults in the United States older than 50 years (43.4 million people) have low bone mass.

In the United States and Canada, one in three women and one in five men with osteoporosis will get a bone fracture during their lifetime. The most common are fractures of the vertebrae of the spine and hips, although fractures of the wrists, feet, toes, and forearm also occur. Fractures caused by osteoporosis are classified according to health outcomes as low-impact or fragility fractures. Low-impact fractures are often caused by falls or another trauma. Fragility fractures may occur in the absence of trauma and can occur from simply coughing or sneezing.

Pathophysiology of Osteoporosis

Primary osteoporosis is associated with the aging process. Up until the age of 30 or 40 years, the percentage of bone formed is greater than the percentage of bone lost. After menopause, women have a dramatic shift in the ratio between bone formation and bone loss, with bone loss exceeding bone formation. In men, this process is more gradual until the age 65 or 70 years; then the rates of bone loss for men and women are approximately equal.

Bone formation and loss is a carefully controlled process and is regulated from birth to death. The process is called *remodeling*. Osteoblasts and osteoclasts are cells that are involved in the bone turnover process. *Osteoblasts* are responsible for bone formation, deposit, and mineralization of the collagen matrix of bone. *Osteoclasts* are responsible for bone resorption. *Bone resorption* is the process whereby bone is broken down into mineral ions (e.g., calcium).

Bone turnover is linked to levels of calcium in the blood. Ninety-nine percent of total body calcium is located in the skeleton; therefore bones are a reservoir for calcium when serum levels are too low. If serum calcium levels are too low, hormones are released to transfer calcium stored in bones back into serum. When blood calcium levels are too high, hormones are released to reduce serum

• **Fig. 14.1** Osteoporosis. Normal bone (left) versus osteoporotic bone (right). (In Nix S: *Williams' basic nutrition and diet therapy*, ed 15, St. Louis, 2017, Elsevier. From Maher AB, Salmond SW, Pellino T: *Orthopaedic nursing*, ed 3, Philadelphia, 2002, Elsevier.)

calcium and deposit excess in bones. The hormones principally responsible for regulation of serum calcium levels are parathyroid hormone (PTH), calcitonin, and vitamin D. PTH is secreted by the parathyroid gland when intestinal absorption of calcium and renal reabsorption of calcium are insufficient to maintain the required calcium balance. Calcitonin reduces serum calcium levels by storing excess in the bone. Vitamin D enhances calcium absorption and is one of the hormones involved in the formation of osteoclasts. PTH and sex hormones are also associated with osteoclast formation. Other hormones linked to the regulation of bone formation and bone loss are estrogen, progesterone, luteinizing hormone, and androgens. Estrogen and progesterone levels are lowered in postmenopausal women, and testosterone levels are reduced in men as part of the normal aging process, which in part explains why osteoporosis increases with age.

Conditions That Produce Osteoporosis

Osteoporosis can be classified as primary or secondary. Secondary osteoporosis may be related to another disease process or can be drug induced. Some of the diseases that can produce secondary osteoporosis include hyperthyroidism, rheumatoid arthritis, inflammatory bowel disease, renal insufficiency, Parkinson's disease, multiple sclerosis, chronic obstructive pulmonary disease, and HIV/AIDS. Some of the conditions associated with bone loss are shown in Box 14.1.

Drugs that can induce osteoporosis are administered for a wide variety of diseases. They are used in the treatment of autoimmune diseases of the musculoskeletal system, seizures, prostate cancer, bipolar disorder, hypothyroidism, kidney disease, and other conditions. Alcohol abuse can also produce osteoporosis. Examples of some of the drugs that can produce bone loss leading to osteoporosis are shown in Box 14.2.

Prevention Tips

It is best to lay the foundation for healthy dense bones early in life, although bone health can be improved at any age. Mild weight-bearing exercise, such as walking, climbing stairs, or stretching with elastic exercise bands or weights, along with a diet rich in vitamin D and calcium, is key to strong bones. Lifestyle changes that reduce alcohol consumption and smoking are also important.

Recommended daily allowances (RDAs) for calcium are listed in Table 14.1. The Osteoporosis Society of Canada and the US

• **BOX 14.1** Diseases and Conditions That May Cause Bone Loss

- HIV/AIDS
- Ankylosing spondylitis
- Blood and bone marrow disorders
- Chronic obstructive pulmonary disease
- Cushing syndrome
- Cystic fibrosis
- Diabetes
- Eating disorders, especially anorexia nervosa and malnutrition
- Female athlete triad: loss of menstrual periods, an eating disorder, and excessive exercise
- Gastrectomy, including gastrointestinal bypass procedures
- Hyperparathyroidism
- Hyperthyroidism
- Hypocalcemia and hypophosphatemia
- Inflammatory bowel disease, including Crohn's disease and ulcerative colitis
- Kidney disease that is chronic and long-lasting
- Liver disease, including biliary cirrhosis
- Malignancies, including lymphoma, leukemia, and multiple myeloma
- Malabsorption syndromes, including celiac disease
- Organ transplants
- Ovarian failure
- Polio and postpolio syndrome
- Premature menopause (before 45 years old)
- Reduced mobility diseases, including multiple sclerosis, muscular dystrophy, Parkinson's disease, spinal cord injuries, stroke
- Rheumatoid arthritis
- Sickle cell anemia and thalassemia
- Testosterone deficiency
- Thyrotoxicosis

From U.S. Department of Health and Human Services: The 2004 Surgeon General's Report on Bone Health and Osteoporosis: What it Means to You. In U.S. Department of Health and Human Services, editor: Washington, DC, 2004, Office of the Surgeon General. Adapted from National Osteoporosis Foundation. (2011). Diseases and Conditions That May Cause Bone Loss. Retrieved July 8, 2012, http://www.nof.org/.

• **BOX 14.2** Drugs That Can Produce Bone Loss

- Antiandrogens (flutamide and nilutamide)
- Aromatase inhibitors
- Cyclosporine
- Depo-medroxyprogesterone acetate
- Gonadotropin-releasing hormone agonists (leuprolide)
- Glucocorticosteroids
- Lithium
- Methotrexate
- Anticonvulsants (e.g., phenytoin)
- Thiazolidinediones

National Osteoporosis Foundation (NOF) recommend that postmenopausal women and men at risk for fractures ingest 1200 mg of calcium daily. The Canadian guidelines for vitamin D is 800 to 2000 IU daily. The NOF guideline is 800 to 1000 IU daily.

Milk, leafy green vegetables, and soybeans contain calcium. Vitamin D is produced by the skin upon exposure to sunlight. Foods rich in calcium are listed in Table 14.2.

Calcium can be obtained from calcium supplements in addition to food. Calcium supplements are available as calcium chloride, calcium citrate, calcium carbonate, calcium lactate, and calcium gluconate. The amount of elemental calcium contained in these

TABLE 14.1 Your Body Needs Calcium

If This Is Your Age	Then You Need This Much Calcium Each Day[a]
Women: 18–50 years	1,000 mg
Women: Older than 50 years	1,200 mg
Men: 18–70 years	1,000 mg
Men: Older than 71 years	1,200 mg

[a]From National Osteoporosis Foundation. (2018). Calcium/Vitamin D. Retreived July 29, 2018, https://www.nof.org/patients/treatment/calciumvitamin-d/.

calcium salts varies. Calcium citrate is most absorbable and easiest to tolerate; however, calcium carbonate provides the greatest amount of elemental calcium per tablet. Calcium carbonate should be taken on a full stomach. Food increases absorption and decreases upset stomach. Calcium citrate may be taken without regard to food.

> ● **TECH NOTE!**
>
> Aerobic, weight-bearing physical activity (e.g., walking or stairclimbing) up to 20–30 minutes daily or 150 minutes per week, plus strength training with weights at least 2 days per week can improve bone health, but most people are not active enough.

> ● **TECH NOTE!**
>
> Calcium can inhibit absorption of some medicines, such as iron and levothyroxine. Warning labels should instruct patients to avoid calcium within 2–4 h of any other medication taken by mouth.

Paget's Disease of Bone

Paget's disease is a progressive disease of bone. The cause is unknown, yet it is believed that genetics, viral infection, and environmental factors may be a factor. Paget's disease is most common in men older than 55 years. Approximately 2%–3% of Americans and 3% of Canadians have Paget's disease.

Pathophysiology of Paget's Disease of the Bone

The disease produces excessive bone resorption followed by increased bone formation, resulting in enlarged bones that are structurally weak. Effects of the disease tend to be localized and most commonly affect the pelvis, lumbar sacral spine, skull, femur, or tibia; however, Paget's disease may be widespread throughout the body, and the entire skeleton can be affected.

Paget's disease causes deformities such as bowed legs, pain, arthritis, deafness, and (rarely) cranial nerve palsies. Pain may be constant or intermittent. Intermittent pain is typically associated with weight bearing or localized microfractures. Constant pain may even occur at rest.

Drugs Used for the Treatment of Osteoporosis and Paget's Disease of Bone

Treatment goals for osteoporosis are to increase bone density and reduce risks for future fractures. Pharmacologic agents that are

TABLE 14.2 Adapted From NIH With National Osteoporosis Foundation Data

Produce	Serving Size	Estimated Calcium*
Collard greens, frozen	8 oz	360 mg
Broccoli raw	8 oz	200 mg
Broccoli, fresh, cooked	8 oz	60 mg
Kale, frozen	8 oz	180 mg
Soy Beans, green, boiled	8 oz	175 mg
Bok Choy, cooked, boiled	8 oz	160 mg
Oranges	1 whole	55 mg
Seafood Serving Size Estimated Calcium*		
Sardines, canned with bones	3 oz	325 mg
Salmon, canned with bones	3 oz	180 mg
Shrimp, canned	3 oz	125 mg
Dairy Serving Size Estimated Calcium*		
Ricotta, part-skim	4 oz	335 mg
Yogurt, plain, low-fat	6 oz	310 mg
Milk, skim, low-fat, whole	8 oz	300 mg
Yogurt with fruit, low-fat	6 oz	260 mg
Mozzarella, part-skim	1 oz	210 mg
Cheddar	1 oz	205 mg
Feta Cheese	4 oz	140 mg
Cottage Cheese, 2%	4 oz	105 mg
Parmesan	1 tbsp	55 mg
Frozen yogurt, vanilla	8 oz	105 mg
Ice Cream, vanilla	8 oz	85 mg
Fortified Food Serving Size Estimated Calcium*		
Almond milk, rice milk or soy milk, fortified	8 oz	300 mg
Orange juice and other fruit juices, fortified	8 oz	300 mg
Tofu, prepared with calcium	4 oz	205 mg
Waffle, frozen, fortified	2 pieces	200 mg
Oatmeal, fortified	1 packet	140 mg
English muffin, fortified	1 muffin	100 mg
Other Serving Size Estimated Calcium*		
Mac & cheese, frozen	1 package	325 mg
Pizza, cheese, frozen	1 serving	115 mg
Beans, baked, canned	4 oz	160 mg

*The calcium content listed for most foods is estimated and can vary due to multiple factors. Check the food label to determine how much calcium is in a particular product.
Adapted from National Osteoporosis Foundation. Calcium-Rich Foods (2018) Retrieved July 29, 2018. https://www.nof.org/patients/treatment/calciumvitamin-d/.

Calcium Supplements

Generic Name	US Brand Name(s)	Dosage Forms and Strengths
	Canadian Brand Name(s)	
calcium carbonate[a] (oyster shell calcium)—various manufacturers—some products listed contain vitamin D	Caltrate Bone & Joint, Caltrate Soft Chews, Citracal Pearls, Os Cal + D₃, TUMS Chewies, TUMS E-X Extra Strength, TUMS Ultra Strength	**Tablets:** 500 mg, 600 mg, 750 mg, 1200 mg **Chewable tablets:** 400 mg, 500 mg, 600 mg, 750 mg, 1000 mg, 1200 mg **Suspension:** 500 mg/5 mL
	Caltrate, Caltrate Select, Caltrate Plus Chewables, TUMS Chewies, TUMS Smoothies Extra Strength, TUMS Ultra Strength	
calcium citrate[a] (plus vit D)	Citracal Maximum, Citracal Petites	**Tablet:** 300 mg, 500 mg, 630 mg[b] **Chewable tablets:** 1000 mg
	Citracal, Citracal Petites	
calcium gluconate[a]	Generics	**Injection:** 10%
	Generics	
calcium chloride[a]	Generics	**Injection:** 10%
	Generics	
calcium, mixed forms (carbonate, citrate, fumerate, malate, succinate) plus vit. D	Generics	**Tablet:** 600 mg, 650 mg
	Generics	
calcium phosphate or tricalcium phosphate (plus vit D)[a]	Citracal Gummies, Posture-D	**Chewable gummies:** 250 mg **Chewable tablets:** 350 mg **Tablets:** 600 mg **Suspension:** 500 mg/15 mL
	Caltrate Gummies Posture-D	

[a]Generics available.
[b]Available in the United States only.

used to treat osteoporosis are categorized as antiresorptive (inhibit bone resorption) or anabolic (promote bone formation). Drug treatment for Paget's disease is recommended for patients that have symptoms or are at risk for fractures or deafness.

> ### ⊘ TECH ALERT!
> The following drugs have look-alike and sound-alike issues:
> Actonel and Actos

Antiresorptive Agents

The majority of the drugs used to treat osteoporosis and Paget's disease are antiresorptive agents. They suppress bone turnover and loss. Bisphosphonates, calcitonin, and estrogens are antiresorptive agents.

Bisphosphonates

Most of the bisphosphonates are used for the treatment of Paget's disease and osteoporosis. Bisphosphonates that are marketed in the United States and/or Canada are alendronate, etidronate, ibandronate, pamidronate, risedronate, tiludronate, and zolendronic acid. Bisphosphonates inhibit bone resorption. Alendronate, ibandronate, and risedronate have been shown to reduce vertebral fractures by up to 40%–50% and hip fractures by 20%–50%. Ibandronate is approved by the US Food and Drug Administration (FDA) for Paget's disease. Intravenous zoledronic acid is indicated for hypercalcemia due to malignant tumors rather than osteoporosis and Paget's disease.

Mechanism of Action and Pharmacokinetics

Bisphosphonates inhibit bone resorption. There are two groups of bisphosphonates. The nitrogen-containing bisphosphonates (alendronate, pamidronate, risedronate) are more potent than the non–nitrogen-containing agents (etidronate, tiludronate). Pamidronate and zoledronic acid are administered by intravenous infusion.

The bisphosphonates are poorly absorbed in the gastrointestinal tract, and food further reduces absorption. All but ibandronate must be taken on an empty stomach at least 30 minutes before the first meal or beverage of the day. Ibandronate must be taken 60 minutes before the first meal. Between 50% and 80% of the drug is eliminated unchanged in the urine within 24 hours of dosing. The remainder permanently binds to bone. Bisphosphonates are available in dosage forms for daily (alendronate, risedronate, ibandronate), weekly (alendronate, risedronate), monthly (risedronate, ibandronate), and yearly (zoledronic acid) dosing. Patient adherence is improved when the medication is dosed once weekly or monthly. Zoledronic acid is administered as a single dose annually for osteoporosis treatment or once every 2 years for prevention. It is administered as a single dose to induce remission in Paget's disease.

> ### ● TECH NOTE!
> An FDA safety announcement warns that, "The safety and effectiveness of Reclast for the treatment of osteoporosis is based on clinical data of three years' duration. The optimal duration of use has not been determined. Patients should have the need for continued therapy re-evaluated on a periodic basis."

Bisphosphonates

	Generic Name	US Brand Name(s)	Dosage Forms and Strengths
		Canadian Brand(s)	
	alendronate[a]	Binosto, Fosamax	**Effervescent tablet**[b]**:** 70 mg
		Fosamax	**Tablets**[c]**:** 5 mg, 10 mg, 40 mg **Tablets, weekly:** 70 mg
	etidronate[a]	Generics	**Tablets:** 200 mg, 400 mg
		Generics	
	ibandronate[a]	Boniva	**Solution, for injection:** 1 mg/mL
		Not available	**Tablets, monthly:** 150 mg
	pamidronate[a]	Aredia	**Powder, for injection:** 30 mg/vial, 60 mg/vial, 90 mg/vial
		Generics	**Solution, for injection:** 3 mg/mL, 6 mg/mL, 9 mg/mL
	risedronate[a]	Actonel, Atelvia	**Tablets:** 5 mg, 30 mg **Tablets weekly:** 35 mg
		Actonel, Actonel DR	**Tablets, delayed release, weekly:** 35 mg **Tablets, monthly:** 17 mg[b], 150 mg
	zoledronic acid	Reclast, Zometa	**Solution, for injection:** 4 mg/5 mL, 4 mg/100 mL, 5 mg/100 mL
		Aclasta, Zometa	
Combinations			
	alendronate + cholecalciferol	Fosamax Plus D	**Tablets:** 70 mg alendronate + 2800 international units vitamin D
		Fosavance	70 mg alendronate + 5600 international units vitamin D

[a]Generic available.
[b]Available in the United States only.
[c]Available in Canada only.

Adverse Reactions

Common adverse effects associated with bisphosphonates are painful swallowing, heartburn, diarrhea, nausea, and vomiting. Less common adverse reactions are musculoskeletal pain, atypical fractures, osteonecrosis or erosion of the jaw bone, and eye inflammation.

> **• TECH NOTE!**
>
> An FDA safety alert recommends that bisphosphonates be discontinued in patients experiencing a femoral shaft fracture; otherwise, patients should continue with therapy and report any hip or thigh pain.

Precautions

To prevent injury to the esophagus by bisphosphonates, the patient should sit or stand upright for 30 to 60 minutes (depending on the agent) after taking the medication. Each tablet should be taken with 6 to 8 oz of water. Calcium and vitamin D supplementation is recommended in conjunction with bisphosphonates but should not be administered at the same time. Multivitamins with iron, calcium supplements, and antacids should be avoided within 2 hours of administration of the prescribed bisphosphonate dose.

Selective Estrogen Receptor Modulators

Selective estrogen receptor modulators (SERMs) treat and prevent further destruction of bone architecture. They are indicated for treatment in postmenopausal women.

Mechanism of Action and Pharmacokinetics

Raloxifene (Evista) and bazedoxifene + conjugated estrogens (Duavee, Duavive) are indicated for the treatment and prevention of osteoporosis. They reduce new fractures of the vertebrae by 30%–50% over 3 years but have no effect on hip fractures. Only 2% of the amount of raloxifene administered is bioavailable. First-pass metabolism and protein binding limit the amount of drug absorbed to produce a therapeutic effect.

Adverse Reactions

Common side effects are hot flashes, leg cramps, peripheral edema, stroke, and venous thromboembolism (VTE). Patients may be instructed to discontinue raloxifene at least 72 hours before and during prolonged immobilization (e.g., bed rest, after surgery) until fully ambulatory again, to prevent VTE.

Calcitonin

Calcitonin is a hormone that is secreted by the thyroid gland and inhibits the rate of bone turnover stimulated by release of PTH.

Selective Estrogen Receptor Modulators

Generic Name	US Brand Name(s) Canadian Brand(s)	Dosage Forms and Strengths
raloxifene[a]	Evista	**Tablets:** 60 mg
	Evista	
bazedoxifene + conjugated estrogens	Duavee	**Tablets:** 20 mg bazedoxifene + 0.45 mg conjugated estrogens
	Duavive	

[a]Generic available.

It lowers serum calcium levels by decreasing intestinal absorption of calcium and increasing renal elimination of calcium. These actions make calcitonin useful for the treatment of Paget's disease. The effectiveness of calcitonin in the treatment of osteoporosis is related to its ability to increase BMD. It has been shown to reduce vertebral fracture risk by 33%–36% over 3 years but has not proven effective in decreasing hip fractures.

Absorption of calcitonin from intramuscular and subcutaneous injection sites is rapid, and the half-life of calcitonin is short (20 minutes). The bioavailability of calcitonin when administered intranasally is 3%–50%. Local adverse reactions are mainly irritation of the nose or injection site.

Miscellaneous

Generic Name	US Brand Name(s) Canadian Brand(s)	Dosage Forms and Strengths
calcitonin[a]	Miacalcin	**Nasal solution:**[b] 200 units per actuation (spray)
	Calcimar	**Solution, for injection:** 200 units/mL

[a]Generic available.
[b]Available in the United States only.

> ⚠ **TECH ALERT!**
> Calcitonin and calcitriol have look-alike and sound-alike issues.

Hormone Replacement Therapy

Estrogen deficiency occurs with the onset of menopause and increases osteoclast activity. Osteoclasts are responsible for bone resorption. Hormone replacement restores estrogen levels and inhibits the effects of estrogen deficiency on bone. Estrogens with or without progestins are indicated for prevention of osteoporosis, decreasing bone turnover, bone loss, and fractures. Hormone replacement therapy (HRT) is not a first-line therapy for the prevention of osteoporosis because of the increased risk for coronary heart disease, stroke, thromboembolism, as well as breast and uterine cancers. HRT also has beneficial effects on BMD and reduces the relative risk for vertebral and hip fractures up to 34%. Increases in BMD are dose dependent; higher doses produce increased BMD. Increases in BMD occur with oral and transdermal dosage forms.

Estrogens (conjugated estrogens, esterified estrogens, estradiol, estropipate) with and without progestins (levonorgestrel, medroxyprogesterone, norethindrone, or norgestimate) are prescribed for HRT in the treatment of osteoporosis. HRT is also indicated for the treatment of menopausal symptoms (hot flashes, vaginal dryness, and atrophy), postmenopausal urogenital symptoms (urgency, dysuria), abnormal uterine bleeding, hypoestrogenism, and breast and prostate cancer (palliation). These drugs are discussed in detail in Chapter 27. Adverse reactions include headache, nausea, rash at the site of patch application, coronary heart disease, depression, stroke, thromboembolism, and breast and uterine cancer.

> ⚠ **TECH ALERT!**
> The following drugs have look-alike and sound-alike issues:
> Alora and Aldara;
> Estratest and Estratest HS

Anabolic Agents

PTH analogues increase the rate of bone remodeling, thicken structural units of bone (ostens), and produce bone architecture that closely resembles normal bone. They decrease osteoblast cell death, allowing the balance between bone formation and bone resorption to shift toward bone formation. This is an improvement over bisphosphonates, because alendronate, risedronate, and etidronate only prevent further destruction of bone architecture. They do not restore normal structure. Teriparatide is a genetically engineered form of human PTH and the only drug currently available in this category. It is administered subcutaneously and injected daily. It is indicated for postmenopausal women and men at high risk for fracture. Common adverse reactions are orthostatic hypotension, dizziness, headache, hypercalcemia, leg cramps, nausea, arthralgias, hyperuricemia, and gout. Safety when used longer than 2 years has not been determined.

> ⚠ **TECH ALERT!**
> Because of the potential risk for osteosarcoma, the FDA requires a boxed warning for teriparatide stating that its use is limited to patients for whom the benefit outweighs the risk.

Hormone Replacement Therapy

Generic Name	US Brand Name(s) / Canadian Brand(s)	Dosage Forms and Strengths
estradiol[a]	Alora, Climara, Estrace, Estraderm, Menostar, Vivelle, Vivelle-Dot Climara, Estrace, Estraderm, Estradot, Oesclim	**Solution for injection:**[b] 5 mg/mL **Tablets, oral (Estrace):** 0.5 mg, 1 mg, 2 mg (Estrace) **Transdermal patch, biweekly (Alora, Estraderm, Estradot, Oesclim, Vivelle, Vivelle Dot):** 0.025 mg/24 h, 0.0375 mg/24 h, 0.05 mg/24 h, 0.075 mg/24 h, 0.1 mg/24 h **Transdermal patch, weekly (Climara):** 0.025 mg/24 h, 0.0375 mg/24 h[b], 0.05 mg/24 h, 0.06 mg/24 h[b], 0.075 mg/24 h, 0.1 mg/24 h and 0.014 mg/24 h (Menostar)[b]
estradiol + levonorgestrol	Climara Pro Not available	**Transdermal patch:** estradiol, 0.045 mg + levonorgestrel, 0.015 mg per 24 h
estradiol + norethindrone[a]	Activella Activelle, Activelle LD	**Tablets:** 0.5 mg estradiol + 0.1 mg norethindrone; 1 mg estradiol + 0.5 mg norethindrone
conjugated estrogens[a]	Premarin Premarin	**Tablets:** 0.3 mg, 0.45 mg[b], 0.625 mg, 1.25 mg
estrogens + medroxyprogesterone	Premphase, Prempro Not Available	**Tablets (Premphase 14/14):** conjugated estrogens 0.625 mg (14 maroon tablets) and 0.625 mg conjugated estrogen + 5 mg medroxyprogesterone (14 blue tablets) **Tablets (Prempro):** 0.3 mg conjugated estrogen + 1.5 mg medroxyprogesterone[b]; 0.45 mg conjugated estrogen + 1.5 mg medroxyprogesterone[b]; 0.625 mg conjugated estrogen + 2.5 mg medroxyprogesterone; 0.625 mg conjugated estrogen + 5 mg medroxyprogesterone
estropipate[a]	Ogen Not available	**Tablets:** 0.625 mg (0.75 mg estropipate), 1.25 mg (1.5 mg estropipate), 5 mg (6 mg estropipate)

[a]Generics available.
[b]Available in the United States.

Anabolic Agents

Generic Name	US Brand Name(s) / Canadian Brand(s)	Dosage Forms and Strengths
teriparatide	Forteo Forteo	**Solution, for injection:** 250 mcg/mL

Monoclonal Antibody

Generic Name	US Brand Name(s) / Canadian Brand(s)	Dosage Forms and Strengths
denosumab	Prolia, Xgeva Prolia, Xgeva	**Solution, for injection:** 60 mg/mL (Prolia), 70 mg/mL (120 mg/1.7 mL) (Xgeva)

Receptor Activator of Nuclear Factor Kappa-Beta Ligand Inhibitors

Denosumab is a monoclonal antibody that improves trabecular bone mass and strength. It produces its effects by inhibiting osteoclast activation and decreasing bone resorption. Bone remodeling is reversed from bone destruction to bone formation. It improves trabecular bone mass and strength. Denosumab is administered subcutaneously twice a year. Adverse reactions include increased risk for infection, hypocalcemia, skin rashes, osteonecrosis of the jaw, and fracture healing complications.

Usual Dosage and Warnings for Drugs Used in the Treatment of Osteoporosis and Paget's Disease

	Generic Name	US Brand Name	Usual Adult Oral Dose and Dosing Schedule	Warning Labels
Bisphosphonates				
	alendronate	Fosamax	**Osteoporosis, prevention:** 5 mg once a day or 35 mg once weekly **Osteoporosis, treatment:** 10 mg once a day or 70 mg once weekly **Paget's disease:** 40 mg once daily for 6 months	STAND OR SIT UPRIGHT FOR AT LEAST 30 MIN AFTER TAKING DOSE; DO NOT LIE DOWN—alendronate, etidronate, risedronate. STAND OR SIT UPRIGHT FOR A LEAST 1 H AFTER TAKING DOSE; DO NOT LIE DOWN—ibandronate. TAKE 30 MIN BEFORE THE FIRST MEAL OF THE DAY WITH 6–8 OZ OF WATER. TAKE 1 H BEFORE FIRST MEAL OF THE DAY—ibandronate. AVOID DAIRY PRODUCTS AND ANTACIDS CONTAINING CALCIUM, MAGNESIUM, OR IRON WITHIN 2 H OF DOSE. TAKE ON AN EMPTY STOMACH (TAKE 2 H BEFORE FOOD)—etidronate.
	ibandronate	Boniva	**Osteoporosis:** 150 mg once monthly or administer 3 mg IV bolus every 3 months	
	etidronate	Didronel	**Paget's disease:** 5 mg to 10 mg/kg/day for up to 6 months or 11 mg to 20 mg/kg/day up to 3 months; re-treat if needed after a drug-free period of 90 days	
	pamidronate	Aredia	**Paget's disease:** 30 mg infused intravenously over 4 h for 3 days in a row	
	risedronate	Actonel	**Osteoporosis:** 5 mg once a day, 35 mg once weekly, 75 mg once daily for 2 days a month, or 150 mg once a month **Paget's disease:** 30 mg once a day for 2 months; re-treat if needed after a 2-month drug-free period	
Bisphosphonate Combinations				
	alendronate + cholecalciferol	Fosamax Plus D	1 tablet once weekly	
Selective Estrogen Receptor Modulators				
	raloxifene	Evista	60 mg/day	TAKE WITH OR WITHOUT FOOD.
Hormone Replacement Therapy				
	estradiol	Estrace	**Prevention of osteoporosis:** **Oral:** 0.5 mg/day (3 weeks on and 1 week off) **Transdermal patch, as Climara, Menostar:** 1 patch once weekly **Transdermal patch, as Alora, Estraderm, Estradot, Vivelle-Dot:** 1 patch twice weekly	TAKE WITH FOOD. ROTATE SITE OF APPLICATION—patch.
	estradiol + levonorgestrel	Climara Pro	**Prevention of osteoporosis:** Apply 1 patch weekly to the lower abdomen.	
	estradiol + norethindrone	Activella	**Prevention of osteoporosis:** **Tablets (Activella):** 1 tablet daily	
	conjugated estrogens	Premarin	**Prevention of osteoporosis:** 0.3 mg cyclically or daily	
	estropipate	Ogen	**Prevention of osteoporosis:** 0.75 mg daily for 25 days of a 31-day cycle	

Continued

Usual Dosage and Warnings for Drugs Used in the Treatment of Osteoporosis and Paget's Disease—cont'd

Generic Name	US Brand Name	Usual Adult Oral Dose and Dosing Schedule	Warning Labels
estrogens + medroxy-progesterone	Premphase, Prempro	**Prevention of osteoporosis:** **Premphase:** Take maroon tablets on days 1 through 14 (0.625 mg conjugated estrogen) and blue tablets on days 15 through 28 (estrogens + 5 mg medroxyprogesterone) **Prempro:** Take 1 tablet daily	

Calcitonin Hormone

calcitonin	Miacalcin	**Osteoporosis:** Inject 100 units/day (IM, subcut) or 1 spray in 1 nostril (200 units/day) (intranasal) **Paget's disease:** Start 100 units/day (IM, subcut); maintenance 50 to 100 units every 1–3 days	1 spray intranasally daily, alternating nostrils each day

Monoclonal Antibody

denosumab	Prolia, Xgeva	**Osteoporosis:** 60 mg subcut every 6 months	REFRIGERATE. DO NOT SHAKE. PROTECT FROM LIGHT.

Parathyroid Hormone Analogue

teriparatide	Forteo	**Osteoporosis:** 20 mcg subcut once a day Not recommended for use beyond 2 years.	REFRIGERATE; DO NOT FREEZE. DISCARD AFTER 28 DAYS OF OPENING.

FDA, Food and Drug Administration; *IM,* Intramuscular; *IV,* Intravenous; *subcut,* Subcutaneous.

TECHNICIAN'S CORNER

1. Mild weight-bearing exercise, along with a diet rich in vitamin D and calcium, is key to strong bones that resist fractures. Come up with a 10-day plan of meals and exercises for a client who is menopausal and overweight.
2. Why are lifestyle changes that reduce alcohol consumption and smoking so important to prevent osteoporosis or Paget's disease?

Key Points

- Osteoporosis is a chronic, progressive disease of bone characterized by loss of bone density and bone strength and resulting in increased fracture risk.
- People that have osteoporosis are at risk for fractures.
- Secondary osteoporosis may be caused by diseases or drugs (e.g., prednisone).
- After menopause, women's rate of bone loss exceeds the rate of bone formed. The rate of bone loss for men and women is equal after age 65 to 70 years.
- Ninety-nine percent of total body calcium is located in the skeleton; therefore bones are a reservoir for calcium when serum levels are too low.
- The hormones principally responsible for regulation of serum calcium levels are parathyroid hormone, calcitonin, and vitamin D.
- Other hormones linked to the regulation of bone formation and bone loss are estrogen, progestins, luteinizing hormone, and androgens.
- Paget's disease is also a progressive disease of bone.
- Paget's disease is characterized by excessive bone resorption in focal areas followed by increased bone formation that results in enlarged bones that are structurally weak.

- Paget's disease can cause bone deformities, pain, fractures, and deafness.
- Prevention and treatment osteoporosis includes lifelong nutritional calcium and vitamin D intake, exercise (weight bearing and strength training), lifestyle changes (e.g., reduce alcohol and smoking), and pharmacotherapy.
- Pharmacologic agents used in the treatment of osteoporosis or Paget's disease are categorized as antiresorptive (inhibit bone resorption) or anabolic (promote bone formation).
- Bisphosphonates, calcitonin, SERMs, and estrogen are antiresorptive agents.
- Parathyroid hormone is an anabolic agent.
- Bisphosphonates must be taken on an empty stomach at least 30 to 60 minutes (depending on the agent) before the first meal or beverage of the day.
- Patients taking oral bisphosphonates must sit upright or stand for at least 30 to 60 minutes after dosing to avoid possible esophageal ulceration.
- Calcium and vitamin D supplementation is recommended in conjunction with bisphosphonate and Receptor Activator of Nuclear Factor Kappa-Beta Ligand (RANKL) therapy.

Review Questions

1. A chronic, progressive disease of bone characterized by loss of bone density and bone strength and resulting in increased fracture risk is called _____.
   a. rheumatoid arthritis
   b. osteoporosis
   c. brittle bone disease
   d. osteosarcoma

2. Alcohol abuse can also produce osteoporosis.
   a. True
   b. False

3. You receive a prescription for alendronate 70 mg take 1 tablet daily, 30 minutes before meals. You consult the pharmacist because _____.
   a. alendronate 70 mg should be taken with food
   b. alendronate 70 mg should be taken once weekly
   c. alendronate should be taken twice weekly
   d. alendronate should be taken once monthly

4. The goals of osteoporosis treatment are to _____ bone density and to _____ risks for future fractures.
   a. decrease, reduce
   b. increase, reduce
   c. reduce, remove
   d. decrease, reduce

5. The majority of the drugs used to treat osteoporosis and Paget's disease are _____ agents.
   a. absorption
   b. antifracture
   c. antiresorptive
   d. anticalcium

6. Only some of the bisphosphonates are indicated for the treatment of Paget's disease.
   a. True
   b. False

7. _____ is a selective estrogen receptor modulator (SERM) indicated for the treatment and prevention of osteoporosis in postmenopausal women and prevents further destruction of bone architecture.
   a. Fosamax
   b. Evista
   c. Boniva
   d. Osteo-cal

8. Hormone replacement therapy is the first-line therapy for the prevention of osteoporosis because of the increased risk for coronary heart disease, stroke, thromboembolism, and breast and uterine cancer.
   a. True
   b. False

9. A diet rich in vitamin _____ and _____ is key to strong bones.
   a. C, calcium
   b. D, sodium
   c. D, calcium
   d. B, iron

10. You receive a prescription for Miacalcin, directions 1 spray in each nostril once daily. You consult with the pharmacist because _____.
   a. Miacalcin is not marketed as a nasal spray
   b. Miacalcin is used twice daily
   c. Miacalcin should be used in only one nostril per dose
   d. Miacalcin is a tablet

Bibliography

Alibhai S, Rahman S, Warde P, et al: Prevention and management of osteoporosis in men receiving androgen deprivation therapy: a survey of urologists and radiation oncologists, *Urology* 68:126–131, 2006.

American Pharmacists Association: New approaches to the management of osteoporosis, *Pharmacy Today* 13(1):1–12, 2010.

Cosman F, Beur SJd, LeBoff MS, et al: Clinician's guide to prevention and treatment of osteoporosis, *Osteoporos Int* 25:2359–2381, 2014.

Cranney A, Papaioannou A, Zytaruk N, et al: For the Clinical Guidelines Committee of Osteoporosis Canada: parathyroid hormone for the treatment of osteoporosis: a systematic review, *CMAJ* 175:52–59, 2006.

FDA: Drugs@FDA: FDA Approved Drug Products: U.S. Department Health and Human Services, nd. Available from: http://www.accessdata.fda.gov/scripts/cder/daf/. (Retrieved July 29, 2018).

FDA: FDA Joint Reproductive Health Drugs Advisory Committee and Drug Safety and Risk Management Advisory Committee Meeting on the long-term use of bisphosphonates for the treatment and prevention of osteoporosis, 2011. From: http://www.fda.gov/downloads/AdvisoryCommittees/CommitteesMeetingMaterials/Drugs/DrugSafetyandRiskManagementAdvisoryCommittee/UCM270963.pdf. (Retrieved 6 May 2012).

FDA: FDA Drug Safety Communication: Ongoing safety review of oral osteoporosis drugs (bisphosphonates) and potential increased risk of esophageal cancer, 2011. From: http://www.fda.gov/Drugs/DrugSafety/ucm263320.htm. (Retrieved 5 May 2011).

Gold D, Alexander I, Ettinger M: How can osteoporosis patients benefit more from their therapy? Adherence issues with bisphosphonate therapy, *Ann Pharmacother* 40:1143–1150, 2006.

Health Canada: Drug Product Database, 2018. Available from: https://health-products.canada.ca/dpd-bdpp/index-eng.jsp. (Retrieved July 29, 2018).

Kalant H, Grant D, Mitchell J: *Principles of medical pharmacology*, ed 7, Toronto, 2007, Elsevier Canada, A Division of Reed Elsevier Canada, pp 860–861. 878–889.

Langston A, Ralston S: Management of Paget's disease of bone, *Rheumatology* 43:955–959, 2004.

Mauck K, Clarke B: Diagnosis, screening, prevention, and treatment of osteoporosis, *Mayo Clin Proc* 81:662–672, 2006.

Osteoporosis Canada: Osteoporosis Facts & Statistics, 2017. Available from: www.osteoporosis.ca. (Cited 10 May 2017).

Osteoporosis Canada: Calcium: An important nutrient that builds stronger bones, 2017. Available from: www.osteoporosis.ca. (Retrieved 10 May 2017).

Reid I, Miller P, Lyles K, et al: Comparison of a single infusion of zoledronic acid with risedronate for Paget's disease, *N Engl J Med* 353:898–908, 2005.

U.S. Department of Health and Human Services: *The 2004 Surgeon General's Report on bone health and osteoporosis: what it means to you*, Washington, DC, 2004, U.S. Department of Health and Human Services, Office of the Surgeon General.

Walsh J: Paget's disease of bone: clinical update, *MJA* 181:262–265, 2004.

Wright NC, Looker AC, Saag KG, et al: The recent prevalence of osteoporosis and low bone mass in the United States based on bone mineral density at the femoral neck or lumbar spine, *J Bone Miner Res* 29(11):2520–2526, 2014.

UNIT **IV**

Drugs Affecting the Ophthalmic and Otic Systems

The eye and the ear are sense organs that have specialized structures to maintain vision, balance, and hearing. The eyes provide visual input about an ever-changing environment that is important for identifying danger, language, learning, communicating, working, performing work or activities of daily living. The ear is divided into three anatomical parts—the external ear, middle ear, and inner ear. The ear has dual sensory functions, hearing and balance, or equilibrium. The stimulation or trigger for hearing and balance is the activation of hair cells, receptors that transmit nerve impulses and are perceived in the brain as sound or balance.

In Unit IV, pharmacotherapy for glaucoma, dry eye, and eye infections is presented. Pharmacotherapy for disorders of the ear, such as Meniere's disease, vertigo, and ear infections, is also described. A brief description of each disorder is provided, followed by a description of the drugs indicated for treatment that includes mechanisms of action, adverse reactions, strength(s), and dosage forms. Antibiotics that are used for the treatment of eye and ear infections are discussed in Unit IV chapters. Antibiotics that are used in the treatment of other types of infection are presented in Unit X.

15

Treatment of Diseases of the Eye

LEARNING OBJECTIVES

1. Learn the terminology associated with the eye and the treatment of glaucoma and ophthalmic infections.
2. List and categorize medications used in the treatment of ophthalmic infections and glaucoma.
3. Describe the mechanism of action for each class of drugs used in the treatment of ophthalmic infections and glaucoma.
4. Identify significant drug look-alike and sound-alike issues.
5. Identify warning labels and precautionary messages associated with medications used in the treatment of ophthalmic infections and glaucoma.

KEY TERMS

Angle-closure glaucoma Sudden increase in intraocular pressure caused by obstruction of the drainage portal between the cornea and iris (angle); that can rapidly progress to blindness.

Aqueous humor Fluid made in the front part of the eye.

Blepharitis Chronic disease of the eye that produces distinctive flaky scales that form on the eyelids and eyelashes.

Conjunctivitis (pink eye) Common, self-limiting ailment that causes itching, burning, and teary outflow.

Cytomegalovirus retinitis Viral opportunistic infection of the eye that can cause pain and blindness.

Dry eye disease Occurs when the eye does not produce tears properly, or when the tears are not of the correct consistency and evaporate too quickly.

Herpes simplex keratitis Painful eye infection caused by herpes virus that can lead to blindness.

Herpes zoster ophthalmicus Painful eye infection caused by herpes virus that can lead to blindness.

Intraocular pressure Inner pressure of the eye. Normal intraocular pressure ranges from 12 to 22 mm Hg.

Iritis Condition associated with inflammation of the iris.

Keratitis Severe infection of the cornea that may be caused by bacteria or fungi.

Open-angle glaucoma Disorder characterized by elevated pressure in the eye that can lead to permanent blindness.

Peripheral vision Sometimes called "side vision," this is usually the first area of vision to be lost with glaucoma.

Photopsia Condition similar to floaters and associated with flashes of light.

Stye Painful lump located on the eyelid margin caused by an acute self-limiting infection of the oil glands of the eyelid.

Uveitis Serious eye condition that produces inflammation of the uvea and can cause scarring of the eye and blindness if untreated.

Vitreous floaters Particles that float in the vitreous and cast shadows on the retina and appear as spots, cobwebs, or spiders.

Dry Eye Disease

Dry eye occurs when the eye does not produce tears properly, or when tears are not of the correct consistency and evaporate too quickly. Inflammation of the surface of the eye may occur along with dry eye, and if left untreated, this condition can lead to pain, ulcers, or scars on the cornea, and some loss of vision. Permanent loss of vision from dry eye is uncommon.

Dry eye can make it more difficult to perform some activities, such as using a computer or reading for an extended period of time. It can decrease tolerance for dry environments such as the air inside an airplane. *Dry eye disease* is treated with prescription and over-the-counter (OTC) eye drops. Restasis (cyclosporine) and Xiidra (lifitegrast ophthalmic solution) are prescription ophthalmics that treat moderate to severe dry eye disease. OTC lubricating eye drops (e.g., TheraTears, Tears Naturale, and HYLO) provide relief of mild symptoms.

Prescription Ophthalmics Used to Treat Dry Eye Disease

Generic Name	US Brand Name(s) / Canada Brand Name(s)	Dosage Forms and Strengths
cyclosporine[a]	Restasis	**Ophthalmic emulsion:** 0.05%
	Restasis	
lifitegrast	Xiidra	**Ophthalmic solution:** 5%
	Xiidra	

[a]Generic available in Canada.

• **Fig. 15.1** Stye. (Courtesy of the Cogan Collection, National Eye Institute/ National Institutes of Health.)

• **Fig. 15.2** Psoriatic blepharitis. (Courtesy of the Cogan Collection, National Eye Institute/National Institutes of Health.)

Bacterial Infections of the Eye

Stye

A *stye* (hordeolum) is a small, painful lump located on the eyelid margin (Fig. 15.1). It is caused by an acute, self-limiting infection of the oil glands of the eyelid and typically resolves on its own in a few days. When more than one stye is present at the same time, the condition is called blepharitis.

Blepharitis

Blepharitis is also known as granulated eyelids because of the distinctive flaky scales found on the eyelids and eyelashes produced by the condition. There are two forms of blepharitis, anterior blepharitis and posterior blepharitis. Anterior blepharitis affects the outside of the eyelid where the eyelashes are attached and is caused by bacteria *(Staphylococcus)* and dandruff—a mild, noninflammatory form of seborrhoeic dermatitis. (See Chapter 36.) Posterior blepharitis affects the inside of the eyelid and is caused by dysfunction of the oil glands in the eyelid, seborrhea, psoriasis (Fig. 15.2), and acne rosacea. The symptoms of blepharitis are eye pain or burning, excessive tearing, feeling of "something in the eye," light sensitivity, blurred vision, dry eye, and flaky scales on the eyelids and eyelashes.

Blepharitis is self-treated by applying clean warm compresses to the eyelids to loosen the scales followed by cleansing the eyelids with a mild eyelid scrub. Antiinfective ointments, corticosteroid eye drops, and artificial tears may also be used to manage the symptoms of blepharitis. Aminoglycoside antiinfectives are used in the treatment of blepharitis and include gentamicin, neomycin, and tobramycin.

Conjunctivitis

Conjunctivitis (pink eye) is a common ailment that causes itching, burning, and teary outflow and is caused by allergies, bacteria, or a virus. Viral and allergic conjunctivitis is typically self-limiting and resolves without treatment with antiinfective agents. Conjunctivitis of bacterial origin is contagious and is treated with antibiotic eye drops or orally administered antiinfectives. Conjunctivitis in newborns may be caused by exposure to a sexually

• **Fig. 15.3** Viral conjunctivitis. (Courtesy of the Cogan Collection, National Eye Institute/National Institutes of Health.)

transmitted infection and is treated preventively by administering antibiotic drops at birth. Antibacterial agents that are used in treatment include aminoglycosides, sulfonamides, quinolones, and macrolides. The antiviral trifluridine is used to treat keratoconjunctivitis caused by herpes simplex type 1 virus (Fig. 15.3).

Iritis

Iritis is a condition associated with inflammation of the iris. Most causes of iritis are unknown; known causes are herpes virus, autoimmune disease, eye trauma, infectious disease (histoplasmosis, toxoplasmosis, syphilis, tuberculosis), and juvenile rheumatoid arthritis.

Symptoms of iritis include redness, blurred vision, inflammation, pain, and light sensitivity. Iritis is treated with the administration of corticosteroids (to reduce inflammation) and mydriatics (to reduce painful swelling). Mydriatics act on the dilator muscle and arterioles of the conjunctiva to produce vasoconstriction and dilation of the pupil. Antivirals are administered when iritis is caused by a viral infection.

Keratitis

Keratitis is a severe infection of the cornea and may be caused by bacteria or fungi. If untreated, the infection can cause permanent loss of vision. The most common causes of microbial keratitis and fungal keratitis are trauma, immunodeficiency, and chronic eye surface disease. Contact lens use can also cause microbial and fungal keratitis. Soft contact lens wearers, especially those who wear their contact lenses overnight, are at greater risk for eye infection. Of the approximately 30 million soft contact lens wearers in the United States, up to 21 persons out of 10,000 will develop microbial keratitis. The incidence of fungal keratitis varies according to geographic region. The incidence is higher in the southern United States (up to 35% of microbial keratitis cases) and lowest in the northeastern United States (up to 2% of microbial keratitis cases).

Uveitis

Uveitis is a serious eye condition that produces inflammation of the uvea and can cause scarring of the eye and blindness if untreated.

There are three kinds of uveitis, each associated with a different part of the eye.

Uveitis may be caused by the herpes virus, histoplasmosis (fungus), toxoplasmosis (parasite), or autoimmune disease, but most of the time the cause is unknown. Symptoms of uveitis include redness, blurred vision, pain, inflammation, and light sensitivity. These symptoms may develop suddenly or can develop over a prolonged time period.

Uveitis is treated with the administration of corticosteroids (to reduce inflammation); mydriatics (to reduce painful swelling); and antiinfectives, antivirals, or antifungals as appropriate.

Most drugs used to treat eye infections are applied topically. Humira (adalimumab) and injectable drug was approved in 2016 by the US Food and Drug Administration (FDA) to treat uveitis. Topical agents used in the treatment of eye infections are listed in the drug tables in this chapter.

Topical Ophthalmics Used to Treat Bacterial Infections

Generic Name	US Brand Name(s) / Canadian Brand(s)	Dosage Forms and Strengths
Aminoglycosides		
gentamicin[a]	Genoptic	Solution, ophthalmic: 0.3%,
	Not available	
tobramycin[a]	Tobrex	Ointment, ophthalmic: 0.3%
	Tobrex	Solution, ophthalmic: 0.3%
neomycin sulfate + bacitracin zinc + polymyxin B sulfate[a]	Neosporin	Ointment, ophthalmic: 400 units/g bacitracin zinc + 3.5 mg/g neomycin + 10,000 units/g polymyxin B
	Not Available	
neomycin sulfate + polymyxin B sulfate + gramicidin[a]	Neosporin	Solution, ophthalmic: 1.75 mg/mL neomycin + 10,000 units/mL polymyxin B + 0.025 mg/mL gramicidin
	Not available	
polymyxin B sulfate + bacitracin[a]	Generics	Ointment, ophthalmic: 10,000 units polymyxin B + 500 units bacitracin/Gm
	Optimyxin Ophthalmic Ointment	
Sulfonamides		
sulfacetamide Na[+a]	Bleph-10	Ointment, ophthalmic: 10%
	Not available	Solution, ophthalmic: 10%
trimethoprim + polymyxin B sulfate[a]	Polytrim	Solution, ophthalmic: 1 mg trimethoprim + 10,000 units polymyxin B/mL
	Polytrim	
Quinolones		
besifloxacin	Besivance	Suspension, ophthalmic: 0.6%
	Besivance	
ciprofloxacin[a]	Ciloxan	Ointment, ophthalmic: 0.3%
	Ciloxan	Solution, ophthalmic: 0.3%
gatifloxacin	Zymar, Zymaxid	Solution, ophthalmic: 0.3% (Zymar), 0.5% (Zymaxid)
	Zymar	
levofloxacin[a]	Generics	Solution, ophthalmic: 0.5%
	Not available	

Continued

Topical Ophthalmics Used to Treat Bacterial Infections—cont'd

Generic Name	US Brand Name(s) / Canadian Brand(s)	Dosage Forms and Strengths
moxifloxacin[a]	Moxeza, Vigamox / Vigamox	**Solution, ophthalmic:** 0.5%
ofloxacin[a]	Ocuflox / Ocuflox	Solution, ophthalmic: 0.3%
Macrolides		
azithromycin	AzaSite / Not available	**Solution, ophthalmic:** 1%
erythromycin[a]	Generics / Generics	**Ointment, ophthalmic:** 0.5%
Anti-infective + Corticosteroid		
neomycin + bacitracin + polymyxin B + hydrocortisone[a]	Generics / Not available	**Ointment, ophthalmic:** 3.5 mg/g neomycin + 400 units/g bacitracin + 10,000 units/g polymyxin B + 1% hydrocortisone
neomycin + dexamethasone + polymyxin	Maxitrol / Maxitrol	**Suspension, ophthalmic:** 3.5 mg neomycin + 0.1% dexamethasone + 6000 units polymyxin/mL[b]; 3.5 mg/mL neomycin + 0.1% dexamethasone + 10,000 units polymyxin/mL[c] **Ointment, ophthalmic:** 3.5 mg neomycin + 0.1% dexamethasone + 6000 units polymyxin/Gm[b]; 3.5 mg neomycin + 0.1% dexamethasone + 10,000 units polymyxin/Gm[c]
neomycin + polymyxin B + hydrocortisone[a]	Generics / Not available	**Suspension, ophthalmic:** 0.35% neomycin + 10,000 units polymyxin B + 1% hydrocortisone/mL
gentamicin + prednisolone[a]	Pred-G / Not available	**Suspension, ophthalmic:** 0.3% gentamicin + 1% prednisolone **Ointment, ophthalmic:** 0.3% gentamicin + 0.6% prednisolone
sulfacetamide + prednisolone acetate[a]	Blephamide / Blephamide	**Ointment, ophthalmic:** 10% sulfacetamide + 0.2% prednisolone **Solution, ophthalmic:** 10% sulfacetamide + 0.2% prednisolone
tobramycin + dexamethasone	Tobradex Tobradex ST / Tobradex	**Ointment, ophthalmic:** 0.3% tobramycin + 0.1% dexamethasone **Suspension, ophthalmic:** 0.3% tobramycin + 0.1% dexamethasone 0.3% tobramycin + 0.05% dexamethasone
tobramycin + loteprednol	Zylet / Not available	**Suspension, ophthalmic:** 0.3% tobramycin + 0.5% loteprednol

[a]Generic available.
[b]Available in Canada only.
[c]Available in the United States only.

Viral Infections of the Eye

Cytomegalovirus Retinitis

Cytomegalovirus retinitis is an opportunistic infection in the eye that occurs in patients who have HIV infection/AIDS or take immunosuppressive drugs. The most common symptoms of CMV retinitis are decreased vision, eye pain, floaters, and photopsia. If untreated, CMV retinitis can lead to blindness. *Vitreous floaters* are particles that cast shadows on the retina and appear as spots, cobwebs, or spiders. *Photopsia* is a condition similar to floaters and is associated with flashes of light.

Cytomegalovirus retinitis is treated by administration of antivirals such as ganciclovir, valganciclovir, foscarnet, and cidofovir.

Herpetic Eye Disease

The herpes virus is the cause of more than 500,000 cases of blindness annually. The two strains of the virus that cause eye infections are *herpes zoster ophthalmicus* and *herpes simplex keratitis*. Other common viral infections caused by the herpes virus are chicken pox and shingles *(herpes varicella-zoster)* and cold sores on the lips and mouth *(herpes simplex* 1).

Both herpes zoster ophthalmicus and herpes simplex keratitis produce eye pain because the virus lives around nerve fibers that, when activated, produce pain. Symptoms specifically associated with herpes zoster ophthalmicus are swelling and rash or sores around the eye, eyelids, or forehead. Symptoms of herpes simplex keratitis are excessive tearing, decreased vision, a gritty feeling in the eye, and pain when looking at bright light.

Viral infections of the eye are treated with antivirals. They may be administered topically in the eye, by mouth or IV infusion according to the drug and condition being treated. Antivirals that are used in the treatment of herpetic eye disease are listed the following table. A detailed discussion of antivirals is found in Chapter 30.

Corticosteroids may also be prescribed to reduce inflammation of the trabecular meshwork. Inflammation can impede the outflow of eye fluids and lead to increased intraocular pressure (IOP) and pain. The use of corticosteroids must be carefully monitored because the drugs sometimes increase IOP. Mydriatics may be administered to maintain the normal flow of eye fluids and prevent buildup of IOP.

Drugs Used to Treat Viral Infections in the Eye

Generic Name	US Brand Name(s) Canadian Brand(s)	Dosage Forms and Strengths
cidofovir[a]	Generics	Solution, for injection: 75 mg/mL
	Generics	
foscarnet	Foscavir	Solution, for injection: 24 mg/mL
	Not available	
ganciclovir[a]	Cytovene, Zirgan	Gel, ophthalmic (Zirgan): 0.15% Powder, for injection (Cytovene): 500 mg per vial
	Cytovene	
trifluridine[a]	Viroptic	Solution, ophthalmic: 1%
	Viroptic	
valganciclovir[a]	Valcyte	Solution, oral: 50 mg/mL Tablet: 450 mg
	Valcyte	

[a]Generic available.

Fungal and Protozoal Infections of the Eye

Fusarium keratitis is a rare fungal infection of the eye that occasionally occurs in people who wear soft contact lenses. If untreated, it can lead to blindness. See the discussion of keratitis for more information. *F. keratitis* and other fungal infections of the eye are treated with antifungals such as natamycin.

Ocular *toxoplasmosis* is caused by protozoa and is transmitted by handling or eating raw and undercooked meat or by handling cat feces. According to the Centers for Disease Control and Prevention, there may be as many as 1.26 million people in the United States with ocular toxoplasmosis. Exposure to the protozoa causes the development of antigens that can cause ocular inflammation, vasculitis, uveitis, and retinal edema.

Drugs used in the treatment and management of toxoplasmosis are pyrimethamine and sulfonamides (sulfadiazine and trimethoprim + sulfamethoxazole).

Ophthalmic Antifungals

Generic Name	US Brand Name(s) Canadian Brand(s)	Dosage Form and Strength
natamycin	Natacyn	Suspension, ophthalmic: 5%
	Not available	

Helminthic Infections

Helminthes are parasitic worms that can cause eye infections and blindness. Three species can cause infection in the human eye. *Onchocerca volvulus* is a round worm that causes onchocerciasis. Onchocerciasis is also known as river blindness and is the second leading cause of infectious blindness in the world, according the World Health Organization. *Taenia solium* is a flat worm that causes cysticercosis, an infection caused by eating undercooked pork. Toxocariasis is the fifth leading cause of uveitis worldwide. Dogs, cats, wolves, and foxes are carriers of the worm that causes toxocariasis. Toxocariasis is an infection that is contracted by eating soil that is infested with feces containing the worm eggs, and is most common in children. Infections can cause loss of vision in the affected eye and strabismus. The dog is also the carrier of another roundworm *(Ancylostoma caninum)* that produces inflammation in the retina that progresses to atrophy of the optic nerve and blindness.

Ivermectin kills the living worms that cause ochocerciasis infection and prevents inflammation and scarring. A single dose of ivermectin is administered yearly. Cysticercosis and toxocariasis are treated by the administration of topical corticosteroids and systemic anthelminthics such as albendazole and thiabendazole. Surgical removal of the living worms may be necessary for cysticercosis to reduce damage to the eye that might occur when drug therapy is used.

❗ TECH ALERT!

valGANcyclovir and valACYclovir have look-alike and sound-alike issues.

■ TECH NOTE!

Ophthalmic drugs can be used in the ear, but otic drugs cannot be used in the eye. All ophthalmic drugs must be sterile.

Summary of Treatments of Bacterial, Fungal, and Viral Infections of the Eye

Usual Dosage for Drugs Used to Treat Infections of the Eye

Generic Name	Brand Name	Usual Dosage
Aminoglycosides		
gentamicin 0.3%	Genoptic, Diogent	Instill 1–2 drops every 4 h while awake until resolved (solution) *or* Apply ½-inch ribbon of ointment 2–3 times a day to eyelid margin
tobramycin 0.3%	Tobrex	Instill 1–2 drops in eye(s) every 4 h *or* Apply ointment 2–3 times a day (every 3–4 h for severe infection)
neomycin + bacitracin + polymyxin B	Neosporin Ophthalmic ointment	Apply small amount to conjunctival sac every 3–4 h for 7–10 days
neomycin + polymyxin B + gramicidin	Neosporin Ophthalmic solution	Instill 1–2 drops in eye(s) every 4 h (or up to 2 drops every hour for severe infection)
Sulfonamides		
sulfacetamide Na⁺ 10%	Sodium Sulamyd, Bleph-10	Instill 1–2 drops every 1 h while awake until resolved (solution)
trimethoprim 1 mg + polymyxin B 10,000 units	Polytrim	Instill 1 drop into eye(s) every 3 h up to 6 doses/day for 7–10 days
Quinolones		
besifloxacin	Besivance	Instill 1 drop in the affected eye(s) 3 times daily, 4–12 h apart, for 7 days
ciprofloxacin 0.3%	Ciloxan	Instill 1–2 drops in eye(s) every 2 h while awake for 2 days; then 1–2 drops every 4 h for 5 days *or* Apply ½-inch ribbon to conjunctival sac 3 times a day for 2 days; then twice daily for 5 days
gatifloxacin	Zymaxid, Zymar	On day 1–2, instill 1 drop in each affected eye every 2 h while awake up to 8 times daily; on days thereafter 1 drop in each affected eye 2–4 times daily while awake (3–7 days)
levofloxacin	generics	Instill 1–2 drops in eye(s) every 2 h while awake days 1–2; then instill every 4 h days 3–7 (up to 4 times a day)
moxifloxacin	Vigamox, Moxeza	Instill 1 drop in affected eye(s) 3 times a day for 7 days (Vigamox); instill 1 drop in affected eye(s) 2 times a day for 7 days (Moxeza)
ofloxacin	Ocuflox	Instill 1 drop in affected eye every 2–4 h for 2 days; then use 1–2 drops 4 times a day for 5 days more
Macrolides		
azithromycin	AzaSite	Instill 1 drop in the affected eye(s) twice daily (8–12 h apart) for the first 2 days followed by 1 drop in the affected eye(s) once daily for the next 5 days
Erythromycin	Generics	Apply ½-inch (1.25 cm) 2–6 times a day until resolved
Antiinfective + Corticosteroid		
neomycin + bacitracin + polymyxin B + hydrocortisone	generics, Cortimyxin	Apply a ½-inch ribbon of ointment every 3–4 h to lower eyelid margin until improvement
neomycin + polymyxin B + dexamethasone	Maxitrol	Apply a ½-inch ribbon of ointment 3–4 times a day or at bedtime *or* Instill 1–2 drops into eye(s) every 4–6 h (up to every 1 h if severe disease)

Usual Dosage for Drugs Used to Treat Infections of the Eye—cont'd

Generic Name	Brand Name	Usual Dosage
gentamicin + prednisolone	Pred-G	Instill 1 drops into eye(s) 2–4 times a day (up to every 1 h during 1st 24–48 h) *or* Apply a ½-inch ribbon of ointment 1–3 times a day
sulfacetamide + prednisolone	Blephamide	Apply to lower conjunctival sac up to 6 times a day *or* Instill 2 drops every 4 h during the day and at bedtime
tobramycin + dexamethasone	Tobradex	Instill 1–2 drops in eye(s) every 4–6 h *or* Apply ointment every 6–8 h
tobramycin + loteprednol	Zylet	Instill 1–2 drops into the conjunctival sac of the affected eye(s) every 4–6 h (up to every 1–2 h during 1st 24–48 h)
Antivirals		
cidofovir	Generics	**CMV:** Infuse 5 mg/kg IV over 1 h once weekly for 2 weeks, then once every other week
ganciclovir	Cytovene, Zirgan	**CMV retinitis:** Infuse 5 mg/kg IV every 12 h for 14–21 days; then once daily 7 days/week (or 6 mg/kg/day for 5 days/week)
foscarnet	Foscavir	**CMV retinitis:** Infuse 60 mg/kg/dose every 8 h or 90 mg every 12 h for 14–21 days; then 90–120 mg/kg/day every 24 h
trifluridine	Viroptic	**Herpes simplex keratoconjunctivitis:** Instill 1 drop in eye(s) every 2 h while awake up to 9 drops/day until corneal ulcer heals; then 1 drop every 4 h for 7 days
valganciclovir	Valcyte	**CMV retinitis:** 900 mg twice a day for 21 days; then take once daily thereafter
Antifungal		
natamycin	Natacyn	**Keratitis:** Instill 1 drop into conjunctival sac every 1–2 h for 3–4 days; then 1 drop every 3–4 h for 14–21 days or until resolved. **Blepharitis & conjunctivitis:** 1 drop every 4–6 h until resolved.

CMV, Cytomeglovirus.

Glaucoma

It is estimated that more than 70 million people worldwide have glaucoma. This number is expected to increase to 80 million by 2020, making glaucoma the second leading cause of blindness worldwide. More than 4 million Americans and 400,000 Canadians older than 20 years have the disease. The prevalence of glaucoma increases with age, growing steadily after age 60 years. Having a family history for glaucoma also increases the risk. Diabetes, which is discussed in Chapter 26, is a risk factor for neurovascular glaucoma.

Pathophysiology

There are actually several types of glaucoma, and all are associated with progressive damage to the structures in the eye responsible for vision. *Peripheral vision* is first to be lost. The person gradually loses the ability to see images from the sides, top, or bottom of the eye(s). Eventually, only central vision remains (Fig. 15.4).

Open-angle glaucoma is the most common and results from abnormal accumulation of *aqueous humor* (Fig. 15.5). This in turn causes excessive *intraocular pressure* (IOP) that produces degeneration of the optic nerve. Sometimes damage to the optic nerve can occur in the absence of increased IOP. When this happens, low-tension or normal-tension glaucoma is said to be the cause. The unit of measure for IOP is millimeters of mercury (mm Hg).

IOP rises rapidly to dangerously high levels when a person has narrow-angle or *angle-closure glaucoma*. Normally, aqueous fluids drain from the eye through an opening in the eye where the cornea and iris meet. This region is called the angle (see Fig. 15.5). When the angle becomes obstructed, as occurs with inflammation or partial blockage of the trabecular meshwork, aqueous humor drainage is impaired and there is a sudden increase in eye pressure. Pain and nausea may occur. If untreated, blindness can result in as little as a few days. Children born with defects in the structure of the angle of the eye may develop congenital glaucoma. Children with congenital glaucoma often have cloudy eyes, light sensitivity, and excessive tearing. If treated promptly, impaired vision may be avoided.

• **Fig. 15.4** Glaucoma. (A) Normal vision. (B) Glaucoma. (Courtesy of U.S. National Institutes of Health National Eye Institute.)

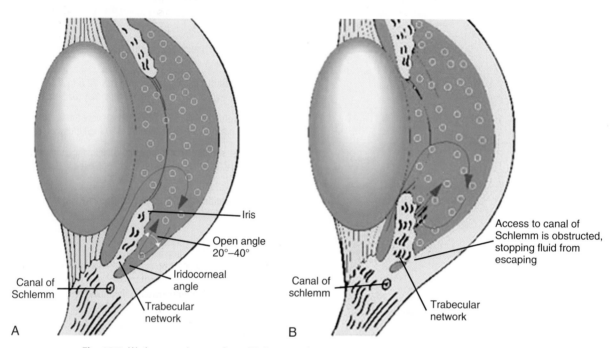

• **Fig. 15.5** (A) Aqueous humor: flow. (B) Aqueous humor: obstruction. (From Clayton BD, Stock YN, Harroun RD: *Basic pharmacology for nurses*, ed 14, St. Louis, 2007, Mosby.)

Treatment

Drugs used in the treatment of glaucoma can be divided into two main classifications according to their method of action. Drugs lower IOP by decreasing the formation of fluids that build up in the eye, or they promote drainage of fluids that accumulate. This is accomplished by actions on parasympathetic or sympathetic nerves that control secretion of fluids and contraction of muscles that block fluid drainage. More than a single agent may be administered for the treatment of glaucoma. When two drops are administered, the second drop should be placed in the eye at least 5 minutes after the first agent. This will give the first eye drop time to "soak in" and avoid being washed away by the second drop.

> **● TECH NOTE!**
>
> -"lol" is a common ending for beta-adrenergic antagonists (also known as beta blockers).

Drugs That Decrease Aqueous Humor Formation

Beta-Adrenergic Antagonists

Most drugs used to treat open-angle glaucoma are beta-adrenergic antagonists, also called beta blockers. They are also administered for the treatment of intraocular hypertension. Stimulation of beta-adrenergic receptors on ciliary cells increases secretion of aqueous humor. Beta-adrenergic antagonists decrease aqueous humor formation by inhibiting the action of epinephrine and norepinephrine on beta-adrenergic receptors located on the muscle and on blood vessels within the ciliary body. However, betaxolol is the only beta-adrenergic antagonist that is selective for $beta_1$-receptor sites. This means that betaxolol may be safer for use in patients who have asthma, congestive heart failure, or other conditions in which blockade of $beta_2$-receptor sites are undesirable. Adverse reactions produced by betaxolol are blurred vision, light sensitivity (photophobia), dizziness, and nausea. Local adverse reactions to carteolol, levobunolol, metipranolol, and timolol include burning, pain, and itching in addition to blurred vision.

Systemic effects are less common and include dizziness, weakness, depression, hypotension, decreased heart rate, and difficulty breathing. Systemic absorption may be reduced by applying finger pressure to the lacrimal sac for 1 to 2 minutes after placing the drops in the eyes.

Beta-Adrenergic Antagonists

Generic Name	US Brand Name(s) Canadian Brand(s)	Dosage Forms and Strengths
betaxolol[a]	Betoptic, Betoptic S Betoptic S	**Solution, ophthalmic (Betoptic):** 0.5% **Suspension, ophthalmic (Betoptic S):** 0.25%
carteolol[a]	Generics Not available	**Solution, ophthalmic:** 1%
levobunolol[a]	Betagan Betagan	**Solution, ophthalmic:** 0.25%[b], 0.5%
metipranolol[a]	Optipranolol Not available	**Solution, ophthalmic:** 0.3%
timolol hemihydrate[a]	Betimol Not available	**Solution, ophthalmic:** 0.25%, 0.5%
timolol maleate[a]	Istalol, Timoptic, Timoptic in OcuDose, Timoptic XE Timoptic, Timoptic XE	**Solution, gel forming (Timoptic XE):** 0.25%, 0.5% **Solution, ophthalmic (Timoptic):** 0.25%, 0.5% **Solution, preservative free (Timoptic in OcuDose):** 0.25%, 0.5%
Combinations		
timolol + brimonidine[a]	Combigan Combigan	**Solution, ophthalmic:** 0.2% brimonidine + 0.5% timolol

[a]Generic available.
[b]Available in the United States only.

> ● **TECH NOTE!**
>
> To minimize systemic side effects, patients are advised to apply gentle pressure to the lacrimal sac for 1 to 2 minutes after the administration of eye drops.

Alpha-Adrenergic Agonists

Alpha-adrenergic receptor agonists are used for the prevention and treatment of increased IOP. There are two alpha-adrenergic receptors in the eye (alpha$_1$ and alpha$_2$). Administration of alpha$_1$-adrenergic receptor agonists reduces blood flow in the ciliary body, and administration of alpha$_2$-adrenergic receptor agonists reduces the formation of aqueous humor. Administration of alpha$_2$-adrenergic agonists produces effects similar to administration of alpha-adrenergic antagonists. Adverse reactions produced by apraclonidine

and brimonidine may be systemic as well as local. Local reactions include blurred vision, decreased night and distance vision, dry eyes, and irritated eyelids. Systemic effects are drowsiness and headache.

Alpha-Adrenergic Agonists

Generic Name	US Brand Name(s) Canadian Brand(s)	Dosage Forms and Strengths
apraclonidine[a]	Iopidine Iopidine	**Solution, ophthalmic:** 0.5%, 1%
brimonidine[a]	Alphagan P, Lumify[b], Mirvaso, Qoliana Alphagan, Alphagan P	**Gel, ophthalmic (Mirvaso):** 0.33% **Solution, ophthalmic:** 0.1%,[c] 0.15%, 0.2% 0.025% (Lumify)[d]

[a]Generic available.
[b]Available without a prescription to reduce eye redness.
[c]Available in the United States only.
[d]Available in Canada only.

> ● **TECH NOTE!**
>
> Generic brimonidine 0.2% is *not* substitutable for Alphagan P, which is currently only available in 0.1% and 0.15% strengths.

Carbonic Anhydrase Inhibitors

Carbonic anhydrase inhibitors are indicated for the treatment of open-angle glaucoma. Acetazolamide and methazolamide tablets are also indicated for prevention of secondary acute angle-closure glaucoma, short-term treatment of angle-closure glaucoma when surgery must be delayed, reduction of IOP after cataract surgery, edema, and prevention of altitude sickness. Carbonic anhydrase inhibitors inhibit the enzyme carbonic anhydrase. The enzyme is involved in the process of converting carbon dioxide and water to bicarbonate. The enzyme is found in many parts of the body, including the ciliary structures of the eye. The production of aqueous humor depends on the transport of bicarbonate and sodium ions. Administration of carbonic anhydrase inhibitors decreases the rate of production of aqueous humor, thereby decreasing IOP. Adverse effects of acetazolamide and methazolamide include dizziness, drowsiness, potassium loss, frequent urination, kidney stones, a tingling sensation in the fingers and toes, bitter or metallic taste, nausea, impotence, and depression. Brimzolamide and dorzolamide produce local adverse effects that include blurred vision; a bitter taste in the mouth; and burning or stinging, dry eyes. Less common reactions are irritation, discharge from the eyes, soreness, headache, and dizziness.

> ● **TECH NOTE!**
>
> "-zolamide" is a common ending for carbonic anhydrase inhibitors.

> ● **TECH NOTE!**
>
> Carbonic anhydrase inhibitors may cause allergic reactions in people who have allergies to sulfonamide antiinfective agents.

Carbonic Anhydrase Inhibitors

Generic Name	US Brand Name(s) Canadian Brand(s)	Dosage Forms and Strengths
acetazolamide[a]	Diamox / Generics	Capsule, sustained release (Diamox): 500 mg[b] Powder, for IV use: 500 mg/vial Tablets: 125 mg,[b] 250 mg
brinzolamide	Azopt / Azopt	Suspension, ophthalmic: 1%
dorzolamide[a]	Trusopt / Trusopt, Trusopt PF	Solution, ophthalmic: 2%
methazolamide[a]	Generics / Generics	Tablets: 25 mg,[b] 50 mg
Carbonic Anhydrase Inhibitor Combination		
brinzolamide + brimonidine	Simbrinza / Simbrinza	Solution, ophthalmic: 0.2% brimonidine + 1% brinzolamide
brinzolamide + timolol	Not available / Azarga	Suspension, ophthalmic: 1% brinzolamide + 0.5% timolol
dorzolamide and timolol[a]	Cosopt, Cosopt PF / Cosopt, Cosopt PF	Solution, ophthalmic: 2% dorzolamide and 0.5% timolol

[a]Generic available.
[b]Available in the United States only.

❶ TECH ALERT!

AcetaZOLAMIDE and acetoHEXAMIDE have look-alike and sound-alike issues.

Drugs That Increase Aqueous Humor Drainage

Miotics are drugs that promote drainage of the aqueous humor. They produce this effect via a variety of mechanisms of action. Cholinergic agonists, acetylcholinesterase inhibitors, and prostaglandin analogues all promote drainage of accumulated levels of aqueous humor and reduce IOP.

Cholinergic Agonists and Cholinesterase Inhibitors

Cholinergic agonists (pilocarpine, carbachol, and echothiophate) are used to reduce IOP caused by glaucoma and cataract surgery. Cholinergic agonists bind to receptor sites and produce effects that mimic the neurotransmitter acetylcholine. Binding produces parasympathetic nervous system effects in the eye, such as contraction of ciliary muscles, and results in miosis. Pilocarpine is a cholinergic agonist that is used in the treatment of open- and closed-angle glaucoma. Cholinergic agonists also produce dilation of the trabecular meshwork to decrease IOP. Pilocarpine (Salagen) is also used to treat xerostomia (dry mouth).

• BOX 15.1 Directions for Preparing Echothiopate Iodide Eye Drops

- Use aseptic technique.
- Tear off aluminum seals and remove and discard rubber plugs from both the drug and diluent containers.
- Pour the diluent into the drug container.
- Remove the dropper assembly from its sterile wrapping. Holding the dropper assembly by the screw cap and WITHOUT COMPRESSING RUBBER BULB, insert it into drug container and screw down tightly.
- Shake for several seconds to ensure mixing.

Echothiophate iodide is a cholinesterase inhibitor. Cholinesterase inhibitors block the enzyme that deactivates acetylcholine (see Chapter 12). This prolongs the effects of acetylcholine and administered cholinergic agonists. Adverse reactions include blurred vision, change in near or distance vision, difficulty in seeing at night or in dim light, headache, twitching of the eyelids, and watering of the eyes. For preparation instructions, see Box 15.1.

Cholinergic Agonists

Generic Name	US Brand Name(s) Canadian Brand(s)	Dosage Forms and Strengths
carbachol[a]	Miostat / Miostat	Solution, ophthalmic: 0.01%
pilocarpine[a]	Isopto Carpine / Isopto Carpine	Solution, ophthalmic (Isopto Carpine): 1%[b], 2%, 4%
Cholinesterase Inhibitor		
echothiophate iodide	Phospholine iodide / Not available	Powder for reconstitution: 0.125% (6.25 mg)

[a]Generic available.
[b]Available in the United States only.

Prostaglandin Analogues

Bimatoprost, latanoprost, and travoprost are prostaglandin analogues that are prodrugs. They mimic the action of prostaglandin F2α and relax the ciliary muscles to permit drainage of aqueous humors. Prostaglandin analogues directly dilate the trabecular meshwork to promote drainage. The use of prostaglandin analogues can cause changes in the color or pigmentation of the eyes and may thicken eyelashes. Latisse (bimatoprost) is marketed as a topical solution to increase the growth of eyelashes in patients that have hypotrichosis, a condition whereby they have no eyelashes. Bimatoprost, latanoprost, and travoprost may decrease vision and produce eye irritation, eye pain, itchy eyes, redness of eye, dry eyes, sun sensitivity, or watery eyes.

● TECH NOTE!

"-prost" is a common ending for drugs that are prostaglandin analogues.

Prostaglandin Analogues

Generic Name	US Brand Name(s) / Canadian Brand(s)	Dosage Forms and Strengths
bimatoprost	Latisse, Lumigan / Latisse, Lumigan, Lumigan RC, Vistitan	Solution, Topical: 0.03% Solution, ophthalmic: 0.01%, 0.03%
latanoprostene bunod	Vyzulta	Solution, ophthalmic: 0.024%
latanoprost[a]	Xalatan / Monoprost, Xalatan	Solution, ophthalmic: 0.005%
tafluprost	Zioptan / Not available	Solution, ophthalmic: 0.0015%
travoprost[a]	Travatan Z / Izba, Travatan Z	Solution, ophthalmic: 0.003% (Izba), 0.004% (Travatan Z)
Combination		
latanoprost + timolol[a]	Not available / Xalacom	Solution, ophthalmic: 0.5% timolol + 0.005% latanoprost
travoprost + timolol	Not available / DuoTrav PQ	Solution, ophthalmic: 0.5% timolol + 0.004% travoprost

[a]Generic available.

Miscellaneous

The use of marijuana is controversial. Although smoking marijuana has been shown to reduce IOP, it is an illicit substance in Canada and the United States, according to federal legislation. Possession is a federal crime despite passage of regulation authorizing medical use in some states.

Nondrug Treatment

Laser Surgery

Laser surgery may be performed to reduce IOP. There are three forms of laser surgery for glaucoma. Laser peripheral iridotomy creates a new drainage hole in the iris, permitting fluids to drain out of the eye. Laser trabeculoplasty unblocks existing channels, and laser cyclophotocoagulation, a type of laser surgery that is performed to reduce the amount of fluid entering the eye, is indicated for people who have severe glaucoma and have not responded to standard glaucoma surgery. Laser cyclophotocoagulation partially destroys the tissues that make the fluid in the eye.

TECHNICIAN'S CORNER

1. The medical use of marijuana is controversial. What are your views on this subject? Give three pros and three cons for the medical use of marijuana.
2. The prevalence of glaucoma in a person with diabetes is greater than in persons without diabetes. What can be done to help diabetic patients decrease the chance of developing glaucoma?
3. How can nonsterile colored contact lenses cause eye infections?

Summary of Drugs Used to Treat Glaucoma

Generic	Brand Name	Usual Dose	Warning Labels
Decrease Aqueous Humor Formation			
Beta-Adrenergic Antagonists			
betaxolol	Betoptic-S	Open-angle glaucoma: Instill 1 drop twice a day in affected eye(s)	SHAKE WELL—betaxolol suspension. WASH HANDS BEFORE USE; AVOID CONTAMINATION OF TIP—all. REMOVE CONTACT LENSES BEFORE USE; WAIT AT LEAST 15 MIN BEFORE REINSERTING—all. STORE AT ROOM TEMPERATURE—all. PROTECT FROM LIGHT—all. DO NOT DISCONTINUE WITHOUT MEDICAL SUPERVISION—all.
carteolol	Generics	Open-angle glaucoma: Instill 1 drop twice a day in affected eye(s)	
levobunolol	Betagan	Open-angle glaucoma: Instill 1–2 drops in affected eye(s) 2 times a day 0.25% or once daily 0.5%.	
metipranolol	Optipranolol	Open-angle glaucoma: Instill 1 drop in affected eye(s) twice daily	
timolol maleate	Timoptic, Timoptic XE	Open-angle glaucoma: Timoptic: Instill 1 drop twice daily in affected eye(s) Timoptic XE, Istalol: Instill 1 drop daily in the morning	
timolol hemihydrate	Betimol	Open-angle glaucoma: Instill 1 drop twice daily in affected eye(s)	

Continued

Summary of Drugs Used to Treat Glaucoma—cont'd

Generic	Brand Name	Usual Dose	Warning Labels
Alpha-Adrenergic Agonists			
apraclonidine	Iopidine	Instill 1–2 drops in affected eye(s) 3 times a day	STORE AT ROOM TEMPERATURE—all. PROTECT FROM LIGHT—all. WASH HANDS BEFORE USE; AVOID CONTAMINATION OF TIP—all. REMOVE CONTACT LENSES BEFORE USE; WAIT AT LEAST 15 MIN BEFORE REINSERTING—all. DO NOT DISCONTINUE WITHOUT MEDICAL SUPERVISION—all.
brimonidine	Alphagan	Instill 1 drop in affected eye(s) 3 times a day	
brimonidine + timolol	Combigan	Instill 1 drop in affected eye(s) 2 times a day	
Carbonic Anhydrase Inhibitors			
acetazolamide	Diamox	**Oral (sustained release):** 500 mg twice daily **Oral (immediate release):** 250 mg 1–4 times a day	TAKE WITH FOOD—acetazolamide, methazolamide. SWALLOW WHOLE; DO NOT CRUSH OR CHEW—sustained-release capsule. MAY CAUSE DIZZINESS OR DROWSINESS—acetazolamide, methazolamide. SHAKE WELL—brinzolamide, brinzolamide + timolol. REMOVE CONTACT LENSES BEFORE USE; WAIT AT LEAST 15 MIN BEFORE REINSERTING—brinzolamide, dorzolamide, dorzolamide + timolol. WASH HANDS BEFORE USE; AVOID CONTAMINATION OF TIP—brinzolamide, dorzolamide, dorzolamide + timolol. STORE AT ROOM TEMPERATURE—brinzolamide, dorzolamide, dorzolamide + timolol. PROTECT FROM LIGHT—brinzolamide, dorzolamide, dorzolamide + timolol. DO NOT DISCONTINUE WITHOUT MEDICAL SUPERVISION—brinzolamide, dorzolamide, dorzolamide + timolol.
brinzolamide	Azopt	Instill 1 drop 3 times a day	
dorzolamide	Trusopt	Instill 1 drop 3 times a day	
brinzolamide + timolol	Azarga	Instill 1 drop 2 times a day	
dorzolamide + timolol	Cosopt	Instill 1 drop twice a day	
methazolamide	Generics	**Oral:** 50–100 mg 2–3 times a day	
Increase Drainage of Aqueous Humor			
Cholinergic Agonists			
carbachol	Miostat	Instill 1–2 drops up to 3 times a day	WASH HANDS BEFORE USE; AVOID CONTAMINATION OF TIP—all. DO NOT DISCONTINUE WITHOUT MEDICAL SUPERVISION—all. STORE AT ROOM TEMPERATURE—carbachol. DO NOT WEAR CONTACT LENSES—carbachol.
pilocarpine	Isopto Carpine	**Solution:** Instill 1 drops up to 3 times a day	
Cholinesterase Inhibitor			
echothiophate	Phospholine Iodide	**Open-angle glaucoma:** Instill 1 drop twice a day	REFRIGERATE OR STORE RECONSTITUTED SOLUTION FOR UP TO 4 WEEKS AT ROOM TEMPERATURE.
Prostaglandin Analogs			
bimatoprost	Lumigan	Instill 1 drop once daily in the evening	WASH HANDS BEFORE USE; AVOID CONTAMINATION OF TIP—all. REMOVE CONTACT LENSES BEFORE USE; WAIT AT LEAST 15 MIN BEFORE REINSERTING—all. DO NOT DISCONTINUE WITHOUT MEDICAL SUPERVISION—all. REFRIGERATE; DO NOT FREEZE—latanoprost, latanoprost + timolol. STORE AT ROOM TEMPERATURE—bimatoprost, travoprost, travoprost + timolol.
latanoprost	Xalatan	Instill 1 drop once daily in the evening	
travoprost	Travatan	Instill 1 drop in affected eye(s) once daily in the evening	
latanoprost + timolol	Xalacom	**Open-angle glaucoma:** Instill 1 drop in affected eye(s) once daily	
travoprost + timolol	DuoTrav	**Open-angle glaucoma:** Instill 1 drop in affected eye(s) once daily	

Key Points

- Glaucoma is the second leading cause of blindness worldwide.
- The percentage of the population that will develop glaucoma increases with advancing age.
- There are actually several types of glaucoma: open-angle, angle-closure, low-tension, and secondary glaucoma.
- The most common form of glaucoma is open-angle glaucoma.
- Increased IOP is caused by a buildup of aqueous humor and is a symptom of glaucoma.
- Drugs used in the treatment of glaucoma can be divided into two main classifications according to their method of action: drugs that decrease formation of aqueous humor and drugs that promote drainage of aqueous humor.
- Drug classifications that decrease formation of the aqueous humor are beta blockers, alpha-adrenergic agonists, and carbonic anhydrase inhibitors.
- Drug classifications that promote drainage of the aqueous humor are cholinergics, cholinesterase inhibitors, and prostaglandin analogues.
- Miotics are drugs that cause contraction of the pupil. Drugs that promote drainage of the aqueous humor produce miosis.
- Blepharitis is self-treated by applying clean warm compresses. In some cases, antiinfective ointments, corticosteroid eye drops, and artificial tears may be administered to manage the symptoms.
- Conjunctivitis (pink eye) may be caused by a virus or bacteria.
- Uveitis is treated with the administration of corticosteroids (to reduce inflammation), mydriatics (to reduce painful swelling), and antiinfectives or antivirals as appropriate.
- Soft contact lens wearers, especially those who wear their contact lenses overnight, are at risk for fungal keratitis.
- A stye is a small, painful lump on the eyelid that is caused by an acute self-limiting infection of the oil glands of the eyelid.
- CMV retinitis is an opportunistic infection in the eye that occurs in patients who have HIV infection/AIDS or who take immunosuppressive drugs and if untreated can cause blindness.
- CMV retinitis is treated by administration of antivirals such as ganciclovir, valganciclovir, foscarnet, and cidofovir.
- Herpetic corneal disease is the cause of more than 500,000 cases of blindness annually.
- Herpes zoster ophthalmicus and herpes simplex keratitis are treated by administering antiviral eye drops, orally administered drugs, or both.
- Ocular toxoplasmosis is caused by protozoa and is transmitted by handling or eating raw and undercooked meat or by handling cat feces.
- Toxoplasmosis can cause ocular inflammation, vasculitis, uveitis, and retinal edema and is treated by administering pyrimethamine and sulfonamides (sulfadiazine and trimethoprim + sulfamethoxazole).
- Onchocerciasis (river blindness) is caused by a roundworm.
- Onchocerciasis is treated by administering a single dose of ivermectin yearly.
- Cysticercosis is treated with praziquantel, corticosteroids, and surgical removal of the living worms.
- Toxocariasis is treated by administering topical corticosteroids and systemic anthelminthics such as thiabendazole.

Review Questions

1. Keratitis is a severe infection of the iris and may be caused by bacteria or fungi.
   a. True
   b. False
2. The medical term for "granulated eyelids" is
   a. uveitis
   b. keratitis
   c. blepharitis
   d. iritis
3. A stye (hordeolum) is a small, painful lump located on the
   a. eyelid
   b. iris
   c. conjunctiva
   d. pupil
4. The most common form of glaucoma is _____.
   a. open angle
   b. closed angle
   c. narrow angle
   d. wide angle
5. The mechanism of action of drugs used in the treatment of glaucoma is_____.
   a. lower intraocular pressure by decreasing the formation of fluids
   b. promote drainage of fluids that accumulate
   c. lower intraocular pressure by increasing the formation of fluids
   d. a and b

6. The classification of the drug(s) most commonly used for the treatment of glaucoma is _____.
   a. alpha-adrenergic antagonists
   b. beta-adrenergic antagonists
   c. carbonic anhydrase inhibitors
   d. prostaglandins
7. Miotics are drugs that are used to decrease the drainage of the aqueous humor.
   a. True
   b. False
8. This drug is a beta-adrenergic antagonist indicated for the treatment of open-angle glaucoma.
   a. latanoprost
   b. acetazolamide
   c. epinephrine
   d. timolol
9. Select the FALSE statement about latanoprost.
   a. It must be stored in the refrigerator.
   b. It may increase pigmentation in the eye.
   c. It must be metabolized to its biologically active form.
   d. It must be premixed before use.
10. Laser surgery is not recommended to reduce intraocular pressure.
    a. True
    b. False

Bibliography

Ament C, Young L: Ocular manifestations of helminthic infections: onchocerciasis, cysticercosis, toxocariasis, and diffuse unilateral subacute neuroretinitis, *Int Ophthalmol Clin* 46:1–10, 2006.

Bourne R: Worldwide glaucoma through the looking glass, *Br J Ophthalmol* 90:253–254, 2006.

Centers for Disease Control and Prevention: Conjunctivitis Treatment, 2010. Retrieved May 15, 2011, from http://www.cdc.gov/conjunctivitis/about/treatment.html.

Centers for Disease Control and Prevention: Pink Eye: Usually Mild and Easy to Treat, 2010. Retrieved May 15, 2011, from http://www.cdc.gov/Features/Conjunctivitis/.

Centers for Disease Control and Prevention: Fusarium keratitis—multiple states, *MMWR Morb Mortal Wkly Rep* 55:1–2, 2006. Retrieved from: http://www.cdc.gov/mmwr/preview/mmwrhtml/mm55d410a1.htm.

Chabner D: *The language of medicine*, ed 8, Philadelphia, 2007, WB Saunders.

Glaucoma Research Foundation: Glaucoma Facts & Stats, 2011. Retrieved May 1, 2011, from http://www.glaucoma.org/glaucoma/glaucoma-facts-and-stats.php.

Green L, Pavan-Langston D: Herpes simplex ocular inflammatory disease, *Int Ophthalmol Clin* 46:27–37, 2006.

FDA: Drugs@FDA: FDA Approved Drug Products, nd. Retrieved August 29, 2018, from http://www.accessdata.fda.gov/scripts/cder/daf/.

Glaucoma Research Foundation: Glaucoma Medications and Their Side Effects, 2016. Retrieved February 20, 2017, from http://www.glaucoma.org/gleams/glaucoma-medications-and-their-side-effects.php.

Glaucoma Research Foundation: Understanding and Living with Glaucoma, 2016. In A. Jackson (Ed.). Retrieved from http://www.glaucoma.org/GRF_Understanding_Glaucoma_EN.pdf.

Health Canada: Drug Product Database, 2018. Retrieved August 29, 2018, from https://health-products.canada.ca/dpd-bdpp/index-eng.jsp.

Institute for Safe Medication Practices: FDA and ISMP Lists of Look-Alike Drug Names with Recommended Tall Man Letters, 2016.

Kolko M: Present and New Treatment Strategies in the Management of Glaucoma, *Open Ophthalmol J* 9(Suppl 1:M5):89–100, 2015.

National Eye Institute: Fact About Dry Eye, 2013. Retrieved February 17, 2017, from https://nei.nih.gov/health/dryeye/dryeye.

Page C, Curtis M, Sutter M, et al: *Integrated pharmacology*, Philadelphia, 2005, Mosby, pp 523–534.

Patton K: *Survival guide for anatomy and physiology*, St Louis, 2006, Mosby.

Quigley H, Broman A: The number of people with glaucoma worldwide in 2010 and 2010, *Br J Ophthalmol* 90:262–267, 2006.

Raffa R, Rawls S, Beyzarov E: *Netter's illustrated pharmacology*, Philadelphia, 2005, WB Saunders, p 48.

Thibodeau GA, Patton KT: *Anatomy and physiology*, ed 6, St Louis, 2007, Mosby. http://www.americanglaucomasociety.net/patients/position_statements/marijuana_glaucoma.

16

Treatment of Disorders of the Ear

LEARNING OBJECTIVES

1. Learn the terminology associated with the ear and ear infections.
2. Describe factors that influence the sense of balance.
3. Describe disorders of the ear and ear infections.
4. List and categorize medications used in the treatment of disorders of the ear and fear infections.
5. Identify significant drug look-alike and sound-alike issues.
6. Identify warning labels and precautionary messages associated with medications used in the treatment of disorders of the ear and ear infections.

KEY TERMS

Cerumen Waxlike substance that is secreted by modified sweat glands in the ear.

Emollient A softening agent, such as an ointment or lotion. Used in the ear to soften ear wax.

Equilibrium Steadiness or balance accompanied by a sense of knowing where the body is in relationship to surroundings.

Labyrinth Bony structure in the inner ear consisting of three parts (vestibule, cochlea, and semicircular canals) and involved in balance.

Ménière disease Chronic inner ear disease associated with intermittent buildup of fluid in the inner ear that causes hearing loss and vertigo.

Otitis Inflammation of the ear.

Otitis externa Inflammation of the ear canal or external ear.

Otitis media Inflammation of the middle ear typically caused by viral or bacterial infection.

Tinnitus Intermittent or continuous whistling, crackling, squeaking, or ringing noise in the ears.

Tympanic membrane Eardrum.

Vertigo Feeling of spinning in space (dizziness and loss of balance).

Disorders Affecting Hearing

Hearing loss can be caused by otosclerosis, autoimmune disease, or sudden sensorineural hearing loss (SSHL). *Otosclerosis* is a disorder that causes destruction of bones in the ear. Hearing loss is typically caused by the immobilization of bones in the ear called stapes (Fig. 16.1 for the anatomy of the ear). Symptoms such as tinnitus may appear in childhood or early adulthood.

SSHL progresses rapidly (hours to days) and typically causes hearing loss in only one ear. Vertigo and tinnitus are other symptoms. The exact cause of SSHL is unknown. It is believed it may be caused by a viral infection, vascular disorder, tumor, or rupture of the inner ear membrane or may be drug induced. Medications that can cause SSHL include loop diuretics, aminoglycoside antibiotics, and antineoplastic agents. Drug-induced SSHL may disappear when the drug is stopped. SSHL that is not drug induced is treated with vasodilating drugs and plasma expanders (e.g., normal saline, 5% glucose). Symptoms such as mild hearing loss resolve spontaneously without treatment. Moderate hearing loss is treated with glucocorticosteroids (see Chapter 13). Patients who have severe hearing loss may have no benefits from the administration of glucocorticosteroids.

Autoimmune diseases such as multiple sclerosis can also cause hearing loss, but sometimes autoimmune hearing loss occurs in the absence of any other disease. Progression occurs over several months, and hearing loss may occur in both ears.

Glucocorticosteroids such as prednisone are used in treatment (see Chapter 13).

Disorders Resulting in Impaired Perception of Sound

Tinnitus is a condition that can cause intermittent or continuous whistling, crackling, squeaking, or ringing noise in the ears. Sometimes it is described as ringing in the ear. It may be caused by disease or bilateral hearing loss caused by normal aging, or it may be induced by drugs or noise. Tinnitus may be the first sign of ototoxicity. Alcohol and salicylates (aspirin) are the most common causes of drug-induced tinnitus.

Nonpharmacologic treatment for tinnitus includes masking the noise using a noise generator or stress management and avoiding alcohol or things that make tinnitus worse. Medications may produce some symptom relief if tinnitus is severe. Drugs that have been used are benzodiazepines (see Chapter 5) and tricyclic antidepressants (see Chapter 6).

Disorders Resulting in Impaired Perception of Motion

The sense organs involved in balance or *equilibrium* are found in the vestibule and the three semicircular canals of the *labyrinth*

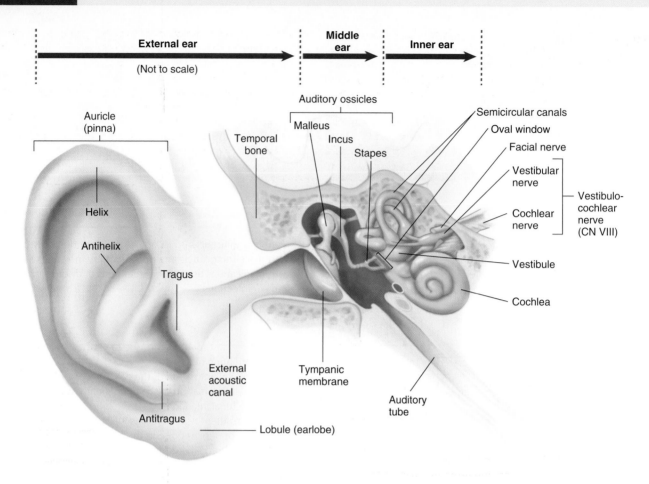

• **Fig. 16.1** The ear. (From Patton KT, Thibodeau GA: *The human body in health and disease*, ed 7, St. Louis, 2018, Elsevier.)

(see Fig. 16.1). The sense organs associated with the semicircular canals function in dynamic equilibrium to maintain balance when the head or body itself is rotated or suddenly moved. Fluids in the semicircular canals shift when the body is in motion to inform the direction and speed of rotation. The superior, posterior, and horizontal semicircular canals inform whether movement is up or down and side to side.

Vertigo

Vertigo and other balance disorders produce symptoms of dizziness or spinning, nausea and vomiting, blurred vision, disorientation, and a feeling of falling because of sense of balance being impaired. Our perception of balance and movement is a function of input from our eye, inner ear, and sense receptors on the skin and skeleton. The body integrates the input it gets from these sources and compares it with previous experience. *Vertigo* is caused by a neural mismatch or sensory conflict, infection, and/or inflammation. A sensory conflict occurs when our eyes tell us that our body should be moving yet our body remains still, such as when we watch a movie of a roller coaster. Similarly, when we read a book in a car that is moving, our inner ear and skin receptors tell us we are in motion, yet our eyes are fixed on the book that is not moving. Again, a sensory conflict occurs. Sensory conflicts may also occur from an inner ear infection, especially if only one ear is involved and one ear receives motion signals and the other ear receives none or a different signal. Head trauma, degeneration of otolith organs (benign positional vertigo), inflammation of the vestibular nerve,

bacterial infection of the labyrinths, brainstem or cerebral pathology, Ménière disease, or motion sickness may also produce vertigo.

Benign Paroxysmal Positional Vertigo

Benign paroxysmal positional vertigo (BPPV) is the number one cause of vertigo, accounting for approximately 20% of all cases. It can occur after trauma to the inner ear, infection, or normal aging. Dizziness or vertigo occurs when otoliths (calcium carbonate crystals) dislodge and shift in the semicircular canals of the ear with changes in the head's position. Impaired structures in the semicircular canals send misinformation about the head's position, resulting in dizziness.

Ménière Disease

Ménière disease is the second most common cause of vertigo. It is a chronic inner ear disease associated with intermittent buildup of fluid in the inner ear. It is characterized by tinnitus, progressive nerve deafness, and vertigo. The cause is unknown. Nonpharmacologic treatment for Ménière disease includes diet and lifestyle changes. Reducing sodium, caffeine, nicotine, and alcohol consumption may be helpful.

Treatment of Disorders of the Ear

Vertigo and Ménière Disease

Many of the treatments for vertigo, Ménière disease, and other balance disorders do not involve drug therapy. Physical therapy is the treatment of choice for BPPV. Physical therapy is used to manipulate the head and shift otoliths that have dislodged. A low-sodium diet and lifestyle changes that restrict alcohol consumption are useful for the treatment of Ménière disease.

When drug therapy is indicated, antihistamines are most widely used and may be prescribed in tablet, transdermal patches, and rectal suppository dosage forms. This is most likely because centrally acting antihistamines have anticholinergic actions that can moderate symptoms of motion sickness. Acetylcholine and histamine are excitatory neurotransmitters involved in the control of vomiting (emesis). Nausea and vomiting are common symptoms of vertigo. Moreover, antihistamines and anticholinergics are vestibular suppressants. Vestibular suppression is useful because it reduces the eye activity responsible for symptoms of vertigo. Administration of vestibular suppressants is not recommended when treatment for vertigo involves physical manipulation of the head and "retraining" of vestibular pathways.

Betahistine, dimenhydrinate, diphenhydramine, and meclizine are antihistamines used to manage vertigo and Ménière disease. Side effects common to all of these drugs are sedation, dry mouth, urinary retention, and blurred vision. Transdermal patches may produce local irritation, burning, or pain at the site where the patch is applied. Dry mouth, thickened bronchial secretions, and urinary retention may be produced, limiting their use in patients with prostate disease, asthma, and other conditions. Use should be limited in lactating women because the drugs may reduce the supply of breast milk. Aminoglycoside antiinfectives such as gentamicin and streptomycin may be prescribed for Ménière disease, but their use is controversial because they can cause ototoxicity. Diuretics may also be prescribed to reduce fluid accumulation in the ear and other body fluids. Diuretics are discussed in Chapter 18.

⊘ TECH ALERT!

Dimenhydrinate and diphenhydramine have look-alike/sound-alike issues.

Bacterial Infections of the Ear

Otitis Externa

Otitis externa, also known as swimmer's ear, is an inflammation of the external auditory canal. It may be caused by bacterial infection, fungal infection, seborrheic dermatitis, psoriasis, and lupus erythematosus. The most common cause is bacterial infection. Fungi (*Candida* spp.) account for only 10% of the cases of otitis externa. Risk factors for development of otitis externa are

(1) exposure to excessive moisture (swimming, humidity, sweating), (2) high environmental temperature, (3) irritation caused by earwax removal, (4) insertion of objects into the ear, and (5) chronic dermatologic disease.

The most common symptoms of otitis externa are ear discomfort or pain, itchiness, and discharge (otorrhea). Topical and systemic drugs are used to treat and control the symptoms of otitis externa. Antiinfectives used in treatment are listed in the drug tables in this chapter.

Agents Used to Manage Vertigo and Ménière Disease

Generic Name	US Brand Name(s) / Canadian Brand(s)	Dosage Forms and Strengths
betahistine[a]	Not available / Serc	**Tablets:** 8 mg, 16 mg, 24 mg
dimenhydrinate[a]	Dramamine (OTC), Trip Tone (OTC) / Gravol (OTC)	**Capsule:** 50 mg **Solution:** 3 mg/mL, 15 mg/5 mL (Gravol) **Solution, for injection (Gravol):** 10 mg/mL, 50 mg/mL **Suppositories (Gravol):** 25 mg, 100 mg **Tablets:** 50 mg **Tablets, chewable:** 15 mg,[b] 25 mg[c] (Dramamine), 50 mg **Tablets, Combined release:** 100 mg[b]
meclizine[a]	Bonine, Dramamine Less Drowsy Formula (OTC) / Not Available	**Tablets:** 12.5 mg, 25 mg **Tablets, chewable:** 25 mg
scopolamine[a]	Transderm Scōp / Transderm V	**Transdermal patch:** 1 mg/72 h,[c] 1.5 mg/72 h[b]

[a]Generic available.
[b]Available in Canada only.
[c]Available in the United States only.
OTC, Over the counter.

Usual Dosage and Warning Labels for Agents Used to Treat Vertigo and Ménière Disease

Generic	Brand	Usual Dose	Warning Labels
betahistine	Serc (Canada only)	**Vertigo:** 8–16 mg 3 times a day or 24 mg twice daily	MAY CAUSE DROWSINESS; MAY IMPAIR ABILITY TO DRIVE. AVOID ALCOHOL. MAINTAIN ADEQUATE FLUID INTAKE. OBSERVE GOOD ORAL HYGIENE. ROTATE SITE OF PATCH APPLICATION—scopolamine. TAKE WITH FOOD—betahistine.
dimenhydrinate	Dramamine, Gravol	**Vertigo, motion sickness, nausea, and vomiting:** 50–100 mg every 4–6 h (maximum, 400 mg/day)	
meclizine	Generics	**Motion sickness:** 25–50 mg 1 h before travel; repeat in 12–24 h as needed **Vertigo:** 25–100 mg/day in divided doses	
scopolamine	Transderm Scōp	**Motion sickness:** Place patch behind ear at least 4 hours before it is needed; replace every 72 h as needed	

Treatment of Otitis Externa

Topical Antiinfectives Used to Treat Otitis Externa

Generic Name	US Brand Name(s) / Canadian brand name(s)	Usual Dosage
Quinolones		
ciprofloxacin	Cetraxal 0.2%	Instill contents of the single use container into affected ear twice daily for 7 days
ciprofloxacin	Otiprio 6%	Insert a single dose into the external ear canal(s) or intratympanically
finafloxacin	Xtoro 0.3%	Instill 4–8 drops in affected ear(s) twice a day for 7 days
ofloxacin 0.3%[a] otic drops	Generics / Not available	Instill 5–10 drops in affected ear(s) once daily for 7 days
Anti-Infective + Corticosteroid		
ciprofloxacin 0.3% + dexamethasone 1%	Ciprodex / Ciprodex	Instill 4 drops in ear(s) 2 times a day for 7 days.
ciprofloxacin 0.2% + hydrocortisone 1%	Cipro HC otic suspension / Not available	Instill 3 drops in affected ear(s) 2 times a day for 7 days
ciprofloxacin 0.3% + fluocinolone 0.025%	Otovel / Otixal	Instill contents of single use vial (0.25 mL) into the affected ear canal every 12 h for 7 days.
gramicidin 025 mg + polymyxin B 10,000 units	Polysporin Eye and Ear drops	Instill 1–2 drops in affected eye or ear 4 times a day for 7 days.
polymyxin B 10,000 units + lidocaine 50 mg	Polysporin + Pain Relief Ear drops	Instill 3–4 drops in affected ear(s) 4 times a day for 5–7 days.
neomycin 0.35% + polymyxin B 10,000 units + hydrocortisone 1%[a]	Cortisporin Otic, Oticair / Not available	Instill 4 drops into ear(s) 3–4 times a day

[a]Generic available.

• **BOX 16.1** **Oral Antiinfectives Used to Treat Otitis Media**

Penicillins
amoxicillin[a]
amoxicillin + clavulanate[a] (Augmentin,[b] Clavulin[c])

Macrolides
azithromycin[a] (Zithromax)
clarithromycin[a] (Biaxin)

Sulfonamides
sulfisoxazole + erythromycin ethylsuccinate[a] sulfamethoxazole (SMX) + trimethoprim (TMP)[a] (Bactrim DS, Septra DS, Sulfatrim DS)

Cephalosporins
cefaclor[a] (Ceclor)
cefdinir[a] (Omnicef)
cefixime (Suprax)
cefpodoxime[a]
cefprozil[a] (Cefzil)
ceftibuten (Cedax)
cefuroxime[a] (Ceftin)
cephalexin[a] (Keflex)

[a]Generic available.
[b]Available in the United States only.
[c]Available in Canada only.

Otitis Media

Otitis media is an inflammation in the middle ear. It may accompany an upper respiratory infection. Children are more susceptible to otitis media than are adults because their eustachian tubes are shorter and straighter. When the eustachian tube is blocked by swelling or mucus from a cold, fluids accumulate and collect in the normally air-filled middle ear. Bacteria may collect in the fluid, along with white blood cells released by the body to fight the infection. Hearing becomes impaired because the eardrum and middle ear bones are unable to move as freely. Pain and pressure builds, and finally the eardrum may tear to release the pressure.

Historically, otitis media has been treated aggressively with orally administered antiinfective drugs; however, new evidence shows that the infection is self-limiting in many cases and will resolve on its own without treatment. Excessive use of antiinfective agents may increase the risk of the development of bacterial resistance. Watchful waiting (up to 48 to 72 hours to see if symptoms disappear) rather than antimicrobial treatment is endorsed by the American Academy of Pediatrics 2013 guidelines for children 6 to 23 months without severe illness.

Evidence shows that prophylactic use of antihistamines and decongestants is ineffective in preventing or treating acute otitis media. It is not recommended and can be harmful in children younger than 2 years of age. Oral antiinfective agents used in the treatment of otitis media are listed in Box 16.1. These agents are described fully in Unit 10.

Auralgia

Ear pain, also called auralgia or otalgia, is a symptom of *otitis* externa, *otitis media*, swimmer's ear, and many other disorders, including viral inflammation of the *tympanic membrane*, temporomandibular joint disorders, referred pain from abscessed teeth, and others. It is treated by administration of topical analgesics, local anesthetics, or oral analgesics. Corticosteroids such as hydrocortisone are combined with otic agents to reduce inflammation and pain. Local anesthetics numb or anesthetize the ear canal and tympanic membrane, further reducing pain and irritation.

When the ear is inflamed, otic drops can produce stinging. This can be minimized by administering suspensions rather than solutions containing alcohol, if this option is available. Otic drops should also be warmed to room temperature before administering into the ear. Sweet olive oil is a home remedy for ear pain. The oil has no analgesic properties, but the warmed oil may be soothing and dislodge cerumen, which may be the cause of the pain.

> **⊗ TECH ALERT!**
>
> Over-the-counter ear products that contain benzocaine and hydrocortisone are no longer marketed in the United States.

Pharmacologic Treatments for Miscellaneous Ear Conditions

Generic Name	US Brand Name(s) / Canadian Brand(s)	Dosage Forms and Strengths
Analgesics		
antipyrine and benzocaine[a]	Not Available	**Solution, otic:** antipyrine 5.4% and benzocaine 1.4%
	Auralgan	

[a]Generic available.

Water-Clogged Ears and Swimmer's Ear

Water-clogged ears and swimmer's ear are different conditions that are sometimes confused. Water-clogged ears are caused by fluids that accumulate in the ear after swimming or showering. Swimmer's ear produces inflammation and infection of the external ear after prolonged exposure to water, along with damage to the lining of the ear canal. Damage to the lining typically occurs when the person uses a rigid object to remove water from the ears. Swimmer's ear produces acute pain, itching, and a foul-smelling discharge from the ear.

Both conditions cause earache. Nonprescription drying agents are safe and effective for treatment of water-clogged ears. Alcohol (Auro-Dri) and mild acidic solutions of vinegar (acetic acid) dry excess water and soothe the eardrum. Alcohol-containing eardrops may produce stinging if the ears are inflamed.

> **⊗ TECH NOTE!**
>
> A common ending for local anesthetics is "-caine."

Treatments for Water-Clogged Ears and Swimmer's Ear

Generic Name	US Brand Name(s) / Canadian Brand Name(s)	Dosage Forms and Strengths
acetic acid solution[a]	Vosol	**Solution, otic:** 2%
	Not Available	
Combination Otic Drops		
acetic acid + hydrocortisone solution[a]	Acetasol HC, Vosol HC	**Solution, otic:** 2% acetic acid + 1% hydrocortisone
	Not available	
isopropyl alcohol + glycerin[a]	Auro-Dri Ear-Water Drying Aid (OTC), Swim-Ear Ear-Water Drying Aid (OTC)	**Solution, otic:** 95% isopropyl alcohol and glycerin 5%
	Auro-Dri Ear-Water Drying Aid (OTC)	

[a]Generic available.
OTC, Over the counter.

> **⊗ TECH NOTE!**
>
> The pH is a measure of how acidic or alkaline (or basic) a solution is. A pH of 1 indicates that the solution is very acidic (e.g., stomach acids [HCl]). A pH of 7 is neutral. Plasma pH ranges between 7.35 and 7.45. A pH of greater than 7 is considered alkaline.

Cerumen Impaction

Cerumen (earwax) is a normal and necessary substance produced by the ear. It functions to reduce the risk for bacterial infections in the ear because earwax has a pH of 6.5 and is bactericidal. Cerumen repels water and helps keep the ear dry during swimming and bathing. It lubricates the skin of the external ear canal and provides a barrier to entry of airborne substances (dust, insects) into the ear canal.

The healthy ear continuously replaces old cerumen. If cerumen becomes impacted, it can produce hearing loss, pressure, and ear pain. This condition is more common in people who wear hearing aids or regularly place earplugs and earphones in the ear. A cotton-tipped applicator or other small sharp object should never be used to remove earwax. These objects can cause accidental perforation of the eardrum (tympanic membrane).

Agents used to remove excess cerumen are called cerumenolytics. Emollients and carbamide peroxide are the principal ingredients found in cerumenolytics. *Emollients* are used to soften the wax, enabling it to slide out of the ear. Olive oil, mineral oil, and glycerin are emollients found in otics for earwax removal.

Peroxide-based products are used to break up the earwax and bubble away the debris. Carbamide peroxide 6.5% (over the counter [OTC]) and triethanolamine polypeptide oleate-condensate (OTC in Canada) are agents available to remove earwax.

After administration of emollients or peroxide-based agents, the affected ear is gently cleansed (irrigated) with warm water to remove cerumen that has become dislodged. Ear irrigation is performed using a bulb syringe.

Cerumenolytics Used to Aid in Earwax Removal

Generic Name	US Brand Name(s) Canadian Brand Name(s)	Dosage Forms and Strengths
carbamide peroxide (also known as urea hydrogen peroxide)[a]	Murine EAR Wax Removal System Debrox (OTC) Murine EAR Wax Removal System (OTC)	**Solution, otic:** 6.5%
paradichlorobenzene + chlorbutol + oil of terebinth + peanut oil	Not available Cerumol (OTC)	**Solution, otic:** Paradichlorobenzene 2% + chlorbutol 5% + oil of terebinth 10% + peanut oil 57%

[a]Generic available.
OTC, Over the counter.

Summary of Drugs Used to Treat Miscellaneous Conditions of the Ear

Generic	Brand	Usual Dose	Warning Labels
Analgesics			
antipyrine and benzocaine	Auralgan	Instill 1–2 drops in ear canal 3–4 times a day or up to every 1–2 h until pain relieved	FOR THE EAR.
Drying Agents			
acetic acid solution	Generics	Instill 4–6 drops in ear canal. Repeat every 2–3 h as needed	FOR THE EAR.
isopropyl alcohol and glycerin	Auro-Dri Ear-Water Drying Aid	**Water-clogged ears:** Instill 4–5 drops in affected ear(s)	
Cerumenolytics			
carbamide peroxide	Debrox (OTC)	**Earwax removal:** Instill 5–10 drops twice daily for up to 4 days	FOR THE EAR.
triethylanolamine polypeptide oleate-condensate	Generics	**Earwax removal:** Fill ear canal; insert cotton pledget; leave in for 15–30 min; then flush with warm water	FOR THE EAR.

OTC, Over the counter.

TECHNICIAN'S CORNER

1. How does ear candling work to remove unwanted cerumen or debris from the ear? What risks are associated with this practice?
2. How can putting a baby to bed with a bottle of milk contribute to otitis media?

Key Points

- Perception of balance and movement is a function of input from the eyes, inner ear, and sense receptors on the skin and skeleton.
- The semicircular canals located in the inner ear control the sense of equilibrium or balance.
- Otosclerosis and autoimmune diseases such as multiple sclerosis and SSHL are conditions that can cause hearing loss.
- Sudden sensorineural hearing loss is treated with glucocorticosteroids.
- Otosclerosis also causes ringing in the ears (tinnitus).
- Tinnitus is a condition that produces ringing in the ear.
- Tinnitus may be drug induced. Aspirin and alcohol are common drugs that can cause tinnitus.
- Aminoglycoside antiinfectives (gentamicin) and loop diuretics can cause ototoxicity.

- Vertigo is a balance disorder that is caused by a neural mismatch or sensory conflict.
- Vertigo can occur from head trauma or degeneration of otolith organs, inflammation of the vestibular nerve, bacterial infection of the labyrinths, brainstem or cerebral pathology, or Ménière disease.
- Vertigo and other balance disorders produce symptoms of dizziness or spinning, nausea and vomiting, blurred vision, disorientation, and a feeling of falling.
- Treatment of balance disorders may involve physical therapy, diet, and lifestyle changes.
- When drug therapy is indicated, antihistamines are most widely used.
- Antihistamines have anticholinergic actions that can moderate symptoms of motion sickness but produce urinary retention

and other side effects that limit their use in patients with prostate disease or asthma or in women who are lactating.

- Other side effects that are common to all antihistamine drugs are sedation, dry mouth, and blurred vision.
- One scopolamine transdermal patch placed behind the ear prevents motion sickness for up to 3 days.
- Ear pain, also called auralgia or otalgia, is a symptom of otitis externa otitis media.
- Ear pain is treated by administration of topical analgesics, local anesthetics, or oral analgesics.
- When the ear is inflamed, otic suspensions are more soothing than solutions that contain alcohol.
- Water-clogged ears and swimmer's ear are different conditions that are sometimes confused.
- Swimmer's ear produces inflammation and infection of the external ear.
- Nonprescription drying agents are safe and effective for treatment of water-clogged ears.
- Cerumen (earwax) is bactericidal and water repellent, and it provides a barrier to entry of airborne substances and lubricates the skin of the external ear canal.

- A cotton-tipped applicator or other small sharp object should never be used to remove earwax.
- Emollients and carbamide peroxide are the principal ingredients found in cerumenolytics.
- After administration of emollients or peroxide-based agents, the affected ear is gently cleansed (irrigated) with warm water to remove cerumen that has become dislodged.
- Otitis externa is inflammation of the external auditory canal and is most commonly caused by a bacterial infection.
- Risk factors for development of otitis externa are (1) exposure to excessive moisture (swimming, humidity, sweating), (2) high environmental temperature, (3) irritation caused by earwax removal, (4) insertion of objects into the ear, and (5) chronic dermatologic disease.
- Otitis media is an inflammation in the middle ear.
- Excessive use of antiinfective agents to treat otitis media may increase the risk of development of bacterial resistance.
- Decongestants and antihistamines are not recommended for prophylaxis or treatment of otitis media in children.

Review Questions

1. Otitis media is an inflammation in the _____ ear.
   a. inner
   b. outer
   c. middle
   d. cochlea
2. Prophylactic use of _____ is ineffective in preventing otitis media.
   a. antihistamines
   b. decongestants
   c. both a and b
   d. none of the above
3. The most common cause of otitis externa is _____
   a. viral infection
   b. bacterial infection
   c. psoriasis
   d. lupus
4. The most common cause for drug-induced tinnitus is _____.
   a. noise
   b. aspirin
   c. alcohol
   d. b and c
5. Which drug treatment for vertigo is available in a "patch" form?
   a. diphenhydramine
   b. scopolamine
   c. dimenhydrinate
   d. betahistine
6. Corticosteroids such as hydrocortisone are combined with _____ agents to reduce inflammation and pain in the ear.
   a. optic
   b. otic
   c. glaucoma
   d. ocular

7. Swimmer's ear produces inflammation and infection of the _____ ear after prolonged exposure to water along with damage to the lining of the ear canal.
   a. internal
   b. inner
   c. external
   d. semicircular canals
8. Children are more susceptible to otitis media than are adults because their eustachian tubes are longer and straighter than those of adults.
   a. True
   b. False
9. Olive oil, mineral oil, and glycerin are emollients found in otics for removal of _____.
   a. ear wax
   b. fluid
   c. bacteria
   d. foreign material
10. Carbamide peroxide 6.5% is an approved agent for _____ removal.
    a. earwax
    b. fluid
    c. bacteria
    d. foreign material

Bibliography

Alberta Medical Association: Guideline for the Diagnosis and Management of Acute Otitis Media: Alberta Medical Association, 2008.

Hain T, Uddin M: Pharmacological treatment of vertigo, *CNS Drugs* 17:85–100, 2003.

Hoberman A, Paradise JL, Rockette HE, et al: Treatment of acute otitis media in children under 2 years of age, *NEJM* 364(2):105–115, 2011.

Koo L, Young L: Management of ocular toxoplasmosis, *Int Ophthalmol Clin* 46:183–193, 2006.

Mayo Clinic: Ménière's Disease: Treatment and Drugs. Retrieved May 15, 2011, from http://www.mayoclinic.com/health/menieres-disease/DS00535/DSECTION=treatments-and-drugs, 2015.

Mayo Clinic: Tinnitus. Retrieved May 16, 2017, from http://www.nlm.nih.gov/medlineplus/tinnitus.html, 2017.

National Institute on Deafness and Other Communication Disorders: NIDCD Fact Sheet: Ear Infections in Children. NIH Publication No.13-4799, Bethesda, MD, NIDCD, National Institutes of Health, US Department of Health and Human Services. Retrieved from https://www.nidcd.nih.gov/health/ear-infections-children, 2013.

National Institute on Deafness and Other Communication Disorders: Balance disorders, Bethesda, MD, 2017, NIDCD, National Institutes of Health, US Department of Health and Human Services. Retrieved from https://www.nidcd.nih.gov/health/balance-disorders.

Page C, Curtis M, Sutter M, et al: *Integrated pharmacology*, Philadelphia, 2005, Mosby, pp 539–544.

Patton K: *Survival guide for anatomy and physiology*, St Louis, 2006, Mosby.

Sander R: Otitis externa: a practical guide to treatment and prevention, *Am Fam Physician* 63:927–936, 941–942, 2001.

Thibodeau GA, Patton KT: *Anatomy and physiology*, ed 6, St Louis, 2007, Mosby.

Uppal S, Bajaj Y, Coatesworth AP: Otosclerosis 2: the medical management of otosclerosis, *Int J Clin Pract* 64(2):256–265, 2010.

Vartiainen E, Karjalainen S, Nuutinen J, et al: Effect of drinking water fluoridation on hearing of patients with otosclerosis in a low fluoride area: a follow-up study, *Am J Otol* 15(4):545–548, 1994.

UNIT V

Drugs Affecting the Cardiovascular System

Maintaining the body's internal environment (homeostasis), depends on the continual transport of oxygen, nutrients, and biochemical messengers among the body's cells. Blood is a complex transport medium that performs vital pickup and delivery services for the body. It is the keystone of the body's heat-regulating mechanism and can absorb large quantities of heat without an appreciable increase in its own temperature, transferring it from the body's core to the surface to be dissipated.

Heart health is maintained by lifestyle factors that include healthy eating and moderate to strenuous exercise. When the heart fails, numerous types of drugs are used in the treatment of heart disease. For example, anticoagulants prevent clot formations, beta-adrenergic drugs reduce the workload of the heart, calcium channel blockers reduce vascular contractions and improve coronary blood flow, digitalis slows and increases the strength of cardiac contractions, nitroglycerin dilates coronary blood vessels, and tissue plasminogen activator (t-PA) helps dissolve clots.

In Unit V, the pharmacotherapy for diseases of the cardiovascular system are described. Angina, hypertension, arrhythmias, coronary heart disease, and stroke are covered. A brief description of each disorder is provided, followed by a description of the drugs indicated for treatment that includes mechanisms of action, adverse reactions, strength(s), and dosage forms. Lifestyle changes that are important in preventing and managing heart disease are also described in Unit V.

17

Treatment of Angina

LEARNING OBJECTIVES

1. Learn the terminology associated with the treatment of angina.
2. List the symptoms of and risk factors for angina.
3. Explain the role of coronary artery disease in the development of angina.
4. Identify lifestyle changes that reduce the risk for angina.
5. List and categorize medications used to treat angina.
6. Describe mechanism of action for each classification of drugs used to treat angina.
7. Identify significant drug look-alike and sound-alike issues.
8. List common endings for drug classes used in the treatment of angina.
9. Identify warning labels and precautionary messages associated with medications used to treat angina.

KEY TERMS

Angina pectoris Symptomatic manifestation of ischemic heart disease characterized by a severe squeezing or pressure-like chest pain and brought on by exertion or stress.

Arteriosclerosis Thickening and loss of elasticity of arterial walls; sometimes called "hardening of the arteries."

Atheromas Hard plaque formed within an artery.

Atherosclerosis Process in which plaques (atheromas) containing cholesterol, lipid material, and lipophages are formed within arteries.

Coronary artery disease Condition that occurs when the arteries that supply blood to the heart muscle become hardened and narrowed.

Embolus A moving blood clot.

Hyperlipidemia Increased concentration of cholesterol and triglycerides in the blood that is associated with the development of atherosclerosis.

Ischemia Deficient blood supply to an area of the body. Myocardial ischemia results in angina and myocardial infarction.

Ischemic heart disease Any condition in which heart muscle is damaged or works inefficiently because of an absence or relative deficiency of its blood supply.

Necrosis Cell death that may be caused by lack of blood and oxygen to the affected areas.

Myocardial infarction Also referred to as a "heart attack." Results in heart muscle tissue death and is caused by the occlusion (blockage) of a coronary artery.

Thrombus Stationary blood clot.

Vasospasm Spasms that constrict blood vessels and reduce the flow of blood and oxygen.

Overview

The word "angina" is derived from the Latin word *ango,* which means "to choke." *Angina pectoris* occurs when there is an imbalance between the heart's demand for oxygen and the oxygen supply (Fig. 17.1). The symptoms of angina are described as severe squeezing or pressure-like chest pain, sometimes radiating to the arms, shoulders, neck, or jaw. The pain is sometimes described as severe heartburn or indigestion. Angina is a symptom of *ischemic heart disease. Ischemia* is caused by loss of blood supply to a region of the body. As many as 10 million people in the United States have angina. People with a history of heart disease, hypertension, and diabetes are at risk for angina.

Lifestyle can also be a risk factor for the condition. In fact, angina is often classified as a chronic disease of lifestyle because many of the risks for developing the condition are related to lifestyle. Risk factors associated with lifestyle include smoking, overeating, a diet high in cholesterol and salt, excessive alcohol consumption, obesity, and lack of exercise. Stress is also a risk factor for angina.

High dietary cholesterol is a contributing factor for the development of *coronary artery disease* (CAD) and myocardial ischemia. Cholesterol, lipid material, and lipophages are deposited within arteries. The lipid streaks harden into plaques (atheromas); this process is called *atherosclerosis.* An *atheroma* can increase in size and reduce blood flow and has the potential to result in thrombus (blood clot) formation (Fig. 17.2). Thrombi can further occlude the artery in which it was formed. A thrombus that breaks off is called an embolus (moving blood clot); it can travel to a smaller artery, where it completely blocks the blood vessel, causing ischemia (inadequate blood supply.) Prolonged ischemia can result in tissue necrosis (death), leading to *myocardial infarction* (heart attack) or stroke. *Arteriosclerosis,* sometimes called "hardening of the arteries," is a condition in which arterial walls thicken and lose elasticity. Arteriosclerosis may occur as part of the normal aging process. Other risk factors are smoking tobacco, obesity, diabetes

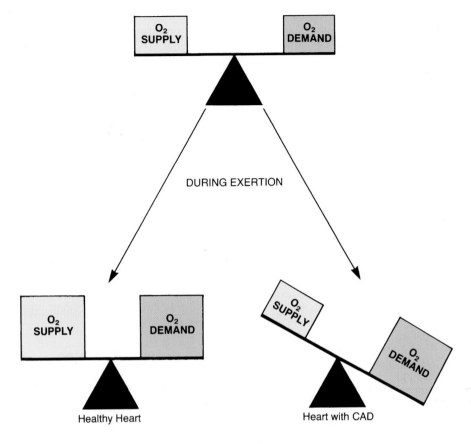

DURING REST
Healthy Heart and Heart with CAD

DURING EXERTION

Healthy Heart

Heart with CAD

• **Fig. 17.1** Effect of exertion on the balance between oxygen supply and oxygen demand in the healthy heart and the heart with CAD. (From Burchum JR, Rosenthal LD, Jones BO: *Lehne's pharmacology for nursing care*, ed 9, St. Louis, 2016 Elsevier.)

• **Fig. 17.2** Plaque buildup in an artery. A, Normal artery without plaque build-up. B, Narrowed artery with plaque build-up. (Courtesy of National Institutes of Health Bethesda, MD.)

and hypertension. When arteriosclerosis occurs in the coronary arteries, the arteries become less able to dilate and increase the heart's blood supply when needed.

> **TECH NOTE!**
>
> A *thrombus* is a stationary blood clot; an *embolus* is a moving blood clot.

Types of Angina

There are three types of angina, which vary according to their pattern and ability to be relieved by medication. They are called stable angina, unstable angina, and variant angina, also known as Prinzmetal or vasospastic angina. In all types of angina, there is an imbalance between blood supplied to the heart muscle and the need for blood and oxygen. The symptoms of angina occur when the blood supplied to the heart is insufficient to meet the heart's need for oxygen.

Stable (Exertional) Angina

Symptoms of stable angina are predictable and are typically brought on by physical exertion, smoking, eating heavy meals, exposure to extreme changes in temperature (hot or cold), and emotional stress. Physical exertion is the most common reason for the onset of angina. Although the amount of blood and oxygen that is supplied to the heart meets its needs under typical conditions, it is insufficient during periods of physical exertion. Rest and antianginal medications such as nitroglycerin adequately treat the acute symptoms of stable angina. Symptoms often subside within 5 minutes.

Unstable Angina

Unstable angina is a serious condition requiring evaluation because it may precede a myocardial infarction (heart attack). It may occur at rest without physical exertion and may result when an embolus partially or completely blocking an artery. Myocardial ischemia causes the symptoms of pain and chest pressure. Symptoms are not relieved by rest or antianginal medicine and may last for up to 30 minutes.

Variant Angina

Variant (Prinzmetal) angina is also known as vasospastic angina because it is caused by *vasospasm* of the coronary arteries. Spasms reduce the opening of the artery, decreasing the blood supply and oxygen to the heart. Similar to unstable angina, the pain typically occurs at rest and during the night or early morning. Unlike unstable angina, it is relieved by medications (e.g., nitrates and calcium channel blockers). Symptoms often persist longer than stable angina and may exceed 5 minutes.

Microvascular Angina

Microvascular angina or cardiac syndrome X is a form of stable angina that may produce greater chest pain and last longer. This type of angina may be a symptom of coronary microvascular disorder that occurs when the tiny blood vessels that nourish the heart do not function well. It differs from other forms of angina because some patients have no CAD risk factors. Microvascular angina most often occurs during exercise but can occur at rest.

Nonpharmacologic Treatment of Angina

Lifestyle Change

Change in modifiable lifestyle practices is an important part of the treatment and prevention of angina and other cardiovascular diseases. Lifestyle changes can reduce the risk for angina, as well as decrease the frequency and severity of symptoms and prevent or slow the progression of angina to myocardial infarction or death.

We may not be able to limit our exposure to stressful situations, but we can control the volume of food we consume and lose weight if necessary. Increasing our level of daily activity, while avoiding overexertion, is another modifiable lifestyle change that we can make. If you smoke, you should quit.

Other lifestyle changes that should be implemented if possible include:

- Taking frequent rest breaks if necessary to avoid angina that is caused by exertion
- Avoiding foods high in salt and cholesterol
- Eating small portions rather than a heavy meal
- Learning techniques to manage stress
- Being an advocate for workplace and community-wide changes that facilitate lifestyle change (e.g., nutritious food choices in school and workplace cafeterias).

Drugs Used in the Treatment of Angina

The primary cause of angina is an imbalance between oxygen supply and oxygen demand in the heart. Drugs used in the treatment of angina are administered to increase the blood and oxygen supply to the heart and/or decrease the heart's demand for oxygen (workload). Nitrates, some beta blockers, and the late sodium current blocker ranolazine are specifically US Food and Drug Administration or Health Canada approved as antianginals. Some calcium channel blockers are also indicated for the treatment of angina. The mechanisms of action of the drugs vary. They produce their effects by dilating blood vessels (veins and arteries), decreasing heart rate, reducing cardiac contractility, or reducing vasospasms.

Current drug therapy for angina has shifted to focus on decreasing cardiovascular events by treating and preventing the cardiovascular diseases that often accompany angina. Previously, treatment was focused primarily on prevention of acute symptoms. Drugs may be administered to persons who have angina to treat comorbid conditions such as hypertension (see Chapter 18), hyperlipidemia, atherosclerosis, atherothrombosis, and myocardial infarction. The following drug classes are used to treat angina: nitrates, beta blockers, calcium channel blockers, and late sodium current blockers.

Nitrates

The organic nitrates are the oldest class of drugs used to treat acute symptoms of angina. Nitrates reduce oxygen demand and increase oxygen supply. They dilate blood vessels (arteries and veins) and increase supply of oxygen to the heart. Nitrates that are commonly used for treatment and prevention of angina are nitroglycerin, isosorbide dinitrate, and isosorbide mononitrate. Nitrates are also indicated for the treatment of congestive heart failure, pulmonary hypertension, and hypertensive emergencies.

● **TECH NOTE!**

Sublingual nitroglycerin is packaged by manufacturers in amber glass bottles and should be dispensed in the manufacturer's original container. Dispense without a safety cap for easy access. It is one of the few drugs exempted from the Poison Prevention Packaging Act.

Mechanism of Action

Nitrates dilate the veins that carry blood away from the heart and dilate the coronary arteries, which supply blood to the heart. When nitrates dilate veins, they reduce heart muscle tension and decrease oxygen demand. Most nitrates are prodrugs that are converted in the body to nitric oxide. Nitric oxide acts at the cellular level to reduce intracellular calcium, block muscle contraction, and relax blood vessels.

Nitrates relax and dilate medium- to large-size coronary arteries. This increases oxygen to the heart. Nitrates also relax smooth muscles in the veins, which reduces fluid backup in the ventricles and the work needed to pump blood out of the ventricles. In the case of obstruction of a coronary artery, nitrates may cause the dilation of adjacent arteries, shifting blood supply away from the blocked region.

● **TECH NOTE!**

Isosorbide dinitrate is also available in unit dose packaging.

● **TECH NOTE!**

It is important for the patients using patches to rotate the sites on the skin to prevent skin irritation.

Pharmacokinetics

Nitrates are formulated for a variety of dosage delivery systems. Nitroglycerin dosage forms include parenteral, sublingual tablets, lingual spray, capsules, sublingual powder, ointments, and transdermal patches. Some dosage delivery systems are designed to deliver nitroglycerin quickly and are used to treat acute symptoms. These include parenteral solution, sublingual tablets, and lingual spray. The other dosage forms of nitroglycerin deliver medication over an extended period (up to 24 hours) and are intended to prevent symptoms of angina. BiDil is a fixed dose combination of isosordil dinitrate (20 mg) (a vasodilator that affects both arteries and veins) and hydralazine HCl (37.5 mg), a predominantly arterial vasodilator.

Nitroglycerin is lipid soluble and readily crosses cell membranes. It is subject to extensive first-pass metabolism, and only 10% of an oral dose is available to produce effects. This explains why parenteral and sublingual dosage forms produce actions more quickly and are more potent than enteral dosage forms (capsules).

Nitroglycerin is volatile and loses its potency on exposure to air, light, and moisture. Potency can also be lost if it is repackaged in plastic prescription vials. Sublingual nitroglycerin is packaged by manufacturers in amber glass bottles and should be dispensed in the manufacturer's original container.

Isosorbide dinitrate and isosorbide mononitrate are not used to treat acute symptoms. They are formulated for prevention (immediate-release and extended-action tablets). Isosorbide mononitrate is a long-acting metabolite of isosorbide dinitrate.

Isosorbide dinitrate and isosorbide mononitrate are more stable than nitroglycerin and do not need to be dispensed in the manufacturer's original container.

❶ **TECH ALERT!**

A warning label may be placed on prescriptions for sildenafil (Viagra), vardenafil (Cialis), and tadalafil (Levitra) (treatment for erectile dysfunction), warning that use with nitroglycerin may cause a fatal drop in blood pressure.

Adverse Reactions

Some of the adverse reactions to nitrates are dosage form dependent, and other effects are common regardless the dosage delivery system. Adverse reactions associated with vasodilation are the most common and include hypotension, facial flushing, dizziness, and headache. Nausea and vomiting, weakness, and fatigue are additional side effects produced by nitroglycerin, isosorbide dinitrate, and isosorbide mononitrate. Sublingual dosage forms can cause stinging or burning under the tongue, and adhesives used in patches can produce allergic reactions.

● **TECH NOTE!**

All nitrates have "nitro" or "nitra" in their brand or generic name.

● **TECH NOTE!**

Nitroglycerin ointment is also marketed for the treatment of anal fissure pain. RECTIV nitroglycerin ointment is applied rectally.

Precautions

Patients who use nitrates can develop tolerance to their effects. This means the drug actions are less effective over time. Tolerance is most common with long-acting nitrates. To minimize the risk for development of tolerance, it is important to avoid continuous exposure to the drug. Transdermal patches are designed to deliver their effects for 24 hours; however, the patch should never be worn for the entire 24-hour period. Patients should be instructed to remove the patch after 10 to 12 hours. Patients must be nitrate free for at least 10 to 12 hours per day.

Late Sodium Channel Current Blockade

Ranexa (ranolazine) is used to treat adult patients with chronic angina. It is classified as a late sodium channel current blocker. It is the only drug in its class. Ranolazine improves coronary blood flow. It works by reducing the sodium-calcium exchange, which ultimately decreases calcium ions. The overall effect of this is to relax heart muscle by decreasing contractility.

Common side effects of Ranexa are dizziness, headache, nausea, and constipation. Ranexa may cause serious side effects such as changes in the electrical activity of the heart. It may also cause kidney failure in people with severe kidney problems. Ranexa is an extended-release tablet that must be swallowed whole. It should not be taken with grapefruit juice, because this will cause an increase of the drug in the blood. Ranolazine may be used at the same time with beta blockers, calcium channel blockers, nitrates, angiotensin-converting enzyme (ACE) inhibitors, and angiotensin receptor blockers (ARBs).

Nitrates Used in the Treatment of Angina

Generic Name	US Brand Name(s) / Canadian Brand(s)	Dosage Forms and Strengths
isosorbide dinitrate[a]	Dilatrate-SR, Isordil	**Capsule, sustained release (Dilatrate-SR):** 40 mg **Tablets, extended release:** 40 mg[b] **Tablets, immediate release (Isordil):** 5 mg, 10 mg, 20 mg,[b] 30 mg, 40 mg[b]
	Generics	
isosorbide mononitrate[a]	Monoket	**Tablets (Monoket):** 10 mg, 20 mg **Tablets, extended release** **(Imdur):** 60 mg (30 mg, 120 mg generic only[b])
	Imdur	
isosorbide dinitrate + hydralazine	BiDil	**Tablets:** 20 mg (isosorbide) + 37.5 mg (hydralazine)
	Not available	
nitroglycerin[a]	GoNitro, Minitran, Nitro-Dur, Nitrolingual, Nitromist, Nitrostat	**Ointment[b]:** 2%, **Powder, sublingual (GoNitro):** 0.4 mg packets **Solution, for injection:** 50 mg/10 mL **Tablets, sublingual (Nitrostat):** 0.3 mg (gr1/200), 0.4 mg (gr1/150), 0.6 mg (gr1/100) **Transdermal patch (Minitran, Nitro-Dur):** 0.1 mg/h (5 cm²),[b] 0.2 mg/h (10 cm²), 0.4 mg/h (20 cm²), 0.6 mg/h, 0.8 mg (40 cm²) **Translingual spray (Nitrolingual, Nitromist,** **Rho-Nitro Pumpspray):** 0.4 mg/spray (200 sprays/canister)
	Minitran, Nitro-Dur, Nitrostat, Nitrolingual, Rho-Nitro Pump spray, Transderm-Nitro, Trinipatch	

[a]Generic available.
[b]Available in the United States only.
[c]Available in Canada only.
gr, grain

Sodium Channel Current Blockers

Generic Name	US Brand Name(s)	Dosage Forms and Strengths
ranolazine	Ranexa	**Tablets, extended release:** 500 mg, 1 Gm extended release

---

❗ TECH ALERT!

The following drugs have look-alike and sound-alike issues:
metoprolol and miSOPROStol;
Inderal, Isordil, Adderall

Beta-Adrenergic Blockers

Beta-adrenergic blockers are administered to reduce the heart's demand for oxygen. This is achieved by decreasing the heart rate and thereby reducing the workload of the heart. There are many beta-adrenergic blockers; however, only four are currently approved for the management of angina. They are atenolol, metoprolol, nadolol, and propranolol. Beta-adrenergic blockers are also indicated for the management of hypertension and postmyocardial infarction (see Chapters 18 and 19) and for the prevention of migraine headache (see Chapter 10).

Mechanism of Action

Beta-adrenergic blockers decrease the frequency and severity of stable (exertional) angina. They bind to beta-receptor sites and block activity of the sympathetic nervous system on cardiac muscle. Heart contractility is reduced and the heart rate is slowed, thereby reducing the workload of the heart. When the heart works less, its need for oxygen and blood supply is reduced.

Beta-adrenergic blocking drugs, used to treat stable angina, include cardioselective beta₁-adrenergic blockers and nonselective mixed beta₁/beta₂ blockers (e.g., propranolol and nadolol). More discussion is found in Chapter 18.

▶ TECH NOTE!

Beta-adrenergic blockers are easily identified because their generic name ends in "-lol."

Pharmacokinetics

Beta-adrenergic blockers are formulated in immediate- and long-acting dosage forms. The elimination half-life varies for specific agents and ranges from as short as 3 to 4 hours (propranolol) to as long as 24 hours (nadolol). Most agents are dosed once to twice a day except short-acting propranolol, which is dosed two to four times a day.

Adverse Reactions

Beta-adrenergic blockers can produce dizziness, fatigue, bradycardia, hypotension, impotence, heart block (a heart beat that is prolonged

Beta-Adrenergic Blockers

Generic Name	US Brand Name(s)	Dosage Forms and Strengths
	Canadian Brand(s)	
atenolol[a]	Tenormin	**Tablets:** 25 mg, 50 mg, 100 mg
	Tenormin	
metoprolol tartrate[a]	Lopressor	**Tablets:** 25 mg, 50 mg, 100 mg **Tablets, slow release (Lopressor SR):** 100 mg, 200 mg
	Lopressor, Lopressor SR	
metoprolol succinate ER[a]	Toprol XL	**Tablets, extended release:** 25 mg,[b] 50 mg,[b] 100 mg, 200 mg
	Generics only	
nadolol[a]	Corgard	**Tablets:** 20 mg,[b] 40 mg, 80 mg, 160 mg[c]
	Generics	
propranolol[a]	Inderal, Inderal-LA, InnoPran XL	**Capsules, extended release (InnoPran XL):** 80 mg, 120 mg **Capsules, sustained release (Inderal LA):** 60 mg, 80 mg, 120 mg, 160 mg **Injection, solution (Inderal):** 1 mg/mL **Solution, oral (United States only):** 20 mg/5 mL, 40 mg/5 mL **Tablet:** 10 mg, 20 mg, 40 mg, 60 mg,[b] 80 mg
	Inderal-LA	

[a]Generic available.
[b]Available in United States only.
[c]Available in Canada only.

and the rhythm is too slow), and occasionally insomnia. Beta-adrenergic blockers can produce bronchospasm, so their use is cautioned in persons with asthma. They should be used cautiously in persons with asthma and diabetes because they can produce bronchospasm and their action to decrease heart rate mask one of the principal signs of hypoglycemia. Patients with diabetes using beta blockers should be educated about other symptoms of hypoglycemia to be aware of. Abrupt discontinuation of beta-adrenergic blockers should be avoided because it can produce tachycardia and a sudden increase in the workload of the heart.

> **● TECH NOTE!**
>
> Hyperlipidemia is a risk factor for angina. Caduet is a combination drug that combines the calcium channel blocker amlodipine with the lipid-lowering drug atorvastatin.

Calcium Channel Blockers

Calcium channel blockers are used in the treatment of variant and stable angina. They are effective in the treatment of variant angina because of their ability to reduce vasospasms that restrict the flow of blood and oxygen. Calcium channel blockers improve exercise tolerance by decreasing the workload of the heart. Calcium channel blockers are effective in the treatment of stable angina alone and in combination with nitrates or beta blockers.

> **❶ TECH ALERT!**
>
> The following drugs have look-alike and sound-alike issues:
> Cardizem, Cardizem SR, Cardizem LA, and Cardizem CD;
> Tiazac and Ziac;
> nicardipine, nifedipine;
> Procardia, Procardia XL, and Cartia XT

Mechanism of Action

Calcium channel blockers block L-type voltage-dependent calcium channels, suppress depolarization, and reduce contraction of the heart muscle. There are two classes of Ca^{2+} channel blockers, dihydropyridines (amlodipine, nifedipine, nicardipine, nimodipine, nisoldipine) and nondihydropyridines, which include phenylalkylamines (verapamil) and benzothiazepines (diltiazem).

Verapamil and diltizem reduce heart oxygen consumption during exercise by decreasing heart rate and heart contractions. Amlodipine, nifedipine, nicardipine, nimodipine, and nisoldipine are more selective for blood vessels, so they are able to increase blood and oxygen supply without slowing heart rate or contractions or increasing the risk of heart block.

> **● TECH NOTE!**
>
> Calcium channel blockers classified as dihydropyridines are easily identified because their generic name ends in "-dipine."

Adverse Reactions

Some adverse drug reactions are common to all calcium channel blockers; other side effects are specific to drug classification. All calcium channel blockers produce hypotension. The dihydropyridines (e.g., nifedipine) produce vasodilation that can lead to dizziness, flushing, and headache. Peripheral edema is caused by venodilation. Verapamil and diltiazem may produce heart failure, bradycardia, and heart block because they slow conduction through the atrioventricular node.

> **● TECH NOTE!**
>
> Grapefruit juice decreases the metabolism of calcium channel blockers. Apply the warning label AVOID GRAPEFRUIT JUICE.

Calcium Channel Blockers

Generic Name	US Brand Name(s) Canadian Brand(s)	Dosage Forms and Strengths
amlodipine[a]	Norvasc	**Tablets:** 2.5 mg, 5 mg, 10 mg
	Norvasc	
diltiazem[a]	Cardizem, Cardizem CD, Cardizem LA, Cartia XT, Diltzac, Tiamate, Taztia XT, Tiazac	**Capsules, extended release:** 120 mg, 180 mg, 240 mg 300 mg, 360 mg, 420 mg (Tiazac only)[b] **Tablets, immediate release (Cardizem):** 30 mg, 60 mg, 90 mg,[b] 120 mg[b] **Tablets, extended release (Cardizem LA, Tiazac XC):** 120 mg, 180 mg, 240 mg, 300 mg, 360 mg, 420 mg[b] (Cardizem LA only)
	Cardizem CD, Tiazac, Tiazac XC	
nicardipine[a]	Generics only	**Capsules:** 20 mg, 30 mg
	Not available	
nifedipine[a]	Adalat CC, Afeditab CR, Procardia, Procardia XL	**Capsule (Procardia):** 5 mg,[c] 10 mg, 20 mg **Tablets, extended release (Adalat CC, Adalat XL SRT, Afeditab CR, Procardia XL):** 20 mg,[c] 30 mg, 60 mg, 90 mg[b]
	Adalat XL SRT	
verapamil[a]	Calan SR, Verelan, Verelan PM	**Capsules, extended release (Verelan PM):** 100 mg, 200 mg, 300 mg **Capsules, extended release (Verelan):** 120 mg, 180 mg, 240 mg, 360 mg[b] **Tablets, immediate release (Calan):** 40 mg,[b] 80 mg, 120 mg, 160 mg **Tablets, sustained release (Calan SR, Isoptin SR):** 120 mg, 180 mg,[c] 240 mg
	Isoptin SR	

Calcium Channel Blocker Combinations (Only Combinations Approved for the Treatment of Angina Are Listed)

amlodipine + atorvastatin[a]	Caduet	**Tablets:** amlodipine 2.5 mg + atorvastatin 10 mg,[b] amlodipine 2.5 mg + atorvastatin 20 mg,[b] amlodipine 2.5 mg + atorvastatin 40 mg,[b] amlodipine 5 mg + atorvastatin 10 mg, amlodipine 5 mg + atorvastatin 20 mg, amlodipine 5 mg + atorvastatin 40 mg, amlodipine 5 mg + atorvastatin 80 mg, amlodipine 10 mg + atorvastatin 10 mg, amlodipine 10 mg + atorvastatin 20 mg, amlodipine 10 mg + atorvastatin 40 mg, amlodipine 10 mg + atorvastatin 80 mg
	Caduet	

[a]Generic available.
[b]Available in the United States only.
[c]Available in Canada only.

Summary of Drugs Used in the Treatment of Angina

	Generic	Brand	Usual Dose	Warning Labels
Nitrates				
	isosorbide dinitrate	Isordil	**Angina:** 5–40 mg 2–3 times a day or up to 160 mg SR (1–4 capsules) not less than once every 18 hours	TAKE ON AN EMPTY STOMACH— isosorbide dinitrate. SWALLOW WHOLE; DO NOT CRUSH OR CHEW— sustained and extended release. AVOID ALCOHOL.
	isosorbide mononitrate	Imdur	**Angina:** 5–20 mg twice a day (7 h apart), 30–60 mg/day (extended release) up to maximum, 240 mg/day	

Summary of Drugs Used in the Treatment of Angina—cont'd

Generic	Brand	Usual Dose	Warning Labels
nitroglycerin	Nitrostat	**Oral:** 2.5–6.5 mg 2–4 times a day (maximum, 26 mg 4 times a day) **Ointment:** 1/2–2 inches (1.25–5.08 cm) of 2% ointment (7.5–30 mg) twice a day (6 h apart) **Powder:** 1–2 packets at onset of symptoms. May take 1 additional packet every 5 minutes until symptoms subside up to a maximum of 15 minutes (3 doses). **Transdermal patch:** Wear 1 patch (0.2–0.8 mg/h) for 12–14 h/day; patch off for 10–12 h/day **Sublingual:** Dissolve 1 tablet sublingually as needed for chest pain; may repeat 1 tablet every 5 min if no relief up to 3 tablets (15 min) or dissolve 1 tablet sublingually 5 min before strenuous activity **Translingual spray:** Place 1–2 sprays in mouth as needed for chest pain; may repeat every 5 min if no relief up to 3 doses (15 min) or use 5–10 min before strenuous activity	STORE IN MANUFACTURER'S ORIGINAL CONTAINER—sublingual, capsules. REPLACE VIALS 3–6 MONTHS AFTER OPENING—sublingual. ROTATE SITE OF APPLICATION—transdermal patch. HOLD SPRAY IN MOUTH FOR UP TO 10 S BEFORE SWALLOWING—translingual spray. IF NO RELIEF OF SYMPTOMS AFTER 3 DOSES OF SUBLINGUAL TABS OR LINGUAL SPRAY (OR 15 MIN), CALL 911—all immediate-release dosage forms. SWALLOW WHOLE; DO NOT CRUSH OR CHEW—sustained and extended release.

Late Sodium Channel Blocker

Generic	Brand	Usual Dose	Warning Labels
ranolazine	Ranexa	The initial dose is 500 mg twice a day and maybe increased to 1000 mg twice a day if needed,	AVOID GRAPEFRUIT JUICE

Beta-Adrenergic Blockers

Generic	Brand	Usual Dose	Warning Labels
atenolol	Tenormin	**Angina**: 50 mg/day (may increase to 100–200 mg once daily)	MAY CAUSE DIZZINESS; USE CAUTION WHEN DRIVING OR PERFORMING TASKS REQUIRING ALERTNESS. AVOID ABRUPT DISCONTINUATION. TAKE WITH FOOD—metoprolol (immediate release). SWALLOW WHOLE; DO NOT CRUSH OR CHEW—sustained release.
metoprolol tartrate	Lopressor	**Angina (immediate release):** Start with 50 mg twice daily increasing to 100–400 mg/day in 2–3 divided doses	
metoprolol succinate	Toprol XL	**Angina (extended release):** 100–400 mg/day as a single dose	
nadolol	Corgard	**Angina:** Begin at 40–80 mg/day; increase to 240 mg once daily	
propranolol	Generics, Inderal LA	**Angina:** 80–320 mg/day in 2–4 divided doses or 80–320 mg once daily (extended release)	

Calcium Channel Blockers

Generic	Brand	Usual Dose	Warning Labels
amlodipine	Norvasc	**Angina:** 5–10 mg once daily	MAY CAUSE DIZZINESS; USE CAUTION WHEN DRIVING OR PERFORMING TASKS REQUIRING ALERTNESS. AVOID ABRUPT DISCONTINUATION. SWALLOW WHOLE; DO NOT CRUSH OR CHEW—extended and sustained release. TAKE WITH FOOD—nicardipine (sustained release).
diltiazem	Cardizem, Cardizem CD	**Extended release, caps:** 120–180 mg once daily (maximum, 540 mg/day) **Immediate release, tablet:** 30 mg 4 times a day (maximum, 180–360 mg/day)	

Continued

Summary of Drugs Used in the Treatment of Angina—cont'd

	Generic	Brand	Usual Dose	Warning Labels
	nicardipine	Generics,	**Immediate release:** 20–40 mg 3 times a day	
	nifedipine	Procardia, Procardia XL	**Immediate release:** 10–30 mg 3–4 times a day (maximum 180 mg/day) **Sustained release:** 30–60 mg once daily (maximum, 120–180 mg per day)	
	verapamil	Calan, Calan SR, Verelan, Isoptin SR	**Extended-release:** Begin 180 mg orally once daily at bedtime; may increase up to 480 mg once daily. **Immediate release:** Begin 80–120 mg 3 times a day; may increase to 240–480 mg/day	
Calcium Channel Blocker Combinations				
	amlodipine + atorvastatin	Caduet	5–10 mg amlodipine once daily	MAY CAUSE DIZZINESS. AVOID GRAPEFRUIT JUICE.

> **● TECH NOTE!**
>
> Be careful when retrieving Cardizem from the shelf because of the many types of dosage forms available (XR, CD, LA, SR).

> **TECHNICIAN'S CORNER**
>
> 1. What is the major difference between arteriosclerosis and atherosclerosis?
> 2. Both nitroglycerin and sildenafil have vasodilating effects on blood vessels. Why is it so important not to use these drugs at the same time?

Other Drug Classifications

ACE inhibitors, anticoagulants, antiplatelet drugs, glycoprotein IIb/IIIa drugs, and antihyperlipidemics may be administered to patients who have angina, especially when comorbid conditions (simultaneous chronic diseases, e.g., angina plus hypertension and dyslipidemia). Drugs used to treat hypertension and dyslipidemia are discussed in Chapters 18 and 19.

Key Points

- Angina is a symptom of ischemic heart disease.
- The symptoms of angina are described as severe squeezing or pressure-like chest pain; sometimes radiating to the arms, shoulders, neck, or jaw.
- Angina pain is sometimes described as severe heartburn or indigestion.
- People with a history of heart disease, hypertension, and diabetes are at risk for angina; however, lifestyle is a significant risk for the condition.
- Risk factors associated with lifestyle include smoking, overeating, a diet high in cholesterol and salt, excessive alcohol consumption, obesity, lack of exercise, and stress.
- Coronary artery disease causes myocardial ischemia.
- Atherosclerosis is a disease of the coronary arteries that results in the buildup of lipid streaks in arteries.
- Atherosclerosis can block the flow of blood through the artery, producing ischemia and cell death *(necrosis)*.
- There are three types of angina: stable, unstable, and variant.
- In all types of angina, there is an imbalance between blood supplied to the heart muscle and the need for blood and oxygen.
- Symptoms of stable angina are typically brought on by physical exertion, smoking, eating heavy meals, exposure to extreme changes in temperature (hot or cold), and emotional stress.
- Unstable angina may occur at rest without physical exertion and results when an embolus partially or completely occludes an artery.
- Variant angina is also known as vasospastic angina because it is caused by vasospasm of the coronary arteries.
- Variant angina may occur at rest similar to unstable angina.
- Lifestyle changes can reduce the risk, frequency, and severity of symptoms and prevent or slow the progression of angina to myocardial infarction or death.
- Recommended lifestyle changes are to (1) take frequent rest breaks, (2) avoid eating foods high in salt and cholesterol, (3) eat smaller portions, (4) learn techniques to manage stress, and (5) become an advocate for workplace and community-wide changes that facilitate lifestyle change.
- Drugs used in the treatment of angina are administered to increase the blood and oxygen supply to the heart and to decrease the workload of the heart.

- Drug therapy for angina is focused on treatment and prevention of symptoms, treatment and prevention of cardiovascular diseases that often accompany angina.
- The organic nitrates are the oldest class of drugs used to treat acute symptoms of angina. They dilate blood vessels (arteries and veins) and increase the supply of oxygen to the heart.
- Nitrates that are commonly used in the treatment and prevention of angina are nitroglycerin, isosorbide dinitrate, and isosorbide mononitrate.
- Nitroglycerin is formulated for parenteral, oral, sublingual, and topical use.
- Dosage delivery systems that are designed to deliver nitroglycerin quickly are used to treat acute symptoms; they include parenteral solution, sublingual tablets, and lingual spray.
- Nitroglycerin in the form of extended release capsules, patches, and ointments delivers medication over an extended period (up to 24 h) to prevent symptoms of angina.
- Isosorbide dinitrate and isosorbide mononitrate are administered for prevention.
- Adverse reactions of nitrates include hypotension, facial flushing, dizziness, headache, nausea and vomiting, weakness, and fatigue.

- To minimize the risk for development of tolerance to nitrates, it is important to have a 10- to 12-hour drug-free period each day.
- A fatal drop in blood pressure can occur when drugs used to treat erectile dysfunction (sildenafil [Viagra], vardenafil [Cialis], and tadalafil [Levitra]) are administered to patients who are taking nitroglycerin.
- The beta blockers are easily identified because their generic name ends in "-lol."
- The beta blockers decrease the heart rate and workload of the heart, thereby reducing the heart's demand for oxygen.
- The beta blockers decrease the frequency and severity of stable (exertional) angina.
- Adverse reactions of the beta blockers are dizziness, fatigue, bradycardia, hypotension, impotence, heart block, and occasionally insomnia.
- Calcium channel blockers classified as dihydropyridines are easily identified because their generic name ends in "-dipine."
- Calcium channel blockers are used in treatment of variant and stable angina.
- Calcium channel blockers reduce vasospasms and improve exercise tolerance by decreasing the workload of the heart and improving blood flow.

Review Questions

1. Thickening and loss of elasticity of arterial walls that is sometimes called "hardening of the arteries" characterizes _____.
   a. atherosclerosis
   b. arteriosclerosis
   c. angiosclerosis
   d. vasosclerosis
2. People with what kind of health history are at risk for angina?
   a. heart disease
   b. hypertension
   c. diabetes
   d. all of the above
3. You receive a prescription for nitroglycerin 0.4 mg SL #30 1 tablet SL PRN chest pain. Refill X3. After consulting the pharmacist, you _____
   a. dispense the prescription as written in a plastic prescription vial
   b. place the tablets in a compliance pack (bubble pack) to improve adherence
   c. dispensed 100 tablets in the manufacturer's original container.
   d. Tell the patient that nitroglycerin is not marketed as a sublingual tablet
4. A common drug ending for beta blockers is
   a. "dipine"
   b. "prolol"
   c. "olol"
   d. "orbide"
5. The organic nitrates are the oldest class of drugs used to treat acute symptoms of angina.
   a. True
   b. False

6. Nitroglycerin is available in all of the dosage forms except?
   a. ointment
   b. transdermal patch
   c. cream
   d. oral spray
7. Stable angina may occur at rest without physical exertion and results when an embolus partially or completely occludes an artery.
   a. True
   b. False
8. Calcium channel blockers are used in treatment of what types of angina?
   a. variant
   b. stable
   c. unstable
   d. a and b
9. The generic name for Tenormin is _____.
   a. atenolol
   b. nifedipine
   c. nadolol
   d. amlodipine
10. Which drug must be dispensed in the manufacturer's original container?
    a. isosorbide dinitrate
    b. isosorbide mononitrate
    c. sublingual nitroglycerin
    d. diltiazem

Bibliography

Banerjee K, Ghosh RK, Kamatam S, et al: Role of Ranolazine in cardiovascular disease and diabetes: Exploring beyond angina, *Int J Cardiol* 227:556–564, 2017. doi: http://dx.doi.org/10.1016/j.ijcard.2016.10.102.

FDA: Drugs@FDA: FDA Approved Drug Products, nd. Retrieved August 6, 2018, from http://www.accessdata.fda.gov/scripts/cder/daf/.

Health Canada: Drug Product Database, 2018. Retrieved August 6, 2018, from https://health-products.canada.ca/dpd-bdpp/index-eng.jspInstitute for Safe Medication Practices. (2016). FDA and ISMP Lists of Look-Alike Drug Names with Recommended Tall Man Letters.

Kalant H, Grant D, Mitchell J: *Principles of medical pharmacology*, ed 7, Toronto, Ontario, Canada, 2007, Elsevier Canada, A Division of Reed Elsevier Canada, pp 451–453, 458–460.

Kloner RA, Chaitman B: Angina and its management, *J Cardiovasc Pharmacol Ther* 2016. doi:10.1177/1074248416679733.

Lanza GA: Cardiac syndrome X: a critical overview and future perspectives, *Heart* 93:159–166, 2007. Retrieved from: http://heart.bmj.com/content/93/2/159.full.pdf.

National Heart, Lung, and Blood Institute: Angina, Bethesda, MD, 2011, National Heart and Blood Institute, National Institutes of Health, US Department of Health and Human Services. Retrieved from http://www.nhlbi.nih.gov/health/dci/Diseases/Angina/Angina_All.html.

Page C, Curtis M, Sutter M, et al: *Integrated pharmacology*, Philadelphia, 2005, Mosby, pp 377–383.

18

Treatment of Hypertension

LEARNING OBJECTIVES

1. Learn the terminology associated with the treatment of hypertension.
2. List risk factors for development of hypertension.
3. List complications associated with untreated or poorly controlled hypertension.
4. Explain the role of coronary heart disease in the development of hypertension.
5. Identify lifestyle changes that reduce the risk for hypertension.
6. List and categorize medications used to treat hypertension.
7. Describe mechanism of action for each class of drugs used to treat hypertension.
8. List common endings for drug classes used in the treatment of hypertension.
9. Identify significant drug look-alike and sound-alike issues.
10. Identify warning labels and precautionary messages associated with medications used to treat hypertension.

KEY TERMS

Aldosterone Hormone that promotes sodium and fluid reabsorption.

Angiotensin II Potent vasoconstrictor that is produced when the renin–aldosterone–angiotensin system is activated.

Angiotensin-converting enzyme Enzyme that catalyzes the conversion of angiotensin I to angiotensin II.

Cardiac output Volume of blood ejected from the left ventricle in 1 minute.

Diastolic blood pressure Measure of blood pressure when the heart is at rest (diastole).

Diuretic Drug that produces diuresis (urination).

Hyperkalemia Elevated serum potassium levels.

Hypertension High blood pressure. Elevated diastolic blood pressure, systolic blood pressure or both.

Isolated systolic hypertension Elevated systolic blood pressure only. Diastolic blood pressure is within the normal range.

Metabolic syndrome Important risk factor for hypertension that promotes the development of atherosclerosis and cardiovascular disease.

Orthostatic hypotension Sudden drop in blood pressure that occurs when arising from lying down or sitting to standing.

Peripheral vascular resistance Resistance to the flow of blood in peripheral arterial blood vessels that affects blood vessel diameter, vessel length, and blood viscosity.

Renin–aldosterone–angiotensin system System that is activated when there is a drop in renal blood flow. Activation increases blood volume, blood flow to the kidneys, vasoconstriction, and blood pressure.

Systolic blood pressure Measure of the pressure when the heart's ventricles are contracting (systole).

Blood Pressure

Blood pressure is necessary to circulate blood, oxygen (O_2), and nutrients to body organs and to remove carbon dioxide (CO_2) and waste products. Without blood pressure, circulatory collapse, and death would result.

When blood pressure is taken, two pressures are measured. They are the systolic pressure and the diastolic pressure.

$$BP = \frac{Systole}{Diastole}$$

The *systolic blood pressure* (SBP) is a measure of the pressure when the heart's ventricles are contracting (systole). The *diastolic blood pressure* (DBP) is a measure of the heart at rest (diastole).

Average normal blood pressure is $\frac{120 \text{ (systole)}}{80 \text{ (diastole)}}$

Hypertension

Hypertension is the most diagnosed medical condition in the United States, affecting one in three adults. Nearly one in four Canadian adults (23%) 25 years or older have high blood pressure. Blood pressure that exceeds 135 to 140 mm HG/85 to 90 mm Hg, depending on whether or not an automated office blood pressure (BP) was taken, is considered hypertension according to Canadian Hypertension Education Program (CHEP) and Joint National Commission (JNC) 8 guidelines. In 2017, the American College of Cardiologists (ACC) and American Heart Association (AHA) redefined hypertension as

• **BOX 18.1** Hypertension Risk Factors

- Age (men older than 55 years; women older than 65 years)
- Diabetes mellitus
- Family history of heart disease
- Metabolic syndrome
- Obesity
- Tobacco usage
- Decreased physical activity
- Dyslipidemia
- Diet high in salt and saturated fats
- Excessive alcohol consumption

• **BOX 18.2** Select Drugs That Can Increase Blood Pressure

- Nonsteroidal antiinflammatory drugs (cyclooxygenase-2 inhibitors)
- Cocaine, amphetamines
- Decongestants
- Diet pills
- Oral contraceptives
- Glucocorticosteroids (e.g., prednisone, hydrocortisone, methylprednisolone)
- Mineralocorticoids (aldosterone)
- Cyclosporine and tacrolimus
- Erythropoietin
- Licorice
- Herbals (ma huang, ephedra, bitter orange)

130 mm Hg/80 mm Hg. *Isolated systolic hypertension* is a condition where only the SBP is elevated; DBP is within the normal range.

What Causes Hypertension?

In more than 90% of cases, the actual cause for hypertension is unknown, yet some risk factors for chronic elevated high blood pressure are known. *Metabolic syndrome*, a condition characterized by abdominal obesity, high blood pressure, high blood sugar, and hyperlipidemia, is an important risk factor for hypertension because it promotes the development of atherosclerosis and cardiovascular disease. Diabetes and dyslipidemia (abnormal amounts of lipids in blood) are other risk factors for hypertension. Box 18.1 lists additional risk factors for high blood pressure.

Drugs may also induce high blood pressure (Box 18.2).

Blood Pressure Classifications

Elevated Blood Pressure

Elevated blood pressure is defined as SBP ranging between 120 and 129 mm Hg and DBP less than 80 mm Hg. Reduction of blood pressure to normal levels is beneficial for persons with elevated blood pressure with and without preexisting disease. Lifestyle modification is often sufficient; however, drug therapy should be added to the treatment program in people who have diabetes or kidney disease if lifestyle changes do not bring blood pressure down to the normal range.

Gestational Hypertension

Hypertension during pregnancy is dangerous to the pregnant woman and the fetus. Gestational hypertension typically occurs after 20 weeks of pregnancy in susceptible women.

TABLE 18.1 Summary of Blood Pressure Classifications and Target Blood Pressure Goals

	2017 ACC/AHA	2018 CHEP
Normal	<120/<80	<120/<80
Elevated Blood Pressure	120–129/<80	
Hypertension		
Stage 1	130–139/80–89	135/85 AOBP or Out of office BP measurement
Stage 2	≥140/≥90	140/90 Non-AOBP
Isolated Systolic Hypertension	Systolic ≥ 140 Diastolic ≤ 90	Systolic ≥ 140 Diastolic ≤ 90
Diabetes or Chronic Kidney Disease	130/80	130/80

AOBP: Automated Office Blood Pressure (without physician present)

Masked Hypertension

Patients whose blood pressure is elevated in measurements taken outside of the physician office but controlled according to measurements taken in the physician's office have "masked hypertension."

White Coat Hypertension

"White coat hypertension" is the opposite of masked hypertension. People that have white coat hypertension have abnormally high blood pressure when the measurement is taken by a health care professional, but blood pressure measurements taken in a nonclinic setting are within normal range (Table 18.1).

Complications Associated With Untreated or Poorly Controlled Hypertension

Hypertension is sometimes called the "silent killer" because it can cause damage to the body without any obvious symptoms. Hypertension can cause damage to the kidneys, heart, brain, arteries, and eyes. Hypertension can weaken arteries and cause aneurysms that can bleed and cause death if they occur in the brain, aorta, or abdomen. Hypertension can cause blindness when blood vessels to the retina are damaged and scarred. For each 20 mm Hg increase in SBP and 10 mm Hg increase in DBP, there is a twofold increase in risk of death from ischemic heart disease (IHD) and stroke. This is because hypertension can damage arteries and make them stiff and thick.

Nonpharmacological Management of Hypertension

Hypertension poses a serious public health challenge because of the risks for death and long-term disability. It is categorized as a chronic disease of lifestyle because it is associated with obesity, excess dietary sodium intake, physical inactivity, excessive alcohol consumption, and inadequate consumption of fruits and vegetables.

TABLE 18.2 Lifestyle Modifications for Management and Prevention of Hypertension

Modification	Recommendation
Weight loss	Maintain normal body weight Body mass index (18.5–24.9 kg/m²)
Diet	Reduce salt (sodium) intake (≤2 g sodium)[b] Increase potassium rich foods (e.g., bananas) Reduce saturated and total fats Eat five or more servings of fruits and vegetables/day
Physical activity	Engage in 30–60 min of aerobic physical activity 4–7 days per week
Alcohol consumption	Drink no more than 2 alcoholic beverages[a] per day—men (women and lightweight persons, 1 drink/day)
Tobacco usage	Stop smoking cigarettes and cigars

[a]Alcoholic beverage = 24 oz of beer, 10 oz of wine, or 3 oz of whiskey (80 proof).
[b]American Heart Association recommends < 1500 mg/day.
Adapted from: Hypertension Canada's 2018 Guidelines for Diagnosis, Risk Assessment, Prevention, and Treatment of Hypertension in Adults and Children 2018 American College of Cardiology/American Heart Association Task Force on Clinical Practice Guidelines.

More than 122 million Americans are overweight, and fewer than 20% engage in regular physical activity or consume adequate fruits and vegetables (five servings per day).

Lifestyle modification is an important strategy for prevention and management of hypertension and can reduce SBP between 4 and 20 mm Hg. A reduction of as little as 5 mm Hg can lower the risk of death from stroke by 14% and death from coronary heart disease (CHD) by 9%. The US Joint National Committee on the Prevention, Detection, Evaluation, and Treatment of High Blood Pressure recommendations for lifestyle changes are listed in Table 18.2.

> ● **TECH NOTE!**
>
> Natural licorice may aggravate hypertension and interfere with the effects of antihypertensive drugs. It increases sodium and water retention and potassium depletion.

> ● **TECH NOTE!**
>
> Processed foods contain "hidden sodium" and account for nearly 80% of the daily sodium consumed.

Drugs Used in the Treatment of Hypertension

Lifestyle modification is the first step in prevention and management of hypertension in people with normal blood pressure or who have elevated blood pressure; however, most people with hypertension will require drug therapy with one or more drugs and lifestyle modification. Pharmaceutical management of hypertension can be challenging because medications prescribed to reduce blood pressure can sometimes produce more symptoms than the disease, resulting in poor adherence to drug therapy.

Drugs used in the treatment of hypertension work at the sites for blood pressure regulation, which are the kidneys, heart, blood vessels, brain, and sympathetic nerves.

Diuretics

The kidneys play a major role in regulating blood pressure. *Diuretics* exert their effects on the kidneys where they increase the elimination of water, sodium, and selected electrolytes (K^+, Cl^-, HCO_3^-). The diuretics lower blood pressure by decreasing blood volume, peripheral resistance in blood vessels, and *cardiac output*. There are several classifications of diuretics. They are thiazide, loop, and potassium (K^+) sparing. *Aldosterone* antagonists are K^+ sparing and are sometimes classified as diuretics because their site of action is the kidney.

Thiazide Diuretics

Thiazide diuretics are a first-line therapy for hypertension. They promote the elimination of water, sodium, potassium, magnesium, and chloride ions. Fluid loss decreases blood volume, yet this is not the primary mechanism of action for their effectiveness in decreasing blood pressure.

Thiazides act at the distal convoluted tubule, where they block the sodium–chloride cotransporter (Fig. 18.1). This interferes with calcium transport into arterioles, decreasing vasoconstriction. Peripheral resistance is lowered along with blood pressure. Thiazides indirectly stimulate aldosterone secretion, causing potassium excretion.

> ● **TECH NOTE!**
>
> Most thiazide diuretics share the common ending "-thiazide."

> ● **TECH NOTE!**
>
> Patients taking thiazides may be advised to eat potassium-rich foods to replenish potassium depleted by the diuretics.

> ● **TECH NOTE!**
>
> Hydrochlorothiazide is commonly abbreviated HCTZ.

Pharmacokinetics

Thiazide diuretics are readily absorbed orally. They are weak acids and are highly protein bound. Their lipid solubility permits reabsorption along the distal nephron. Their duration of effect varies from as little as 6 hours to as long as 48 hours depending on the drug. Most thiazide diuretics are dosed once a day.

Adverse Reactions and Precautions

Thiazide diuretics can cause dehydration, hyponatremia (sodium loss), and electrolyte deficiency including hypokalemia (potassium loss), hypomagnesemia (magnesium loss), and hypochloremia (chloride loss).

The thiazide diuretics can precipitate a flare-up of gout because they can cause hyperuricemia (excess uric acid). They should be used with caution in patients with diabetes because they may produce hyperglycemia and glucose intolerance. The thiazides have direct and indirect effects on insulin release. Other adverse drug reactions are gastrointestinal upset, impotence, and photosensitivity. Diuretics should be taken in the morning to avoid the need to urinate in the middle of the night.

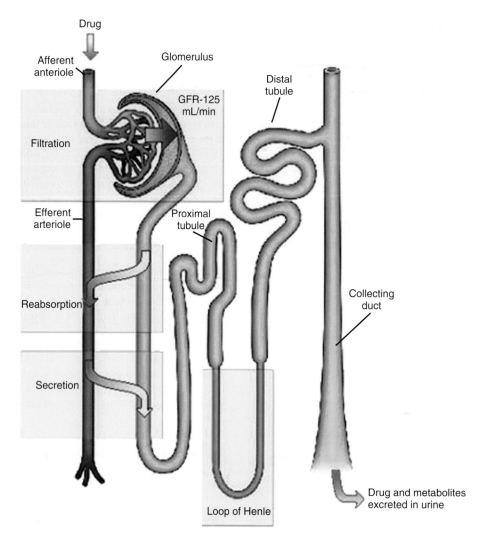

• **Fig. 18.1** Nephron. *GFR*, Glomerular Filtration Rate. (From Patton KT, Thibodeau GA: *The human body in health and disease*, ed 7, St. Louis, 2018, Elsevier.)

❶ TECH ALERT!

The following drugs have look-alike and sound-alike issues: hydroCHLOROthiazide, hydrOXYzine, and hydrALAZINE; metolazone and methimazole.

Loop Diuretics

The loop diuretics are the most potent diuretics. They inhibit the reabsorption of 20% to 30% of sodium load; the thiazides inhibit only 5% to 10%, and the potassium-sparing diuretics inhibit only 1% to 3% of the sodium load. Loop diuretics increase potassium excretion and are often administered with a potassium supplement to reduce the risk of hypokalemia. They also stimulate aldosterone secretion, similar to the thiazides, and increase calcium excretion.

❶ TECH ALERT!

The following drugs have look-alike and sound-alike issues: Lasix and Luvox.

Pharmacokinetics

The loop diuretics are readily absorbed from the gastrointestinal tract. They are up to 98% protein bound. Differences among the loop diuretics are associated with their degree of metabolism in the liver and the extent to which they are eliminated unchanged in the urine. Whereas bumetanide is partially metabolized in the liver, and 50% is excreted unchanged in the urine, torsemide's metabolism in the liver is greater and 20% is excreted unchanged. Torsemide's long half-life permits once-daily dosing.

Adverse Reactions and Precautions

The loop diuretics can cause dehydration, severe hypotension, hypokalemia, hyperuricemia, and photosensitivity. Deafness has occurred when large doses are infused rapidly. Patients taking loop diuretics should take the last dose of the day in early evening to avoid the need to urinate in the middle of the night.

Potassium Supplements

Potassium supplement may be prescribed to reduce the risk for hypokalemia or to treat hyperkalemia.

Thiazide Diuretics

Generic Name	US Brand Name / Canadian Brand(s)	Dosage Forms and Strengths
chlorothiazide[a]	Diuril	**Injection, powder for reconstitution[b]:** 500 mg vial
	Not available	**Suspension, oral** 250 mg/5 mL **Tablets:** 250 mg, 500 mg (generic only)
chlorthalidone[a]	Generics	**Tablets:** 25 mg,[b] 50 mg
	Generics	
hydrochlorothiazide[a]	Microzide	**Capsules (Microzide):** 12.5 mg
	Generics	**Tablets:** 12.5 mg, 25 mg, 50 mg
indapamide[a]	Generics	**Tablets:** 1.25 mg, 2.5 mg
	Lozide	
metolazone[a]	Zaroxolyn	**Tablets, slow acting (Zaroxolyn):** 2.5 mg, 5 mg,[b] 10 mg[b]
	Zaroxolyn	

[a]Generic available.
[b]Available in the United States only.

Loop Diuretics

Generic Name	US Brand Name / Canadian Brand(s)	Dosage Forms and Strengths
bumetanide[a]	Bumex	**Injection, solution[b]:** 0.25 mg/mL
	Burinex	**Tablets:** 0.5 mg,[b] 1 mg, 2 mg,[b] 5 mg[c]
furosemide[a]	Lasix	**Injection, solution:** 10 mg/mL
	Lasix, Lasix Special	**Solution, oral:** 10 mg/mL, 40 mg/5 mL[b] **Tablets:** 20 mg, 40 mg, 80 mg, 500 mg (Lasix Special)[c]
torsemide[a]	Demadex	**Tablets:** 5 mg, 10 mg, 20 mg, 100 mg
	Not available	

[a]Generic available.
[b]Available in the United States only.
[c]Available in Canada only.

Electrolyte Replacement Therapy: Potassium

Generic Name	US Brand Name(s) / Canadian Brand Name(s)	Dosage Forms and Strengths
potassium chloride[a]	Klor Con, Klor Con M10, Klor Con M15, Klor Con M20, Klor-Con Sprinkle, K-Tab	**Capsule (Klor Con, Micro-K)[b]:** 8 mEq, 10 mEq **Tablet, effervescent (K-Lyte):** 25 mEq
	K-Lyte, Slow K	**Tablet, wax matrix (Slow K, K-Tab):** 8 mEq, 10 mEq,[b] 20 mEq[b] **Tablet, microdispersed (Klor Con M)[b]:** 10 mEq, 15 mEq, 20 mEq **Solution, oral:** 20 mEq/15 mL, 40 mEq/15 mL **Solution, for intravenous use (in D₅W):** 20 mEq/mL, 30 mEq, 40 mEq

[a]Generic available.
[b]Available in the United States only.

• BOX 18.3 Management of Hyperkalemia

- Restrict dietary intake of potassium in mild cases.
- Administer a cation exchange resin (e.g., sodium polystyrene sulfonate) to exchange sodium and hydrogen ions for potassium ions in the large intestine and eliminate the potassium resin in feces.
- Dialysis to remove the excess potassium can be instituted to correct severe hyperkalemia.

Potassium-Sparing Diuretics

The potassium-sparing diuretics inhibit sodium reabsorption while avoiding potassium loss. They are less effective than loop and thiazide diuretics. Combining K⁺-sparing diuretics with a thiazide diuretic increases their effectiveness. Examples are amiloride–hydrochlorothiazide and triamterene–hydrochlorothiazide.

Triamterene is readily absorbed in the gastrointestinal tract, and amiloride is 50% absorbed. The duration of effect ranges from 7 to 9 hours (triamterene) and 24 hours (amiloride).

Adverse Reactions and Precautions

Hyperkalemia occurs when serum potassium levels are elevated higher than 5.5 mEq/L. It is the most serious adverse reaction of the potassium-sparing diuretics, and the risk is increased if they are prescribed concurrently with angiotensin-converting enzyme (ACE) inhibitors. They may also cause nausea or vomiting. Hyperkalemia may produce cardiac arrhythmias; and the risk is increased in patients with heart failure that take digoxin. Patients should be advised to avoid salt substitutes because they contain potassium chloride (KCl). Strategies to manage hyperkalemia are list in Box 18.3.

Aldosterone Receptor Antagonists

Aldosterone is a hormone that is released when the kidney perceives a decrease in blood flow and blood pressure. Aldosterone causes sodium and water reabsorption to increase blood pressure.

Spironolactone is an aldosterone antagonist. Spironolactone is sometimes classified as a potassium-sparing diuretic because it conserves potassium. In addition to its use in treating hypertension, spironolactone is used to treat primary aldosteronism, hypokalemia, and heart failure. It can take several weeks to see maximal effect, which differs from loop diuretics, which work immediately.

Spironolactone is about as effective as triamterene and amiloride (sodium reabsorption is approximately 1% to 3%). It is readily absorbed orally and is eliminated in urine. It has a long half-life and is dosed once daily. Eplerenone is a selective aldosterone receptor antagonist (SARA). It is indicated for the treatment of hypertension as monotherapy or used with other antihypertensive drugs. It is also indicated for the treatment of heart failure. Eplerenone increases the excretion of renin and aldosterone.

Adverse Reactions and Precautions

Eplerenone and spironolactone may cause hyperkalemia. Other adverse reactions are nausea, an unpleasant aftertaste, gynecomastia (breast enlargement in males), hirsutism (excessive hair growth in women), impotence, and menstrual irregularities. Potassium containing salt substitutes should be avoided when eplerenone and spironolactone are administered.

Angiotensin-Converting Enzyme Inhibitors

The ACE inhibitors lower blood pressure by blocking the action of *angiotensin-converting enzyme*. ACE converts angiotensin I to its active metabolite angiotensin II. *Angiotensin II* is a potent vasoconstrictor. It stimulates the release of aldosterone and promotes the release of norepinephrine from sympathetic neurons. The ACE inhibitors are first-line therapy for treatment of hypertension in patients with chronic kidney disease (CKD), diabetes, and coronary artery disease, according the CHEP and JNC 8 guidelines.

> **TECH NOTE!**
>
> The ACE inhibitors share the common ending "-pril."

Aldosterone Receptor Antagonists

Generic Name	US Brand Name / Canadian Brand(s)	Dosage Forms and Strengths
eplerenone[a]	Inspra	**Tablets:** 25 mg, 50 mg
	Inspra	
spironolactone[a]	Aldactone, Carospir	**Oral Suspension (Carospir):** 25 mg/mL
	Aldactone	**Tablets:** 25 mg, 50 mg,[b] 100 mg

Combination Aldosterone Receptor Antagonists

Generic Name	US Brand Name / Canadian Brand(s)	Dosage Forms and Strengths
spironolactone + hydrochlorothiazide[a]	Aldactazide	**Tablets:** 25 mg spironolactone + 25 mg HCTZ
	Aldactazide	50 mg spironolactone + 50 mg HCTZ

[a]Generic available.
[b]Available in the United States only.
HCTZ, Hydrochlorothiazide.

⊘ TECH ALERT!

The following drugs have look-alike and sound-alike issues: benazepril and Benadryl; Capoten and Catapres; Accupril and Aciphex.

Mechanism of Action

The ACE inhibitors reduce the level of angiotensin II and aldosterone. They also decrease reabsorption of sodium in the renal tubules. In addition, they cause the accumulation of bradykinins (peptides that produce dilation of arteries). This reduces peripheral resistance, further lowering blood pressure.

Pharmacokinetics

The ACE inhibitors differ in activity, metabolism, and elimination, which may influence which ACE is prescribed. For example, enalapril, perindopril, quinapril, ramipril, and trandolapril are prodrugs. They would not be drugs of first choice for patients with decreased liver function because prodrugs have limited activity until they undergo metabolism. Enalaprilat, perindoprilat, quinaprilat, ramiprilat, and trandolaprilat are their active metabolites. Captopril and lisinopril are already active compounds. Fosinopril is a good choice for patients with decreased kidney function because 50% is eliminated by the kidney and 50% by the liver. All other ACE inhibitors are 90% eliminated by the kidney and can accumulate if kidney disease is present.

▎ TECH NOTE!

The contents of Altace capsules may be sprinkled on food or dissolved in liquid.

Adverse Reactions and Precautions

Dry cough is a characteristic side effect that is caused by the accumulation of bradykinins. Other adverse drug reactions are hyperkalemia, lightheadedness, hypotension, diarrhea, and skin rashes. Angioedema is a rare but potentially lethal allergic reaction that can cause swelling of the throat or airways. The ACE inhibitors are contraindicated in pregnancy because they can interfere with fetal development of the kidneys. Fetal death has been reported. Salt substitutes should be avoided to reduce risks for hyperkalemia.

Angiotensin-Converting Enzyme Inhibitors

	Generic Name	US Brand Name / Canadian Brand(s)	Dosage Forms and Strengths
	benazepril[a]	Lotensin Generics	**Tablets:** 5 mg, 10 mg, 20 mg, 40 mg[b]
	captopril[a]	Generics Generics	**Tablets:** 6.25 mg,[c] 12.5 mg, 25 mg, 50 mg, 100 mg
	enalapril maleate[a]	Epaned, Vasotec Generics	**Injection, solution (as enalaprilat):** 1.25 mg/mL **Solution, oral:** 1 mg/mL **Tablets:** 2.5 mg, 5 mg, 10 mg, 20 mg
	enalapril sodium[a]	Not available Vasotec	**Tablets:** 2 mg, 4 mg, 8 mg, 16 mg
	fosinopril[a]	Generics Generics	**Tablets:** 10 mg, 20 mg, 40 mg[b]
	lisinopril[a]	Prinivil, Qbrelis, Zestril Prinivil, Zestril	**Solution, oral (Qbrelis):** 1 mg/mL **Tablets:** 2.5 mg,[b] 5 mg, 10 mg, 20 mg, 30 mg,[b] 40 mg
	moexipril[a]	Generic Not available	**Tablet, film-coated:** 7.5 mg, 15 mg
	perindopril[a]	Aceon Coversyl	**Tablets:** 2 mg, 4 mg, 8 mg
	quinapril[a]	Accupril Accupril	**Tablets:** 5 mg, 10 mg, 20 mg, 40 mg

Continued

Angiotensin-Converting Enzyme Inhibitors—cont'd

	Generic Name	US Brand Name / Canadian Brand(s)	Dosage Forms and Strengths
	ramipril[a]	Altace Altace	**Capsules:** 1.25 mg, 2.5 mg, 5 mg, 10 mg, 15 mg[c]
	trandolapril[a]	Generics Mavik	**Tablets:** 0.5 mg,[c] 1 mg, 2 mg, 4 mg

Combination Angiotensin-Converting Enzyme Inhibitors and Diuretics

	Generic Name	US Brand Name / Canadian Brand(s)	Dosage Forms and Strengths
	benazepril + hydrochlorothiazide[a]	Lotensin HCT Not available	**Tablets:** benazepril 10 mg + hydrochlorothiazide 12.5 mg benazepril 20 mg + hydrochlorothiazide 12.5 mg benazepril 20 mg + hydrochlorothiazide 25 mg
	captopril + hydrochlorothiazide[a]	Generics Not available	**Tablets:** captopril 25 mg + hydrochlorothiazide 15 mg captopril 25 mg + hydrochlorothiazide 25 mg captopril 50 mg + hydrochlorothiazide 15 mg captopril 50 mg + hydrochlorothiazide 25 mg
	enalapril + hydrochlorothiazide[a]	Vaseretic Vaseretic	**Tablets:** enalapril 5 mg + hydrochlorothiazide 12.5 mg enalapril 10 mg + hydrochlorothiazide 25 mg enalapril 8 mg + hydrochlorothiazide 25 mg[c]
	lisinopril + hydrochlorothiazide[a]	Zestoretic Zestoretic	**Tablets:** lisinopril 10 mg + hydrochlorothiazide 12.5 mg lisinopril 20 mg + hydrochlorothiazide 12.5 mg lisinopril 20 mg + hydrochlorothiazide 25 mg
	moexipril + hydrochlorothiazide[a]	Generics Not available	**Tablets:** moexipril 7.5 mg + hydrochlorothiazide 12.5 mg moexipril 15 mg + hydrochlorothiazide 12.5 mg moexipril 15 mg + hydrochlorothiazide 25 mg
	quinapril + hydrochlorothiazide	Accuretic, Quinaretic Accuretic	**Tablets:** quinapril 10 mg + hydrochlorothiazide 12.5 mg quinapril 20 mg + hydrochlorothiazide 12.5 mg quinapril 20 mg + hydrochlorothiazide 25 mg
	ramipril + hydrochlorothiazide	Not available Altace HCT	**Tablets:** ramipril 2.5 mg + hydrochlorothiazide 12.5 mg ramipril 5 mg + hydrochlorothiazide 12.5 mg ramipril 10 mg + hydrochlorothiazide 12.5 mg ramipril 5 mg + hydrochlorothiazide 25 mg ramipril 10 mg + hydrochlorothiazide 25 mg

Combination Angiotensin-Converting Enzyme Inhibitor and Calcium Channel Blocker

	Generic Name	US Brand Name / Canadian Brand(s)	Dosage Forms and Strengths
	benazepril + amlodipine[a]	Lotrel Not available	**Capsules:** benazepril 10 mg + amlodipine 2.5 mg benazepril 10 mg + amlodipine 5 mg benazepril 20 mg + amlodipine 5 mg benazepril 40 mg + amlodipine 5 mg benazepril 20 mg + amlodipine 10 mg benazepril 40 mg + amlodipine 10 mg
	trandolapril + verapamil[d]	Tarka Tarka	**Tablets, extended release:** trandolapril 1 mg + verapamil 240 mg[b] trandolapril 2 mg + verapamil 180 mg[b] trandolapril 2 mg + verapamil 240 mg trandolapril 4 mg + verapamil 240 mg

[a]Generic available.
[b]Available in the United States only.
[c]Available in Canada only.
[d]Generic available in the United States only.

Angiotensin II Receptor Antagonists

The angiotensin II receptor blockers (ARBs) lower blood pressure by competitively binding at the angiotensin II receptor site. ARBs also reduce ventricular and arterial hypertrophy that is associated with chronic hypertension because the drugs inhibit angiotensin II–stimulated growth of smooth muscle.

The ARBs are similar to ACE inhibitors in effectiveness but produce less dry cough, perhaps because they do not increase bradykinin levels like the ACE inhibitors. The ARBs are first-line therapy for treatment of hypertension, especially in patients with diabetes and coronary artery disease who cannot tolerate ACE inhibitors.

> ### TECH NOTE!
> Angiotensin II antagonists share the common ending "-sartan."

Pharmacokinetics

The plasma half-life of individual ARBs vary. Losartan, one of the first ARBs to be marketed, has a relatively short half-life (only 2 hours), but it has an active metabolite with a plasma half-life of up to 6 to 9 hours. Losartan has an active metabolite that is 10 to 40 times more potent than the parent compound. The duration of action for irbesartan, candesartan, and telmisartan is longer (12 to 18 hours). The drugs are administered as a single daily dose.

Adverse Reactions and Precautions

Common adverse drug reactions associated with the ARBs are fatigue, abdominal pain, dizziness, dry mouth, constipation, impotence, and muscle cramps. The ARBs are contraindicated in the second and third trimesters of pregnancy because they can interfere with fetal development of the kidneys, and fetal death has been reported.

> ### ❶ TECH ALERT!
> The following drugs have look-alike and sound-alike issues: Cozaar, Colace, and Zocor; Diovan, Dioval, Darvon, and Zyban.

Angiotensin II Receptor Antagonists

Generic Name	US Brand Name / Canadian Brand(s)	Dosage Forms and Strengths
azilsartan	Edarbi	**Tablet:** 40 mg, 80 mg
	Edarbi	
candesartan[a]	Atacand	**Tablets:** 4 mg, 8 mg, 16 mg, 32 mg
	Atacand	
eprosartan[b]	Generic only	**Tablets:** 400 mg, 600 mg
	Teveten	
irbesartan[a]	Avapro	**Tablets:** 75 mg, 150 mg, 300 mg
	Avapro	
losartan[a]	Cozaar	**Tablets:** 25 mg, 50 mg, 100 mg
	Cozaar	
olmesartan[a]	Benicar	**Tablets:** 5 mg,[c] 20 mg, 40 mg
	Olmetec	
telmisartan[a]	Micardis	**Tablets:** 20 mg,[c] 40 mg, 80 mg
	Micardis	
valsartan[a]	Diovan	**Tablets:** 40 mg, 80 mg, 160 mg, 320 mg
	Diovan	

Continued

Angiotensin II Receptor Antagonists—cont'd

Generic Name	US Brand Name / Canadian Brand(s)	Dosage Forms and Strengths
Combination Angiotensin II Receptor Antagonists and Diuretics		
azilsartan + chlorthalidone	Edarbyclor / Edarbyclor	**Tablets:** azilsartan 40 mg + chlorthalidone 12.5 mg azilsartan 40 mg + chlorthalidone 25 mg
candesartan + hydrochlorothiazide[a]	Atacand HCT / Atacand Plus	**Tablets:** candesartan 16 mg + hydrochlorothiazide 12.5 mg candesartan 32 mg + hydrochlorothiazide 12.5 mg candesartan 32 mg + hydrochlorothiazide 25 mg
eprosartan + hydrochlorothiazide	Not available / Teveten Plus	**Tablets:** eprosartan 600 mg + hydrochlorothiazide 12.5 mg
irbesartan + hydrochlorothiazide[a]	Avalide / Avalide	**Tablets:** irbesartan 150 mg + hydrochlorothiazide 12.5 mg irbesartan 300 mg + hydrochlorothiazide 12.5 mg
losartan + hydrochlorothiazide[a]	Hyzaar / Hyzaar, Hyzaar DS	**Tablets:** losartan 50 mg + hydrochlorothiazide 12.5 mg losartan 100 mg + hydrochlorothiazide 12.5 mg losartan 100 mg + hydrochlorothiazide 25 mg
olmesartan + hydrochlorothiazide[a]	Benicar HCT / Olmetec Plus	**Tablets:** olmesartan 20 mg + hydrochlorothiazide 12.5 mg olmesartan 40 mg + hydrochlorothiazide 12.5 mg olmesartan 40 mg + hydrochlorothiazide 25 mg
telmisartan + hydrochlorothiazide[a]	Micardis HCT / Micardis Plus	**Tablets:** telmisartan 40 mg + hydrochlorothiazide 12.5 mg[c] telmisartan 80 mg + hydrochlorothiazide 12.5 mg telmisartan 80 mg + hydrochlorothiazide 25 mg
valsartan + hydrochlorothiazide[a]	Diovan HCT / Diovan HCT	**Tablets:** valsartan 80 mg + hydrochlorothiazide 12.5 mg valsartan 160 mg + hydrochlorothiazide 12.5 mg valsartan 160 mg + hydrochlorothiazide 25 mg valsartan 320 mg + hydrochlorothiazide 12.5 mg valsartan 320 mg + hydrochlorothiazide 25 mg

[a]Generic available.
[b]Generic available in the United States only.
[c]Available in the United States only.

Beta-Adrenergic Blockers (Beta Blockers)

Beta blockers used in the treatment of hypertension block the effect of norepinephrine and epinephrine on the heart and blood vessels to reduce heart rate and blood pressure.

> ### ▪ TECH NOTE!
> Blockers share the common ending "-olol."

Mechanism of Action

Beta-adrenergic blockers used in the treatment of hypertension may be selective (β_1) or nonselective (β_1, β_2). β_1-Selective agents are first-line therapy for patients who have hypertension and angina or after myocardial infarction.

All beta blockers decrease blood pressure, reduce the heart rate and decrease the force of contractions in the heart which lowers the cardiac output. Chronic use produces vasodilation. This may be caused by decreased renin release. Renin acts to convert the hormone angiotensinogen to angiotensin I, a precursor to angiotensin II, a potent vasoconstrictor.

Adverse Reactions and Precautions

Adverse drug reactions associated with beta-adrenergic blockers are dizziness, lethargy, nausea, palpitations, impotence, bradycardia, hypoglycemia, cardiac rhythm disturbance, congestive heart failure, and depression. They may also produce bronchospasm, although selective β_1-adrenergic blockers are less likely to produce this effect.

Beta blockers should not be discontinued abruptly because this may cause the onset of arrhythmias or angina. Beta-adrenergic blockers should be used with caution in patients with diabetes because they mask the signs of hypoglycemia.

> ### ⚠ TECH ALERT!
> The following drugs have look-alike and sound-alike issues:
> Inderal and Adderall;
> Zebeta, Zetia, and Diabeta;
> metoprolol succinate and metoprolol tartrate;
> Toprol XL and Topimax;
> Carvedilol and captopril.

Beta-Adrenergic Blockers

Generic Name	US Brand Name / Canadian Brand(s)	Dosage Forms and Strengths
Beta Blockers: Nonselective		
nadolol[a]	Corgard	**Tablets:** 20 mg,[b] 40 mg, 80 mg, 160 mg[c]
	Generics	
pindolol[a]	Generics	**Tablets:** 5 mg, 10 mg, 15 mg[c]
	Visken	
propranolol[a]	Hemangeol*, Inderal, Inderal LA, InnoPran XL	**Capsules, extended release (InnoPran XL):**[b] 80 mg, 120 mg **Capsules, sustained release (Inderal LA):** 60 mg, 80 mg, 120 mg, 160 mg **Injection, solution:** 1 mg/mL **Solution, oral:** 20 mg/5 mL **Tablets:** 10 mg, 20 mg, 40 mg, 60 mg,[b] 80 mg
	Inderal LA	
timolol[a]	Generics	**Tablets:** 5 mg, 10 mg, 20 mg
	Generics	
Beta Blockers: β-1 Selective		
acebutolol[a]	Generics	**Capsules:**[b] 200 mg, 400 mg **Tablets:**[c] 100 mg, 200 mg, 400 mg
	Sectral	
atenolol[a]	Tenormin	**Tablets:** 25 mg, 50 mg, 100 mg
	Tenormin	
betaxolol[a]	Generics	**Tablets:** 10 mg, 20 mg
	Not available	
bisoprolol[a]	Generics	**Tablets:** 5 mg, 10 mg
	Generics	
metoprolol[a]	Kapspargo Sprinkle, Lopressor, Toprol XL	**Capsule, extended release (Kapspargo Sprinkle):** 25 mg, 50 mg, 100 mg, 200 mg **Injection, solution (Lopressor):** 1 mg/mL **Tablets, immediate release (Lopressor):** 25 mg, 50 mg, 100 mg **Tablets, extended release (Toprol XL):** 25 mg, 50 mg, 100 mg, 200 mg **Tablets, extended release (Lopressor SR):** 100 mg, 200 mg
	Lopressor, Lopressor SR	
nebivolol	Bystolic	**Tablet:** 2.5 mg, 5 mg, 10 mg, 20 mg
	Bystolic	
Combination Beta Blockers and Diuretics		
atenolol + chlorthalidone	Tenoretic 50, Tenoretic 100	**Tablets:** atenolol 50 mg + chlorthalidone 25 mg, atenolol 100 mg + chlorthalidone 25 mg
	Tenoretic 50/25, Tenoretic 100/25	
bisoprolol + hydrochlorothiazide[a]	Ziac	**Tablets:** bisoprolol 2.5 mg + hydrochlorothiazide 6.25 mg, bisoprolol 5 mg + hydrochlorothiazide 6.25 mg, bisoprolol 10 mg + hydrochlorothiazide 6.25 mg
	Not available	
metoprolol + hydrochlorothiazide[a]	Lopressor HCT	**Tablets:** metoprolol 50 mg + hydrochlorothiazide 25 mg, metoprolol 100 mg + hydrochlorothiazide 25 mg, metoprolol 100 mg + hydrochlorothiazide 50 mg
	Not available	
nadolol + bendroflumethiazide[a]	Corzide	**Tablets:** nadolol 40 mg + bendroflumethiazide 5 mg nadolol 80 mg + bendroflumethiazide 5 mg
	Not available	
pindolol + hydrochlorothiazide	Not available	**Tablets:** pindolol 10 mg + hydrochlorothiazide 25 mg, pindolol 10 mg + hydrochlorothiazide 50 mg
	Viskazide	
propranolol + hydrochlorothiazide[a]	Generics	**Tablets:** propranolol 40 mg + hydrochlorothiazide 25 mg, propranolol 80 mg + hydrochlorothiazide 25 mg
	Not available	

*Used for the treatment of proliferating infantile hemangioma, a condition causing benign vascular tumors.
[a]Generic available.
[b]Available in the United States only.
[c]Available in Canada only.

Combination Beta$_1$- and Alpha$_1$-Blockers

| | Generic Name | US Brand Name | Dosage Forms and Strengths |
		Canadian Brand(s)	
	carvedilol[a]	Coreg, Coreg CR	**Tablets:** 3.125 mg, 6.25 mg, 12.5 mg, 25 mg
		Generics	**Capsules, extended release (Coreg CR):**[b] 10 mg, 20 mg, 40 mg, 80 mg
	labetalol[a]	Trandate	**Injection, solution, and prefilled syringe:** 5 mg/mL
		Trandate	**Tablets:** 100 mg, 200 mg, 300 mg[b]

[a]Generic available.
[b]Strength available in the United States only.

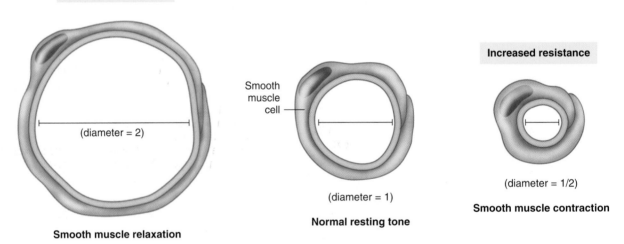

Decreased resistance

(diameter = 2)

Smooth muscle relaxation

Smooth muscle cell

(diameter = 1)

Normal resting tone

Increased resistance

(diameter = 1/2)

Smooth muscle contraction

• **Fig. 18.2** Peripheral vascular resistance. (From Patton KT, Thibodeau GA: *The human body in health and disease*, ed 7, St. Louis, 2018, Elsevier.)

Alpha$_1$-Blockers

The arteries have an abundance of α_1 receptors that mediate vasoconstriction. Administration of alpha$_1$-blockers produces vascular relaxation, which reduces *peripheral vascular resistance* and lowers blood pressure (Fig. 18.2). The α_1-adrenergic antagonists also reduce low-density lipoprotein cholesterol levels, making them useful in the treatment of IHD. The α_1-adrenergic antagonists doxazosin and terazosin have the ability to reduce urethral resistance and increase urine flow, making them effective in the treatment of benign prostatic hyperplasia.

> **❗ TECH ALERT!**
>
> The following drugs have look-alike and sound-alike issues: Cardura and Coumadin.

Alpha$_1$-Blockers

| Generic Name | US Brand Name | Dosage Forms and Strengths |
	Canadian Brand(s)	
doxazosin[a]	Cardura, Cardura XL	**Tablets:** 1 mg, 2 mg, 4 mg, 8 mg[b]
	Cardura-1, Cardura-2, Cardura-4	**Tablets, extended release (Cardura XL):**[b] 4 mg, 8 mg
prazosin[a]	Minipress	**Capsules:** 1 mg, 2 mg, 5 mg
	Generics	
terazosin[a]	Generics	**Capsules:**[b] 1 mg, 2 mg, 5 mg, 10 mg
	Generics	**Tablets:**[c] 1 mg, 2 mg, 5 mg, 10 mg

[a]Generic available.
[b]Available in the United States only.
[c]Available in the Canada only

Adverse Reactions

Adverse drug effects are postural hypotension, dizziness, reflex tachycardia, headache, weakness, and fatigue.

Calcium Channel Blockers

There are two classes of calcium channel blockers. The dihydropyridines are selective for blood vessels and are effective at lowering blood pressure because of their ability to relax blood vessels. Examples of drugs in this class are amlodipine, felodipine, isradipine, nicardipine, nifedipine, and nisoldipine. The phenylalkylamines (e.g., verapamil) and benzothiazepines (e.g., diltiazem) decrease cardiac workload, heart rate, and heart contractions. Verapamil is more selective for the heart muscle (myocardium) than blood vessels. Diltiazem's action is intermediate between verapamil and dihydropyridines.

Adverse Effects

Dihydropyridines (e.g., nifedipine) may produce dizziness, flushing, and headache. Phenylalkylamines and benzothiazepines (e.g., diltiazem) can produce bradycardia and constipation. The exact mechanism of action, pharmacokinetics, and more adverse reactions are discussed in Chapter 17.

> **❶ TECH ALERT!**
> Carvedilol and captopril have look-alike and sound-alike issues.

Calcium Channel Blockers

Generic Name	US Brand Name / Canadian Brand(s)	Dosage Forms and Strengths
amlodipine[a]	Norvasc	**Tablets:** 2.5 mg, 5 mg, 10 mg
	Norvasc	
diltiazem[a]	Cardizem, Cardizem CD, Cardizem LA, Cartia XT, Diltzac, Tiamate, Tiazac, Taztia XT	**Capsules, extended release (Cardizem CD, Cartia XT, Diltzac, Taztia XT):** 120 mg, 180 mg, 240 mg, 300 mg, 360 mg, 420 mg[b] (Tiazac only)
		Injection, powder for reconstitution:[b] 100 mg
		Solution for injection: 5 mg/mL
	Cardizem CD, Tiazac, Tiazac XC	**Tablets:** 30 mg, 60 mg, 90 mg, 120 mg
		Tablets, extended release (Cardizem LA, Tiamate, Tiazac XC): 120 mg, 180 mg, 240 mg, 300 mg, 360 mg, 420 mg[b]
felodipine[a]	Generics	**Tablets, extended release:** 2.5 mg, 5 mg, 10 mg
	Plendil	
isradipine[a]	Generics	**Capsules:** 2.5 mg, 5 mg
	Not available	
nicardipine[a]	Generics	**Capsules:** 20 mg, 30 mg
	Not available	**Solution for injection:** 2.5 mg/mL
		Solution for injection, premixed: 0.1 mg/mL in NaCl 0.9%
		0.2 mg/mL in NaCl 0.9%
nifedipine[a]	Afeditab CR, Adalat CC, Procardia, Procardia XL	**Capsules (Procardia):** 5 mg,[c] 10 mg, 20 mg[b]
		Tablets, extended release (Adalat XL): 20 mg, 30 mg, 60 mg
	Adalat XL	**Tablets, extended release (Adalat CC):** 30 mg, 60 mg, 90 mg
nisoldipine[a]	Sular ER	**Tablets, extended release:** 8.5 mg, 17 mg, 20 mg, 25.5 mg, 30 mg, 34 mg, 40 mg
	Not available	
verapamil[a]	Calan SR, Verelan	**Capsules, extended release (Verelan):** 120 mg, 180 mg, 240 mg, 360 mg
	Isoptin SR	**Capsules, extended release (Verelan PM):** 100 mg, 200 mg, 300 mg
		Solution for injection: 2.5 mg/mL
		Tablets: 40 mg,[b] 80 mg, 120 mg, 160 mg
		Tablets, extended release (Calan SR, Isoptin SR): 120 mg, 180 mg, 240 mg

Continued

Calcium Channel Blockers—cont'd

Generic Name	US Brand Name Canadian Brand(s)	Dosage Forms and Strengths
Combination Calcium Channel Blocker and ACE Inhibitors		
amlodipine + benazepril[a]	Lotrel	**Capsules:** amlodipine 2.5 mg + benazepril 10 mg amlodipine 5 mg + benazepril 10 mg amlodipine 5 mg + benazepril 20 mg amlodipine 5 mg + benazepril 40 mg amlodipine 10 mg + benazepril 20 mg amlodipine 10 mg + benazepril 40 mg
	Not available	
amlodipine + perindopril	Prestalia	**Tablets:** amlodipine 2.5 mg + perindopril 3.5 mg amlodipine 5 mg + perindopril 7 mg amlodipine 10 mg + perindopril 14 mg
	Viacoram	
Combination Calcium Channel Blocker and Angiotensin II Receptor Blockers		
amlodipine + olmesartan[a]	Azor	**Tablets:** amlodipine 5 mg + olmesartan 20 mg amlodipine 5 mg + olmesartan 40 mg amlodipine 10 mg + olmesartan 20 mg amlodipine 10 mg + olmesartan 40 mg
	Not available	
amlodipine + olmesartan + hydrochlorothiazide[a]	Tribenzor	**Tablets:** amlodipine 5 mg + olmesartan 20 mg + hydrochlorothiazide 12.5 mg amlodipine 5 mg + olmesartan 40 mg + hydrochlorothiazide 12.5 mg amlodipine 5 mg + olmesartan 20 mg + hydrochlorothiazide 25 mg amlodipine 10 mg + olmesartan 20 mg + hydrochlorothiazide 12.5 mg amlodipine 10 mg + olmesartan 20 mg + hydrochlorothiazide 25 mg
	Not Available	
amlodipine + telmisartan[a]	Twynsta	**Tablets:** amlodipine 5 mg + telmisartan 40 mg[b] amlodipine 5 mg + telmisartan 80 mg amlodipine 10 mg + telmisartan 40 mg amlodipine 10 mg + telmisartan 80 mg
	Twynsta	
amlodipine + valsartan[a]	Exforge	**Tablets:** amlodipine 5 mg + valsartan 160 mg amlodipine 5 mg + valsartan 320 mg amlodipine 10 mg + valsartan 160 mg amlodipine 10 mg + valsartan 320 mg
	Not available	
amlodipine + valsartan + hydrochlorothiazide[a]	Exforge HCT	**Tablets:** amlodipine 5 mg + valsartan 160 mg + HCTZ 12.5 mg amlodipine 5 mg + valsartan 160 mg + HCTZ 25 mg amlodipine 10 mg + valsartan 160 mg + HCTZ 12.5 mg amlodipine 10 mg + valsartan 160 mg + HCTZ 25 mg amlodipine 10 mg + valsartan 320 mg + HCTZ 25 mg
	Not available	
Combination Calcium Channel Blocker + Anticholesterol		
amlodipine + atorvastatin[a]	Caduet	**Tablets:** amlodipine 2.5 mg + atorvastatin 10 mg[b] amlodipine 2.5 mg + atorvastatin 20 mg[b] amlodipine 2.5 mg + atorvastatin 40 mg[b] amlodipine 5 mg + atorvastatin 10 mg amlodipine 5 mg + atorvastatin 20 mg amlodipine 5 mg + atorvastatin 40 mg amlodipine 5 mg + atorvastatin 80 mg amlodipine 10 mg + atorvastatin 10 mg amlodipine 10 mg + atorvastatin 20 mg amlodipine 10 mg + atorvastatin 40 mg amlodipine 10 mg + atorvastatin 80 mg
	Caduet	

[a]Generic available.
[b]Available in the United States only.
[c]Available in Canada only.
ACE, Angiotensin-converting enzyme; HCTZ, hydrochlorothiazide.

Central-Acting α₂-Agonists

Blood pressure is controlled by a complex feedback mechanism. Increased adrenergic stimulation in the brain leads to decreased sympathetic nervous system messages flowing from the central nervous system (CNS). Methyldopa is a prodrug that acts like a false neurotransmitter. It is metabolized to α-methylnorepinephrine, which the body thinks is norepinephrine; however, it is selective in mimicking the autoinhibitory effects of norepinephrine. When methyldopa binds to receptors, efferent sympathetic activity is reduced, blood vessels dilate, and peripheral resistance is decreased. Clonidine inhibits norepinephrine release from the CNS and peripheral sites.

> **⦸ TECH ALERT!**
>
> The following drugs have look-alike and sound-alike issues: clonidine, clonazepam and klonopin; guanfacine and guaifenesin.

Adverse Reactions

Common adverse drug effects of centrally acting α₂-agonists are sedation, dry mouth, *orthostatic hypotension*, impotence, and constipation. Methyldopa can also cause depression, nasal stuffiness, and gastrointestinal upset. Methyldopa may produce galactorrhea, hemolytic anemia, and liver dysfunction.

Direct Vasodilators

Hydralazine and minoxidil decrease peripheral resistance and reduce blood pressure by relaxing vascular smooth muscle. Minoxidil works by activating adenosine triphosphate–sensitive K^+ channels, setting in motion a chain of events that decrease calcium influx (through L-type calcium channels) into vascular smooth muscle. This decreases arterial blood vessel contractions.

Neither hydralazine nor minoxidil are first-line drugs for the treatment of hypertension. Hydralazine is recommended for hypertensive emergencies (parenteral use) and is safe for the treatment of preeclampsia in pregnant women.

> **⦸ TECH ALERT!**
>
> The following drugs have look-alike and sound-alike issues: hydRALAZINE, hydROXYzine, and hydroCHLOROthiazide; Loniten and Lipitor.

Adverse Reactions

The adverse drug reactions for hydralazine and minoxidil include orthostatic hypotension, headache, gastrointestinal upset, sodium and fluid retention, palpitations, and arrhythmia. Hydralazine can cause a lupus-like syndrome, and minoxidil causes facial hair growth. The discovery that minoxidil increases hair growth resulted in the drug being formulated for topical use for the treatment of baldness.

Direct Renin Inhibitors

Aliskiren is the first of a new class of drugs called direct renin inhibitors. It acts to block the conversion of angiotensinogen to angiotensin I, the first step in the *Renin–Aldosterone–Angiotensin System* (RAAS) system cascade (Fig. 18.3). Renin inhibitors block the formation of both angiotensin I and angiotensin II (vasoconstrictor) and aldosterone release by interrupting the RAAS system at the beginning. Aliskiren may be used as monotherapy or in combination with other antihypertensive agents.

α₂-Agonists

Generic Name	US Brand Name Canadian Brand(s)	Dosage Forms and Strengths
clonidine[a]	Catapres, Catapres-TTS, Duraclon, Kapvay Generics	**Injection, epidural solution (Duraclon):**[b] 0.1 mg/mL, 0.5 mg/mL **Patch, transdermal:** 0.1 mg/24 h (Catapres TTS-1) 0.2 mg/24 h (Catapres TTS-2) 0.3 mg/24 h (Catapres TTS-3) **Tablets:** 0.025 mg,[c] 0.1 mg, 0.2 mg, 0.3 mg[b] **Tablet, extended release (Kapvay):**[b] 0.1 mg
guanfacine[d]	Intuniv Intuniv XR	**Tablets:** 1 mg, 2 mg **Tablets, extended release (Intuniv, Intuniv XR):** 1 mg, 2 mg, 3 mg, 4 mg
methyldopa[a]	Generics Generics	**Tablets:** 125 mg,[c] 250 mg, 500 mg
Combination α₂-Agonist and Diuretic		
methyldopa + hydrochlorothiazide[a]	Generics Generics	**Tablets:** methyldopa 250 mg + hydrochlorothiazide 15 mg methyldopa 250 mg + hydrochlorothiazide 25 mg

[a]Generic available.
[b]Available in the United States only.
[c]Available in Canada only.
[d]Generic available in the United States only.

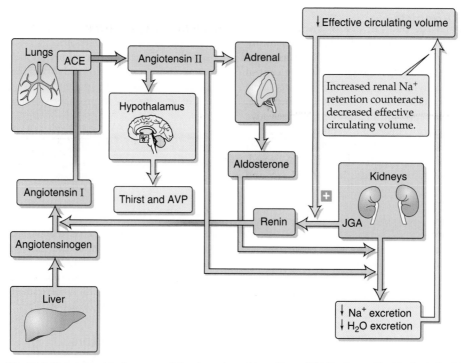

• **Fig. 18.3** The renin–aldosterone–angiotensin system. (From Boron WF, Boulpaep EL: *Medical physiology*, ed 3, Philadelphia, 2017, Elsevier.)

Vasodilators

Generic Name	US Brand Name / Canadian Brand(s)	Dosage Forms and Strengths
hydralazine[a]	Generics / Apresoline	**Injection, solution (Apresoline):** 20 mg/mL (1 mL) **Tablets:** 10 mg, 25 mg, 50 mg, 100 mg[b]
hydralazine + hydrochlorothiazide[a]	Generics / Not available	**Capsule:** hydralazine 25 mg + hydrochlorothiazide 25 mg hydralazine 50 mg + hydrochlorothiazide 50 mg
minoxidil[a]	Generics / Loniten	**Tablets:** 2.5 mg, 10 mg

[a]Generic available.
[b]Available in the United States only.

Renin Inhibitors

Generic Name	US Brand Name / Canadian Brand(s)	Dosage Forms and Strengths
aliskiren	Tekturna / Rasilez	**Tablets:** 150 mg, 300 mg
Combination Renin Inhibitors		
aliskiren + hydrochlorothiazide	Tekturna HCT / Rasilez HCT	**Tablets:** aliskiren 150 mg + hydrochlorothiazide 12.5 mg aliskiren 150 mg + hydrochlorothiazide 25 mg aliskiren 300 mg + hydrochlorothiazide 12.5 mg aliskiren 300 mg + hydrochlorothiazide 25 mg

Adverse Reactions and Precautions

The most common side effect of aliskiren is diarrhea (2.3%). The drug may also cause dizziness, headache, hyperkalemia, aggravate gout, or, in rare cases, cause acute renal failure.

Concurrent use of ACE inhibitors and ARBs with Aliskiren is contraindicated, especially in patients with diabetes. The FDA requires a boxed warning in the package labeling regarding the risk for fetal toxicity when aliskiren is taken during pregnancy.

TECHNICIAN'S CORNER

1. Patients with hypertension are often advised to "cut your salt intake in half" as part of their treatment. How much salt is too much, and what is the daily healthy limit?
2. When a patient has been prescribed antihypertensive medications, can he or she ever be released from taking them?

Summary of Drugs Used in the Treatment and Management of Hypertension

	Drug Name	Usual Dose and Dosing Schedule	Warning Label(s)
Diuretics			
Thiazides			
	chlorothiazide	500–1000 mg 1–2 times a day	TAKE WITH FOOD. MAY BE ADVISABLE TO EAT BANANAS OR DRINK ORANGE JUICE. AVOID PROLONGED EXPOSURE TO SUNLIGHT. SOME OTC DRUGS CAN AGGRAVATE YOUR CONDITION.
	chlorthalidone	12.5–50 mg once daily	
	hydrochlorothiazide (HCTZ)[a]	12.5–50 mg once daily	
	indapamide	1.25–2.5 mg once daily	
	metolazone	2.5–10 mg once daily	
Loop			
	bumetanide	0.5–2 mg once daily (typically 1 mg/day for hypertension)	MAY BE ADVISABLE TO EAT BANANAS OR DRINK ORANGE JUICE. MAY CAUSE DIZZINESS OR LIGHTHEADEDNESS. AVOID PROLONGED EXPOSURE TO SUNLIGHT. SOME OTC DRUGS CAN AGGRAVATE YOUR CONDITION.
	furosemide[a]	20–80 mg daily in 1–2 divided doses	
	torsemide	5–10 mg once daily	
Aldosterone Receptor Antagonists			
	spironolactone[a]	25–100 mg daily in single or divided doses	TAKE WITH FOOD. MAY CAUSE DIZZINESS OR LIGHTHEADEDNESS. AVOID SALT SUBSTITUTES. AVOID GRAPEFRUIT JUICE.
	eplerenone	50 mg 1–2 times daily	
Aldosterone Receptor Antagonist Combination			
	spironolactone + HCTZ	1–4 tablets daily in 1–2 divided doses (25–100 mg spironolactone + 25–100 mg HCTZ once daily)	AVOID SALT SUBSTITUTES AND POTASSIUM-RICH DIETS. MAY CAUSE DIZZINESS OR LIGHTHEADEDNESS. AVOID PROLONGED EXPOSURE TO SUNLIGHT.
Potassium-Sparing Combination			
	amiloride + HCTZ	10 mg amiloride + 100 mg HCTZ once daily	AVOID SALT SUBSTITUTES. MAY CAUSE DIZZINESS OR LIGHTHEADEDNESS. AVOID PROLONGED EXPOSURE TO SUNLIGHT.
	triamterene + HCTZ[a]	37.5–75 mg triamterene + 25–50 mg HCTZ once daily	
Beta Blockers			
	atenolol[a]	25–100 mg daily	DO NOT DISCONTINUE WITHOUT MEDICAL SUPERVISION. MAY CAUSE DIZZINESS OR LIGHTHEADEDNESS. TAKE WITH FOOD—immediate-release metoprolol. SWALLOW WHOLE; DO NOT CRUSH OR CHEW—sustained release.
	acebutolol	200–600 mg twice daily	
	betaxolol	10–20 mg once daily	
	bisoprolol	2.5–10 mg once daily	
	metoprolol[a]	50–100 mg 1–2 times a day	
	metoprolol extended release[a]	25–100 mg once daily	
	nadolol	40–320 mg once daily (Typically 40-80 mg daily)	
	nebivolol[a]	5–40 mg once daily	

Continued

Summary of Drugs Used in the Treatment and Management of Hypertension—cont'd

	Drug Name	Usual Dose and Dosing Schedule	Warning Label(s)
	propranolol[a] propranolol long acting	40–120 mg twice daily (Maximum up to 640 mg daily) 80–180 mg once daily	
	timolol	20–60 mg daily in 2 divided doses	
Combined Alpha and Beta Blockers			
	carvedilol[a] carvedilol CR[a]	6.25–25 mg twice daily 20–80 mg once daily	TAKE WITH FOOD. DO NOT DISCONTINUE WITHOUT MEDICAL SUPERVISION. MAY CAUSE DIZZINESS OR LIGHTHEADEDNESS.
	labetalol	200–400 mg twice daily (Up to 2400 mg/day)	
Beta Blockers + Diuretic Combination			
	atenolol + chlorthalidone	50–100 mg atenolol + 25 mg chlorthalidone once daily	Same warnings for thiazides plus beta blockers.
	bisoprolol + HCTZ	2.5–20 mg bisoprolol + 6.25–12.5 mg HCTZ once daily	
	metoprolol + HCTZ	100–200 mg metoprolol + 25–50 mg HCTZ once daily	
	nadolol + bendroflumethiazide	40–80 mg nadolol + 5 mg bendroflumethiazide once daily	
	pindolol + HCTZ	1–2 tablets once daily	
	propranolol + HCTZ	40–80 mg propranolol + 50 mg HCTZ twice daily	
Angiotensin-Converting Enzyme Inhibitors			
	benazepril[a]	10–40 mg once a day or 2 divided doses	DO NOT DISCONTINUE WITHOUT MEDICAL SUPERVISION. MAY CAUSE DIZZINESS OR LIGHTHEADEDNESS. AVOID SALT SUBSTITUTES. DO NOT TAKE THIS DRUG IF YOU BECOME PREGNANT. MAY CAUSE A DRY COUGH; IF IT PERSISTS, REPORT IT TO YOUR DOCTOR. TAKE ON AN EMPTY STOMACH—captopril, moexipril. TAKE WITH FOOD—perindopril.
	captopril	25–50 mg 2–3 times a day	
	enalapril[a]	5–40 mg daily in single or divided doses	
	fosinopril	10–40 mg once a day or 2 divided doses (Up to 80 mg daily if needed)	
	lisinopril[a]	10–40 mg once a day	
	moexipril	7.5–30 mg once a day or 2 divided doses	

Summary of Drugs Used in the Treatment and Management of Hypertension—cont'd

	Drug Name	Usual Dose and Dosing Schedule	Warning Label(s)
	perindopril	4–8 mg once a day or 2 divided doses (Up to 16 mg daily if needed)	
	quinapril	10–80 mg once a day or 2 divided doses	
	ramipril[a]	2.5–20 mg once a day or 2 divided doses	
	trandolapril	1–4 mg once or twice a day	
Angiotensin-Converting Enzyme Inhibitor + Diuretic Combination			
	benazepril + HCTZ	10–40 mg benazepril + 12.5–50 mg HCTZ once daily	Same warnings for thiazides plus ACE inhibitors.
	captopril + HCTZ	25–50 mg captopril + 15–50 mg HCTZ 2–3 times a day	
	enalapril + HCTZ	10–20 mg enalapril + 12.5–50 mg HCTZ once daily	
	fosinopril + HCTZ	10–20 mg fosinopril + 12.5 mg HCTZ once daily	
	lisinopril + HCTZ[a]	10–80 mg lisinopril + 12.5–50 mg HCTZ once daily	
	moexipril + HCTZ	7.5–30 mg moexipril + 12.5–50 mg HCTZ once daily	
	quinapril + HCTZ	10–40 mg quinapril + 12.5–25 mg HCTZ once daily	
Angiotensin II Antagonists			
	candesartan	16–32 mg once daily or 2 divided doses	DO NOT DISCONTINUE WITHOUT MEDICAL SUPERVISION.
	eprosartan	400–800 mg once daily or 2 divided doses	MAY CAUSE DIZZINESS OR LIGHTHEADEDNESS.
	irbesartan[a]	150–300 mg once daily	DO NOT TAKE THIS DRUG IF YOU BECOME PREGNANT.
	losartan[a]	50–100 mg once daily or 2 divided doses	AVOID SALT SUBSTITUTES.
	olmesartan[a]	20–40 mg once daily	
	telmisartan	20–80 mg once daily	
	valsartan[a]	80–320 mg once daily	

Continued

Summary of Drugs Used in the Treatment and Management of Hypertension—cont'd

Drug Name	Usual Dose and Dosing Schedule	Warning Label(s)
Angiotensin II Antagonist + Diuretic Combination		
candesartan + HCTZ	8–32 mg candesartan + 12.5–50 mg HCTZ once daily or 2 divided doses	Same warnings as for ARBs and thiazide diuretics.
eprosartan + HCTZ	600 mg eprosartan + 12.5 mg HCTZ once daily	
irbesartan + HCTZ	150–300 mg irbesartan + 12.5–25 mg HCTZ once daily	
losartan + HCTZ[a]	50–100 mg losartan + 12.5–25 mg HCTZ once daily	
olmesartan + HCTZ	20–40 mg olmesartan + 12.5–25 mg HCTZ once daily	
telmisartan + HCTZ	80–160 mg telmisartan + 12.5–25 mg HCTZ once daily	
valsartan + HCTZ	160–320 mg valsartan + 12.5–25 mg HCTZ once daily	
Calcium Channel Blockers		
diltiazem extended release[a]	240–360 mg once daily	MAY CAUSE DIZZINESS.
diltiazem long acting	120–540 mg once a day	USE CAUTION WHEN DRIVING OR PERFORMING TASKS REQUIRING ALERTNESS.
verapamil immediate release[a]	80 mg 3 times a day	SWALLOW WHOLE; DO NOT CRUSH OR CHEW— sustained release.
verapamil long acting[a]	180–240 mg 1–2 times a day	AVOID GRAPEFRUIT JUICE
verapamil extended release[a]	120–480 mg once daily	TAKE ON AN EMPTY STOMACH—nisoldipine
amlodipine[a]	2.5–10 mg once a day	
felodipine	2.5–10 mg once a day	
isradipine	2.5–10 mg twice a day	
nicardipine sustained release	30–60 mg twice a day	
nicardipine IV	5–15 mg/h IV	
nifedipine long acting[a]	30–60 mg once daily	
nisoldipine	17–34 mg once daily	
Calcium Channel Blockers + Angiotensin-Converting Enzyme Inhibitor Combination		
amlodipine + benazepril[a]	2.5–10 mg amlodipine + 10–40 mg benazepril once daily	Same warnings as CCBs plus ACE inhibitors.
verapamil + trandolapril	1–4 mg trandolapril + 120–480 mg verapamil daily in 1 or 2 divided doses	

Summary of Drugs Used in the Treatment and Management of Hypertension—cont'd

Drug Name	Usual Dose and Dosing Schedule	Warning Label(s)
Centrally Acting α₂-Agonist and Other Central-Acting Drugs		
clonidine[a]	0.1–0.3 mg twice a day	ROTATE SITE OF APPLICATION—patch.
clonidine patch	0.1–0.3 mg once a week	DO NOT DISCONTINUE WITHOUT MEDICAL SUPERVISION.
methyldopa	250–1000 mg 2–3 daily	MAY CAUSE DIZZINESS OR LIGHTHEADEDNESS.
guanfacine[a]	1–2 mg once daily at bedtime	
Central-Acting Drug + Diuretic Combination		
250 mg methyldopa + 15 mg HCTZ	1 tablet 2–3 times daily	Same warnings as α₂-agonist and thiazide diuretics.
250 mg methyldopa + 25 mg HCTZ	1 tablet twice daily	
500 mg methyldopa + 50 mg HCTZ	1 tablet daily	
α1-Antagonists		
doxazosin	1–16 mg once a day	DO NOT DISCONTINUE WITHOUT MEDICAL SUPERVISION.
prazosin	1–20 mg 2–3 times a day (Maximum 40 mg/day)	MAY CAUSE DIZZINESS OR LIGHTHEADEDNESS.
terazosin[a]	1–5 mg 1–2 times a day (Maximum 20 mg/day)	
Direct Vasodilators		
hydralazine[a]	10–50 mg 4 times a day / 20–40 mg IM or IV bolus as needed	DO NOT DISCONTINUE WITHOUT MEDICAL SUPERVISION.
minoxidil	4–40 mg daily in 1–2 doses	TAKE WITH FOOD. MAY CAUSE DIZZINESS OR LIGHTHEADEDNESS.
enalaprilat	1.25–5 mg over 5 minutes every 6 hours IV	FOR HYPERTENSIVE EMERGENCIES.
Renin Inhibitors		
aliskiren	150–300 mg once daily	MAY CAUSE DIZZINESS. AVOID SALT SUBSTITUTES.
aliskiren + HCTZ	1 tablet once daily; begin with 150 mg aliskiren/12.5 mg HCTZ and increase to 300 mg aliskiren/25 mg HCTZ as needed	AVOID PROLONGED EXPOSURE TO SUNLIGHT—Tekturna HCT. MAY CAUSE PERSISTENT COUGH. MAY UPSET STOMACH.

[a]Top 200 Drugs From Kane SP. ClinCalc DrugStats Database, Version 18.0. ClinCalc: http://clincalc.com/DrugStats. Updated February 3, 2018. Accessed July 24, 2018.

ACE, Angiotensin-converting enzyme; *CCBs*, Calcium Channel Blockers; *HCTZ*, hydrochlorothiazide; *IM*, intramuscular; *OTC*, Over-the Counter.

Key Points

- Blood pressure is a ratio of the pressure when the heart's ventricles are contracting (systole) and the pressure measured when the heart is at rest (diastole).
- Normal blood pressure is less than 120 mm Hg (systolic)/less than 80 mm Hg (diastolic).
- Sites for blood pressure control are the kidneys, heart, blood vessels, CNS, and sympathetic nerves.
- The CNS senses changes in blood pressure and signals sympathetic nerves to release neurotransmitters that control heart rate and blood flow through the arteries.

- Risk factors for high blood pressure are age (older than 55 years in men and 65 years in women), diabetes mellitus, family history of heart disease, metabolic syndrome, obesity, tobacco usage, decreased physical activity, increased total low-density lipoprotein or low high-density lipoprotein, diet high in salt and saturated fats, and excessive alcohol consumption.
- Reduction of blood pressure to normal levels is beneficial for persons with elevated blood pressure with and without preexisting disease.

- Isolated systolic hypertension is a condition whereby SBP is elevated and DBP is within the normal range.
- White coat hypertension is an abnormally high blood pressure when the measurement is taken by a health care professional.
- Hypertension is sometimes called the "silent killer" because it can cause damage to the body without any obvious symptoms. Hypertension can weaken arteries and cause aneurysms in the brain, aorta, or abdomen; blindness; kidney disease; and IHD.
- Adoption of a healthy lifestyle can reduce blood pressure in patients with elevated blood pressure.
- Lifestyle modifications to reduce blood pressure include weight loss, a diet low in salt and cholesterol, increased physical activity, and decreased alcohol and tobacco consumption.
- The diuretics are classified as thiazide, loop, and potassium sparing.
- The thiazide diuretics promote water, sodium, potassium, and chloride ion elimination; decrease blood volume; and lower peripheral resistance.
- The loop diuretics block the sodium–potassium cotransporter in the ascending loop of Henle and are the most potent diuretics.
- The diuretics should be taken in the morning to avoid the need to urinate in the middle of the night.
- The effect of the loop diuretics and thiazides is reduced if they are taken concurrently with NSAIDs.
- The potassium-sparing diuretics inhibit sodium reabsorption while avoiding potassium loss. They are less effective than the loop and thiazide diuretics.
- Patients taking potassium-sparing diuretics should be advised to avoid salt substitutes because they contain potassium chloride.

- Spironolactone and eplerenone are aldosterone receptor antagonists. Spironolactone is sometimes classified as a potassium-sparing diuretic.
- The ACE inhibitors decrease blood pressure by blocking the conversion of angiotensin I to angiotensin II, a potent vasoconstrictor.
- Dry cough is a common side effect of the ACE inhibitors.
- The ACE inhibitors are contraindicated in pregnancy because they can interfere with fetal development of the kidneys.
- The ARBs are competitive antagonists at the angiotensin II receptor site.
- The beta-adrenergic blockers (beta blockers) lower blood pressure by decreasing heart rate and peripheral resistance.
- The alpha$_1$-blockers lower blood pressure by producing vascular relaxation, which reduces peripheral resistance.
- The calcium channel blockers are effective at lowering blood pressure because of their ability to relax blood vessels. They also decrease heart rate and force of contractions, lowering the cardiac output.
- Methyldopa is a prodrug that mimics the autoinhibitory effects of norepinephrine.
- Clonidine inhibits norepinephrine release from the CNS and peripheral sites.
- Hydralazine and minoxidil decrease peripheral resistance and reduce blood pressure by relaxing vascular smooth muscle.
- Hydralazine is recommended for hypertensive emergencies (parenteral use) and is safe for use in pregnant women.
- The direct renin inhibitors (e.g., aliskiren) prevent the formation of both angiotensin I and angiotensin II. They have a lower risk for dry cough and angioedema than ACE inhibitors.

Review Questions

1. _____ is the most often diagnosed medical condition in the United States.
   a. Myocardial infarction
   b. Hypertension
   c. Diabetes
   d. Cancer
2. Lifestyle modification is not an important strategy for the prevention and management of hypertension.
   a. True
   b. False
3. The _____ play(s) a major role in regulating blood pressure and is (are) the site of action for diuretics.
   a. liver
   b. brain
   c. heart
   d. kidneys
4. There are several classifications of diuretics. Which of the following is *not* a class of diuretics?
   a. thiazide
   b. loop
   c. sodium sparing
   d. potassium sparing

5. Diuretics should be taken in the _____ to avoid the need to urinate in the middle of the night (nocturia).
   a. evening
   b. morning
   c. afternoon
   d. night
6. Spironolactone blocks the effect of _____.
   a. aldosterone
   b. antidiuretic hormone
   c. epinephrine
   d. norepinephrine
7. A common ending for ACE inhibitors is
   a. -pine
   b. -statin
   c. -pril
   d. -olol
8. Doxazosin and terazosin are examples of what class of drugs?
   a. ACE inhibitors
   b. Beta blocker
   c. Alpha$_1$-blocker
   d. calcium channel blocker

9. Calcium channel blockers are effective at lowering blood pressure because of their ability to constrict blood vessels.
   a. True
   b. False

10. _____ is recommended for hypertensive emergencies (parenteral use) and is safe for use in pregnant women.
   a. Hydralazine
   b. Hydroxyzine
   c. Hydrodiuril
   d. Hydrocodone

Bibliography

Centers for Disease Control and Prevention: High Blood Pressure, 2017. From: https://www.cdc.gov/bloodpressure/index.htm. (Retrieved 17 June 2017).

FDA: Drugs@FDA: FDA Approved Drug Products, nd. From: http://www.accessdata.fda.gov/scripts/cder/daf/. (Retrieved 17 June 2017.)

Grundy SM, Cleeman JI, Daniels SR, et al: Diagnosis and management of the metabolic syndrome: an American Heart Association/National Heart, Lung, and Blood Institute scientific statement. *Cardiol Rev* 13:2005. doi:10.1161/CIRCULATIONAHA.105. American Heart Association. Available at: http://www.circulationaha.org.

Health Canada: Drug Product Database, 2017. From: https://health-products.canada.ca/dpd-bdpp/index-eng.jsp. (Retrieved 17 June 2017).

Institute for Safe Medication Practices: FDA and ISMP Lists of Look-Alike Drug Names with Recommended Tall Man Letters, 2016.

James PA, Oparil S, Carter BL, et al: 2014 evidence-based guideline for the management of high blood pressure in adults report from the panel members appointed to the eighth Joint National Committee (JNC 8), *JAMA* 311(5):507–520, 2014. doi:10.1001/jama.2013.284427.

Kalant H, Grant D, Mitchell J: *Principles of medical pharmacology*, ed 7, Toronto, 2007, Elsevier Canada, A Division of Reed Elsevier Canada, pp 157–169. 449–464.

Klabunde RE: Cardiovascular Pharmacology Concepts. Calcium Channel Blockers (CCBs), 2015. From: http://www.cvpharmacology.com/vasodilator/CCB.htm. (Retrieved 17 June 2017).

Leung AA, Nerenberg K, Daskalopoulou SS, et al: Hypertension Canada's 2016 Canadian hypertension education program guidelines for blood pressure measurement, diagnosis, assessment of risk, prevention, and treatment of hypertension, *Can J Cardiol* 32:569–588, 2016.

Nerenberg KA, Zarnke KB, Leung AA, et al: Hypertension Canada's 2018 guidelines for diagnosis, risk assessment, prevention, and treatment of hypertension in adults and children, *Can J Cardiol* 34(5):506–525, 2018.

Page C, Curtis M, Sutter M, et al: *Integrated pharmacology*, Philadelphia, 2005, Mosby, pp 395–408.

Whelton PK, Carey RM, Aronow WS, et al: 2017 ACC/AHA/AAPA/ABC/ACPM/AGS/APhA/ASH/ASPC/NMA/PCNA Guideline for the prevention, detection, evaluation, and management of high blood pressure in adults: a report of the American College of Cardiology/American Heart Association Task Force on clinical practice guidelines, *Hypertension* 71(6):e13–e115, 2018. (Retrieved from: http://hyper.ahajournals.org. 17 July 2018).

19

Treatment of Heart Disease and Stroke

LEARNING OBJECTIVES

1. Learn the terminology associated with heart failure, myocardial infarction, and stroke.
2. List the risk factors for heart failure, myocardial infarction, and stroke.
3. List the symptoms of heart failure, myocardial infarction, and stroke.
4. List and categorize medications used to treat heart failure, myocardial infarction, stroke, and hyperlipidemia.
5. Describe mechanism of action for each class of drugs used to treat heart failure, myocardial infarction, stroke, and hyperlipidemia.
6. Identify warning labels and precautionary messages associated with medications used to treat heart failure, myocardial infarction, stroke, and hyperlipidemia.

KEY TERMS

Anticoagulant Drug that prolongs coagulation time and is used to prevent clot formation.

Antiplatelet drug Drug that prevents accumulation of platelets, thereby blocking an important step in the clot formation process.

Antithrombotic Drug that inhibits clot formation by reducing the coagulation action of the blood protein thrombin.

Atherosclerosis Buildup of lipids and plaque inside artery walls, impeding the flow of blood and oxygen.

Atherothrombosis Formation of a blood clot in an artery.

Automaticity is the spontaneous depolarization (contraction) of heart cells.

Cardioglycosides Class of drugs, most commonly derived from the foxglove plant, that have the ability to alter cardiovascular function. Digitalis is representative of this class of drugs.

Cerebral infarction is also known as a stroke. An infarction is a sudden loss of blood supply to an area that results in cell death

Cholesterol Naturally occurring, waxy substance produced by the liver and found in foods that maintains cell membranes and is needed for vitamin D production. Excess cholesterol can cause atherosclerosis.

Ejection fraction Percentage of blood ejected from the left ventricle with each heartbeat.

Heart failure Clinical syndrome in which the heart is unable to pump blood at a rate necessary to meet the body's metabolic needs.

Hemostasis Process of stopping the flow of blood.

High-density lipoprotein "Good cholesterol"; lipoproteins that transport cholesterol, triglycerides, and other lipids from blood to body tissues.

Hyperlipidemia Excess lipids or fatty substances in the blood.

Ischemia Reduction of blood supplied to tissues that is typically caused by blood vessel obstruction due to atherosclerosis, stenosis, or plaque.

Low-density lipoprotein Compound consisting of a lipid and a protein that carries the majority of the total cholesterol in the blood and deposits the excess along the inside of arterial walls; also known as "bad cholesterol."

Myocardial infarction Sudden loss of blood supply in the heart. Also known as a heart attack.

Natriuretic peptides Hormones that play a role in cardiac homeostasis.

Partial thromboplastin time Test given to determine effectiveness of heparin in reducing antithrombotic activity.

Plaque Fatty cholesterol deposits.

Platelets Structures found in the blood that are involved in the coagulation process.

Positive inotropic effect Increase in the force of myocardial contractions.

Prothrombin time Test given to determine the effectiveness of warfarin in reducing clotting time.

Rhabdomyolysis Breakdown of muscle fibers and release of contents into the circulation.

Thrombolytic Drug used to dissolve blood clots.

Tissue plasminogen activator Naturally occurring thrombolytic substance.

Transient ischemic attack Stroke that typically lasts for a few minutes; also known as a mini-stroke.

Triglycerides Storage form of energy found in fat tissue muscle; metabolize to very-low-density lipoproteins.

Overview

Heart disease is the number one cause of death in the United States and the second leading cause of death in Canada. Coronary heart disease (CHD) is the leading cause of heart attack and is a risk factor for stroke and heart failure.

Heart Failure

Heart failure (HF) is a clinical syndrome in which the heart is unable to pump blood at a rate necessary to meet the body's metabolic needs. Heart failure affects nearly 6 million people in the United States and is responsible for more than 1 million hospital visits and nearly 300,000 deaths annually. The syndrome affects 1% to 2% of the adult population worldwide and is rapidly rising to about 10% of the population older than 70 years old up to age 75 years; the prevalence of heart failure is higher in men, but after age 75 years, the prevalence is higher in women.

Disease, lifestyle, and drugs can contribute to the onset or aggravation of heart failure. Kidney dysfunction, diabetes, metabolic syndrome, ischemic heart disease, hypertension, hypothyroidism, hyperthyroidism, bradyarrhythmia, tachyarrhythmia, pulmonary embolism, HIV/AIDS, and myocardial infarction can contribute to heart failure. Obesity, cocaine abuse, excessive salt, and alcohol consumption as well of lack of physical activity can worsen heart failure. Nonsteroidal antiinflammatory drugs, for example, worsen edema and interfere with the effect of drugs used to treat heart failure (e.g., angiotensin-converting enzyme [ACE] inhibitors). Many other medications associated with causing edema can likewise contribute to the development or exacerbation of heart failure.

Heart Attack

More than 7.6 million Americans have had a heart attack and 356,000 Americans annually experience sudden cardiac arrest. Approximately 1 in 20 people die from heart attacks. Heart attack (*myocardial infarction*) produces symptoms that are similar to those of angina. More than 40,000 Canadians will have a heart attack annually. Prompt treatment is essential to persons experiencing the symptoms listed in Table 19.1. If symptoms persist beyond 15 minutes, emergency assistance (dialing 911) should be sought.

Stroke

Stroke is the third leading cause of death in Canada and the fifth highest cause of death in the United States. Strokes occur when brain cells are deprived of oxygen or are damaged by sudden bleeding into the brain. Approximately 795,000 Americans have a stroke annually; however, stroke is on the decline. Between 2003 and 2013 the number of people that had a stroke annually in the United States declined, moving stroke from the fourth leading cause of death to the fifth cause of death in America. Approximately 50,000 will have a mini-stroke (*transient ischemic attack* [TIA]). Persons who have had one stroke and recover are more likely to have another. All strokes produce similar symptoms. Symptoms (Table 19.2) appear suddenly.

Ischemic strokes are caused by oxygen deprivation. Anoxia (absence of oxygen) occurs when arteries are obstructed, causing brain infarcts. *Thrombotic stroke* is caused by an enlarged thrombus or blood clot. *Embolic stroke* is caused by an embolus (traveling clot) or *plaque* that has been dislodged. Blood clots (thrombi, emboli) are the most common cause of strokes.

Hemorrhagic strokes are caused by bleeding in the brain. It may be the result of an aneurysm, a weakened spot of the artery wall that has stretched or burst, filling the area with blood and causing damage. TIAs are also known as mini-strokes. They typically last only a few minutes and symptoms usually resolve within 1 hour.

Pathophysiology of Heart Failure, Heart Attack, and Stroke

Heart failure may affect the left side of the heart, the right side of the heart, or both sides. Left-sided heart failure reduces the volume of oxygen and nutrient-rich blood pumped from the left ventricle to the rest of the body. The *ejection fraction*, the percentage of blood ejected from the left ventricle with each heartbeat, is reduced. Right-sided heart failure reduces the capacity of the heart to fill with sufficient blood and pump the blood to the lungs to pick up oxygen. Persons with right-sided heart failure may have swelling in the legs and ankles. Fluid accumulation can result in weight gain and increased urination. Persons with right- and left-sided heart failure may experience shortness of breath and feelings of fatigue.

In heart failure, the ejection fraction may be reduced (≤40%) or preserved (≥50%). In HF with reduced ejection fraction (HFrEF), left ventricular contractions are reduced causing a decrease in the

TABLE 19.1	Characteristics of Myocardial Infarction Versus Angina	
Characteristics	Myocardial Infarction	Angina
Timing	Sudden onset Lasts longer than 30 min May occur at rest	Often occurs after exercise Lasts 1–5 min Rest may relieve symptoms
Location	Mid-chest radiating to jaw, neck, arms, and epigastric area	Mid-chest radiating to jaw, neck, arms, and epigastric area
Quality	Severe squeezing or heaviness in chest area	Heaviness, chest tightness, indigestion

Mild

TABLE 19.2	Symptoms of Stroke
Limbs	Numbness or weakness of arms or legs Difficulty walking Loss of balance or coordination
Ears, eyes, nose, and throat	Facial numbness or weakness Impaired speech Impaired vision
Cognitive	Confusion Difficulty understanding speech
Other	Dizziness Severe headache

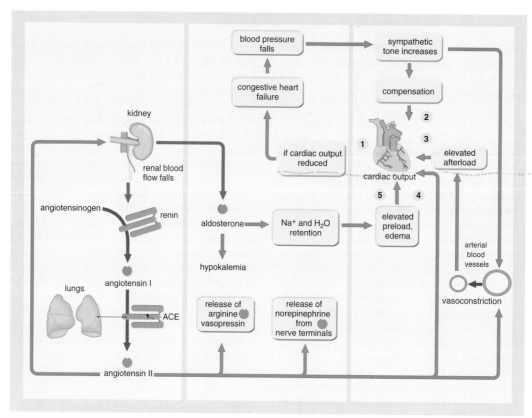

• **Fig. 19.1** Compensatory mechanisms in congestive heart failure. *ACE,* Angiotensin-converting enzyme. (From Page C, Curtis M, Sutter M, et al: *Integrated pharmacology,* ed 3, Philadelphia, 2005, Mosby.)

volume of blood ejected from the ventricles (stroke volume). In heart failure with preserved ejection fraction (HF*p*EF), stroke volume is reduced because the left ventricle is unable to accept a sufficient volume of blood during diastole. Cardiac output is reduced, causing fatigue, dyspnea, and pulmonary hypertension.

Compensatory mechanisms are "switched on" when heart function fails (Fig. 19.1). In an attempt to satisfy the metabolic needs of the body, the renin–aldosterone–angiotensin system (RAAS) is activated. RAAS activation increases blood volume and cardiac output by increasing sodium and fluid retention. The sympathetic nervous system is activated to increase HR, heart contractility and blood vessel relaxation in an effort to increase cardiac output. Unfortunately, while compensatory mechanisms are initially helpful, heart function progressively worsens over time.

Natriuretic peptides are hormones that also play a role in cardiac physiology. Atrial natriuretic peptide (ANP) and brain natriuretic peptide (BNP) are both found in cardiac tissue and are released in response to excessive stretching of heart muscle cells. Atrial stretching causes ANP release. Fluid accumulation and filling pressure in the left ventricle stimulates BNP release. Elevated BNP levels may be used to confirm a diagnosis of heart failure.

Stages of Heart Failure

There are four stages of heart failure. Heart failure may also be described by functional class. American College of Cardiology/American Heart Association (ACC/AHA) descriptions and New York Heart Association (NYHA) functional classifications are compared in Table 19.3.

Stroke and myocardial infarction occur when the blood supply to the brain (stroke) or heart (myocardial infarction) is interrupted. Cells become damaged from *ischemia* (reduction of blood supplied to tissues) or die when they are deprived of oxygen and nutrients. Vascular inflammation is a cause of atherosclerosis. Chronic inflammation of the arteries that supply the heart and brain can also lead to stroke and myocardial infarction. The risk for chronic vascular inflammation increases with age. *Atherosclerosis* (a buildup of lipids and plaque inside of artery walls) can block blood flow through arteries. *Atherothrombosis* (the formation of a blood clot in the artery) can clog arteries and is triggered by atherosclerosis.

Risk Factors for Cardiovascular Disease

Risk factors for stroke and heart attack are categorized as modifiable and nonmodifiable. Nonmodifiable risk factors are age, gender, and family history. In addition, chronic diseases such as hypertension, ischemic heart disease, and diabetes place patients at increased risk for stroke.

Nonmodifiable Risk Factors

Age

Age is a significant risk factor for stroke and myocardial infarction. Although stroke can occur at any age, the risk increases exponentially with each increasing decade. Approximately 66% of strokes occur in persons older than 65 years. Strokes that occur in persons older than 65 years old are more likely to be fatal.

TABLE 19.3 | **Classification[a] and Management of Heart Failure**

ACC/AHA stage A	NYHA class I	• No symptoms
		• High risk for developing heart failure because of:
		  • Hypertension
		  • Coronary artery disease
		  • Diabetes mellitus
		  • History of cardiotoxic drug therapy
		  • Alcohol abuse
		  • History of rheumatic fever
		  • Family history of cardiomyopathy
			• Lifestyle modification
			• Diuretics if patient has fluid retention
			• ACE inhibitors
			• Beta blockers
			• Treatment of underlying disease (diabetes, hypertension, etc.)
			• Antihyperlipidemics
			• Antiarrhythmics

ACC/AHA stage B	NYHA class II	• Structural heart disease but no prior symptoms of heart failure • Prior myocardial infarction • Left ventricular hypertrophy • Asymptomatic valvular disease • Left ventricular dilation or hypocontractility	• All of stage A treatment options, plus • Structural repairs (e.g., heart valve replacement) if needed
ACC/AHA stage C	NYHA class II and III	Current or prior symptoms of heart failure associated with structural heart disease	Treatment of symptoms as per stage A and B recommendations plus digoxin
ACC/AHA stage D	NYHA class IV	Advanced structural heart disease plus heart failure symptoms at rest despite medical therapy	Treatment of symptoms as per stage A and B recommendations plus digoxin

[a]American College of Cardiology/American Heart Association guidelines for evaluation and management and NYHA functional classes.
ACC/AHA, American College of Cardiology/American Heart Association; *ACE*, angiotensin-converting enzyme; *NYHA*, New York Heart Association.

Gender

Gender is an important risk factor for stroke. Men are 1.25 times more likely to have a stroke than are women, yet strokes in men are less likely to be fatal. This is probably because men are often younger than women when they have a stroke. As with stroke, men have a greater risk for heart attack than do women; however, older women are more likely to die within 3 weeks of a heart attack than are men.

Modifiable Risk Factors

Modifiable risk factors for stroke and myocardial infarction are smoking, alcohol consumption, and diet. Smoking promotes atherosclerosis, increases clotting factors in the blood (fibrinogen), stimulates vasoconstriction, and weakens the endothelial wall. These factors contribute to the risk for ischemic stroke and hemorrhagic stroke. Excessive alcohol consumption and binge drinking lead to an increase in blood pressure and can reduce *platelets*, which increase the risk for hemorrhagic stroke. After heavy drinking, a rebound effect occurs that increases platelets and thickens the blood significantly, increasing the risk of ischemic stroke. A diet high in *cholesterol* may increase the risk for atherosclerosis, and a diet high in salt can aggravate hypertension.

Hypertension

Hypertension increases the risk for stroke four to six times above that of persons without hypertension, and 90% of persons who have had a stroke have hypertension.

Atrial Fibrillation

Atrial fibrillation (see Chapter 20), a rapid and irregular beating of the atrium chamber of the heart, can increase the risk for clots. If the clots are dislodged, they can block an artery, leading to stroke or myocardial infarction. Malformations of the heart valves (e.g., mitral valve stenosis) can also lead to clot formation, increasing the risk of stroke or myocardial infarction.

High Cholesterol

High cholesterol levels are a risk factor for stroke and myocardial infarction. Cholesterol may be in the form of *high-density lipoproteins* (HDLs) and *low-density lipoproteins* (LDLs). LDLs can build up within artery walls and harden. This hardened material is called plaque, and it can impede blood supply to the heart and brain. Plaque can become dislodged, interrupting blood supply and causing stroke or myocardial infarction. Diabetes also increases the development of atherosclerosis and therefore is a risk factor for stroke and myocardial infarction.

Infection and Inflammation

Infection is a risk factor for stroke and myocardial infarction. The immune system response to bacterial and viral infections is to release cytokines, leukotrienes, macrophages, and other infection-fighting substances that increase inflammation. Inflammation can increase the risk for ischemic and embolic stroke.

Drugs Used to Treat Heart Disease

Most of the treatments used in heart failure focus on treating symptoms, underlying causes, and factors that worsen heart failure. Many of the same drugs administered in the treatment of hypertension are also used in the treatment of heart failure. They include diuretics, aldosterone antagonists, beta blockers, ACE inhibitors, and angiotensin II receptor blockers (ARBs). These drugs are covered in detail in Chapter 18.

Atherosclerosis and atherothrombosis are important risk factors for stroke and myocardial infarction. Drugs that control the buildup of lipids and plaque and drugs that reduce the formation of blood clots are administered to prevent stroke, myocardial infarction, and acute coronary syndrome.

• BOX 19.1 Lifestyle Modifications Recommended for People With Heart Failure

- Follow a diet low in salt.
- Limit the amount of fluids that you drink.
- Increase physical activity.
- Lose weight if you are overweight.
- Quit smoking if you smoke.
- Limit alcohol consumption.

Cardioglycosides

The *cardioglycosides* are the oldest class of drugs used in the treatment of heart failure. Digitalis is a cardioglycoside derived from the foxglove plant. Digoxin is the only commercially available cardioglycoside in the United States and Canada. Despite its historical use, studies by the Digitalis Investigation Group (DIG) trial show that although digoxin reduces hospitalization and improves exercise tolerance in symptomatic patients with HF*r*EF, it fails to increase survival in patients with heart failure. In fact, digoxin may actually increase mortality in women.

> **• TECH NOTE!**
>
> Lifestyle modification is recommended for people with heart failure to reduce symptoms and complications (see Box 19.1).

Mechanism of Action

Cardioglycosides such as digoxin have a *positive inotropic effect* on the heart; they increase the force of myocardial contractions. The greater force of contractions increases the cardiac output and reduces heart size. As end-diastolic pressures decrease, pulmonary and systemic venous pressures are reduced.

The positive inotropic effect is produced by the inhibition of the Na^+/K^+ ATPase pump. Digoxin-induced inhibition of the Na^+/Ca^{2+} exchanger leads to increased intracellular calcium, an electrolyte involved in the contraction of cardiac smooth muscle.

Digoxin increases cardiac output and decreases compensatory sympathetic activity, which slows the heart rate. The heart rate is also slowed by stimulation of parasympathetic nervous system activity (increased vagal tone). Digoxin decreases intracellular potassium. Potassium depletion can increase automaticity and can cause arrhythmias. *Automaticity* is the spontaneous depolarization (contraction) of heart cells. Digoxin produces significant effects on the heart's conduction system. It decreases conduction velocity through the atrioventricular (AV) node, prolonging the time between contractions (refractory period). The number of depolarizations is reduced, too. A further description of digoxin's effect on the conduction system is described in Chapter 20.

Pharmacokinetics

Digoxin is marketed in several dosage forms. They are tablets, oral solution, and parenteral solution. Oral absorption is good (60% to 85%), and the bioavailability of orally administered digoxin is between 70% and 85%. The bioavailability of digoxin differs among commercial manufacturers, so attempts should be made to consistently dispense the same manufacturer's product each time. Food can decrease absorption.

The peak effect of digoxin occurs 1.5 to 5 hours after administration, and the half-life of digoxin is approximately 36 hours. Between 30% and 50% is eliminated unchanged by the kidneys, and clearance is reduced in heart failure.

Adverse Reactions

Adverse drug reactions produced by digoxin include diarrhea, constipation, nausea, vomiting, fatigue, weakness, visual disturbances (altered color perception, hazy vision), photophobia, impotence, and gynecomastia. Signs of digitalis toxicity are arrhythmia, dizziness, headache, convulsions, delusions, and coma.

Precautions

Digitalis has a narrow therapeutic index, the dosage range between the therapeutic dose and lethal dose is narrow; therefore patients should watch for signs of digitalis toxicity. According to current AHA/ACC recommendations, digoxin is not recommended for the treatment of HF*r*EF in men or women who also have sinoatrial or AV block.

> **• TECH NOTE!**
>
> DigiFab (digoxin immune Fab) is an antidote for digoxin toxicity.

Diuretics

The diuretics are administered to treat volume overload. They also lower blood pressure and reduce pulmonary edema and swelling in the ankles, legs, and feet (peripheral edema). When diuretics are administered, potassium levels should be monitored, because loop and thiazide diuretics can cause hypokalemia (see Chapter 18). Hypokalemia can increase the effects of digoxin, leading to toxicity. The drug summary table provides doses used for the treatment of heart failure.

Aldosterone Antagonists

Aldosterone is a hormone that promotes Na^+ retention and water accumulation. Spironolactone and eplerenone are aldosterone antagonists. They are administered with other drugs to decrease Na^+ and water levels. Both drugs can increase K^+ levels in the body (hyperkalemia). Excess potassium may produce arrhythmias, so potassium levels should be monitored. Spironolactone is recommended to treat moderate to severe heart failure when the ability to pump blood out of the left ventricle is compromised. Eplerenone is specifically marketed for reducing cardiovascular risk in patients after myocardial infarction.

Beta Blockers

The beta blockers reduce the heart rate, lower peripheral arterial resistance, lower blood pressure, and decrease the workload of the heart. They also reduce left ventricular hypertrophy. Studies show that beta blockers can lower the risk of mortality associated with HF*r*EF type heart failure. Beta blockers block excess sympathetic stimulation induced by heart failure as a result of compensatory mechanisms. The beta blockers drug table in this chapter shows doses used for the treatment of heart failure. Adverse reactions requiring management are fluid retention and worsening HF; fatigue; bradycardia or heart block; and hypotension.

Cardioglycosides

	Generic Name	US Brand Name(s) / Canadian Brand(s)	Dosage Forms and Strengths
	digoxin[a]	Lanoxin, Lanoxin Pediatric / Toloxin	**Elixir/solution, oral:** 0.05 mg/mL **Solution for Injection:** 0.1 mg/mL[c], 0.25 mg/mL **Tablets (Lanoxin):** 0.0625 mg, 0.125 mg, 0.25 mg

Digoxin Antidote

	Generic Name	US Brand Name(s) / Canadian Brand(s)	Dosage Forms and Strengths
	digoxin immune Fab	Not available / DigiFab	**Injection:** 40 mg (Digifab) lyophilized powder for reconstitution

[a]Generic available.
[b]Available in Canada only.
[c]Available in the United States only.

Angiotensin-Converting Enzyme Inhibitors and Angiotensin II Receptor Blockers

The ACE inhibitors are one of the few classes of drugs used in the treatment of HF*r*EF-type heart failure that have been shown to reduce mortality (prolong life). They reduce left ventricular hypertrophy, improve diastolic filling, increase cardiac output, and reduce peripheral vascular resistance. When angiotensin II levels are decreased, sympathetic tone and aldosterone-mediated sodium increase and blood volume expansion are also reduced. The ARBs are also administered for the treatment of heart failure. The ARBs improve exercise tolerance and diastolic filling in patients with HF. In this chapter, dosages for ACE inhibitors used in heart failure are shown.

Vasodilators

Isosorbide dinitrate and hydralazine are used in combination for the treatment of heart failure for their vasodilating effects. This reduces peripheral resistance along with cardiac preload and afterload. Moreover, hydralazine has been shown to indirectly increase the force of myocardial contractions (positive inotropic effect). When combined with nitrates such as isosorbide dinitrate, hydralazine can decrease mortality and effectively reduce cardiac congestion.

Miscellaneous Agents for Treatment of Heart Failure

The two newest agents marketed for the treatment of HF are the angiotensin receptor neprilysin inhibitor sacubitril/valsartan (Entresto) and ivabradine (Corlanor, Lancora), an I*f*-channel blocker. Sacubitril is a prodrug that slows the degradation of natriuretic peptides and bradykinin. Diuresis, natriuresis, and myocardial relaxation and antiremodeling are enhanced. Valsartan, an ARB, inhibits angiotensin II and aldosterone. Hypotension and hyperkalemia are side effects of sacubitril/valsartan. ARBs are described in detail in Chapter 18.

Ivabradine slows the heart rate through inhibition of the I*f* channel in the sinus node. The most common adverse reactions are bradycardia, hypertension, atrial fibrillation.

Miscellaneous Agents for Treatment of Heart Failure

Generic Name	US Brand Name(s) / Canadian Brand(s)	Dosage Forms and Strengths
sacubitril/ valsartan	Entresto / Entresto	**Tablet:** 24 mg sacubitril + 26 mg valsartan; 49 mg sacubitril + 51 mg valsartan; 97 mg sacubitril + 103 mg valsartan
ivabradine	Corlanor / Lancora	**Tablet:** 5 mg; 7.5 mg

Drugs That Control Hemostasis

Clotting is a normal process without which one would bleed to death if an injury occurs (Fig. 19.2); however, clots that form in arteries may dislodge and obstruct the supply of blood and oxygen to the brain or heart. Drugs that control *hemostasis* (the process of stopping the flow of blood) are administered to patients at risk for heart attack or stroke in order to prevent blood clots from forming in an artery. Drugs that control the rate of clot formation and clot dissolution are classified as *antithrombotics*. Antithrombotic drugs include (1) agents that inhibit platelets; (2) *anticoagulants*, which lessen coagulation; and (3) fibrinolytic agents. Fibrinolytics dissolve existing clots.

Antiplatelet Drugs

Antiplatelet drugs produce their effect by interfering with steps in the clot formation process (Fig. 19.3). When an injury occurs, platelets cluster at the site and start to stick to the damaged cell wall (adhesion). The platelets are activated by natural substances in the blood such as thromboxane A2 (TXA_2), thrombin, and collagen. After platelets are activated, a cascade of events occurs that attracts more platelets to the region (aggregation) and causes fibrin to combine with the platelets. This strengthens the clot.

Sequence of Events		Substances Involved
Stage 1 Blood vessel · Red blood cell · Platelet	• Injury occurs to vessel (intrinsic pathway) or tissue (extrinsic pathway) • Vessel constricts • Platelets release platelet factors	*Intrinsic:* Factor XII: Hageman factor, contact factor High–molecular weight kininogen (HMWK) Prekallikrein Kallikrein Factor XI: Plasma thromboplastin antecedent (PTA) Factor IV (Ca^{++}): Calcium Factor IX: Plasma thromboplastin component (PTC), Christmas factor Factor VII: Serum prothrombin conversion accelerator (SPCA) Factor VIII: Antihemophilic globulin (AHG), antihemophilic factor (AHF) Phospholipid *Extrinsic:* Factor III: Thromboplastin, tissue thromboplastin Factor VII: SPCA Tissue factor Ca^{++}
	• Platelet factors attract more platelets • Platelets aggregate around wound • Prothrombin activator formed	Factor III: Thromboplastin, tissue thromboplastin Factor X: Stuart-Prower factor Factor V: Proaccelerin, labile factor Phospholipid Factor IV (Ca^{++}): Calcium Factor II: Prothrombin
Stage 2 Thromboplastin Prothrombin → Thrombin	• Thromboplastin converts prothrombin to thrombin	Factor II: Prothrombin Factor IV (Ca^{++}): Calcium
Stage 3 Thrombin Fibrinogen → Fibrin	• Thrombin converts fibrinogen to fibrin threads	Factor I: Fibrinogen
	• Fibrin threads tangle with platelets and trap red blood cells, forming a clot • Factor XIII stabilizes clot and it begins to retract and harden	Factor XIII: Fibrin-stabilizing factor, fibrinase Factor IV (Ca^{++}): Calcium
Stage 4 Plasminogen → Plasmin	• Plasminogen converts to plasmin	
	• Plasmin breaks the clot into fibrin split products, dissolving it	

• **Fig. 19.2** Clot formation. *TXA₂*, Thromboxane A_2. (From Lilley LL, Harrington S, Snyder JS: *Pharmacology and the nursing process*, ed 5, St Louis, 2007, Mosby.)

Although aspirin is a nonprescription drug, it is effective for the management of post–myocardial infarction and stroke. In addition to its antiplatelet activity, aspirin blocks the enzyme cyclooxygenase (see Chapter 10), reducing plaque formation. Aspirin inhibits prostaglandin synthesis, which decreases TXA_2.

Abciximab, eptifibatide, and tirofiban are glycoprotein IIb/IIIa inhibitors that block the final pathway of platelet aggregation. They are administered parenterally. Ticlopidine interferes with platelet adhesion and aggregation. Ticlopidine also decreases the thickness or viscosity of blood by reducing the concentration of

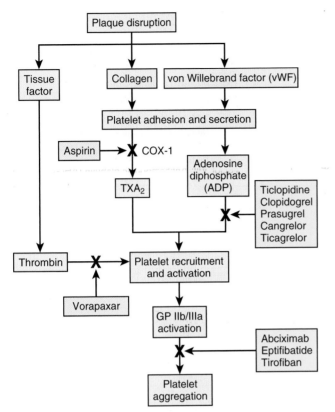

• **Fig. 19.3** Action for antiplatelet drugs. *ADP,* Adenosine diphosphate; *vWF,* von Willebrand factor. (Modified from Lilley LL, Harrington S, Snyder JS: *Pharmacology and the nursing process,* ed 5, St Louis, 2007, Mosby.)

---

fibrinogen. Clopidogrel's mechanism of action is similar to that of ticlopidine. Dipyridamole inhibits platelet aggregation and is a coronary vasodilator.

Pharmacokinetics

Oral absorption of aspirin, clopidogrel, and ticlopidine is good. The bioavailability of ticlopidine is enhanced by administering the drug with food. The peak effect of clopidogrel and ticlopidine is delayed and may take up to 4 days to be reached. The bioavailability of clopidogrel and aspirin is unaffected by food; however, food may decrease the bioavailability of dipyridamole.

A continuous infusion of abciximab must be given to maintain therapeutic blood levels. The effect on platelets lasts longer when abciximab is administered than tirofiban. Tirofiban has an elimination half-life of 2 hours.

Adverse Reactions and Precautions

Bleeding is a common side effect of antiplatelet drugs. Black, tarry stools; blood in vomit, urine, or stools; nosebleeds; and red or purple spots on the skin may indicate bleeding. Many drugs can enhance the effects of antiplatelet drugs and increase the potential for bleeding or hemorrhage. Nonprescription drugs such as nonsteroidal antiinflammatory drugs (NSAIDs, e.g., ibuprofen), vitamin supplements (fish oil), and herbs (feverfew, garlic, ginger) can increase the risk for bleeding.

Other side effects associated with antiplatelet drugs are skin rash or itching, stomach pain, and pain at the injection site (abciximab). Less commonly, patients may experience difficulty breathing, dizziness, weakness, joint pain, and bone marrow toxicity.

⚠ TECH ALERT!

The following drugs have look-alike and sound-alike issues:
Plavix and Paxil;
Ticlid and Tequin.

Anticoagulants

Parenterally Administered Anticoagulants

Heparin is an anticoagulant that is derived from pig intestines or cow lungs. The extraction process results in a mixture of fragments of varied molecular weights. Low-molecular-weight heparins (LMWHs) are produced by separating the heparin fragments.

Heparin and LMWH are administered parenterally to prevent the formation blood clots. Their uses include:

- Treatment of deep venous thrombosis and arterial thromboembolism
- Early treatment and prevention of myocardial infarction
- Prevention of pulmonary embolism
- Prevention of clotting medical devices (e.g., in indwelling catheters, stents, or prosthetic valves)
- Prevention of acute ischemic stroke

Mechanism of Action and Pharmacokinetics

Heparin and LMWH increase the activity of antithrombin III (ATIII). This inhibits clotting factors of the common pathway, Xa and IIa (thrombin), and prevents clot formation (Fig. 19.4). Fondaparinux and tinzaparin also inhibit Xa activity.

To test the effectiveness of heparin and to determine whether dosage adjustments are necessary, an activated *partial thromboplastin time* (aPTT) test is performed. This test measures antithrombic activity. The aPTT is a test of the intrinsic anticoagulation pathway. It tests the time it takes for the blood to clot. If heparin is effective in reducing antithrombotic activity, the clotting time will be prolonged. The test is not performed when LMWH is administered because increases in the aPTT may occur even when antithrombotic activity has not increased. Anti-Xa activity is monitored when tinzaparin or fondaparinux are administered.

Heparin and LMWH are administered by intravenous or subcutaneous injection. Oral absorption is poor. LMWH differs from heparin in a variety of ways. LMWH can be dosed less frequently than heparin, yet they are equally effective. Heparin is dosed two or three times a day, and LMWH is dosed once daily. LMWH has higher bioavailability, increased half-life, fewer side effects (lower risk of thrombocytopenia and osteoporosis), and less protein binding. Higher doses of heparin must be administered because of protein binding.

Adverse Reactions

The most common adverse reaction is bleeding. Heparin and LMWH can cause osteoporosis.

▪ TECH NOTE!

Low-molecular-weight heparins are not substitutable in accordance with product substitution laws. They must be dispensed as written because they differ in manufacturing process, molecular weight, dosage, units, and antithrombotic activity.

Antiplatelet Drugs

	Generic Name	US Brand Name(s)	Dosage Forms and Strengths
		Canadian Brand(s)	
	aspirin[a] (Numerous—see Chapter 10)	Bayer Chewable, Bayer Low Dose, Ecotrin Low Strength, St. Joseph Low Dose	**Tablets:** 81 mg, 325 mg, 500 mg **Tablets, chewable:** 81 mg **Tablets, delayed release:** 81 mg, 325 mg
		Bayer Aspirin 81, Bayer Aspirin 81 Quick Chews	
	clopidogrel[a]	Plavix	**Tablets:** 75 mg, 300 mg
		Plavix	
	dipyridamole[a]	Persantine	**Injection:** 5 mg/mL **Tablets:** 25 mg, 50 mg, 75 mg
		Persantine	
	ticlopidine[a]	Generics	**Tablets:** 250 mg
		Generics	
	vorapaxar	Zontivity	**Tablet:** 2.08 mg
		Zontivity (Approved)	
	dipyridamole + aspirin[ab]	Aggrenox	**Tablets:** 200 mg dipyridamole + 25 mg aspirin
		Aggrenox	

[a]Generic available.
[b]Available in the United States only.
[ab]Generic available in the United States only.

Glycoprotein IIb/IIIa Inhibitors

Generic Name	US Brand Name(s)	Dosage Forms and Strengths
	Canadian Brand(s)	
abciximab	ReoPro	**Solution for injection:** 2 mg/mL
	Not Available	
eptifibatide[ab]	Integrilin	**Solution for injection:** 0.75 mg/mL, 2 mg/mL
	Integrilin	
tirofiban	Aggrastat	**Solution for injection:** 50 µg/mL, 250 µg/mL[b]
	Aggrastat	

[ab]Generic available in the United States only.
[b]Available in the United States only.

Orally Administered Anticoagulants

Warfarin and dabigatran are orally administered anticoagulants. Warfarin is used to prevent pulmonary embolism, thrombotic and embolic stroke, acute myocardial infarction, and atrial fibrillation. Dabigatran is the first oral anticoagulant to become available since the approval of warfarin more than 50 years ago. It is indicated to reduce the risk of stroke and systemic embolism in patients with nonvalvular atrial fibrillation. It is also approved in Canada and Europe to prevent clots in patients that have undergone hip and knee replacement surgeries.

Mechanism of Action and Pharmacokinetics

Dabigatran is an oral direct thrombin inhibitor. Warfarin interferes with the formation of vitamin K–dependent clotting factors. *Prothrombin time* (PT) is a test to determine how well warfarin is working to prevent clotting and to determine whether dosage adjustments are necessary. This test is also called an international normalized ratio (INR) test. The effectiveness of warfarin may be decreased by consumption of foods rich in vitamin K and nutritional supplements with vitamin K. Foods and beverages rich in vitamin K are chickpeas, kale, turnip greens, broccoli, beef and pork liver, parsley, spinach, and green tea.

Warfarin has good oral absorption and bioavailability. The maximum effects of warfarin are not achieved until 4 to 5 days after initiating therapy because warfarin does not block the activity of existing coagulation factors. Stores of existing clotting factors must be depleted before the maximum effect of warfarin on clotting is achieved. Warfarin is highly protein bound, so it interacts with many other drugs. Pharmacy technicians should alert a pharmacist whenever a drug interaction is reported.

TECH NOTE!

Warfarin is the active ingredient in rodent poisons.

Adverse Reactions

The most common adverse reaction is bleeding. Signs of bleeding are bruising; swollen joints, bleeding gums; red spots on the skin or in the eye; nosebleeds; coughing up blood; and heavy menstrual bleeding. In addition to bleeding, dabigatran may cause dyspepsia, gastroesophageal reflux disease, and peptic ulcer.

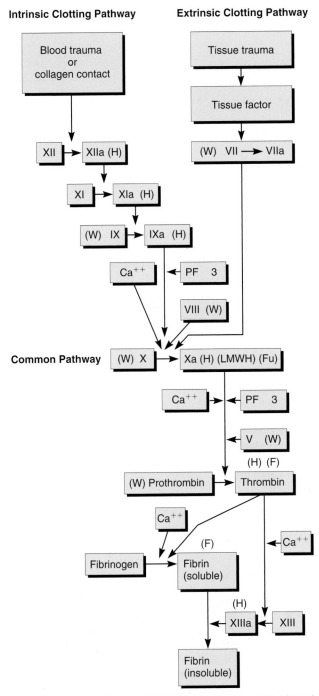

Intrinsic Clotting Pathway

Extrinsic Clotting Pathway

Common Pathway

• Fig. 19.4 Clotting pathways. *LMWHs,* Low-molecular-weight heparins; *PF 3,* platelet factor 3. (From Clayton BD, Willihnganz MJ: *Basic pharmacology for nurses,* ed 17, St Louis, 2017, Elsevier.)

> ❗ **TECH ALERT!**
>
> Warfarin can cause fetal abnormalities, so pharmacy technicians should apply the warning label "AVOID PREGNANCY" to prescription vials.

Precautions

Pharmacy technicians should remind patients taking anticoagulants to seek the advice of a pharmacist before taking prescription and nonprescription drugs. Many drugs interact with anticoagulants, causing serious bleeding or hemorrhage. Anticoagulants should not be combined with antiplatelet drugs, aspirin, NSAIDs, vitamin supplements, and herbs (e.g., feverfew, fish oil supplements, garlic, ginger, ginkgo biloba).

Treating Overdose

Overdose of warfarin or heparin can result in hemorrhage and death. Overdose may be treated by giving a blood transfusion. In some cases, warfarin overdose can be reversed by the administration of vitamin K. Heparin overdose may be treated by the administration of protamine sulfate.

> ▪ **TECH NOTE!**
>
> Warfarin tablets are color coded to reduce medication errors.

> ❗ **TECH ALERT!**
>
> The following drugs have look-alike and sound-alike issues: Coumadin and Cardura.

> ▪ **TECH NOTE!**
>
> Idarucizumab (Praxbind) reverses the effects of dabigatran.

> ❗ **TECH ALERT!**
>
> Argatroban injection must be diluted.

Thrombolytics

Just as the body has a mechanism to form clots at the site of injury to prevent hemorrhage, the body also has a system to stop excessive clot formation, thereby avoiding obstructions to blood flow in blood vessels. *Thrombolytics,* also called fibrinolytics, are drugs that can dissolve blood clots. The drugs are administered in the early stage of stroke to open blood vessels in the brain. They are also used in the treatment of acute myocardial infarction.

Mechanism of Action

Thrombolytic agents currently in use in the United States and Canada are alteplase and tenecteplase. Reteplase is marketed in the United States only. All activate the fibrinolytic system, the body's normal system for preventing excess clotting. Alteplase is a *tissue plasminogen activator* produced by recombinant DNA technology. Tissue plasminogen activator is a naturally occurring thrombolytic substance. Thrombolytics dissolve blood clots that have formed in blood vessels. They increase the activity of plasmin, an enzyme that digests fibrin and other clotting factors. Without fibrin, the structure of the thrombin clot is weakened, and the clot dissolves.

Pharmacokinetics

Thrombolytics work rapidly. They can reopen an obstructed blood vessel within 90 minutes of administration. Alteplase and tenecteplase differ in specificity and half-life. The half-life for alteplase is 30 to 45 minutes; it is 20 to 24 minutes for tenecteplase. All thrombolytics lose shelf life rapidly after reconstitution. They must be stored in the refrigerator and used within 24 hours.

> ▪ **TECH NOTE!**
>
> Thrombolytic agents are very expensive. A single dose can cost more than $1000.

Anticoagulant Drugs

Generic Name	US Brand Name(s) / Canadian Brand(s)	Dosage Forms and Strengths
warfarin[a]	Coumadin, Jantoven / Coumadin	**Tablets:** 1 mg, 2 mg, 2.5 mg, 3 mg, 4 mg, 5 mg, 6 mg, 7.5 mg, 10 mg
dalteparin	Fragmin / Fragmin	**Solution, for injection:** 10,000, 12,500, 25,000 international units/mL **Injection, prefilled syringe:** 2500 units/0.2 mL, 3500 units/0.28 mL, 5000 units/0.2 mL 7500 units/0.3 mL, 10,000 units/0.4 mL[c], 12,500 units/0.5 mL, 15,000 units/0.6 mL, 18,000 units/0.72 mL
enoxaparin[a]	Lovenox, Lovenox Preservative Free / Lovenox, Lovenox HP	**Solution, for injection:** 300 mg/3 mL (100 mg/mL) **Injection, prefilled syringe:** 30 mg/0.3 mL, 40 mg/0.4 mL, 60 mg/0.6 mL, 80 mg/0.8 mL, 100 mg/1 mL, 120 mg/0.8 mL, 150 mg/mL
heparin sodium[a]	Generics / Heparin Leo	**Solution, for irrigation (heparin lock flush):** 100 units/mL **Solution, for injection:** 1000 units/mL, 5000 units/mL, 10,000 units/mL, 20,000 units/mL[b]
tinzaparin	Innohep / Innohep	**Solution, for injection:** 10,000 units/mL,[c] 20,000 units/mL
fondaparinux[a]	Arixtra / Arixtra	**Solution, for injection:** 2.5 mg/0.5 mL, 5 mg/0.4 mL[b], 7.5 mg/0.6 mL, 10 mg/0.8 mL[b]
argatroban[a]	Argatroban / Argatroban	**Solution, for injection:** 100 mg/mL **Solution, for IV infusion[b] (sodium chloride 0.9%):** 1 mg/mL (50 mL, 125 mL)
dabigatran	Pradaxa / Pradaxa	**Capsule:** 75 mg, 110 mg, 150 mg

[a]Generic available.
[b]Available in the United States only.
[c]Available in Canada only.

Adverse Reactions

The thrombolytics must be administered within the first 1 to 3 hours after a stroke occurs. Thereafter the risk of hemorrhage exceeds the benefit of administering clot-dissolving drugs. The risk of intracranial hemorrhage, leading to irreversible damage or death, increases exponentially over time. Thrombolytics can cause bruising and bleeding in the gastrointestinal tract, genitourinary tract, and mouth (gums) in addition to bleeding in the brain. Other adverse reactions are nausea, vomiting, hypotension, transient arrhythmia, allergic reaction, and fever.

> **⊘ TECH ALERT!**
> Activase and Altace have look-alike and sound-alike issues.

Drugs That Treat Hyperlipidemia

Hyperlipidemia is a disorder associated with dysfunctional fat metabolism. While fats are necessary to form steroid hormones, bile, prostaglandins, and cell membranes, excessive buildup in the blood (hyperlipidemia) is a significant risk factor for stroke and myocardial infarction. A principal focus for prevention of cardiovascular disease is treatment of hyperlipidemia. The emphasis is on reducing LDLs and raising HDL levels.

Thrombolytic Agents

Generic Name	US Brand Name(s) / Canadian Brand(s)	Dosage Forms and Strengths
alteplase (t-PA)	Activase, Cathflo Activase / Activase, Cathflo Activase	**Injection, powder for reconstitution (Activase):** 50 mg vial, 100 mg vial; 2 mg vial (Cathflo Activase)
reteplase (r-PA)	Retavase / Not Available	**Injection, powder for reconstitution:** 10 units per vial
tenecteplase	TNKase / TNKase	**Injection, powder for reconstitution:** 50 mg vial

LDL is known as "bad cholesterol" because elevated LDL cholesterol levels promote plaque buildup in arteries, atherothrombosis, and vasoconstriction. All increase the risk of cardiovascular disease and stroke. HDL controls excessive levels of LDL by transporting cholesterol from cells in the artery wall back to the

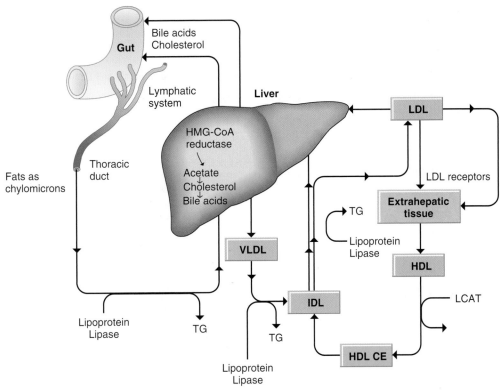

• **Fig. 19.5** Lipid metabolism pathways. *HDL,* High density lipoprotein; *LDL,* low density lipoprotein; *VLDL,* Very low density lipoprotein; *IDL,* intermediate density lipoprotein; *LCAT,* Lecithin–cholesterol acyltransferase; *TG,* triglyceride. (From Lilley LL, Harrington S, Snyder JS: *Pharmacology and the nursing process,* ed 5. St Louis, 2007, Mosby.)

liver for removal. Atherosclerosis is a chronic inflammatory disorder and heart failure is also linked to inflammation. HDL has protective antiinflammatory properties and acts as an antioxidant to diminish LDL oxidation, thereby reducing inflammation and oxidative stress. HDL also has antithrombotic, vasodilatory, and antiinfectious properties, all of which protect against cardiovascular disease.

Recent evidence has shown that increasing HDL ("good cholesterol") in addition to reducing LDL cholesterol can lower the risk for cardiovascular disease even in persons who have normal HDL levels before starting HDL drug therapy. Lipid-lowering drugs interfere with steps in the lipid metabolism pathway (Fig. 19.5). They may affect cholesterol synthesis or elimination in bile or act on LDL metabolism. Although the mechanisms of action may vary, all lipid-lowering drugs reduce LDL and *triglyceride* levels.

Hydroxymethylglutaryl CoA Reductase Inhibitors

Hydroxymethylglutaryl (HMG) CoA reductase inhibitors are also called "statins." Atorvastatin, lovastatin, pravastatin, rosuvastatin, and simvastatin are all HMG CoA reductase inhibitors. HMG CoA reductase is an enzyme that is involved in the final step of cholesterol synthesis.

> **● TECH NOTE!**
>
> All hydroxymethylglutaryl CoA inhibitors have the common ending "-statin."

Mechanism of Action and Pharmacokinetics

Statins increase LDL clearance. They are more effective than other lipid-lowering drugs at lowering LDL (up to 60%). They have been shown to only minimally elevate HDL (up to 16%) above pre-drug levels. Simvastatin and lovastatin are prodrugs and must undergo metabolic changes before they are pharmacologically active.

Adverse Reactions

Common side effects include diarrhea, gas, headache, joint pain, nausea, vomiting, stomach upset or pain, and tiredness. Serious, life-threatening muscle disorders that may be caused by statins are myositis (inflammation of muscle) and *rhabdomyolysis* (breakdown of muscle fibers and release of contents into the circulation). Statins can also elevate liver enzymes, resulting in liver dysfunction.

> **TECHNICIAN'S CORNER**
>
> The following drugs have look-alike and sound-alike issues: Lipitor and Loniten.

Fibric Acid Derivatives

Fibric acid derivatives or fibrates are regarded as broad-spectrum lipid-lowering drugs. Fibrates increase the clearance of very low-density lipoprotein (VLDL). Fibrates are less effective than statins at reducing LDL (≈10%) and in elevating HDL (up to 10% above pretherapy levels).

Mechanism of Action

Fibrates appear to activate the protein Peroxisome proliferator-activated receptor-alpha (PPAR-α). PPAR-α activates the enzyme lipoprotein lipase. Activating these enzymes decreases VLDL cholesterol (which is converted into LDL cholesterol) and triglycerides. Fibrates also increase HDL cholesterol.

Statins (Hydroxymethylglutaryl CoA Inhibitors)

	Generic Name	US Brand Name(s) / Canadian Brand(s)	Dosage Forms and Strengths
	atorvastatin[a]	Lipitor / Lipitor	**Tablets:** 10 mg, 20 mg, 40 mg, 80 mg
	fluvastatin[a]	Lescol XL / Lescol, Lescol XL	**Capsules (Lescol):** 20 mg, 40 mg **Tablets, extended release (Lescol XL):** 80 mg
	lovastatin[a]	Altoprev / Generics	**Tablets:** 10 mg,[b] 20 mg, 40 mg **Tablets, extended release (Altoprev):** 20 mg, 40 mg, 60 mg
	pravastatin[a]	Pravachol / Pravachol	**Tablets:** 10 mg, 20 mg, 40 mg, 80 mg[b]
	rosuvastatin[a,c]	Crestor / Crestor	**Tablets:** 5 mg, 10 mg, 20 mg, 40 mg
	simvastatin[a]	FloLipid Zocor / Zocor	**Solution, oral:** 20 mg/5 mL, 40 mg/5 mL **Tablets:** 5 mg, 10 mg, 20 mg, 40 mg, 80 mg
	pitavastatin	Livalo Zypitamag / Not available	**Tablets:** 1 mg, 2 mg, 4 mg
	ezetimibe + simvastatin[a]	Vytorin / Not available	**Tablets:** 10 mg ezetimibe + 10 mg simvastatin 10 mg ezetimibe + 20 mg simvastatin 10 mg ezetimibe + 40 mg simvastatin 10 mg ezetimibe + 80 mg simvastatin
	atorvastatin + amlodipine[a]	Caduet / Caduet	**Tablets:** atorvastatin 10 mg + amlodipine 2.5 mg[b] atorvastatin 10 mg + amlodipine 5 mg atorvastatin 10 mg + amlodipine 10 mg atorvastatin 20 mg + amlodipine 2.5 mg[b] atorvastatin 20 mg + amlodipine 5 mg atorvastatin 20 mg + amlodipine 10 mg atorvastatin 40 mg + amlodipine 2.5 mg[b] atorvastatin 40 mg + amlodipine 5 mg atorvastatin 40 mg + amlodipine 10 mg atorvastatin 80 mg + amlodipine 5 mg atorvastatin 80 mg + amlodipine 10 mg
	atorvastatin + ezetimibe[b]	Generic / Not available	atorvastatin 10 mg + ezetimibe 10 mg atorvastatin 20 mg + ezetimibe 10 mg atorvastatin 40 mg + ezetimibe 10 mg atorvastatin 80 mg + ezetimibe 10 mg

[a]Generic available.
[b]Available in the United States only.
[c]Available in Canada only.

Precautions

If administered together, statins and fibrates produce a drug interaction that may increase the likelihood of development of myopathies.

Bile Acid Sequestrants

Bile acid sequestrants promote intestinal clearance of cholesterol. They are administered to reduce LDL levels. They are not absorbed and therefore are the drugs of choice for use in pregnancy.

Mechanism of Action

Bile acid sequestrants bind to cholesterol-containing bile acids in the intestine. The bound complex is insoluble and is excreted in the feces. Cholesterol depletion increases LDL receptor activity, which increases removal of LDLs from the blood.

Adverse Effects and Precautions

Bile acid sequestrants produce bloating and gas and must be administered at least 1 hour before or 4 hours after other medications to avoid decreasing the absorption of other drugs. Bile acid sequestrants can lower body levels of fat-soluble vitamins such as vitamins A, D, E, and K. Unfortunately, the resins can increase triglyceride levels.

Nicotinic Acid Derivatives

Niacin is vitamin B_3. It is the most effective lipid-lowering agent for increasing HDL (up to 35%).

Mechanism of Action

The mechanism of niacin's antilipemic action is unknown. It is thought that effects may be linked to decreased VLDL synthesis and clearance in the liver; decreased VLDL triglyceride transport; and actions on free fatty acid release, lipoprotein lipase activity, and triglyceride synthesis. Nicotinic acid elevation of HDL is possibly associated with an increase in serum levels of Apo A-I and lipoprotein A-I, and a decrease in serum levels of Apo-B.

Fibric Acid Derivatives

Generic Name	US Brand Name(s) / Canadian Brand(s)	Dosage Forms and Strengths
gemfibrozil[a]	Lopid	**Tablets:** 300 mg[b], 600 mg
	Generic	
fenofibric acid[a]	Fibricor	**Tablets (Fibricor):** 35 mg, 105 mg
	Not available	**Capsule, Extended Release (Trilipix):** 45 mg, 135 mg
fenofibrate[a]	Antara, Fenoglide, Lipofen, Tricor, Triglide	**Capsules (Lipofen):** 50 mg, 150 mg
	Lipidil EZ, Lipidil Supra	**Capsules (micronized):** 30 mg, 43 mg, 90 mg, 130 mg (Antara); 67 mg, 134 mg, 200 mg
		Tablets: 160 mg (Triglide); 40 mg, 120 mg (Fenoglide); 48 mg, 145 mg (Lipidil EZ, Tricor)
		Tablets, micronized: 100 mg, 160 mg (Lipidil Supra)

[a]Generic available.
[b]Available in Canada only.

Bile Acid Sequestrants

Generic Name	US Brand Name(s) / Canadian Brand(s)	Dosage Forms and Strengths
cholestyramine[a]	Prevalite	**Powder, for reconstitution (regular and sugar free):** 4 g/packet or scoop
	Olestyr	
colesevelam	Welchol	**Tablets:** 625 mg
	Lodalis	**Powder, for suspension:** 1.875 g,[b] 3.75 g
colestipol[a]	Colestid	**Granules, for reconstitution:** 5 g/packet or scoop
	Colestid	**Tablets:** 1 g[c]

[a]Generic available.
[b]Available in the United States only.
[c]Available in Canada only.

Miscellaneous Cholesterol-Lowering Agents

Generic Name	US Brand Name(s) / Canadian Brand(s)	Dosage Forms and Strengths
ezetimibe[a]	Zetia Ezetrol	**Tablets:** 10 mg

[a]Generic available.

Nicotinic Acid

Generic Name	US Brand Name(s) / Canadian Brand(s)	Dosage Forms and Strengths
niacin[a]	Niaspan, Niacor, Slo-Niacin Niaspan, Niaspan FCT	**Tablets:** 500 mg (Niacor, various) **Tablets, time released:** 500 mg, 750 mg, 1000 mg (Niaspan, Niaspan FCT, Slo-Niacin)

[a]Generic available.

Usual Dose and Dosing Schedule for Drugs Used in the Treatment of Cardiovascular Diseases

	Drug Name	Usual Dose and Dosing Schedule	
Cardioglycosides	digoxin	0.125–0.25 mg once daily	TAKE AS DIRECTED; DO NOT SKIP OR EXCEED DOSAGE. IF YOU MISS A DOSE, TAKE IT AS SOON AS YOU REMEMBER UNLESS THE NEXT DOSE IS SCHEDULED TO BE TAKEN IN LESS THAN 12 H.
Digoxin Antidote	DigiFab	Varies according to the amount of digoxin to be neutralized	
If-channel Blocker	ivabradine	2.5–7.5 mg two times a day	AVOID PREGNANCY
Thiazides	chlorothiazide	500–1000 mg 1–2 times a day	See Chapter 18
	chlorthalidone	50–100 mg/day (maximum 200 mg/day)	
	hydrochlorothiazide (HCTZ)	25–100 mg 1–2 times/day	
	indapamide	2.5–5 mg/day	
	metolazone	5–20 mg once daily (maximum 20 mg/day)	

Usual Dose and Dosing Schedule for Drugs Used in the Treatment of Cardiovascular Diseases—cont'd

	Drug Name	Usual Dose and Dosing Schedule	
Loop			
	bumetanide	0.5–2 mg typically as a single dose (maximum 10 mg/day)	See Chapter 18
	furosemide	20–80 mg PO 1–2 times per day (maximum, 600 mg/day PO) 20 to 40 mg IM or slow IV, over 1 to 2 minutes; may repeat same dosage 2 hours later	
	torsemide	10–20 mg PO or IV daily (maximum, 200 mg/day)	
Aldosterone Receptor Antagonists			
	eplerenone	25–50 mg once daily	
	spironolactone	25-50 mg once daily	
Beta Blockers			
	bisoprolol	1.25–10 mg once daily	See Chapter 18
	metoprolol extended release	Begin 12.5 mg/day; increase up to 200 mg/day	
Combined Alpha and Beta Blockers			
	carvedilol	**Immediate release:** Begin 3.125 mg twice daily; increase to 25–50 mg twice daily **Controlled release:** Begin 10 mg/day; increase up to 80 mg/day	See Chapter 18
Angiotensin-Converting Enzyme inhibitors			
	benazepril	2–20 mg once daily	See Chapter 18
	captopril	6.25–50 mg 3 times a day	
	enalapril	2.5–20 mg twice daily	
	fosinopril	5–40 mg once daily	
	lisinopril	2.5–40 mg once daily	
	perindopril	2–16 mg once daily	
	quinapril	5–20 mg twice daily	

Continued

Usual Dose and Dosing Schedule for Drugs Used in the Treatment of Cardiovascular Diseases—cont'd

	Drug Name	Usual Dose and Dosing Schedule	
	ramipril	1.25–10 mg/day in 2 divided doses	
	trandolapril	1–4 mg once daily	

Angiotensin II Antagonists

	Drug Name	Usual Dose and Dosing Schedule	
	candesartan	Begin 4 mg once daily; increase to 32 mg/day	See Chapter 18
	losartan	25–150 mg once daily	
	valsartan	40–160 mg twice daily	
	valsartan + sacubitril (Entresto)	1 tablet twice a day	

Vasodilators (Hydralazine + Isosorbide in Combination)

Drug Name	Usual Dose and Dosing Schedule
hydralazine + isosorbide (BiDil)	1–2 tablets 3 times a day
hydralazine	Initiate at 10–25 mg 3 times a day; maintenance 200 mg/day in 2–4 divided doses (maximum, 300 mg/day) for systolic heart failure
isosorbide dinitrate	5–40 mg 2–3 times/day (maximum 240 mg/day)

Antiplatelet Drugs

	Drug Name	Usual Dose and Dosing Schedule	
	abciximab	0.25 mg/kg bolus followed by 0.125 mcg/kg/min infusion for up to 12 h	REPORT SIGNS OF BLEEDING—all.
	aspirin	81–325 mg once daily	DO NOT SHAKE—abciximab, eptifibatide, tirofiban.
	eptifibatide	180 mcg/kg IV bolus (maximum, 22.6 mg); 2 mcg/kg/min continuous IV infusion (maximum, 15 mg/h)	REFRIGERATE AT 2°C–8°C; DO NOT FREEZE—abciximab, eptifibatide, tirofiban.
	tirofiban	25 mcg/kg/min IV for 5 min followed by 0.15 mcg/kg/min IV	AVOID PREGNANCY—aspirin. PROTECT FROM LIGHT—tirofiban. STORE AT ROOM TEMPERATURE— tirofiban.
	clopidogrel	75 mg once daily	TAKE ON AN EMPTY STOMACH— dipyridamole. TAKE WITH FOOD—aspirin, ticlopidine.
	dipyridamole	75—100 mg 4 times/day	SWALLOW WHOLE; DO NOT CRUSH OR CHEW—aspirin + dipyridamole.
	ticlopidine	250 mg twice daily	
	aspirin + dipyridamole	Take 1 capsule twice daily	

Usual Dose and Dosing Schedule for Drugs Used in the Treatment of Cardiovascular Diseases—cont'd

	Drug Name	Usual Dose and Dosing Schedule	
Anticoagulants			
	dalteparin	120 international units/kg/day subcutaneous every 12 h with aspirin (non-Q-wave myocardial infarction)	REPORT SIGNS OF BLEEDING—all. AVOID OTC WITHOUT MEDICAL SUPERVISION—vitamins, herbals, analgesics (aspirin and NSAIDs)—warfarin, dabigatran. AVOID PREGNANCY—warfarin. SWALLOW WHOLE; DO NOT CRUSH OR CHEW—dabigatran. PROTECT FROM MOISTURE—dabigatran. STORE IN MANUFACTURER'S ORIGINAL PACKAGING—dabigatran.
	enoxaparin	30 mg IV bolus followed by 1 mg/kg SC every 12 h for up to 7 days	
	heparin Na+	60 international units/kg IV bolus with initial dose of thrombolytic therapy; then 12 international units/kg/h IV	
	tinzaparin	175 units/kg (or 0.00875 mL/kg) SC once daily	
	dabigatran	75–150 mg orally twice daily	
	warfarin	Individualized	
Thrombolytics			
	alteplase (t-PA)	Based on weight not to exceed 100 mg total dose	REFRIGERATE RECONSTITUTED SOLUTION (2°C–8°C)—all. DO NOT SHAKE—all. STABLE FOR 8 H AFTER RECONSTITUTION—tenecteplase.
	tenecteplase	Based on weight. Not to exceed 50 mg/dose	
	reteplase (r-PA)	10 units IV bolus over 2 min followed by another 10-unit bolus	
HMG CoA Reductase Inhibitors (Statins)			
	atorvastatin	10–80 mg once daily	AVOID GRAPEFRUIT JUICE—atorvastatin, lovastatin, simvastatin. AVOID PREGNANCY—all. SWALLOW WHOLE; DO NOT CHEW—extended release.
	lovastatin	10–80 mg once daily	
	fluvastatin	20–80 mg once daily	
	pravastatin	40–80 mg once daily	
	rosuvastatin	5–40 mg once daily	
	simvastatin	5–40 mg once daily	

Continued

Usual Dose and Dosing Schedule for Drugs Used in the Treatment of Cardiovascular Diseases—cont'd

	Drug Name	Usual Dose and Dosing Schedule	
	pitavastatin	1–4 mg once daily	
Fibric Acid Derivatives			
	fenofibrate	1 capsule/tablet daily; dose varies according to manufacturer's product e.g., 40–120 mg once a day (Fenoglide®), 50–150 mg daily (Lipofen®), 54–160 mg daily (Tricor®, Triglide)	TAKE ON AN EMPTY STOMACH— gemfibrozil.
	fenofibric acid	45–135 mg once daily (Trilipix); 35–105 mg once daily (Fibricor)	
	gemfibrozil	600 mg twice daily	
Bile Acid Sequestrants			
	cholestyramine	4–24 g daily in 1–2 divided doses	TAKE 1 H BEFORE OR 4 H AFTER OTHER DRUGS.
	colestipol	5–30 g in 1–2 divided doses	RECONSTITUTE WITH 2–6 OZ OF LIQUID; SHAKE WELL—all.
	colesevelam	3.75 g daily in 1–2 doses	SWALLOW WHOLE, TAKE WITH HALF GLASS WATER AND FOOD.
Miscellaneous			
	ezetimibe	10 mg once daily	
	niacin (vit. B$_3$)	0.5–2 g 1–3 times/day 1–2 g once daily	TAKE WITH FOOD—niacin
	ezetimibe + simvastatin	1 tablet once daily in the evening	AVOID GRAPEFRUIT JUICE. TAKE WITH FOOD. AVOID PREGNANCY.

NSAIDs, Nonsteroidal antiinflammatory drugs; *SC*, subcutaneous.

TECHNICIAN'S CORNER

1. Research and make a list of over-the-counter medications that should be avoided by patients taking digoxin and warfarin.
2. Patients with cardiovascular disease are always advised to make lifestyle modifications as part of their treatment. Why is that process so important and so difficult to do?

Key Points

- Heart failure is a clinical syndrome in which the heart is unable to pump blood at a rate necessary to meet the body's metabolic needs.
- Heart failure may affect the left side of the heart, the right side of the heart, or both sides.
- Compensatory mechanisms are "switched on" when the heart function fails. Compensatory mechanisms attempt to satisfy the metabolic needs of the body.
- RAAS activation increases blood volume and cardiac output because RAAS activation produces sodium and fluid retention.
- There are four stages of heart failure: stage A, high risk for developing heart failure; stage B, structural changes without symptoms; stage C, symptomatic; and stage D, advanced structural heart disease plus heart failure symptoms.
- The diuretics are administered in heart failure to reduce edema. Diuretics that produce hypokalemia can increase the effects of digoxin, leading to toxicity.
- Drugs used in the treatment of heart failure include the cardioglycosides, diuretics, aldosterone antagonists, beta blockers, ACE inhibitors, ARBs, and vasodilators.
- Digoxin has a positive inotropic effect on the heart; the result is an increase in the force of myocardial contractions.
- Spironolactone and eplerenone are aldosterone antagonists that can increase potassium levels. Potassium levels should be monitored, because hyperkalemia can produce arrhythmias.
- ACE inhibitors and ARBs may reduce mortality. They reduce left ventricular hypertrophy, improve diastolic filling, increase cardiac output, and reduce peripheral vascular resistance.
- Isosorbide dinitrate and hydralazine are used in combination for the treatment of heart failure to decrease mortality and effectively reduce cardiac congestion.
- Strokes occur when brain cells are deprived of oxygen or are damaged by sudden bleeding into the brain.
- Transient ischemic attacks are also known as mini-strokes and last only a few minutes.
- Myocardial infarction produces symptoms that are similar to those of angina.
- Chronic inflammation of arteries that supply the heart and brain can also lead to stroke and myocardial infarction, because vascular inflammation is a cause of atherosclerosis.
- Atherosclerosis (a buildup of lipids and plaque inside of artery walls) can block blood flow through arteries.
- Atherothrombosis (the formation of a blood clot in the artery) is triggered by atherosclerosis and can also cause clogged arteries.
- The risk for heart failure, stroke, and myocardial infarction is increased by nonmodifiable risk factors, modifiable risk factors, and chronic disease.
- Nonmodifiable risk factors are age, gender, and family history of stroke and myocardial infarction.
- Modifiable risk factors are smoking, heavy alcohol consumption, and diet high in cholesterol.
- Drugs administered to prevent stroke and myocardial infarction control the buildup of lipids and plaque; reducing the formation of blood clots.
- Drugs that control hemostasis (the process of stopping the flow of blood) prevent the formation of clots that can obstruct the supply of blood to the brain and heart.
- Antithrombotic drugs include (1) agents that inhibit platelets; (2) anticoagulants, which attenuate coagulation; and (3) fibrinolytic agents. Fibrinolytics dissolve existing clots.
- Antiplatelet drugs interfere with early steps in the clot formation process.
- Aspirin is a nonprescription drug that has antiplatelet activity.
- Dabigatran is an oral direct thrombin inhibitor indicated to reduce the risk of stroke and systemic embolism in patients with nonvalvular atrial fibrillation.
- Abciximab, eptifibatide, and tirofiban are parenteral antiplatelet drugs. They block the final pathway for platelet aggregation.
- Ticlopidine, clopidogrel, and dipyridamole are orally administered antiplatelet drugs.
- Bleeding is a common side effect of all antiplatelet drugs. Other side effects associated with antiplatelet drugs are skin rash or itching, stomach pain, and pain at the injection site (abciximab).
- Nonprescription drugs, vitamin supplements, and herbs can enhance the effects of antiplatelet drugs. These drugs include NSAIDs (e.g., ibuprofen), feverfew, fish oil supplements, garlic, and ginger.
- Heparin and LMWH are anticoagulants that are administered to prevent the formation of blood clots.
- To test the effectiveness of heparin and to determine whether dosage adjustments are necessary, an aPTT test is performed.
- Warfarin interferes with the formation of vitamin K–dependent clotting factors. PT is a test to determine how well warfarin is working to reduce clotting.
- Warfarin can cause fetal abnormalities, so pharmacy technicians should apply the warning label "AVOID PREGNANCY" to prescription vials.
- Warfarin overdose is reversed by the administration of vitamin K. Heparin overdose is treated with protamine sulfate.
- Thrombolytics, also called fibrinolytics, are drugs that can dissolve blood clots and must be administered within the first few hours of a stroke.
- Statins are HMG CoA reductase inhibitors and block the final step of cholesterol synthesis and promote LDL elimination.
- Bile acid sequestrants promote intestinal clearance of cholesterol.
- Niacin is vitamin B_3. It is effective for increasing HDLs.

Review Questions

1. Drugs that control the rate of clot formation and clot dissolution are classified as _____ and can prevent stroke and myocardial infarction.
   a. antihyperlipidemics
   b. antifibrinolytics
   c. antithrombotics
   d. antihemorrhagics

2. The _____ are the oldest class of drugs used in the treatment of heart failure.
   a. aminoglycosides
   b. cardioglycosides
   c. diuretics
   d. antibiotics

3. Digitalis is a cardioglycoside derived from the foxglove plant.
   a. True
   b. False

4. Statin drugs primarily lower what kind of cholesterol?
   a. LDL
   b. bile
   c. HDL
   d. all of the above

5. _____ is a parenteral antiplatelet drug.
   a. ticlopidine
   b. dipyridamole
   c. abciximab
   d. simvastatin

6. Thiazide diuretics can cause
   a. hyperkalemia
   b. hypernatremia
   c. hypokalemia
   d. hypocalcemia

7. The mechanism of action for beta blockers used in the treatment of heart failure is to block excess _____ stimulation induced by heart failure.
   a. sympathetic
   b. parasympathetic

8. Spironolactone may be used in the treatment of moderate to severe heart failure to _____.
   a. reduce water and K^+ accumulation
   b. reduce water and Ca^{++} accumulation
   c. reduce water and Na^+ accumulation
   d. reduce water and Cl^- accumulation

9. Thrombolytics must be administered within the first _____ hours after a stroke has occurred.
   a. 1 to 3
   b. 2 to 4
   c. 3 to 5
   d. 4 to 6

10. Isosorbide dinitrate and hydralazine are used in combination for the treatment of heart failure for their _____ effects.
    a. vasodilating
    b. vasoconstricting
    c. sympathetic
    d. parasympathetic

Bibliography

Aronow W: Epidemiology, pathophysiology, prognosis, and treatment of systolic and diastolic heart failure, *Cardiol Rev* 14:108–124, 2006.

Chapman J: Therapeutic elevation of HDL-cholesterol to prevent atherosclerosis and coronary heart disease, *Pharmacol Ther* 111:893–908, 2006.

Davies M, Gibbs C, Lip G: ABC of heart failure management: diuretics, ACE inhibitors, and nitrates, *BMJ* 320:428–431, 2000.

FDA: Drugs@FDA: FDA Approved Drug Products, nd. Retrieved July 2, 2017, from http://www.accessdata.fda.gov/scripts/cder/daf/.

Felker M, Petersen J, Mark D: Natriuretic peptides in the diagnosis and management of heart failure, *CMAJ* 175:611–617, 2006.

Health Canada: Drug Product Database, 2017. Retrieved July 2, 2017, from https://health-products.canada.ca/dpd-bdpp/index-eng.jsp.

Hoffman R, Benz E, Shattil S, et al: *Hematology: Basic principles and practice*, ed 4, 2005. Figure 130-1, Chapter 130.

Howlett JG, Chan M, Ezekowitz JA, et al: The Canadian Cardiovascular Society Heart Failure Companion: Bridging Guidelines to Your Practice, *Can J Cardiol* 32:296e310, 2016.

Institute for Safe Medication Practices: FDA and ISMP Lists of Look-Alike Drug Names with Recommended Tall Man Letters, 2016.

Kalant H, Grant D, Mitchell J: *Principles of medical pharmacology*, ed 7, Toronto, 2007, Elsevier Canada, A Division of Reed Elsevier Canada, pp 22–27, 451, 453–454, 472–482, 503–504.

May H, Muhlestein J, Carlquist J, et al: Relation of serum total cholesterol, C-reactive protein levels, and statin therapy to survival in heart failure, *Am J Cardiol* 98:653–658, 2006.

National Heart, Lung, and Blood Institute: *Heart attack*, Bethesda, MD, 2015, National Institutes of Health, US Department of Health and Human Services. Available at: http://www.nhlbi.nih.gov/health/dci/Diseases/HeartAttack/HeartAttack_All.html.

National Heart, Lung, and Blood Institute: *High blood cholesterol*, Bethesda, MD, 2016, National Institutes of Health, US Department of Health and Human Services. Available at: http://www.nhlbi.nih.gov/health/dci/Diseases/Hbc/HBC_all.html.

National Institute of Neurological Disorders and Stroke: *Stroke: hope through research*, Bethesda, MD, 2004, National Institute of Mental Health, National Institutes of Health, US Department of Health and Human Services. Available at: http://www.ninds.nih.gov/disorders/stroke/detail_stroke.htm. Last updated December 20, 2006; NIH publication No. 99-2222.

National Heart, Lung, and Blood Institute: *What is heart failure? Diseases and conditions index*, Bethesda, MD, 2015, National Heart, Lung, and Blood Institute, National Institutes of Health, US Department of Health and Human Services. Available at: https://www.nhlbi.nih.gov/health/health-topics/topics/hf/.

Page C, Curtis M, Sutter M, et al: *Integrated pharmacology*, Philadelphia, 2005, Mosby, pp 386–391, 393–395.

Ringleb R: Thrombolytics, anticoagulants, and antiplatelet agents, *Stroke* 37:312–313, 2006. Available at: http://stroke.ahajournals.org/cgi/content/full/37/2/312.

Shammas R, Khan N, Nekkanti R, et al: Diastolic heart failure and left ventricular diastolic dysfunction: what we know, and what we don't know!, *Int J Cardiol* 115(3):284–292, 2006.

Yancy CW, Jessup M, Bozkurt B, et al: 2013 ACCF/AHA Guideline for the Management of Heart Failure: a report of the American College of Cardiology Foundation/American Heart Association Task Force on Practice Guidelines, *Circulation* 128:1–375, 2013.

20

Treatment of Arrhythmia

LEARNING OBJECTIVES

1 Learn the terminology associated with arrhythmias.
2 List risk factors for arrhythmias.
3 Describe the types of arrhythmias.
4 List and categorize medications used to treat arrhythmias.
5 Describe mechanism of action for each class of drugs used to treat arrhythmias.
6 Identify significant drug look-alike and sound-alike issues.
7 Identify warning labels and precautionary messages associated with medications used to treat arrhythmias.

KEY TERMS

Atrial fibrillation Rapid and uncoordinated contractions. The heart may beat between 300 and 400 beats/min.
Atrial flutter Irregular heartbeat in which contractions in atrium exceed the number of contractions in the ventricle. The heart rate is between 160 and 350 beats/min.
Automaticity Spontaneous contraction of heart muscle cells.
Depolarization Process during which the heart muscle conducts an electrical impulse, causing a contraction.
Ectopic Occurring in an abnormal location.
Electrical cardioversion Process of applying an electrical shock to the heart with a defibrillator to convert the heart to a normal rhythm.

Refractory period Time between contractions that it takes for repolarization to occur.
Repolarization Period of time when the heart is recharging and preparing for another contraction.
Supraventricular tachycardia Heart rate up to 200 beats/min that originates in an area above the ventricles.
Ventricular fibrillation Life-threatening arrhythmia during which the heart beats up to 600 beats/min.
Ventricular tachycardia Ventricles beat faster than 200 beats/min.

Overview

The heart normally beats at a rate between 60 and 100 beats/min or approximately 100,000 beats/day. With each beat or contraction, blood is pumped throughout the body, supplying oxygen and nutrients to cells and organs, including the heart. An arrhythmia is defined as an irregular heart rhythm or a heart rate that is too rapid or too slow. Arrhythmias can produce heart rates that exceed 600 beats/min. An arrhythmia can impair the heart's ability to distribute blood. Symptoms of arrhythmia are listed in Box 20.1.

Atrial fibrillation (Afib) is the most common arrhythmia, and although not usually life threatening, it is a risk factor for stroke. Individuals with Afib are at three to five times greater risk for stroke, and one in three persons who have had a stroke have Afib. Afib can lead to stroke because the condition causes uncoordinated contractions that interfere with pumping blood out of the heart. If the blood pools, it may form a clot. Should the clot dislodge, it may travel to the brain and block one of the arteries, which causes the stroke.

Afib affects approximately 1% of the population, and it is estimated that it will affect nearly 15 million Americans by 2050. Nearly 350,000 Canadians are affected. Risk factors for Afib are similar to risk factors for coronary heart disease (CHD) and are similarly categorized as nonmodifiable risk factors, modifiable risk factors, and disease risk factors (Table 20.1). A description of these risk factors is found in chapters on hypertension, heart failure, myocardial infarction, and stroke (see Chapters 18 and 19).

Ventricular fibrillation is the leading cause of sudden cardiac death, killing nearly 600,000 people in the United States and Europe each year.

How Arrhythmias Are Formed

Heart contractions occur when cardiac cells "fire." This is known as *depolarization*. During depolarization, positively charged ions enter heart cells through specialized exchange channels. Sodium entry initiates depolarization of the atria and ventricles, and calcium entry results in depolarization of the sinoatrial (SA) and atrioventricular (AV) nodes. When the heart cells have fired, another contraction cannot occur until repolarization occurs. *Repolarization* is the process of returning the cells to their resting state. The time it takes for repolarization to occur is called the *refractory period*.

Arrhythmias occur when the cardiac ion exchange channels function improperly. This can result in excessive firing, extra currents during the refractory period, and establishment of sinus rhythm by nonpacemaker cells. These conditions may occur after a heart attack because fibrous scar tissue may develop in the healing process. Conduction is poor across fibrous tissue. Inflammation and oxidative stress (see Chapter 19) can also cause arrhythmias. In addition,

TABLE 20.1 Risk Factors for Atrial Fibrillation

Nonmodifiable	Age, gender, low heart rate, emotional stress
Modifiable	Obesity, smoking, excessive alcohol consumption, stimulant use
Disease	Hypertension, heart failure, CHD, stroke, infection, diabetes, thyroid disease, obstructive sleep apnea

CHD, Coronary heart disease.

• BOX 20.1 Symptoms of Arrhythmia

- Palpitations or fluttering in the chest
- Rapid, irregular heart rate
- Sweating or nausea
- Chest pain
- Shortness of breath
- Lightheadedness or dizziness
- Fainting

TABLE 20.2 Antiarrhythmic Drugs

Class	Category	Generic Name
Class IA	Na$^+$ channel blocker	quinidine sulfate, quinidine gluconate, procainamide, disopyramide
Class IB	Na$^+$ channel blocker	lidocaine, mexiletine, tocainide
Class IC	Na$^+$ channel blocker	flecainide, propafenone
Class II	Beta blocker	propranolol, esmolol, acebutolol
Class III	K$^+$ channel blocker	amiodarone, dofetilide, dronedarone, ranolazine, sotalol, tilide, vernakalant
Class IV	Ca^{2+} channel blocker	verapamil

after an arrhythmia occurs, it may stimulate the formation of other arrhythmias.

Types of Arrhythmias

Atrial Flutter

Atrial flutter refers to an irregular heartbeat in which contractions in the atrium exceed the number of contractions in the ventricle. The heart rate may be between 160 and 350 beats/min. It usually occurs in the right atrium and is treated by inserting a catheter into the atrium (catheter ablation) rather than by drug therapy.

Atrial Fibrillation

Atrial fibrillation is defined as rapid and uncoordinated contractions of the atria. The heart may beat between 300 and 400 beats/min. There are three forms of Afib. They are temporary, recurrent (paroxysmal), persistent (>7 days), and permanent (>1 year).

Supraventricular Tachycardia

Supraventricular tachycardia (SVT) occurs in areas of the heart that lay above the ventricles. SVT may occur intermittently (paroxysmal) or frequently. The heartbeat may increase up to 200 beats/min and last several seconds to a few hours.

Ventricular Tachycardia

Ventricular tachycardia causes the ventricles to beat faster than 200 beats/min. It may occur when the spread of electrical impulses between heart chambers is "short-circuited" across scar tissue caused by a heart attack.

Ventricular Fibrillation

Ventricular fibrillation may cause the ventricles to beat faster than 600 beats/min. Ventricular fibrillation is life threatening because the ventricles are unable to fill with blood and blood is not effectively pumped throughout the body. Ventricular fibrillation is typically reversed only after electrical cardioversion. *Electrical cardioversion* is the process of applying an electrical shock to the heart with a defibrillator to return the heart to a normal rhythm.

Multiple mechanisms are involved in ventricular fibrillation, such as self-generated reentry of unstable wavelets and rapid, intermittent excitation alternating of the heart muscle with conduction block.

Treatment of Arrhythmia

Afib is treated with antiarrhythmic drugs to treat irregular heart rhythms and rate, as well as drugs that reduce clot formation, such as antiplatelet drugs (e.g., aspirin, clopidogrel) or anticoagulants (e.g., warfarin, dabigatran). The use of antiarrhythmic drug to treat other arrhythmias has declined because studies have shown that they may produce secondary cardiac arrhythmias.

Mechanism of Action

Antiarrhythmic drugs are categorized into four classes (classes I, II, III, and IV) according to their mechanisms of action and structural similarities. Class I antiarrhythmics are further subdivided into classes IA, IB, and IC. Antiarrhythmic drugs are listed in Table 20.2. All antiarrhythmic agents are proarrhythmic (can cause other arrhythmias).

Class I Antiarrhythmic Drugs

Quinidine is the prototype class IA antiarrhythmic and has been widely used since the 1920s. It is the active ingredient in cinchona bark. Class I agents act on sodium channels and slow the rate of depolarization. They also reduce *automaticity* (spontaneous contraction of heart muscle cells), delay conduction, and prolong the time between contractions (refractory period). Class IA agents have a moderate effect on depolarization and intermediate effects on the sodium channel. Class IB agents have a minimal effect on depolarization, and their effect on the sodium channel is rapid. The effect of class IC antiarrhythmic drugs on sodium channels is very slow, and they produce marked effects on depolarization. They are 80% to 90% effective at suppressing arrhythmias. All class I antiarrhythmic agents may be administered orally except lidocaine.

❶ TECH ALERT!

The following drugs have look-alike and sound-alike issues:
Procan SR and Proscar;
quinidine and quinine

Adverse Reactions and Precautions

Common side effects of antiarrhythmic agents are bradycardia, hypotension, and dizziness. Most antiarrhythmic agents cause nausea and vomiting, diarrhea, or constipation. Class I antiarrhythmic agents can produce local anesthesia and itchy, flaky rashes. Quinidine and procainamide can also produce a lupus-like syndrome, causing arthritis and chest pain. Tinnitus (ringing in the ears) is a sign of quinidine toxicity.

Class IA Antiarrhythmic Drugs

Generic Name	US Brand Name(s) / Canadian Brand(s)	Dosage Forms and Strengths
disopyramide[a]	Norpace, Norpace CR	**Capsules:** 100 mg, 150 mg[b] **Capsules, extended release (Norpace CR)**[b]: 100 mg, 150 mg
	Rythmodan	
procainamide[a]	Generics	**Solution, injection:** 100 mg/mL
	Not Available	
quinidine gluconate[a]	Generics	**Solution, injection:** 80 mg/mL **Tablets, extended release:** 324 mg
	Not available	
quinidine sulfate[a]	Generics	**Tablet**[b]: 200 mg, 300 mg
	Not Available	

[a]Generic available.
[b]Available in the United States only.
[c]Available in Canada only.

Class IB Antiarrhythmic Drugs

Generic Name	US Brand Name(s) / Canadian Brand(s)	Dosage Forms and Strengths
lidocaine[a]	Generics	**Solution, injection**[b]: 20 mg/mL (Xylocard) **Solution, in dextrose 5%:** 0.2%, 0.4%, 0.8%[c]
	Xylocard	
mexiletine[a]	Generic	**Capsules:** 100 mg[b], 150 mg[c], 200 mg, 250 mg[c]
	Generic	

[a]Generic available.
[b]Available in Canada only.
[c]Available in the United States only.

Class IC Antiarrhythmic Drugs

Generic Name	US Brand Name(s) / Canadian Brand(s)	Dosage Forms and Strengths
flecainide[a]	Tambocor	**Tablets:** 50 mg, 100 mg, 150 mg[b]
	Generic only	
propafenone[a]	Rythmol, Rythmol SR	**Capsules, extended release (Rythmol SR)**[b]: 225 mg, 325 mg, 425 mg **Tablets:** 150 mg, 225 mg,[b] 300 mg
	Rythmol	

[a]Generic available.
[b]Strength available in the United States only.

Class II Antiarrhythmic Drugs

Class II antiarrhythmic agents are beta-adrenergic antagonists. Beta blockers antagonize stimulation of the AV and SA nodes. They increase the refractory period, decrease automaticity, and slow conduction velocity. Beta blockers are indicated for primary management of ventricular arrhythmias. They are effective in suppressing *ectopic* (occurring in an abnormal location) beats and arrhythmias.

Adverse Reactions and Precautions

Adverse reactions for class II antiarrhythmics (beta blockers) are described in detail in Chapter 18. They should be used with caution in patients with asthma, diabetes, and heart failure because they can cause bronchospasm, mask the signs of hypoglycemia, and may increase or decrease blood sugar levels.

❶ TECH ALERT!

The following drugs have look-alike and sound-alike issues:
Brevibloc and Brevital

Class III Antiarrhythmic Drugs

Amiodarone, dofetilide, dronedarone, ibutilide, ranolazine, sotalol, and vernakalant are class III antiarrhythmic agents. Class III antiarrhythmics prolong depolarization and prolong the refractory period by their action on ion channels. Ibutilide promotes the influx of sodium through slow inward sodium channels. All other class III drugs block potassium channels. Dronedarone is a multichannel ion blocker that also inhibits sodium and calcium ion channels. Ranolazine and vernakalant primarily act on the atria. Amiodarone can suppress both supraventricular and ventricular arrhythmias, notably by increasing reentry time. Dofetilide, ibutilide, ranolazine, sotalol, and vernakalant are indicated for the treatment of Afib. Dronedarone is only indicated for the treatment of Afib. Sotalol is also indicated for ventricular tachycardia and atrial flutter.

Class II Antiarrhythmic Drugs

Generic Name	US Brand Name(s)	Dosage Forms and Strengths
	Canadian Brand(s)	
acebutolol[a]	Generic only	Capsules: 100 mg,[b] 200 mg, 400 mg
	Sectral	
esmolol[a]	Brevibloc, Brevibloc Double Strength	Solution, injection: 10 mg/mL (Brevibloc), 20 mg/mL (Brevibloc Double Strength)[c]
	Brevibloc	
propranolol[a]	Inderal LA, InnoPran XL	Capsules, extended release (Inderal LA): 60 mg, 80 mg, 120 mg, 160 mg
	Inderal LA	Solution, injection: 1 mg/mL
		Solution, oral[c]: 20 mg/5 mL, 40 mg/5 mL
		Tablets: 10 mg, 20 mg, 40 mg, 60 mg[c], 80 mg

[a]Generic available.
[b]Available in Canada only.
[c]Available in United States only.

Adverse Reactions and Precautions

Side effects of amiodarone are photosensitivity, skin discoloration, stomach upset, visual disturbances (sun sensitivity, blurred vision, dry eyes), and corneal deposits. Serious side effects of amiodarone include thyroid disease and fatal hepatotoxicity (amiodarone). Vernakalant produces sneezing and taste disturbances. Dofetilide is contraindicated in renal failure (creatine clearance <20 mL/min), and ibutilide should be avoided in women who are pregnant or breastfeeding.

⊘ TECH ALERT!

The following drugs have look-alike and sound-alike issues:
amiodarone and amantadine

Class IV Antiarrhythmic Drugs

Class IV antiarrhythmic agents are calcium channel blockers. The only calcium channel blocker that are effective in treating supraventricular arrhythmias, Afib, and atrial flutter are verapamil and diltiazem. Calcium channel blockers (class IV) produce headache, flushing, and peripheral edema. Additional adverse reactions and precautions are described in Chapters 17 and 18.

Miscellaneous

Digoxin, a drug used to treat heart failure, is also approved for the treatment of Afib. It reduces arrhythmias by slowing the conduction velocity and prolonging the refractory period in the Purkinje fibers and AV node. In the atria and ventricles, digoxin shortens the refractory period. Digoxin also reduces electrical discharges from the SA node. It may be administered intravenously or orally. Digoxin has a narrow therapeutic index, so it is important to avoid excessive doses. The adverse effects of digoxin are described in Chapter 19.

Class III Antiarrhythmic Drugs

Generic Name	US Brand Name(s)	Dosage Forms and Strengths
	Canadian Brand(s)	
amiodarone[a]	Nexterone, Pacerone	Solution, injection (Nexterone): 1.5 mg/mL[b], 1.8 mg/mL[b], 50 mg/mL[c]
	Generic only	Tablets: 100 mg, 200 mg, 400 mg[b]
dofetilide[a]	Tikosyn	Capsules: 0.125 mg, 0.25 mg, 0.5 mg
	Not available	
dronedarone	Multaq	Tablets: 400 mg
	Multaq	
ibutilide[ab]	Corvert	Solution: Injection: 0.1 mg/mL
	Corvert	
ranolazine	Ranexa	Tablets (extended release): 500 mg, 1000 mg
	Not available	
sotalol[a] sotalol AF[a]	Betapace, Betapace AF, Sorine, Sotylize	Tablets: 80 mg, 120 mg,[b] 160 mg, 240 mg[b]
		Tablets (AF)[b]: 80 mg, 120 mg, 160 mg
	Generics	Solution, injection[b]: 150 mg/10 mL
		Solution, oral[b]: 5 mg/mL
vernakalant	Not available	Solution, intravenous: 20 mg/mL
	Brinavess	

[a]Generic available.
[b]Available in the United States only.
[c]Available in Canada only.
[ab]Generic available in the United States only.

Drug Used to Prevent Arrhythmias

Arrhythmia management is currently focused on prevention. Prevention is important because Afib is a risk factor for stroke (see Chapter 19). Hypertension doubles the risk for Afib; therefore hypertension should be treated to reduce the risk. Angiotensin-converting enzyme (ACE) inhibitors and angiotensin II receptor blockers (ARBs) type 1 can significantly reduce the risk for first time Afib in patients with hypertension or heart failure and postmyocardial infarction. The use of these drugs to treat hypertension is discussed in Chapter 18.

Mechanism of Action

The ACE inhibitors lengthen the refractory period and shorten conduction time. The ACE inhibitors also reduce blood pressure. The ARBs have a similar mechanism but also reduce inflammation and structural changes in the atria that can activate Afib.

TECHNICIAN'S CORNER

1. What is the difference between a palpitation and an arrhythmia?
2. How is an arrhythmia diagnosed?

Class IV Antiarrhythmic Drugs

Generic Name	US Brand Name(s) / Canadian Brand(s)	Dosage Forms and Strengths
verapamil[a]	Calan, Calan SR, Verelan, Verelan PM Covera HS / Isoptin SR	**See** Chapter 18

[a]Generic available.

Summary of Drugs Used in the Treatment of Arrhythmia*

Generic Name	Usual Dose and Dosing Schedule	Warning Labels
Antiarrhythmic Drugs		
Class IA		
disopyramide[a]	**Ventricular arrhythmia:** Start with 200–300 mg immediate release; then 400 to 800 mg/day in divided doses (every 6 hr for immediate-release or every 12 hr for controlled-release)	MAY CAUSE DIZZINESS OR DROWSINESS. SWALLOW WHOLE; DO NOT CRUSH OR CHEW—extended release. TAKE ON AN EMPTY STOMACH—procainamide. AVOID GRAPEFRUIT JUICE—quinidine sulfate. REFRIGERATE; DO NOT FREEZE—Diluted quinidine gluconate solution may be stored for up to 48 h at 4°C (39°F) or 24 h at room temperature.
procainamide[a]	**Advanced cardiac life support—Ventricular arrhythmia** 20 to 50 mg/min IV until the arrhythmia is suppressed, or additional conditions met; Maintenance infusion rate is 1 to 4 mg/min; OR 100 mg IV every 5 minutes until arrhythmia is controlled or additional conditions are met **Ventricular arrhythmia, Life-threatening** initial, direct IV injection 100 mg every 5 min to MAX dose 1 g OR IV loading infusion 20 mg/mL at 1 mL/min for 25 to 30 min to MAX dose 1 g; maintenance IV infusion, 2 to 6 mg/min.	
quinidine gluconate[a]	**Atrial flutter/Atrial fibrillation:** 324–648 mg PO every 8–12 h **Ventricular arrhythmia, life threatening:** 0.25 mg/kg/min IV infusion until sinus rhythm restored; MAX total dose 10 mg/kg	
quinidine sulfate[a]	**Atrial flutter/atrial fibrillation/ventricular arrhythmia:** 200–400 mg every 6–8 h (immediate release); 300 mg every 8–12 h (extended release)	
Class IB		
lidocaine[a]	50–100 mg IV infused 25–50 mg/min; may repeat dose in 10 min if necessary **Continuous infusion:** 1–2 mg/min until basic cardiac rhythm is stabilized	MAY CAUSE DIZZINESS OR DROWSINESS. TAKE WITH FOOD—mexiletine.
mexiletine[a]	**Ventricular arrhythmia:** 200–300 mg every 8 h	

Continued

Summary of Drugs Used in the Treatment of Arrhythmia*—cont'd

	Generic Name	Usual Dose and Dosing Schedule	Warning Labels
Class IC			
	flecainide[a] (max daily dose of 400 mg)	**Atrial flutter/atrial fibrillation, Paroxysmal supraventricular tachycardia:** 50–300 mg/day dosed every 12 hr **Ventricular arrhythmia:** 100–400 mg/day dosed every 12 hr	DO NOT SKIP OR EXCEED DOSE.
	propafenone[a]	**Atrial flutter, atrial fibrillation, paroxysmal supraventricular tachycardia, ventricular arrhythmia:** 150–300 mg every 8 h (immediate release) **Atrial flutter, atrial fibrillation:** 225–425 mg every 12 h (extended release)	WEAR SUNGLASSES—propafenone. AVOID GRAPEFRUIT JUICE. SWALLOW WHOLE; DO NOT CRUSH OR CHEW—extended release.
Class II			
	acebutolol[a]	**Ventricular arrhythmia:** 400–1200 mg/day in 2–3 divided doses	MAY CAUSE DIZZINESS OR DROWSINESS.
	esmolol[a]	**Ventricular/supraventricular tachycardia:** 500 mcg/kg IV loading dose over 1 min **May repeat:** 50–200 mcg/kg/min IV every 4 min based on ventricular response.	CONCENTRATE; MUST BE DILUTED—esmolol. ORAL CONCENTRATE; MUST BE DILUTED—propranolol.
	propranolol[a]	**Cardiac dysrhythmia:** 10 to 30 mg 3 to 4 times daily (immediate-release tab) **Cardiac dysrhythmia:** 1 to 3 mg IV (odnèt exceed 1 mg/min), may repeat after 2 minutes; additional doses may be given after 4 hours	SWALLOW WHOLE; DO NOT CRUSH OR CHEW—extended release. DO NOT SKIP DOSES.
Class III			
	amiodarone[a]	**Atrial fibrillation prevention (heart surgery):** Optimal dosage has not established. Off label use. **Supraventricular arrhythmia:** 400 to 600 mg/day orally in divided doses for 2 to 4 weeks, then 100 to 200 mg orally daily (Sinus rhythm maintenance in atrial fibrillation) **Ventricular arrhythmia, life threatening:** various IV; Oral treatment and prophylaxis: Initial, 800 to 1600 mg daily in divided doses for 1 to 3 weeks, then decrease to 600 to 800 mg orally daily for one month. Maintenance, 400–600 mg daily in 1–2 doses.	AVOID PROLONGED EXPOSURE TO SUNLIGHT—amiodarone. MAY CAUSE DIZZINESS OR DROWSINESS. AVOID GRAPEFRUIT JUICE—amiodarone, dofetilide, dronedarone, ranolazine. SHOULD NOT BE ADMINISTERED DURING PREGNANCY—ibutilide. TAKE ON AN EMPTY STOMACH—sotalol.
	ibutilide	**Atrial arrhythmia:** varies, up to 1 mg/IV infused over at least 10 min; Repeat prn	AVOID SALT SUBSTITUTES—sotalol PROTECT FROM MOISTURE—dofetilide.
	dofetilide	**Atrial fibrillation/atrial flutter:** individualized, up to 1000 mcg/day PO; initiation of dofetilide in a hospitalized setting for a minimum of 3 days	SWALLOW WHOLE; DO NOT CRUSH OR CHEW—extended release. DILUTE BEFORE USE— vernakalant
	dronedarone	**Atrial fibrillation:** 400 mg 2 times a day with meals	
	ranolazine	**Atrial fibrillation/cardioversion:** 750–1000 mg twice a day or 1500 mg as a single dose (off label dosage for adjunct therapy with amiodarone or dronedarone)	
	sotalol[a]	**Atrial fibrillation, Ventricular arrhythmia:** 80–160 mg 2 times a day; Betapace is usually taken twice a day, and Betapace AF is taken once or twice a day	
	vernakalant	**Atrial fibrillation:** 3 mg/kg dosed according to body weight	
Class IV			
	verapamil[a]	Paroxysmal supraventricular tachycardia: 240–480 mg/day PO in 3–4 divided doses (immediate release) 2.5–5 mg IV over 2–4 min; may repeat 5–10 mg every 15–30 min up to 20 mg IV Atrial fibrillation/flutter: **or paroxysmal supraventricular tachycardia:** 240–320 mg daily by mouth in 3–4 divided doses (immediate release tabs). Maximum 480 mg/day **Atrial fibrillation/atrial flutter, paroxysmal supraventricular tachycardia:** 0.075 to 0.15 mg/kg (5 to 10 mg) IV over 2–3 minutes; may give additional 10 mg after 30 minutes if necessary	TAKE WITH FOOD.

Summary of Drugs Used in the Treatment of Arrhythmia*—cont'd

Generic Name	Usual Dose and Dosing Schedule	Warning Labels
Angiotensin-Converting Enzyme Inhibitors—See Chapter 18		
Angiotensin II Receptor Antagonists Type 1—See Chapter 18		
Miscellaneous		
digoxin[a]	**Atrial fibrillation (rapid digitalization): Loading dose:** 10–15 mcg/kg PO or IV given in 3 divided doses every 6–8 h **Maintenance:** 125–500 mcg PO or IV once a day	TAKE ON AN EMPTY STOMACH. AVOID HIGH-FIBER DIET. ASK PHARMACIST BEFORE TAKING OTC MEDICINES.

[a]Generic available.
*Dosing can vary significantly based on patient-specific factors and the arrhythmia being treated.
IV, Intravenously; *PO,* orally or "by mouth".

Key Points

- An arrhythmia is defined as an irregular heart rhythm or a heart rate that is too rapid or too slow.
- An arrhythmia can impair the heart's ability to distribute blood.
- Atrial fibrillation is the most common arrhythmia; it can increase the risk for stroke.
- Nonmodifiable risk factors for arrhythmia are age and gender.
- Modifiable risk factors for arrhythmia are obesity, smoking, excessive alcohol consumption, and stimulant use.
- Disease-specific risk factors for arrhythmia are hypertension, heart failure, coronary heart disease, previous stroke, infection, diabetes, thyroid disease, and obstructive sleep apnea.
- Ventricular fibrillation is the leading cause of sudden cardiac death.
- Excessive firing, extra currents during the refractory period, and establishment of sinus rhythm by nonpacemaker cells can lead to arrhythmias.
- Antiarrhythmic drugs are categorized into four classes (classes I, II, III, and IV) according to their mechanisms of action and structural similarities.
- Class I antiarrhythmic drugs produce a sodium channel blockade.
- Class I antiarrhythmic drugs reduce automaticity (spontaneous contraction of heart muscle cells), delay conduction, and prolong the time between contractions (refractory period).
- Class II antiarrhythmic drugs are beta-adrenergic blockers.
- Beta blockers antagonize stimulation at the AV and SA nodes. They increase the refractory period, decrease automaticity, and slow conduction velocity.
- Class III antiarrhythmic drugs produce potassium channel blockade.
- Class III antiarrhythmic drugs prolong depolarization and prolong the refractory period.
- Class IV antiarrhythmic drugs produce calcium channel blockade.
- Digoxin is approved for the treatment of atrial fibrillation. It reduces arrhythmias by slowing the conduction velocity and prolonging the refractory period in the Purkinje fibers and AV node.
- In the atria and ventricles, digoxin shortens the refractory period. Digoxin also reduces electrical discharges from the SA node.
- The ACE inhibitors and ARBs can significantly reduce the risk for first time atrial fibrillation in patients with hypertension or heart failure and postmyocardial infarction.
- The ACE enzyme inhibitors lengthen the refractory period and shorten conduction time.
- The ARBs also reduce inflammation and structural changes in the atria that can activate atrial fibrillation.

Review Questions

1. All of the following antiarrhythmic drugs are marketed as immediate release and extended release dosage forms EXCEPT _____.
   a. verapamil
   b. propafenone
   c. quinidine sulfate
   d. dronederone
2. _____ fibrillation is the most common arrhythmia.
   a. Atrial
   b. Ventricular
   c. Aortic
   d. Pulmonary
3. All of the following antiarrhythmic drugs are marketed as a parenteral dosage form EXCEPT _____.
   a. digoxin
   b. ranolazine
   c. esmolol
   d. amiodarone
4. Select the drug that is NOT indicated for the management of atrial arrhythmias.
   a. ranolazine
   b. propranolol
   c. nitroglycerin
   d. sotalol

5. All antiarrhythmic agents are proarrhythmic (can cause other arrhythmias). They also can cause all of the following symptoms except _____.
   a. bradycardia
   b. hypotension
   c. hypertension
   d. dizziness

6. Digoxin has a narrow therapeutic index, so it is important to avoid excessive doses.
   a. True
   b. False

7. Arrhythmia management is currently focused on _____.
   a. cure
   b. prevention
   c. medication
   d. all of the above

8. Select the drug that is classified as an ion channel blocker _____.
   a. propranolol
   b. verapamil
   c. ranolazine
   d. lidocaine

9. Dofetilide is placed in which class of drugs for arrhythmias?
   a. class I
   b. class II
   c. class III
   d. class IV

10. Select the Brand, generic pair that is INCORRECT.
    a. Cordarone, amiodarone
    b. Corvert, ibutilde
    c. Rhythmol, propranolol
    d. Ranexa, ranolazine

Bibliography

Aksnes T, Flaa A, Strand A, et al: Prevention of new-onset atrial fibrillation and its predictors with angiotensin II-receptor blockers in the treatment of hypertension and heart failure, *J Hypertens* 25(1):15–23, 2007.

FDA: (nd). Drugs@FDA: FDA Approved Drug Products. Retrieved July 16, 2017, from http://www.accessdata.fda.gov/scripts/cder/daf/.

Fragakis N, Vassilikos VP: New antiarrhythmic drugs for atrial fibrillation, *Continuing Cardiology Education* 2(3):2016. doi:10.1002/cce2.34.

Health Canada: Drug Product Database, 2017. Retrieved July 16, 2017, from https://health-products.canada.ca/dpd-bdpp/index-eng.jsp.

Kalant H, Grant D, Mitchell J: *Principles of medical pharmacology*, ed 7, Toronto, 2007, Elsevier Canada, A Division of Reed Elsevier Canada, pp 366–376.

Lance L, Lacy C, Armstrong L, et al: *Drug information handbook for the allied health professional*, ed 12, Hudson, OH, 2005, APhA Lexi-Comp.

Nash M, Mourad A, Clayton R, et al: Evidence for multiple mechanism in human ventricular fibrillation, *Circulation* 114:536–542, 2006. Available at: http://circ.ahajournals.org/cgi/content/full/114/6/536.

Page C, Curtis M, Sutter M, et al: *Integrated pharmacology*, Philadelphia, 2005, Mosby, pp 432–446.

Tveit A, et al: Candesartan in the prevention of relapsing atrial fibrillation, *Int J Cardiol* 1–7, 2006.

Zipes DP, et al: ACC/AHA/ESC practice guidelines, *J Am Coll Cardiol* 48:e268–e270, 2006.

Drugs Affecting the Gastrointestinal System

The organs of the digestive system work together to perform the vital function of preparing food for absorption and for use by the millions of body cells. Digested food must be modified in its chemical composition and physical state so that nutrients can be absorbed and used by the body's cells. Structures of the digestive system are the mouth (lips, cheeks, tongue, and palate), esophagus, stomach, intestines, appendix, liver, gallbladder, and pancreas. To protect itself from self-erosion (autodigestion) by digestive juices, epithelial cells in the stomach produce and secrete a bicarbonate-rich solution that coats the stomach mucosa. Bicarbonate is alkaline, a base, and neutralizes the hydrochloric acid secreted by the parietal cells, producing water in the process. Bicarbonate secretions that neutralize the acid from the stomach are also produced in the intestines and pancreas. The end products such as glucose and amino acids are absorbed and enter cells for use as an energy source or for other metabolic functions.

In Unit VI, the pharmacotherapy for gastroesophageal reflux disease (GERD), peptic ulcer disease (PUD), irritable bowel syndrome (IBS), ulcerative colitis, Crohn's disease, constipation, and diarrhea are described. A brief description of each disorder is provided, followed by a description of the drugs indicated for treatment that includes mechanisms of action, adverse reactions, strength(s), dosage forms, OTC or prescription status, and drug schedules. Laxatives and stool softeners used for the treatment of constipation, and antidiarrheals used for the treatment of diarrhea, are also presented.

21

Treatment of Gastroesophageal Reflux Disease, Laryngopharyngeal Reflux, and Peptic Ulcer Disease

LEARNING OBJECTIVES

1. Learn the terminology associated with gastroesophageal reflux disease (GERD), laryngopharyngeal reflux (LPR), and peptic ulcer disease (PUD).
2. List the symptoms of GERD, LPR, and PUD.
3. List risk factors for GERD and PUD.
4. List and categorize medications used to treat GERD, LPR, and PUD.
5. Describe mechanism of action for drugs used to treat GERD, LPR, and PUD.
6. Identify significant drug look-alike and sound-alike issues.
7. List common endings for drug classes used for the treatment of GERD, LPR, and PUD.
8. Identify warning labels and precautionary messages associated with medications used to treat GERD and PUD.

KEY TERMS

Duodenal ulcer Ulcer located in the upper portion of the small intestine or duodenum.
Gastric ulcer Ulcer located in the stomach.
Gastroesophageal reflux A condition whereby the stomach contents occasionally flow up into the esophagus, producing heartburn.
Gastroesophageal reflux disease Motility disorder associated with impaired peristalsis that results in persistent backflow of gastric contents into the esophagus.
Hiatal hernia Condition in which the lower esophageal sphincter shifts above the diaphragm.
Laryngopharyngeal reflux Reflux of gastric contents into the larynx and pharynx.

Lower esophageal sphincter Sphincter separating the esophagus and the stomach.
Peptic ulcer disease Term used to describe ulcers located in the duodenum or stomach.
Peristalsis Forceful wave of contractions in the esophagus that moves food and liquids from the mouth to the stomach.
Reflux Backflow of gastric contents into esophagus or laryngopharyngeal region.
Ulcer Open wound or sore.
Upper esophageal sphincter Sphincter separating the pharynx and esophagus.

Overview

Gastroesophageal reflux disease (GERD), *peptic ulcer disease* (PUD), and *laryngopharyngeal reflux* are diseases that affect millions of Americans and Canadians. Direct and indirect health care costs (e.g., missed days of work) are estimated to be greater than $10 billion annually.

Gastroesophageal Reflux Disease

Gastroesophageal reflux (GER) is a condition whereby the stomach contents flow up into the esophagus, producing symptoms described as heartburn. Persistent GER, more than twice a week, is a sign of GERD. It is estimated that 20% of Americans have GERD.

GER and GERD may initially produce minor discomfort, such as heartburn and chronic cough. Excessive or chronic exposure to gastric acid and pepsin may produce inflammation, ulceration, or hemorrhage and changes to the epithelial cells that can lead to esophageal or stomach cancer.

Persons of any age can develop GERD. Infants may have GERD because their digestive system is immature, however many will outgrow GERD by their first birthday. Obesity, smoking, and pregnancy are additional risk factors.

What Causes Reflux?

GERD is a motility disorder associated with impaired peristalsis. *Peristalsis* is a forceful wave of contractions in the esophagus that

• **Fig. 21.1** Gastroesophageal junction. (A) Location of the lower esophageal sphincter (*LES*). (B) Hiatal hernia. (Courtesy Dr. J.T. Laitman, Mount Sinai School of Medicine, Center for Anatomy and Functional Morphology, New York.)

moves food and other orally ingested contents from the mouth to the stomach. The *lower esophageal sphincter* (LES) is a muscle located at the junction between the esophagus and upper stomach that relaxes to permit food and liquids to pass from the esophagus into the stomach and then contracts to prevent stomach contents from returning to the esophagus. GER occurs when there is a buildup of pressure in the stomach causing the LES to open and leak stomach contents back up into the esophagus.

Normally the LES lies below the diaphragm, which helps to keep the stomach contents from flowing back into the esophagus. Delayed gastric emptying or transient relaxation of the LES, especially after eating, may also cause reflux.

Hiatal hernia is a significant risk factor for GERD in persons older than 50 years. When a hiatal hernia occurs, the diaphragm muscle is unable to hold the LES in normal position and the sphincter shifts above the diaphragm. Larger hiatal hernias are linked to more severe esophagitis (Fig. 21.1).

Factors Contributing to Gastroesophageal Reflux Disease

Many factors can aggravate GERD; these include foods, lifestyle, prescription and over-the-counter (OTC) medicines, and even body position. Foods that can aggravate GERD are listed in Table 21.1. Lifestyle factors that aggravate GERD include alcohol consumption and cigarette smoking. GERD symptoms are made worse when the body is in a prone position (lying down). Raising the head of the bed 6 to 8 inches can reduce symptoms. Pregnancy and obesity can also aggravate GERD. Many prescription and OTC medicines can worsen GERD (Box 21.1). These drugs impair peristalsis, delay gastric emptying, decrease esophageal sphincter tone, decrease the protective mucosal lining, and/or increase gastric acid levels.

Laryngopharyngeal Reflux

Laryngopharyngeal reflux (LPR) is closely related to GERD and can occur simultaneously. When gastric contents reflux into the larynx and pharynx, located in the head and neck region, inflammation occurs that may cause hoarseness, voice fatigue, laryngitis, sore throat, chronic cough, bad breath, sinusitis, wheezing, aggravation of asthma, and even middle ear infections.

As in GERD, LPR occurs when the normal reflux barriers fail. Anatomic barriers that protect against LPR are the gastroesophageal junction (includes the LES) and the *upper esophageal sphincter* (UES). The UES separates the pharynx and esophagus. It relaxes to permit the passage of food and liquids during swallowing, prevent air from entering the esophagus during breathing, and prevent gastric secretions entering the pharynx via the esophagus. If the UES is damaged by exposure to stomach contents, it can become less sensitive and lose its ability to function properly. This increases the likelihood of reflux and more damage (Fig. 21.2). Laryngeal mucosal resistance protects the larynx from damage caused by reflux.

Peptic Ulcer Disease

An *ulcer* is an open wound or sore. Ulcers can occur anywhere on the body. In the gastrointestinal (GI) tract, *gastric ulcers* form in the stomach (Fig. 21.3), *duodenal ulcers* form in the upper region of the small intestines, and peptic ulcers form in the stomach or duodenum.

Risk Factors for Peptic Ulcer Disease

Helicobacter pylori infection is the primary cause of peptic ulcer disease (PUD). Almost two-thirds of the global population have the infection. More than 90% of people who have duodenal ulcers and 80% of people who have gastric ulcers are infected with *H. pylori*. *H. pylori* infection is also a risk factor for the development of stomach cancer. Worldwide, most people infected with *H. pylori* develop the infection in childhood. Infections are transmitted person to person by the gastric-oral route. Once the bacteria are ingested, they release buffers that enable the bacteria to survive in the acidic contents of the stomach. The bacteria also

TABLE 21.1 Natural Alternatives for Gastroesophageal Reflux Disease

Safe Foods	Food to Avoid	Natural Alternative
Fruits—apples, bananas	Fruits—tomatoes, citrus fruits and juice (e.g., lemon)	Magnesium oxide—increases lower esophageal sphincter tone
Vegetables—broccoli, carrots, cabbage, peas, green beans, baked potato	Juice—orange juice, cranberry juice, grapefruit juice Fried vegetables (e.g., French fries) Raw onion, garlic, mint	Almonds—chew on a few almonds after each meal
Meat products—skinless chicken breast, extra lean ground beef, London broil, egg whites and substitutes, nonfatty fish	Fried and fatty meat products—ground beef, chicken nuggets, buffalo wings, marbled sirloin	Fennel tea or chamomile tea—soothing effect, sip slowly
Dairy—fat-free cream cheese, goat cheese, low-fat soy cheese, fat-free sour cream	Dairy products—regular cottage cheese, sour cream, ice cream, milk shake	Ginger (any form)—reduces acid in stomach
Grains—brown or white rice, multigrain or white bread, cereal (e.g., bran, oatmeal), corn bread, graham crackers, pretzels, rice cakes	Grains—spaghetti (pasta) with tomato sauce, macaroni and cheese	Organic apple cider—shake well; pulp contains enzymes to reduce acid
Salad—low-fat salad dressing	Salad—creamy and oil and vinegar salad dressings	Chewing gum—produces saliva, which dilutes stomach acid
Sweets, fat free (e.g., fat free cookies, jelly beans, red licorice, baked potato chips)	Sweets, high fat (e.g., butter cookies, chocolate, doughnuts, corn chips, brownies)	
Beverage—mineral water	Beverages—wine, liquor, caffeinated beverages (e.g., coffee, tea, cola)	

• **Fig. 21.2** Laryngopharyngeal reflux—direction of backflow into head and neck regions. (Courtesy Dr. J.T. Laitman, Mount Sinai School of Medicine, Center for Anatomy and Functional Morphology, New York.)

• **Fig. 21.3** Gastric ulcer. (From Rosai J: *Rosai and Ackerman's surgical pathology*, ed 9, Philadelphia, 2004, Mosby.)

• BOX 21.1 Prescription Medicines That Worsen Gastroesophageal Reflux Disease

- anticholinergics (e.g., hyoscyamine)
- opioids (e.g., codeine)
- calcium channel blockers (e.g., verapamil)
- nonsteroidal antiinflammatory drugs (e.g., naproxen)
- hormones (e.g., progesterone)
- benzodiazepines (e.g., diazepam)
- antiarrhythmics (e.g., quinidine)
- bisphosphonates (e.g., alendronate)
- xanthines (e.g., theophylline)
- iron supplements
- potassium supplements

release virulence factors that are responsible for inflammation and tissue damage. Fortunately, most people who are infected with *H. pylori* will not develop chronic gastritis or PUD. Researchers are working to develop a vaccine that can be administered in childhood to prevent *H. pylori* infection. Persons with a family history of ulcers or living with close relatives who have PUD; older than 50 years; or who use medicines such as salicylates (e.g., aspirin), nonsteroidal antiinflammatory drugs (NSAIDs) (e.g., naproxen), and corticosteroids (e.g., prednisone) are at increased risk for PUD.

When a person exhibits symptoms of PUD, several simple tests can be performed to see whether the person has an *H. pylori* infection. A sample of blood may be drawn to look for antibodies and other evidence of past or current infection, or a breath test may be done to check for evidence of urease, an enzyme released by *H. pylori*. An endoscopy may be performed to look for ulcers inside the stomach and small intestine using an endoscope, a thin flexible tube with a small video camera and light attached to one end that is passed down the esophagus into the stomach.

Symptoms of Gastroesophageal Reflux Disease, Laryngopharyngeal Reflux, and Peptic Ulcer Disease

Some of the symptoms of GERD, LPR, and PUD are common to all three conditions, whereas others are disease-specific. Symptoms associated with GERD, LPR, and PUD are categorized in Table 21.2.

TABLE 21.2	Symptoms of Gastroesophageal Reflux Disease, Laryngopharyngeal Reflux, and Peptic Ulcer Disease	
Disease	**Unique Symptoms**	**Common Symptoms**
Gastroesophageal reflux disease	Difficulty swallowing Dry cough Bad breath Bloated stomach Rumbling noise in stomach Belching or burping Respiratory problems Hoarseness	Heartburn Stomachache Hunger pains Nausea or vomiting Chest pain
Laryngopharyngeal reflux	Hoarseness Voice fatigue or breaks Sore throat Excessive phlegm or saliva Chronic cough Bad breath Middle ear infection Wheezing Chronic sinusitis	
Peptic ulcer disease	Burning pain in the gut beginning 2–3 h after a meal Weight loss Loss of appetite	

Lifestyle Modification

Lifestyle changes to reduce the risk for GERD and PUD or their symptoms include eating small, frequent meals, avoiding foods that aggravate GERD and PUD, limiting alcohol consumption, and stopping smoking. Cigarette smoking interferes with the healing of an ulcer by constricting blood vessels in the ulcerated area. Alcohol is a gastric irritant. See Box 21.2 for lifestyle modifications recommended for people with GERD and PUD.

Drugs Used in the Treatment of Gastroesophageal Reflux Disease, Laryngopharyngeal Reflux, and Peptic Ulcer Disease

The treatment of GERD, LPR, and PUD is aimed at reducing GI irritants (e.g., volume of gastric acid, digestive enzymes such as pepsin) and increasing protective factors (e.g., mucus secretion by epithelial cells). Drugs used in the treatment of PUD, GERD, and LPR are classified according to their pharmacologic effects: (1) acid-suppressing drugs (e.g., histamine 2 [H2] receptor antagonists, proton pump inhibitors [PPIs]); (2) mucosal protectants (e.g., prostaglandins, sucralfate); (3) prokinetic drugs (e.g., metoclopramide); (4) acid-neutralizing drugs (e.g., antacids); and (5) drugs that eliminate *H. pylori* (e.g., anti-infectives).

> ● **TECH NOTE!**
> It is a myth that stress and spicy foods can cause ulcers; however, some foods can aggravate existing GERD (see Table 21.1).

> ● **TECH NOTE!**
> A common ending for H2 blockers is *-tidine*.

Histamine 2 Receptor Antagonist Drugs

There are four H2 receptor antagonists marketed in the United States and Canada—cimetidine, famotidine, nizatidine, and ranitidine. All H2 receptor antagonists are available in prescription and nonprescription strengths.

Mechanism of Action and Pharmacokinetics

Histamine stimulates acid secretion by gastric parietal cells. H2 receptor antagonists competitively and reversibly bind to H2

> ● **BOX 21.2** Lifestyle Modifications Recommended for People With Gastroesophageal Reflux Disease or Peptic Ulcer Disease
>
> - Avoid lying down after eating (wait at least 3 hours).
> - Elevate the head of the bed 6 to 8 inches.
> - Eat small meals.
> - Lose weight if you are overweight.
> - Quit smoking if you smoke.
> - Do not drink alcohol.
> - Limit use of aspirin and nonsteroidal antiinflammatory drugs.

receptors, blocking histamine-mediated acid secretion. The secretion of pepsin, a digestive enzyme released when the volume of acid in the stomach is high, occurs when food is present in the stomach and decreases as gastric acid levels decrease. Chronic exposure to pepsin can cause inflammation and peptic ulcers.

The effect of H2 receptor antagonists on nocturnal (nighttime) acid secretion is significantly greater than on acid secretion after meals. The duration of effect on nocturnal secretion ranges from 8 hours (cimetidine) to 13 hours (ranitidine). The duration of effect on secretion after meals is reduced to 3 to 5 hours. The most potent H2 receptor antagonists is ranitidine. It is approximately 10 times more effective than cimetidine.

Adverse Reactions

H2 receptor antagonists can produce dizziness or drowsiness, constipation or diarrhea, bloating, headache, and confusion when taken at therapeutic doses. Older adults are more susceptible to these adverse effects. Less common adverse effects include skin rash, agitation, depression, hepatitis, and decreased libido. High-dose cimetidine may produce breast swelling or tenderness in males (gynecomastia).

Precautions

Cimetidine inhibits several metabolic enzymes and is responsible for increasing the elimination of more than 25 different drugs. The pharmacist should be alerted to all drug interactions that are flagged by prescription-filling software.

---

❶ TECH ALERT!

The following drugs have look-alike and sound-alike issues:
raNITIdine, riMANTAdine
Zantac, Xanax, and ZyrTEC

Proton Pump Inhibitor Drugs

There are six PPIs currently marketed in the United States and Canada—dexlansoprazole, esomeprazole, lansoprazole, omeprazole, pantoprazole, and rabeprazole. Esomeprazole is an S isomer (mirror image) of omeprazole. PPIs are effective in treating GERD, LPR, and PUD because they decrease gastric acid levels. They are more potent than H2 receptor antagonists. Omeprazole and lansoprazole are available for OTC use in the United States. All other PPIs are only commercially available in prescription strengths. OTC PPIs are marketed for the treatment of heartburn.

● TECH NOTE!

PPIs have the common ending -prazole.

Mechanism of Action and Pharmacokinetics

PPIs decrease gastric acids by interfering with the final step in gastric acid production. PPIs interfere with hydrogen and potassium

---

Histamine 2 Receptor Antagonists (H2 Blockers)

Generic Name	US Brand Name(s) / Canadian Brand Name(s)	Dosage Forms and Strengths
cimetidine[a]	Tagamet HB[b]	**Tablet:** 100 mg[c], 200 mg,[b] 300 mg, 400 mg, 600 mg[d], 800 mg[c]
	Generics	**Solution, oral:** 300 mg/5 mL **Injection, solution:** 300 mg/2 mL
famotidine[a]	Pepcid, Pepcid AC	**Tablet:** 10 mg,[b] 20 mg,[b] 40 mg **Tablet, chewable:** 20 mg[b,c]
	Pepcid, Pepcid AC,[b] Maximum Strength Pepcid AC[b]	**Injection, solution:** 0.4 mg/mL, 10 mg/mL **Powder for oral suspension:** 40 mg/5 mL[c]
nizatidine[a]	Axid AR[b]	**Capsule:** 150 mg, 300 mg[c]
	Axid	**Tablet:** 75 mg[b] **Oral solution**[c]: 15 mg/mL
ranitidine[a]	Zantac, Zantac-75,[b] Zantac-150,[b] Zantac-300	**Capsule**[c]: 150 mg, 300 mg **Tablet:** 75 mg,[b] 150 mg,[b] 300 mg
	Zantac, Zantac Maximum Strength Nonprescription	**Injection, solution:** 25 mg/mL **Oral solution/syrup:** 15 mg/mL

H2 Receptor Antagonist Combinations

famotidine + calcium carbonate + magnesium hydroxide	Pepcid Complete[b]	10 mg famotidine + 800 mg calcium carbonate + 165 mg magnesium hydroxide
	Pepcid Complete[b]	

[a]Generic available.
[b]Over-the-counter in Canada and the United States.
[c]Available in the United States only.
[d]Available in Canada only.

ion exchange via the H^+/K^+-ATPase proton pump located on parietal cells in the stomach.

PPIs can be destroyed in gastric acids. Zegerid is a formulation combining an antacid with omeprazole to reduce the destruction of omeprazole by gastric acids. PPIs are delayed-release formulations. They must not be crushed or chewed. Delayed-release tablets disintegrate in less than 1 minute.

Adverse Reactions

All the PPIs have a similar side effect profile. More common side effects are abdominal pain, headache, diarrhea or constipation, flatulence (gas), and nausea. Less common side effects are jaundice, skin rash, unusual tiredness or fatigue, agitation, vitamin B_{12} deficiency, dark yellow or brown urine, and vomiting.

Proton Pump Inhibitors

	Generic Name	US Brand Name(s) / Canadian Brand Name(s)	Dosage Forms and Strengths
	dexlansoprazole[a]	Dexilant	**Capsules, delayed release:** 30 mg, 60 mg
		Dexilant	
	esomeprazole	Nexium, Nexium 24 HR[e]	**Capsules, delayed release:** 20 mg[e], 40 mg[b]
		Nexium, Nexium 24 HR[e]	**Powder for oral suspension:** 2.5 mg,[b] 5 mg,[b] 10 mg, 20 mg,[b] 40 mg/packet[b]
			Powder for injection: 40 mg/vial[b]
			Tablet, delayed-release: 20 mg,[d] 40 mg[d]
	lansoprazole[a]	Prevacid, Prevacid 24 HR[e]	**Capsules, delayed-release (Prevacid, Prevacid 24 HR):** 15 mg,[e] 30 mg
		Prevacid, Prevacid FasTab	**Tablets, Disintegrating (Prevacid FasTab):** 15 mg, 30 mg
	omeprazole[a]	Prilosec, Prilosec OTC[e]	**Capsules, delayed-release:** 10 mg[e], 20 mg[e], 40 mg[b]
		Losec OLEX, OMEP	**Granules for suspension[b]:** 2.5 mg, 10 mg
			Tablets, disintegrating[b,e]: 20 mg
			Tablets, delayed-release: 10 mg[e], 20 mg[e]
	pantoprazole sodium,[a] pantoprazole magnesium	Protonix	**Granules, for oral suspension:** 40 mg[b]
		Pantoloc, Tecta	**Powder, for injection:** 40 mg base per vial
			Tablet, delayed release, as sodium salt (Protonix, Pantoloc): 20 mg, 40 mg
			Tablet, enteric-coated, as magnesium salt (Tecta): 40 mg
	rabeprazole[a]	Aciphex	**Sprinkle[b]:** 5 mg, 10 mg
		Pariet	**Tablet, delayed-release:** 10 mg,[c] 20 mg

PPI Combination Products

	Generic Name	US Brand Name(s) / Canadian Brand Name(s)	Dosage Forms and Strengths
	esomeprazole + naproxen	Vimovo	**Tablet:** 20 mg esomeprazole + 375 mg naproxen
		Vimovo	20 mg esomeprazole + 500 mg naproxen[b]
	lansoprazole + amoxicillin + clarithromycin	Generic only	**Combo pack:** 30 mg lansoprazole capsule + 500 mg amoxicillin capsule + 500 mg clarithromycin tablet
		HP-PAC	
	omeprazole + sodium bicarbonate	Zegerid, Zegerid OTC[e]	**Capsule:** 20 mg omeprazole + 1100 mg sodium bicarbonate[e]
		Not available	40 mg omeprazole + 1100 mg sodium bicarbonate
			Powder, for oral suspension: 20 mg omeprazole + 1680 mg sodium bicarbonate[e]
			40 mg omeprazole + 1680 mg sodium bicarbonate

[a]Generic available.
[b]Available in the United States only.
[c]Available in Canada only.
[d]Generic available in Canada only.
[e]Over-the-counter in the United States only.

❶ TECH ALERT!

The following drugs have look-alike and sound-alike issues:
PriLOSEC and PROzac
Losec and Lasix
Protonix, Lotronex, and protamine
RABEprazole and ARIPiprazole
Aciphex, Aricept, and Accupril

Mucosal Protectants

Misoprostol and sucralfate are mucosal protectants. The drugs protect the epithelial cells that line the stomach and small intestine from damage by gastric acids, pepsin, and *H. pylori*. The drug is approved for the prevention of NSAID-induced peptic ulcers. Sucralfate is approved for the treatment and maintenance therapy of duodenal ulcers.

Mechanism of Action

Misoprostol is a synthetic prostaglandin E (PGE). It stimulates the production of protective mucus and bicarbonate in the stomach. It also increases the regeneration of gastric epithelial cells and enhances blood flow to the stomach.

Sucralfate binds to the ulcerated area and forms a protective barrier, much like a bandage protects a sore. It also promotes the regeneration of stomach epithelial cells. It is a weak inhibitor of *H. pylori*.

Adverse Reactions and Precautions

Misoprostol may produce abdominal cramps, diarrhea, menstrual irregularities, headache, and dizziness. It is contraindicated in pregnancy because it stimulates uterine contractions. Sucralfate may produce constipation, gas, dry mouth, and headache.

Sucralfate can block the absorption of several drugs, including H2 receptor antagonists, PPIs, and some antibiotics. To avoid drug interactions, the drugs should not be taken at the same time as sucralfate.

● TECH NOTE!

Misoprostol is labeled with a boxed warning that the drug should not be taken by pregnant women because the drug may stimulate uterine contractions. In the United States, misoprostol must be dispensed in the manufacturer's original container.

Mucosal Protectant Drugs

Generic Name	US Brand Name(s)	Dosage Forms and Strengths
	Canadian Brand Name(s)	
misoprostol[a]	Cytotec	**Tablet:** 0.1 mg; 0.2 mg
	Generics	
sucralfate[a]	Carafate	**Suspension, oral:** 1 g/5 mL,[b] 1 g/10 mL[c]
	Sulcrate, Sulcrate Suspension Plus	**Tablet:** 1 g

[a]Generic available.
[b]Available in Canada only.
[c]Available in the United States only.

❶ TECH ALERT!

The following drugs have look-alike and sound-alike issues:
miSOPROStol and mifepristone

Prokinetic Drugs

Prokinetic drugs are used for the treatment of GERD and LPR. They increase peristalsis (the wavelike movement throughout the GI tract), speed up gastric emptying, and improve LES tone. Metoclopramide is currently the only prokinetic drug approved by the US Food and Drug Administration (FDA). Domperidone is approved in Canada for the symptomatic management of motility disorders associated with chronic gastritis and diabetic gastroparesis.

Mechanism of Action

Metoclopramide increases peristalsis by stimulating the release of acetylcholine in the periphery and increasing cholinergic activity. Domperidone blocks peripheral dopamine receptors to increase peristalsis. Both drugs enhance gastroduodenal coordination. Centrally, metoclopramide and domperidone block dopamine receptors, which decreases nausea.

Adverse Reactions

Common adverse effects associated with metoclopramide and domperidone include diarrhea, abdominal pain, constipation, restlessness, dizziness, and headache. Metoclopramide may cause drowsiness. Less common effects are leg cramps, skin rash, irregular heartbeat, and breast enlargement in men and women.

Prokinetic Drugs

Generic Name	US Brand Name(s)	Dosage Forms and Strengths
	Canadian Brand Name(s)	
metoclopramide[a]	Metozolv ODT, Reglan	**Tablet, oral disintegrating tablet (Metozolv ODT):** 5 mg[b]
	Metonia	**Tablet:** 5 mg, 10 mg
		Solution, for injection: 5 mg/mL
		Solution, oral: 1 mg/mL
domperidone[a]	Not available	**Tablet:** 10 mg
	Generics	

[a]Generic available.
[b]Available in the United States only.

Antacids

Antacids are the oldest drugs used for the treatment of GERD and PUD. Antacid use has declined since more potent drugs, requiring fewer daily doses, have been developed. Antacids can be obtained without prescription.

Mechanism of Action

Antacids neutralize gastric acids and decrease pepsin secretion. The acid-neutralizing capacity (ANC) is a standard used to evaluate the potency of antacids. The ANC is a measure of the ability of an antacid to do the following: (1) neutralize approximately 1 to 2 ounces hydrochloric acid (i.e., the volume of acid normally present between meals) and (2) raise the pH of the stomach to 3.5 within 10 minutes.

Adverse Reactions

The side effects of antacids are related to their active ingredient and are dose related. Magnesium-containing antacids cause diarrhea; aluminum-containing antacids cause constipation and, in high doses, deplete phosphate levels in blood (hypophosphatemia). Calcium-containing antacids cause constipation and, in high doses, produce hypercalcemia and kidney stones. Sodium bicarbonate (baking soda) has been associated with rebound hyperacidity, metabolic alkalosis, edema, and hypertension.

Antimicrobials

Antimicrobials are prescribed for the treatment of PUD to eradicate *H. pylori* infection. Clarithromycin, metronidazole, amoxicillin, and tetracycline are effective for eradicating *H. pylori*. They are prescribed in combination with drugs that decrease gastric acids and protect the gastric mucosa. Antimicrobials will be described in detail in Chapter 29.

TECHNICIAN'S CORNER

1. Describe the function of the lower esophageal sphincter and how it is affected by gastroesophageal reflux disease.
2. Consumption of which two products increases the risk for peptic ulcer disease and can aggravate existing disease? How does it interfere with the healing of an ulcer?

Examples of Selected Antacids

Generic Name	US Brand Name(s) / Canadian Brand Name(s)
aluminum hydroxide[a]	Alternagel, Amphojel
	Not available
aluminum hydroxide + magnesium hydroxide[a]	Mag-Al, Mylanta Ultimate
	Gelusil
aluminum hydroxide + magnesium hydroxide + simethicone	Almacone, Maalox Max, Mintox, Mylanta Maximum Strength, Mylanta Regular Strength, Rulox
	Diovol Plus, Maalox with Anti-gas, Maalox with Anti-gas Extra Strength
calcium carbonate[a]	Caltrate, Alka-Mints, Maalox Antacid Barrier, Pepto Bismol Children's Chewable, Rolaids Extra Strength, TUMS, TUMS EX, TUMS Ultra
	Alka-Seltzer Heartburn Relief Chewable, Caltrate, TUMS, TUMS Ultra, TUMS Extra Strength
calcium carbonate + magnesium hydroxide[a]	Rolaids Chewable, Rolaids Extra Strength Chewable, Mylanta Supreme Suspension, Mylanta Ultra Chewable
	Not available
calcium carbonate + simethicone	Titralac Plus, Tums Plus
	Maalox Extra Strength with Anti-gas, Rolaids Extra Strength Plus Gas
alginic acid + magnesium carbonate	Gaviscon
	Gaviscon, Gaviscon Max Relief

[a]Generic available.

Summary of Drugs Used for Treatment of Gastroesophageal Reflux Disease, Laryngopharyngeal Reflux, and Peptic Ulcer Disease

	Generic Name	US Brand Name	Usual Adult Oral Dosage and Dosing Schedule	Warning Labels
H2 Receptor Antagonists				
	cimetidine	Tagamet	**PUD:** 800 mg daily at bedtime, or 400 mg twice daily or 300 mg 4 times daily for 8–12 weeks Maintenance: 400 mg daily at bedtime **GERD:** 800 mg twice daily or 400 mg 4 times daily for 12 weeks	AVOID ANTACIDS WITHIN 2 H OF DOSE (CIMETIDINE, NIZATIDINE). AVOID ALCOHOL—ALL. SHAKE SUSPENSION WELL. DISCARD FAMOTIDINE ORAL SUSPENSION 30 DAYS AFTER MIXING. STORE INJECTION IN THE REFRIGERATOR (FAMOTIDINE, RANITIDINE). STORE CIMETIDINE INJECTION AT ROOM TEMPERATURE.
	famotidine	Pepcid	**PUD:** 40 mg once daily at bedtime or 20 mg twice daily for 4–8 weeks **GERD:** 20–40 mg twice daily for 6–12 weeks	

Continued

	Generic Name	US Brand Name	Usual Adult Oral Dosage and Dosing Schedule	Warning Labels
	nizatidine	Axid	**PUD:** 150 mg every 12 h or 300 mg at bedtime for up to 8 weeks **GERD:** 150 mg every 12 h for up to 12 weeks **Indigestion/heartburn:** 75 mg 30–60 min prior to food/beverage up to 150 mg/day	
	ranitidine	Zantac	**PUD:** 150 mg twice daily or 300 mg once daily at bedtime for 4–6 weeks **GERD:** 150 mg twice daily for 4–8 weeks **Indigestion/heartburn:** 75 to 150 mg orally 30–60 min before eating or drinking; MAX 300 mg/day	

Proton Pump Inhibitors

	Generic Name	US Brand Name	Usual Adult Oral Dosage and Dosing Schedule	Warning Labels
	dexlansoprazole	Dexilant	**GERD:** 30 mg once or twice daily	SWALLOW WHOLE; DO NOT CRUSH OR CHEW (CAPSULES CAN BE SPRINKLED ONTO FOOD BUT DO NOT CRUSH THE CONTENTS INTO THE FOOD).
	esomeprazole	Nexium	**PUD:** 40 mg daily in 1–2 divided doses as part of H. pylori triple drug therapy regimen. **GERD:** 20–40 mg once daily for up to 4–8 weeks **Indigestion/heartburn:** 20 mg once daily	DELAYED RELEASE—TAKE 30 MIN BEFORE A MEAL (LANSOPRAZOLE). TAKE 60 MIN BEFORE A MEAL (ESOMEPRAZOLE).
	lansoprazole	Prevacid	**PUD:** 15 mg once daily in the morning for up to 4 weeks or 30 mg twice daily as part of H. pylori triple and quadruple drug therapy regimens. **GERD:** 15–30 mg once daily in the morning for up to 8 weeks **Indigestion/heartburn:** 15 mg orally once a day for 14 days	GRANULES FOR ORAL SUSPENSION MUST BE MIXED WITH 1 TO 2 TABLESPOONFULS OF LIQUID. ALLOW MIXTURE TO STAND FOR 2–3 MIN, THEN IMMEDIATELY DRINK ENTIRE MIXTURE. DISSOLVE DISINTEGRATING TABLETS ON TONGUE.
	omeprazole	Prilosec	**PUD:** 40 mg once daily for 4–8 weeks or 20 mg twice daily as part of H. pylori triple drug therapy regimen **GERD:** 20 mg once daily for 4–8 weeks	
	pantoprazole	Protonix	**PUD:** 40 mg once daily after the morning meal for 4–8 weeks **GERD:** 40 mg once daily for up to 8 weeks	
	rabeprazole	Aciphex	**PUD:** 20 mg once daily after the morning meal for 3–6 weeks or 20–40 mg twice daily as part of the H. pylori triple drug therapy regimen. **GERD:** 20 mg once daily for 4 weeks; repeat course of treatment if necessary.	

Prokinetic Drugs

	Generic Name	US Brand Name	Usual Adult Oral Dosage and Dosing Schedule	Warning Labels
	metoclopramide	Reglan	**GERD:** 10–15 mg, up to 4 times a day	MAY CAUSE DROWSINESS. AVOID ALCOHOL. TAKE 15–30 MIN BEFORE MEALS.
	domperidone	Generics	10 mg 3–4 times a day	

Mucosal Protectants

	Generic Name	US Brand Name	Usual Adult Oral Dosage and Dosing Schedule	Warning Labels
	misoprostol	Cytotec	**NSAID-induced PUD prevention:** 100–200 mcg 4 times a day for 4–8 weeks	AVOID PREGNANCY.
	sucralfate	Carafate	**Duodenal ulcer:** 1 g 4 times a day for 4–8 weeks	TAKE ON AN EMPTY STOMACH. SHAKE SUSPENSION WELL.

Antimicrobial Combinations for *H. pylori* Eradication

	Generic Name	US Brand Name	Usual Adult Oral Dosage and Dosing Schedule	Warning Labels
	lansoprazole + amoxicillin + clarithromycin	HP-PAC	***H. pylori*–associated ulcer:** 2 amoxicillin caps + 1 lansoprazole cap + 1 clarithromycin tablet twice daily for 10–14 days	SWALLOW WHOLE; DON'T CRUSH OR CHEW. MAY DECREASE EFFECTIVENESS OF ORAL CONTRACEPTIVES

GERD, Gastroesophageal reflux disease; *NSAID*, nonsteroidal antiinflammatory drug; *PUD*, peptic ulcer disease.

Key Points

- GERD, PUD, and LPR are diseases that affect millions of Americans and Canadians.
- GERD causes a chronic backflow *(reflux)* of acidic stomach contents and digestive enzymes up into the esophagus.
- Excessive or chronic exposure to gastric acids can lead to inflammation, ulceration, and changes to the epithelial cells that can cause stomach cancer.
- GERD may also increase the risk for development of chronic disease, such as asthma.
- Hiatal hernia is a significant risk factor for GERD in persons older than 50 years.
- Fried food, mint, tomato-based foods, and citrus fruits are some foods that can aggravate GERD.
- Consumption of caffeinated beverages and alcohol and cigarette smoking are lifestyle factors that make GERD symptoms worse.
- Prescription and over-the-counter medicines can aggravate GERD.
- LPR occurs when gastric contents reflux into the larynx and pharynx.
- LPR causes hoarseness, voice fatigue, laryngitis, sore throat, chronic cough, bad breath, sinusitis, wheezing, aggravation of asthma, and even middle ear infections.
- Almost two-thirds of the world's population are infected with *H. pylori*, the primary cause of PUD.
- Medicines that can cause the development of ulcers are salicylates (e.g., aspirin), nonsteroidal antiinflammatory drugs (e.g., naproxen), and corticosteroids (e.g., prednisone).
- The treatment of GERD, LPR, and PUD is aimed at reducing GI irritants (e.g., gastric acid, digestive enzymes such as pepsin) and increasing protective factors (e.g., mucus secretion by epithelial cells).
- Acid-neutralizing drugs (antacids), acid-suppressing drugs (PPIs and H2 receptor antagonists), and mucosal protectants (e.g., misoprostol, sucralfate) are used to treat GERD, LPR, and PUD.
- Treatment of PUD also involves eliminating *H. pylori* infection with antimicrobials.
- Prokinetic drugs (e.g., metoclopramide) increase GI motility.
- The four H2 receptor antagonists marketed in the United States and Canada are cimetidine, famotidine, nizatidine, and ranitidine.
- H2 receptor antagonists competitively and reversibly bind to H2 receptors, blocking histamine-mediated acid secretion.
- The six PPIs currently marketed in the United States and Canada are dexlansoprazole, esomeprazole, lansoprazole, omeprazole, pantoprazole, and rabeprazole.
- PPIs decrease gastric acids by interfering with the final step in gastric acid production.
- PPIs are delayed-release formulations and must not be crushed or chewed.
- Misoprostol is synthetic PGE. It stimulates the production of protective mucus and bicarbonate in the stomach.
- Misoprostol is contraindicated in pregnancy.
- Sucralfate binds to the ulcerated area and forms a protective barrier, much like a bandage protects a sore.
- Prokinetic drugs (e.g., metoclopramide, domperidone) increase peristalsis, speed gastric emptying, and improve LES tone.
- Antacids neutralize gastric acids and decrease pepsin secretion.
- Antimicrobials are prescribed in the treatment of PUD to eradicate *H. pylori* infection. Clarithromycin, metronidazole, amoxicillin, and tetracycline are effective for eradicating *H. pylori*.

Review Questions

1. Which sphincter in the digestive system is affected by GERD?
   a. Cardiac sphincter
   b. Pyloric sphincter
   c. Lower esophageal sphincter
   d. Laryngeal sphincter
2. What bacteria contribute to peptic ulcer disease?
   a. Streptococcus
   b. Helicobacter pylori
   c. Staphylococcus
   d. Helicobacter spirella
3. Name two H2 receptor antagonist drugs.
   a. Prilosec and cimetidine
   b. Prevacid and ranitidine
   c. Famotidine and diphenhydramine
   d. Ranitidine and famotidine
4. Proton pump inhibitors are effective in treating GERD, LPR, and PUD because they _____.
   a. Decrease gastric acid
   b. Block histamine
   c. Decrease respiratory mucus
   d. Do none of the above

5. Name two proton pump inhibitor drugs.
   a. Omeprazole and ketoconazole
   b. Esomeprazole and lansoprazole
   c. Pantoprazole and miconazole
   d. Omeprazole and nizatidine
6. _____ is currently the only prokinetic drug approved by the FDA in the United States.
   a. Pantoprazole
   b. Misoprostol
   c. Metoclopramide
   d. Sucralfate
7. _____-containing antacids cause diarrhea; _____-containing antacids cause constipation.
   a. Calcium; aluminum
   b. Magnesium; sodium
   c. Calcium; magnesium
   d. Magnesium; calcium
8. Antacids are the oldest drugs used in the treatment of GERD and PUD. Is this statement true or false?
   a. True
   b. False

9. What is the brand name for esomeprazole?
   a. Aciphex
   b. Protonix
   c. Pepcid
   d. Nexium

10. Which drug binds to the ulcerated area and forms a protective barrier, much like a bandage protects a sore?
   a. Sucralfate
   b. Misoprostol
   c. Axid
   d. Nexium

Bibliography

Archer M, PharmD, Clinical Pharmacist, Oderda G, PharmD, MPH, Professor: University of Utah College of Pharmacy, Copyright © 2012 by University of Utah College of Pharmacy, Salt Lake City, Utah. All rights reserved. Drug Class review: Histamine H2 Receptor Antagonists March 2012.

Food and Drug Administration. Drugs@FDA: FDA Approved Drug Products. nd. From: http://www.accessdata.fda.gov/scripts/cder/daf/. (Retrieved August 13, 2018).

Guimarães E, Marguet C, Moreira Camargos P: Treatment of gastroesophageal reflux disease, *J Pediatr* 82(Suppl):S133–S145, 2006.

Health Canada. Drug Product Database. 2018. From: https://health-products.canada.ca/dpd-bdpp/index-eng.jsp. (Retrieved August 13, 2018).

Howden C, Blume S, de Lissovoy G: Practice patterns for managing *Helicobacter pylori* infection and upper gastrointestinal symptoms, *Am J Manag Care* 13:37–44, 2007.

Institute for Safe Medication Practices. FDA and ISMP Lists of Look-Alike Drug Names with Recommended Tall Man Letters. 2016.

Kabir S: The current status of *Helicobacter pylori* vaccines: a review, *Helicobacter* 12:89–102, 2007.

Kalant H, Grant D, Mitchell J: *Principles of medical pharmacology*, ed 7, Toronto, 2007, Elsevier Canada, pp 557–571.

Lipan M, Reidenberg J, Laitman J: *Anatomy of reflux: a growing health problem affecting structures of the head and neck, the anatomical record. Part B: new anatomy*, New York, 2006, Wiley-Liss, pp 261–270.

Mayo Clinic: GERD: Can certain medications increase severity? 2012. http://www.mayoclinic.com/health/heartburn-gerd/AN00720/METHOD=print.

National Digestive Diseases Information Clearinghouse: *Heartburn, hiatal hernia, and gastroesophageal reflux disease (GERD) (NIH Publ. No. 03-0882)*, Bethesda, MD, 2003, National Institute of Diabetes and Digestive and Kidney Diseases. https://www.niddk.nih.gov/health-information/digestive-diseases.

Pilotto A, Francheschi M, Leandro G, et al: Clinical features of reflux esophagitis in older people: a study of 840 consecutive patients, *J Am Geriatr Soc* 54:1537–1542, 2006.

Web MD: Heartburn/GERD health center, 2012. http://www.webmd.com/heartburn-gerd/guide.

22

Treatment of Irritable Bowel Syndrome, Ulcerative Colitis, and Crohn's Disease

LEARNING OBJECTIVES

1. Learn the terminology associated with irritable bowel syndrome (IBS), ulcerative colitis, and Crohn's disease.
2. List the symptoms of and risk factors for IBS, ulcerative colitis, and Crohn's disease.
3. List and categorize medications used to treat IBS, ulcerative colitis, and Crohn's disease.
4. Describe the mechanisms of action for drugs used to treat IBS, ulcerative colitis, and Crohn's disease.

5. Identify significant drug look-alike and sound-alike issues.
6. List common endings for drug classes used for the treatment of IBS, ulcerative colitis, and Crohn's disease.
7. Identify warning labels and precautionary messages associated with medications used to treat IBS, ulcerative colitis, and Crohn's disease.

KEY TERMS

Antidiarrheals Drugs that prevent or relieve diarrhea
Constipation Abnormally delayed or infrequent passage of dry, hardened feces
Crohn's disease Disease that produces inflammation and damage anywhere along the gastrointestinal tract
Diarrhea Abnormally frequent passage of loose and watery stools
Gastroenteritis Inflammation of the lining membrane of the stomach and the intestines
Inflammatory bowel disease Chronic disorder of the gastrointestinal tract characterized by inflammation of the

intestine, resulting in abdominal cramping and persistent diarrhea
Irritable bowel syndrome Condition that causes abdominal distress and erratic movement of the contents of the large bowel, resulting in diarrhea and/or constipation
Laxative Medicine that induces evacuation of the bowel
Ulcerative colitis Disease that produces inflammation, ulcers, and damage to the colon

Overview

Irritable bowel syndrome (IBS) and *inflammatory bowel disease* (IBD) are conditions of the gastrointestinal (GI) tract. The similar names sometimes cause confusion, but the root causes are not the same. The two major types of IBD are *ulcerative colitis* and *Crohn's disease*. Both conditions are linked to inflammation of the GI tract, unlike IBS. Diagnostic tests that are performed to diagnose ulcerative colitis and Crohn's disease include the testing of stool samples, taking x-rays, and performing a colonoscopy. A colonoscopy is performed by inserting a thin tube with a small light and camera at the end (i.e., an endoscope) into the anus, enabling the physician to examine the colon for inflammation and damage (Fig. 22.1).

Irritable Bowel Syndrome

An estimated 10% to 15% of people in North America have IBS. IBS affects quality of life and productivity for millions of people. Symptoms commonly occur before the age of 35 years. IBS causes

abdominal pain, bloating, and other discomfort. Movement of waste through the colon (large bowel) may occur too slowly, resulting in *constipation*, or it occurs too rapidly, causing *diarrhea*. IBS is sometimes called colitis, but it is not the same condition as ulcerative colitis.

What Causes Irritable Bowel Syndrome?

There is no one specific cause for IBS. Persons with IBS have an overly sensitive colon. Food allergies, stress, antibiotic use, chronic alcohol use, bile acid malabsorption, and infection are possible causes. Some infections may produce stomach and intestinal inflammation (*gastroenteritis*). Postinfectious IBS may follow an acute bout of gastroenteritis. IBS may also be associated with abnormally low levels of the neurotransmitter serotonin. Up to 95% of the body's serotonin (5-HT) is found in the stomach epithelium. The remaining 5% is found in neurons in the brain (see Chapter 6). Low levels of serotonin can cause GI motility problems and increase the sensitivity of pain receptors in the GI tract.

• **Fig. 22.1** Colonoscopy and sigmoidoscopy. (From Chabner DE: *The language of medicine*, ed 10, St. Louis, 2014, Elsevier.)

Inflammatory Bowel Disease

IBD is thought to be an autoimmune disorder whereby the body reacts negatively to its own intestinal tract. The four inflammatory diseases of the bowel are ulcerative colitis, Crohn's disease, ulcerative proctitis, and pouchitis. Ulcerative colitis and Crohn's are the most common and are discussed in this chapter. Ulcerative colitis affects only the colon, and Crohn's can involve any segment of the GI tract. Crohn's may also cause inflammation in the eyes, mouth, or some joints.

Ulcerative Colitis

Ulcerative colitis is one of several irritable bowel diseases that produce inflammation and damage to the colon. Ultimately, *ulcers* (sores) form in the lining of the colon and rectum. Ulcerative colitis can occur at any age but most commonly begins between the ages of 15 and 30 years and affects men and women equally.

Ulcerative colitis differs from Crohn's disease in two important ways. Ulcerative colitis produces inflammation in the upper layers of the lining of the small intestine and colon, whereas Crohn's disease produces inflammation deep in the intestinal wall. Moreover, the inflammation is limited to the small intestine and colon rather than involving other areas of the GI tract.

What Causes Ulcerative Colitis?

The exact cause of ulcerative colitis is unknown, but it is believed to be linked to abnormal functioning of the immune system. When a person has ulcerative colitis, the body's immune system recognizes the bacteria that normally inhabit the GI tract as harmful invaders.

Crohn's Disease

Crohn's disease causes chronic inflammation anywhere along the entire length of the GI tube, from the mouth to the anus, although it typically affects the ileum (the lower part of the small intestine). The inflammation is formed deep within the intestinal wall, causing abdominal pain.

Causes

The root cause of Crohn's disease is not known. The body's immune system is thought to target the bacteria that normally inhabit the GI tract, foods, and other substances, recognizing them as harmful invaders. This produces an inflammatory response, which, if chronic, can lead to ulceration. It is not known whether genes, environmental antigens, microbes, or the body's own immune system triggers the onset of the disease. As with ulcerative colitis, high levels of tumor necrosis factor (TNF) and other substances that are released to fight infection are present in individuals that have Crohn's disease.

Symptoms of Irritable Bowel Syndrome, Ulcerative Colitis, and Crohn's Disease

Many of the symptoms of IBS, ulcerative colitis, and Crohn's disease are similar; however, some of these symptoms are disease-specific. Table 22.1 compares symptoms common to IBS, ulcerative colitis, and Crohn's disease.

Lifestyle Modification

Lifestyle changes can reduce symptoms of IBS, ulcerative colitis, or Crohn's disease. Foods and beverages that aggravate diarrhea, bloating, and gas should be avoided. Stress management may also reduce the frequency of symptoms. A list of lifestyle modifications is given in Box 22.1.

> ● **TECH NOTE!**
> Drinking carbonated beverages and chewing gum can cause gas and bloating.

Drugs Used for the Treatment of Irritable Bowel Syndrome

Drugs used to treat IBS include serotonin receptor antagonists (e.g., alosetron), prostaglandin E1 derivatives (e.g., lubiprostone),

TABLE 22.1 Symptoms of Irritable Bowel Syndrome, Ulcerative Colitis, and Crohn's Dsease

	Irritable Bowel Syndrome	Ulcerative Colitis	Crohn's Disease
Similar symptoms	Abdominal pain Diarrhea (mucus, pus) Cramping	Abdominal pain Diarrhea (bloody) Cramping	Abdominal pain Diarrhea Cramping
Disease-specific symptoms	rratic bowel movements (diarrhea alternating with constipation) Abdominal pain relieved by having a bowel movement Bloating Constipation	Rectal bleeding Aemia Weight loss, loss of appetite Fatigue Loss of vitamins and minerals Skin lesions Joint pain (arthritis) Decreased growth in children Fever	Rectal bleeding Anemia Weight loss, loss of appetite Loss of vitamins and minerals Skin lesions Joint pain (arthritis) Decreased growth in children Fever

---

• BOX 22.1 Lifestyle Modification to Reduce Symptoms of Irritable Bowel Syndrome, Ulcerative Colitis, and Crohn's Disease[a]

- Eat small meals.
- Drink at least six to eight glasses of water daily.
- Avoid alcohol.
- Avoid caffeinated beverages (e.g., coffee, tea, cola drinks).
- Limit carbonated beverages.
- Avoid foods that worsen symptoms.[a]
- Engage in stress-reduction activities.

[a]*Following a diet for celiac disease may reduce symptoms of irritable bowel syndrome. Avoid wheat, rye, barley, dairy, and chocolate.*

---

laxatives, fiber supplements, antidiarrheals, and anticholinergics (e.g., dicyclomine).

Serotonin Receptor Antagonist

New medications have been developed that selectively target the serotonin receptors. The neurotransmitter serotonin controls GI motility. There are a number of types of serotonin receptors. Stimulation of 5-HT$_3$ receptors can cause diarrhea. Stimulation of 5-HT$_4$ receptors produces constipation.

Mechanism of Action

Alosetron acts at the 5-HT$_3$ receptor. The drug decreases gastric motility and regulates transit through the colon, gastric secretions, and visceral pain.

> **TECH NOTE!**
> Alosetron is available only from health care providers who participate in a special prescribing program.

Adverse Reactions

The most common side effects of alosetron therapy are constipation, anxiety, difficulty sleeping or drowsiness, dry mouth, frequent urination, gas, headache, nausea, and restlessness. Alosetron's side effects limit its use. Alosetron may cause severe GI obstruction or impaction, leading to toxic megacolon—a life-threatening condition.

Precautions

Alosetron is only approved for women with severe IBS when other therapies have failed. The US Food and Drug Administration (FDA) requires physicians to obtain special training before prescribing the drug because it can significantly decrease blood flow to the colon, potentially causing ischemic colitis, toxic megacolon, and death.

Serotonin Receptor Antagonist

Generic Name	US Brand Name Canadian Brand Name	Dosage Forms and Strengths
alosetron[a]	Lotronex Not available	**Tablet:** 0.5 mg, 1 mg

[a]Generic available.

Prostaglandin E1 Derivative

Lubiprostone (Amitiza) is FDA-approved for the treatment of IBS in women when constipation is the predominant symptom. Lubiprostone increases intestinal fluid secretion, thus improving the consistency of the stool and reducing straining.

Mechanism of Action

Lubiprostone activates type 2 chloride channels (CIC-2) in the gut, which increases secretions. The increased intestinal fluid volume softens the stool, increases motility in the intestine, and promotes spontaneous bowel movements.

Adverse Reactions

Up to one-third of patients treated with lubiprostone experience nausea. Other side effects are abdominal pain and diarrhea.

Prostaglandin E1 (PGE1) Derivative

Generic Name	US Brand Name Canadian Brand Name	Dosage Forms and Strengths
lubiprostone	Amitiza Not available	**Capsule:** 8 mcg, 24 mcg

Bulk-Forming Laxatives and Fiber Supplements

Bulk-forming laxative and fiber supplements are administered to relieve constipation and diarrhea. Polycarbophil is a bulk-forming laxative that is FDA-approved for the treatment of IBS. It can be obtained without prescription.

Mechanism of Action

Bulk-forming *laxatives* swell in the presence of liquid. Polycarbophil can absorb 60 to 100 times its weight in water to form a gel. Bacteria that normally live in the colon digest the cellulose and polysaccharide fibers. As the bacteria colony grows, colonic bulk increases. The increased bulk causes the bowel to feel full and stimulates peristalsis and transit of contents through the bowel. It also promotes fluid accumulation in the colon.

Adverse Reactions

Bulk-forming laxatives can cause bloating, gas, abdominal cramps, nausea, diarrhea, or constipation.

Opioid Antidiarrheals

Difenoxin, diphenoxylate, and loperamide are opioid *antidiarrheals* that are administered to control watery and frequent stools. Difenoxin and loperamide are more potent than diphenoxylate. Difenoxin and diphenoxylate are Schedule V controlled substance in the United States. Loperamide is available without a prescription.

Mechanism of Action

Opioid antidiarrheals bind to receptors on the smooth muscle cells of the GI tract. They induce spasms that interfere with effective peristalsis. They decrease propulsive contractions by inhibiting the release of acetylcholine. Difenoxin is an active metabolite of diphenoxylate.

Adverse Reactions

Sedation and dizziness are the most common side effects of opioid antidiarrheals. They may also produce constipation. Diphenoxylate and its metabolite difenoxin are controlled substances because they can produce tolerance and dependence.

---

❶ TECH ALERT!

The following drugs have look-alike and sound-alike issues:
difenoxin + atropine
diphenoxylate + atropine

Anticholinergics

Anticholinergic drugs are used for the treatment of IBS when diarrhea is the primary symptom. Atropine and dicyclomine are FDA-approved agents for the treatment of IBS. Atropine and dicyclomine decrease GI muscular tone and motility by producing a nonspecific, direct spasmolytic action on GI smooth muscle.

Bulk-Forming Laxatives

Generic Name	US Brand Names / Canadian Brand Names	Dosage Forms and Strengths	Over the Counter or Prescription
polycarbophil[a]	Equalactin, Fibercon Fiberlax	**Tablet:** 500 mg, 625 mg	OTC
	Equalactin, Fibercon		

[a]Generic available.
OTC, Over-the-counter.

Antidiarrheals

Generic Name	US Brand Names / Canadian Brand Names	Dosage Forms and Strengths	US Controlled Substance Schedule
difenoxin + atropine	Motofen	**Tablet:** 1 mg difenoxin + 0.025 mg atropine	C-IV
	Not available		
diphenoxylate + atropine[a]	Lomotil	**Solution, oral:** 2.5 mg diphenoxylate + 0.025 mg atropine/5 mL	C-V (Schedule I narcotic in Canada)
	Lomotil	**Tablet:** 2.5 mg diphenoxylate + 0.025 mg atropine	
loperamide[a]	Imodium-AD[b]	**Capsule:** 1 mg[b], 2 mg[b]	Not scheduled
	Diarr-Eze,[b] Diarrhea Relief,[b] Imodium Calming Liquid,[b] Imodium Quick Dissolve,[b] Imodium Liqui-gels[b]	**Tablet, ODT[b]:** 2 mg **Tablet[b]:** 2 mg **Solution, oral[b]:** 1 mg/5 mL **Suspension, oral[b]:** 1 mg/7.5 mL	
loperamide + simethicone	Imodium Multi-Symptom Relief[b]	**Tablet[b]:** 2 mg loperamide + 125 mg simethicone	Not scheduled
	Imodium Complete[b]		

[a]Generic available.
[b]Available over-the-counter.

Adverse Reactions

Anticholinergic agents may produce constipation, difficulty sleeping, dry mouth, change in taste, headache, photophobia (increased sensitivity of the eyes to light), nausea, sexual difficulty (e.g., impotence), fast or slow heartbeat, urinary retention, dizziness, or drowsiness. At higher doses, hallucinations may occur.

Anticholinergics

Generic Name	US Brand Name / Canadian Brand Name	Dosage Forms and Strengths
dicyclomine[a]	Bentyl	**Capsule:** 10 mg
	Bentylol, Protylol	**Solution, for injection:** 10 mg/mL **Tablet:** 10 mg,[b] 20 mg **Syrup**[c]**:** 10 mg/5 mL

[a]Generic available.
[b]Available in Canada only.
[c]Available in the United States only.

Drugs Used for the Treatment of Ulcerative Colitis

Medicines administered for the management of ulcerative colitis are used to induce remission, reduce symptoms, and improve quality of life.

Aminosalicylates

Aminosalicylates are administered to patients with ulcerative colitis and Crohn's disease to reduce inflammation. The four aminosalicylate antiinflammatory agents available in the United States and Canada are sulfasalazine, olsalazine, mesalamine (mesalazine in Canada), and balsalazide.

> ### ● TECH NOTE!
> A common ending for aminosalicylates is -salazine.

Mechanism of Action and Pharmacokinetics

Sulfasalazine, olsalazine, and mesalamine (mesalazine in Canada) are all formulations that contain 5-aminosalicylic acid (5-ASA). Sulfasalazine (sulfapyridine+5-ASA) and olsalazine (two 5-ASA molecules) are also prodrugs. Balsalazide is a prodrug of mesalamine. Bacteria in the colon metabolize the drugs and release the active metabolite (5-ASA).

The mechanism of action for aminosalicylates' antiinflammatory action is not completely understood. Sulfasalazine inhibits proinflammatory substances released by the body (e.g., leukotrienes, prostaglandins, cytokines). It also decreases cytokine production. The effectiveness of sulfasalazine and olsalazine is reduced by factors that decrease the bacteria in the colon (e.g., antibiotics) and decrease the gut pH. Delayed-release formulations of 5-ASA are coated with a pH-dependent resin; releasing the active drug in a less acidic environment. The optimal activity of 5-ASA depends on a rise in the pH to greater than 7 in the distal ileum. Pentasa is a time-release formulation.

> ### ● TECH ALERT!
> The following drugs have look-alike and sound-alike issues:
sulfaSALAzine and sulfADIAZINE;
Colazal and Clozaril;
Asacol and Os-Cal

Adverse Reactions

The most common adverse effects of sulfasalazine, olsalazine, mesalamine (mesalazine), and balsalazide are nausea, vomiting, heartburn, headache, and watery diarrhea. Sulfasalazine may also cause sunburn, impaired folic acid absorption, crystalluria, and damage to white blood cells (cytopenias).

Aminosalicylates

Generic Name	US Brand Names / Canadian Brand Names	Dosage Forms and Strengths
balsalazide[a]	Colazal, Giazo	**Capsule (Colazal):** 750 mg
	Not available	**Tablet (Giazo):** 1.1 Gm
mesalamine[a] (known as mesalazine in Canada; 5-aminosalicylic acid [5-ASA])	Apriso, Asacol HD, Canasa, Delzicol, Lialda, Pentasa, Rowasa, sfRowasa	**Capsule, biphasic, extended-release (Apriso):** 0.375 g[b] **Capsule, extended-release:** 250 mg,[b] 400 mg, 500 mg[b] **Suppository:** 500 mg,[c] 1 g
	Asacol, Asacol-800, Mezavant, Pentasa, Salofalk	**Suspension, rectal (Pentasa):** 1 g/100 mL,[c] 4 g/100 mL[c] **Suspension, rectal (Salofalk, Rowasa):** 2 g/60 mL[c]; 4 g/60 mL **Tablet, delayed-release (Asacol HD, Asacol-800):** 400 mg,[c] 800 mg **Tablet, delayed- and extended-release (Lialda, Mezavant):** 1.2 g **Tablet, enteric-coated (Salofalk):** 500 mg[c] **Tablet, extended-release (Pentasa):** 500 mg[c], 1 gm[c]
olsalazine	Dipentum	**Capsule:** 250 mg
	Dipentum	
sulfasalazine[a]	Azulfidine, Azulfidine EN Tabs	**Tablet:** 500 mg **Tablet, enteric-coated:** 500 mg
	Salazopyrin, Salazopyrin EN Tabs	

[a]Generic available.
[b]Available in the United States only.
[c]Available in Canada only.

Corticosteroids

Corticosteroids (e.g., prednisone) are commonly prescribed to suppress inflammation, reduce flare-ups, and treat pain associated with ulcerative colitis and Crohn's disease. They decrease the synthesis of proinflammatory substances such as prostaglandins (see Chapter 10), leukotrienes, cytokines, arachidonic acid, and macrophages that are released as part of the inflammatory response. Corticosteroids have immunosuppressive actions that may inhibit the abnormal immune system activity associated with Crohn's disease and ulcerative colitis. Corticosteroids prescribed to treat ulcerative colitis and Crohn's disease may be administered by mouth or rectally in the form of an enema or suppository.

Adverse Reactions

Oral administration produces systemic effects, described in Chapter 15. Up to 40% of patients treated for Crohn's disease become corticosteroid-dependent. Adverse effects caused by rectal administration may be local (e.g., burning, itching) or systemic (e.g., nausea, constipation or diarrhea, appetite changes, headache). Rectal and "gut-specific" formulations are presented in this chapter.

Corticosteroids

Generic Name	US Brand Names / Canadian Brand Names	Dosage Forms and Strengths
budesonide	Entocort EC, Uceris / Cortiment, Entocort, Entocort Enema	**Capsule (Entocort):** 3 mg **Rectal foam[b]:** 2 mg/actuation **Rectal suspension[b]:** 2.3 mg/115 mL **Tablet, delayed and extended release (Cortiment, Uceris):** 9 mg
hydrocortisone[a]	Colocort, Cortenema, Cortifoam / Cortenema, Cortifoam	**Foam, rectal (Cortifoam):** 10% **Suspension, rectal (Colocort, Cortenema):** 100 mg/60 mL
hydrocortisone + pramoxine	Proctofoam / Proctofoam	**Rectal foam:** 1% hydrocortisone + 1% pramoxine

[a]Generic available.
[b]Available in the United States only.

Drugs Used for the Treatment of Crohn's Disease

Given the similarity of symptoms and the similar mechanism of disease progression of Crohn's disease and ulcerative colitis, many agents used for the treatment of these diseases are the same.

Aminosalicylates, corticosteroids, immunosuppressants, antidiarrheals, and nutritional supplements are used for the treatment of both Crohn's disease and ulcerative colitis. Additional medications used for the treatment of Crohn's disease are immunosuppressants, immunomodulators and antibiotics.

> ❶ *TECH ALERT!*
>
> The following drugs have look-alike and sound-alike issues: azaTHIOprine and AzaCITIDdine;

Immunosuppressants

Azathioprine, 6-mercaptopurine, and methotrexate are classified as antimetabolites. They are used for the treatment of Crohn's disease to induce remission. Azathioprine suppresses the T-cell–mediated

Immunosuppressants

Generic Name	US Brand Names / Canadian Brand Names	Dosage Forms and Strengths
azathioprine[a,b]	Azasan, Imuran / Imuran	**Powder, for injection:** 50 mg/vial,[c] 100 mg/vial[b] **Tablet:** 25 mg,[b] 50 mg, 75 mg,[b] 100 mg[b]
6-mercaptopurine[a,b]	Purinethol, Purixan / Purinethol	**Suspension, oral (Purixan):** 20 mg/mL **Tablet:** 50 mg
methotrexate[a]	Trexall, Otrexup, Rasuvo, Xatmep / Generics	**Tablet:** 2.5 mg, 5 mg,[b] 7.5 mg,[b] 10 mg, 15 mg[b] **Solution, for subcutaneous injection (Otrexup, Metoject, Rasuvo):** 7.5 mg/0.15 mL,[b] 10 mg/0.2 mL,[b] 10 mg/0.4 mL,[b] 12.5 mg/0.25 mL,[b] 15 mg/0.3 mL,[b] 15 mg/0.4 mL,[b] 17.5 mg/0.35 mL, 17.5 mg/0.4 mL,[b] 20 mg/0.4 mL, 22.5 mg/0.4 mL,[b] 22.5 mg/0.45 mL, 25 mg/0.5 mL, 27.5 mg/0.55 mL,[b] 30 mg/0.6 mL[b] **Solution, injection:** 10 mg/mL[c] 25 mg/mL **Solution, oral (Xatmep):** 2 mg/mL

[a]Generic available.
[b]Available in the United States only.
[c]Available in Canada only.

immune system response. Methotrexate decreases cytokine and immunoglobulin production and cyclooxygenase-2 (COX-2) activity. Decreasing these pro-inflammatory substances reduces both inflammation and immune system activity (see Chapter 13).

Immunomodulators

Adalimumab, certolizumab, golimumab, infliximab, and natalizumab are immunomodulators that have been approved for the treatment of moderate to severe Crohn's disease or ulcerative colitis. They are administered to induce remission of active disease and then continued as maintenance therapy in patients who have had unsuccessful results with other therapies.

> ### ● TECH NOTE!
> A common ending for immunomodulators is *-mab*.

Mechanism of Action

Most immunomodulator biologics used for the treatment of Crohn's disease are a genetically engineered TNF-α inhibitors. Infliximab blocks the inflammatory process by preventing cell lysis (destruction) and the release of substances that cause inflammation. A detailed description of the mechanism of action for TNF-α inhibitors is given in Chapter 13. Natalizumab is an α_4 integrin inhibitor. It reduces T-cell–mediated intestinal inflammation. Additional immunomodulators are discussed in Chapter 32.

Adverse Reactions

Common adverse reactions to infliximab are nausea, stomach pain, headache, redness, and itching at the site of infusion. It may also increase susceptibility to opportunistic infections, reactivate dormant infections (e.g., tuberculosis), or worsen of existing infection.

> ### ● TECH NOTE!
> Infliximab package labeling contains a boxed warning that the drug may cause serious infections and malignancies.

> ### ● TECH NOTE!
> Patients taking natalizumab (Tysabri) must be enrolled in an FDA Risk Evaluation and Mitigation Strategy (REMS) program.

Antiinfectives

Patients who have Crohn's disease may develop fistulas. A fistula forms when an ulcer tunnels from the site of origin to surrounding tissues. Fistulas may be located in the bladder, vagina, or skin surrounding the anus and rectum. Antiinfective agents may be prescribed to treat infections that develop in the fistula. Fistulas may be treated with ampicillin, sulfonamides, cephalosporins, tetracycline, or metronidazole; these drugs are described in Chapter 29.

TECHNICIAN'S CORNER

1. Why might bulk-forming laxatives be useful for treating IBS with diarrhea or constipation?
2. Which lifestyle modifications might lessen the symptoms of irritable bowel syndrome?

■ Immunomodulators

Biosimilar Name	US Brand Names / Canadian Brand Names	Dosage Forms and Strengths
adalimumab-ATTO adalimumab-ADBM adalimumab	Amjevita Cyltezo Humira Humira	**Solution, for injection:** 20 mg/0.4 mL,[a] 40 mg/0.8 mL (Amjevita)
certolizumab	Cimzia Cimzia	**Powder, for injection:** 200 mg/vial **Solution, for injection:** 200 mg/mL
golimumab	Simponi, Simponi Aria Simponi, Simponi IV	**Solution, for injection:** 50 mg/0.5 mL; 100 mg/mL **Solution, Intravenous (Simponi Aria, Simponi IV)** 50 mg/4 mL (12.5 mg/mL)
infliximab, infliximab-DYYB, infliximab-QBTX infliximab-ADBA	Remicade, Inflectra, Ixifi Reflexis Remicade, Inflectra, Reflexis	**Powder, for injection:** 100 mg/vial
natalizumab	Tysabri Tysabri	**Solution for injection:** 300 mg/15 mL (20 mg/mL)

[a]Available in the United States only.

■ Summary of Drugs Used for the Treatment of Irritable Bowel Disease, Ulcerative Colitis, and Crohn's Disease

Generic Name	US Brand Name	Usual Adult Oral Dose and Dosing Schedule	Warning Labels
Serotonin Receptor Antagonist			
alosetron	Lotronex	IBS: 0.5–1 mg twice daily	MAY CAUSE DIZZINESS OR DROWSINESS; AVOID DRIVING. AVOID ALCOHOL. TAKE WITH A FULL GLASS OF WATER.

Continued

Summary of Drugs Used for the Treatment of Irritable Bowel Disease, Ulcerative Colitis, and Crohn's Disease—cont'd

Generic Name	US Brand Name	Usual Adult Oral Dose and Dosing Schedule	Warning Labels
Prostaglandin E1 Derivative			
lubiprostone	Amitiza	**IBS:** 8–24 mcg twice daily	TAKE WITH A FULL GLASS OF WATER. TAKE WITH FOOD.
Bulk-Forming Laxatives			
polycarbophil	Equalactin	**IBS:** 2 tablets 1–4 times daily	TAKE WITH A FULL GLASS OF WATER.
Antidiarrheals			
difenoxin + atropine[a]	Motofen	**Acute diarrhea:** 2 tablets immediately; then 1 tablet after each loose stool every 3–4 hr (maximum 8 tabs/day)	MAY CAUSE DIZZINESS OR DROWSINESS; AVOID DRIVING. AVOID ALCOHOL. DRINK LOTS OF FLUIDS.
diphenoxylate + atropine[a]	Lomotil	**Acute diarrhea:** 2 tablets immediately; then 1–2 tablet 4 times daily	
loperamide[a]	Imodium	**Acute diarrhea:** 2 tablets immediately; then 1 tablet after each loose stool (maximum 16 mg/day)	
Anticholinergics			
dicyclomine	Bentyl	**IBS:** 20 mg to 40 mg orally 4 times daily, 10–20 mg IM 4 times a day; maximum 1–2 days	MAY CAUSE DIZZINESS OR DROWSINESS; AVOID DRIVING. AVOID ALCOHOL. DRINK LOTS OF FLUIDS. TAKE ON AN EMPTY STOMACH. AVOID ANTACIDS WITHIN 1–2 H OF DOSE.
Aminosalicylates			
balsalazide	Colazal, Giazo	**Ulcerative colitis (UC):** 3 caps (2250 mg) 3 times daily for 8–12 weeks (Colazal); Men, 3.3 g orally twice daily for up to 8 weeks (Giazo)	SWALLOW WHOLE; DON'T CRUSH OR CHEW. CAPSULE CONTENTS MAY BE SPRINKLED ON APPLESAUCE.
mesalamine (5-ASA)	Canasa	**UC:** Insert one suppository rectally twice daily	REMOVE FOIL AND INSERT (SUPPOSITORY). MAY DISCOLOR CLOTHING OR SKIN (ORANGE-YELLOW, SUPPOSITORY). SHAKE WELL (RECTAL SUSPENSION). SWALLOW WHOLE; DON'T CRUSH OR CHEW (DELAYED RELEASE). TAKE WITH FOOD (DELAYED RELEASE). DO NOT SUBSTITUTE ASACOL HD WITH DELZICOL (not interchangeable)
	Rowasa	**UC:** 4 g enema nightly	
	Asacol-HD, Delzicol	**UC:** 1 tablet 3 times daily	
	Lialda	**UC:** 2–4 tablets once daily for up to 8 weeks	
	Pentasa, Mesasal, Salofalk	**UC:** 1 g 4 times daily	
olsalazine	Dipentum	**UC:** 1 g daily in 2 divided doses	SWALLOW WHOLE; DON'T CRUSH OR CHEW. TAKE WITH FOOD.
sulfasalazine	Azulfidine	**UC:** 1 g 3 or 4 times daily	SWALLOW WHOLE; DON'T CRUSH OR CHEW (ENTERIC-COATED TABLETS). AVOID PROLONGED EXPOSURE TO SUNLIGHT. DRINK LOTS OF FLUIDS.
Corticosteroids			
hydrocortisone	Cortema	**UC:** 100 mg rectal enema nightly for 21 days	SHAKE WELL.
	Anucort	**UC:** 1 suppository rectally 2 to 3 times daily for 2 weeks	REMOVE FOIL AND INSERT.
	Cortifoam	**UC:** 1 applicatorful 1 to 2 times daily for 2 to 3 weeks; then every other day	SHAKE WELL.

Summary of Drugs Used for the Treatment of Irritable Bowel Disease, Ulcerative Colitis, and Crohn's Disease—cont'd

	Generic Name	US Brand Name	Usual Adult Oral Dose and Dosing Schedule	Warning Labels
Immunosuppressants	azathioprine	Azasan, Imuran	Dose not listed in FDA or Health Canada labeling	TAKE WITH FOOD – AZATHIOPRINE. AVOID ALCOHOL. AVOID PREGNANCY.
	6-mecaptopurine	Purinethol	Dose not listed in FDA or Health Canada labeling	
	methotrexate	Trexall	Dose not listed in FDA or Health Canada labeling	
Immunomodulators	adalimumab	Humira	**Crohn's and UC:** 160 mg followed by 80 mg in 2 weeks; then 40 mg maintenance dose every other week starting on day 29 of therapy.	REPORT SIGNS OF INFECTION. DO NOT MISS DOSES.
	certolizumab	Cimzia	**Crohn's:** 400 mg subcutaneously followed by 400 mg at weeks 2 and 4; then every 4 weeks thereafter if necessary.	
	golimumab	Simponi	**UC:** 200 mg subcutaneously followed by 100 mg at week 2 and every 4 weeks thereafter	
	infliximab	Remicade	**Crohn's or UC:** 5 mg/kg IV at weeks 0, 2, and 6; then every 8 weeks	
	natalizumab	Tysabri	**Crohn's:** 300 mg IV infusion given over 1 h every 4 weeks. Revaluate every 3 months	

Key Points

- Irritable bowel syndrome, ulcerative colitis, and Crohn's disease are conditions that are linked to inflammation of the GI tract.
- Abdominal pain, diarrhea, and cramping are common symptoms of IBS, ulcerative colitis, and Crohn's disease.
- Persons with IBS may have diarrhea or constipation.
- In ulcerative colitis and Crohn's disease, the body's immune system recognizes the bacteria that normally inhabit the GI tract as harmful invaders.
- Ulcerative colitis produces inflammation in the upper layers of the lining of the small intestine and colon.
- Crohn's disease may produce inflammation and can occur anywhere along the entire length of the GI tube, from the mouth to the anus, although typically it affects the ileum (the lower part of the small intestine). Inflammation occurs deep in the intestinal wall.
- Lifestyle modification such as stress management, eating small meals, and avoiding alcohol and caffeinated and carbonated beverages can reduce symptoms of IBS, ulcerative colitis, and Crohn's disease. IBS may be treated by administering a serotonin receptor antagonist, antidiarrheal, laxative, fiber supplement, or anticholinergic agent.
- Alosetron is a $5\text{-}HT_3$ receptor antagonist used in women to control diarrhea caused by severe IBS when other types of treatment have failed.
- Alosetron prescriptions cannot be refilled without a follow-up examination by the physician.
- Lubiprostone is a prostaglandin derivative approved for the treatment of IBS with constipation.
- Bulk-forming laxative and fiber supplements are given to relieve constipation and diarrhea.
- Antidiarrheals control watery, frequent stools.
- Diphenoxylate and difenoxin, controlled substances in the United States, may cause tolerance and dependence.
- Loperamide is not habit forming and is sold over the counter.
- Atropine and dicyclomine decrease diarrhea by reducing GI muscular tone and motility.
- The aminosalicylates sulfasalazine, olsalazine, balsalazide, and mesalamine (mesalazine) are administered to patients with ulcerative colitis and Crohn's disease to reduce inflammation.
- All commercially available aminosalicylates are formulated as delayed-release products.
- Glucocorticosteroids are prescribed commonly to suppress inflammation, reduce flare-ups, and treat pain associated with ulcerative colitis and Crohn's disease.
- Glucocorticosteroids have immunosuppressive actions that may inhibit the abnormal immune system activity associated with Crohn's disease and ulcerative colitis.
- Infliximab is an immunomodulator approved for the treatment of Crohn's disease; it is administered to induce remission.
- Infliximab is a TNF-α inhibitor that is genetically engineered to block the inflammatory process.
- Patients who have Crohn's disease may develop fistulas. Antiinfective agents may be prescribed to treat fistula infections.

Review Questions

1. Which disease(s) is/are linked to inflammation of the entire GI tract?
   a. Irritable bowel syndrome
   b. Ulcerative colitis
   c. Crohn's disease
   d. All of the above

2. How must adalimumab (Humira) be stored?
   a. At room temperature
   b. In the refrigerator
   c. Kept frozen in the freezer
   d. Either refrigerated or stored at room temperature

3. Which of the following drugs is marketed as a powder that must be reconstituted prior to administration?
   a. Cimzia
   b. Cortenema
   c. Sulfasalazine suspension
   d. diclomine syrup

4. Name three common symptoms of irritable bowel syndrome, ulcerative colitis, and Crohn's disease:
   a. Bloating, constipation, cramping
   b. Abdominal pain, diarrhea, cramping
   c. Rectal bleeding, bloating, diarrhea
   d. Cramping, abdominal pain, bloating

5. Which of the following drugs is used to treat IBS in which constipation is the primary symptom?
   a. Amitiza
   b. Lotronex
   c. Lovenox
   d. Alosetron

6. _____ are administered to treat the symptoms of irritable bowel syndrome.
   a. Bulk-forming laxatives
   b. Fiber supplements
   c. Bile acid sequestrants
   d. a and b

7. An immunomodulator that has been approved for the treatment of Crohn's disease is _____.
   a. Golimumab
   b. Methotrexate
   c. Lomotil
   d. Budesonide

8. Patients who have Crohn's disease may develop _____, which form when an ulcer tunnels from the site of origin to surrounding tissues.
   a. Ulcers
   b. Fistulas
   c. Diverticuli
   d. None of the above

9. Select corticosteroid that is formulated for rectal use _____.
   a. Enterocort EC
   b. Medrol
   c. prednisone
   d. Cortenema

10. These warning labels should be applied to prescription vials for which class of drugs used for IBS? "May cause dizziness or drowsiness; avoid driving, avoid alcohol, drink lots of fluids, take on an empty stomach."
    a. Anticholinergics
    b. Bulk-forming laxatives
    c. Serotonin antagonists
    d. Corticosteroids

Bibliography

American College of Gastroenterology Task Force on Irritable Bowel Syndrome, Brandt LJ, Chey WD, et al: An evidence-based position statement on the management of irritable bowel syndrome, *Am J Gastroenterol* 104(Suppl 1):S1–S35, 2009.

Bressler B, Marshall J, et al: Clinical practice guidelines for the medical management of nonhospitalized ulcerative colitis: the Toronto consensus, *Gastroenterology* 148(5):1035–1958, 2015.

Chang J, Talley N: Current and emerging therapies in irritable bowel syndrome: from pathophysiology to treatment, *Trends Pharmacol Sci* 31:326–328, 2010.

Crohn's & Colitis Foundation, 2017. Immunomodulators Fact Sheet. Retrieved Aug. 12, 2017, from www.crohnscolitisfoundation.org.

Food and Drug Administration, nd. Drugs@FDA: FDA Approved Drug Products. Retrieved Aug 15, 2018, from http://www.accessdata.fda.gov/scripts/cder/daf/.

Health Canada, 2018. Drug Product Database. Retrieved August 15, 2018, from https://health-products.canada.ca/dpd-bdpp/index-eng.jsp.

Institute for Safe Medication Practices, 2016. FDA and ISMP Lists of Look-Alike Drug Names with Recommended Tall Man Letters.

Kalant H, Grant D, Mitchell J: *Pharmacotherapy of intestinal Motility Disorders and Inflammatory Bowel Disease Principles of medical pharmacology*, ed 7, Toronto, 2007, Elsevier Canada, pp 572–583.

Love BL: Pharmacotherapy for moderate to severe inflammatory bowel disease: evolving strategies, *Am J Manag Care* 22(3):s39–s50, 2016.

National Digestive Diseases Information Clearinghouse: Crohn's disease, 2016. Retrieved 12 August 2017 from http://www.digestive.niddk.nih.gov/ddiseases/pubs/crohns/index.aspx).

National Digestive Diseases Information Clearinghouse: Irritable bowel syndrome, 2015. Retrieved 12 August 2017 from http://www.digestive.niddk.nih.gov/ddiseases/pubs/ibs/index.aspx.

National Digestive Diseases Information Clearinghouse: Ulcerative colitis, 2014. Retrieved 12 August 2017 from http://www.digestive.niddk.nih.gov/ddiseases/pubs/colitis/index.aspx.

Terdiman JP, Gruss CB, Heidelbaugh JJ, et al: American Gastroenterological Association Institute guideline on the use of thiopurines, methotrexate, and anti–TNF-a biologic drugs for the induction and maintenance of remission in inflammatory Crohn's disease, *Gastroenterology* 145:1459–1463, 2013.

Xia H: Post-infectious irritable bowel syndrome, *World J Gastroenterol* 15(29):3591–3596, 2009.

Drugs Affecting the Respiratory System

Respiration involves the exchange of oxygen (O_2) and carbon dioxide ($CO_{2)}$ in the cells in the body. A properly functioning respiratory system ensures that the tissues of the body receive an adequate oxygen supply and carbon dioxide is promptly removed. In addition, the respiratory system effectively filters, warms, and humidifies the air we breathe. Respiratory organs also influence sound reproduction, including speech used in communicating oral language. Specialized epithelia in the respiratory tract make the sense of smell (olfaction) possible. The respiratory system also plays an important role in the regulation, or homeostasis, of pH (acid-base balance) in the body. Functionally, the respiratory system includes the lungs and accessory structures such as the oral cavity, rib cage, and respiratory muscles, including the diaphragm. Diseases of the respiratory tract, such as asthma, chronic obstructive pulmonary disease (COPD), and cystic fibrosis affect the upper and lower respiratory tract. They impair breathing and gas exchange. In Unit VII, the pharmacotherapy for asthma, chronic obstructive pulmonary disease (COPD) and asthma is presented. A brief description of each disorder is provided, followed by a description of the drugs indicated for treatment that includes mechanisms of action, adverse reactions, strength(s), dosage forms and OTC or prescription status.

23

Treatment of Asthma and Chronic Obstructive Pulmonary Disease

LEARNING OBJECTIVES

1. Learn the terminology associated with asthma and chronic obstructive pulmonary disease (COPD).
2. List risk factors for asthma and COPD.
3. List the symptoms of asthma and COPD.
4. List and categorize medications used in the treatment of asthma and COPD.
5. Describe the mechanism of action of drugs used to treat asthma and COPD.
6. Identify significant drug look-alike and sound-alike issues.
7. List common endings for drug classes used for the treatment of asthma and COPD.
8. Identify warning labels and precautionary messages associated with medications used to treat asthma and COPD.

KEY TERMS

Allergic asthma Asthma symptoms induced by a hypersensitivity reaction upon exposure to environmental allergens.

Asthma A chronic disease that affects the airways, producing irritation, inflammation, and difficulty breathing.

Bronchodilator A drug that relaxes tightened airway muscles and improves airflow through the airways.

Chronic obstructive pulmonary disease A progressive disease of the airways that produces a gradual loss of pulmonary function.

Forced expiratory volume The maximum volume of air that can be breathed out in 1 second; also called forced vital capacity.

Metered-dose inhaler A device used for delivering a dose of inhaled medication. A solution or powder is delivered as a mist and inhaled.

Nebulizer A device that converts a liquid drug into a mist that is inhaled.

Peak flow meter A handheld device used to measure the volume of air exhaled and how rapidly the air is moved out.

Spacer A device attached to the end of a metered-dose inhaler that facilitates drug delivery into the lungs (rather than to the back of the throat).

Spirometry A test that measures the volume of air that is expired (blown out of the lungs) after taking a deep breath and how rapidly the volume of air is expired.

Asthma

Overview

Asthma is a chronic disease that affects the airways, producing irritation, inflammation, and difficulty breathing. As many as 25 million adults and 7 million children in the United States have been diagnosed with asthma, making it the number one chronic disease of childhood. Approximately 2.4 million Canadians 12 years of age and older have asthma, according to Statistics Canada. Females are more likely than males to report that they have asthma.

The burden of disease attributed to asthma is great because it is responsible for missed days at school and work and increased health care costs due to emergency department visits, hospitalization, and outpatient doctor visits. Asthma is the reason for more than 13.3 million healthcare visits annually.

Asthma is classified according to the severity of symptoms. The three classifications for asthma are mild, moderate, and severe (Box 23.1).

It is not known exactly why some people develop asthma and others do not; however, there are factors that can increase the risk for asthma. A prime example is a positive family history of asthma or exposure to tobacco smoke. Research suggests that during pregnancy, secondhand smoke exposure may be just as damaging to the unborn baby as to the mother. Chronic exposure to other sources of air pollution and exposure to some allergens and infections early in life may also be risk factors.

Pathophysiology

Symptoms of asthma are linked to a progression of physiologic changes in the airways. Initially, the airways (bronchial tube and

• BOX 23.1 Classification of Asthma*

- **Mild asthma**: Well controlled with "as-needed" reliever medication alone or with low-intensity controller treatment such as low-dose inhaled corticosteroids (ICSs) or leukotriene receptor antagonists
- **Moderate asthma**: Well controlled with low-dose ICS/long-acting beta₂-agonists (LABAs)
- **Severe asthma**: Requires high-dose ICSs/LABAs to prevent it from becoming uncontrolled or asthma that remains uncontrolled despite this treatment

*Asthma classifications adapted from 2016 Global Initiative for Asthma (GINA) guidelines.

• BOX 23.2 Common Symptoms of Asthma

- Cough
- Wheezing
- Shortness of breath
- Chest tightness

• BOX 23.3 Asthma Triggers

Allergens
- Animal dander (from the skin, hair, or feathers of animals)
- Dust mites (contained in house dust)
- Cockroaches
- Pollen from trees and grass
- Mold (indoor and outdoor)

Irritants
- Cigarette smoke
- Air pollution
- Cold air or changes in weather
- Strong odors from painting or cooking
- Scented products
- Strong emotional expression (including crying or laughing hard) and stress

Others
- Medicines such as aspirin and beta blockers
- Sulfites in food (dried fruit) or beverages (wine)
- Gastroesophageal reflux disease and laryngopharyngeal reflux, which can worsen asthma symptoms
- Irritants or allergens that one may be exposed to at work, such as special chemicals or dusts

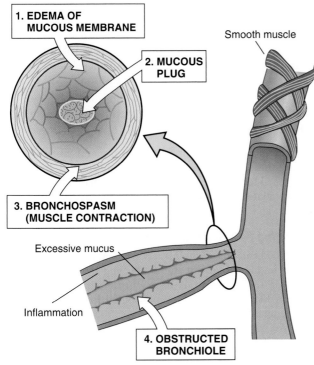

• **Fig. 23.1** Airway changes during an asthma episode. (From VanMeter KC, Hubert RJ: *Gould's pathophysiology for the heart professions*, ed 5, St. Louis, 2014, Elsevier.)

bronchioles) become irritated. This causes airway constriction, which makes the passage of air more difficult. Airways also become inflamed and swollen, further restricting the flow of air through the bronchial passages. Mucus production is increased above normal levels, which can also obstruct breathing passages (Fig. 23.1).

Symptoms

Airway constriction, inflammation, and mucus produce characteristic asthma symptoms (Box 23.2) such as coughing, wheezing, shortness of breath (SOB), and chest tightness. Symptoms may be mild or severe (i.e., life threatening) and vary for each individual. During

an asthma episode (often called an asthma attack), breathing may be noisy and labored. A whistling or creaking sound may be heard with inspiration and expiration. Patients describe chest tightness that feels as though something or someone were "squeezing or sitting on their chest" and the feeling that they cannot get enough air into their lungs. Actually, SOB is associated with reduced expiration rather than decreased inspiration. Breathing may become faster and shallower. Nocturnal asthma is a condition characterized by decreased FEV1 (*forced expiratory volume* in 1 second). The maximal volume of air that can be breathed out in 1 second is reduced. Increased airway inflammation is present, along with exaggerated bronchial constriction (hyperresponsiveness). Cough at night may disrupt sleep. In one study of patients with asthma, as many as 74% reported nocturnal asthma symptoms at least once weekly. In nocturnal asthma, lung function and antiinflammatory hormones (e.g., cortisol) decrease and the release of pro-inflammatory mediators (e.g., leukotrienes, cytokines) increases in the middle of the night, according to the patient's circadian rhythm (biologic clock).

Asthma Triggers

Asthma triggers are things that can precipitate an asthma episode in individuals with asthma (Box 23.3). An asthma episode is also called an asthma attack. Examples of triggers are allergens such as animal dander, environmental pollutants, cleaning fluid, mold, tobacco smoke, and even cold air. Exposure to cockroach droppings and air pollution is linked to the rise of asthma in inner-city youth. Other triggers are upper respiratory infection and strenuous exercise. The risk for exercise-induced asthma can be minimized by taking prescribed medicines prior to exercise.

Managing Asthma Symptoms

Asthma symptoms can be managed with a combination of medication, lifestyle modification, and home monitoring of breathing using a peak flow meter and medication. Asthma has two main components, airway inflammation and acute bronchoconstriction (constriction of the airways). The drugs administered for the treatment and management of asthma are divided into two classes. Rescue medicines treat the acute symptoms and include short-acting β_2-adrenergic agonists such as albuterol (salbutamol in Canada). Maintenance therapy is used to prevent asthma episodes. Maintenance medications include long-acting β_2-adrenergic agonists (e.g., salmeterol), inhaled corticosteroids (e.g., budesonide), leukotriene modifiers (e.g., montelukast), mast cell stabilizers (e.g., ipratropium bromide), and xanthine derivatives (e.g., aminophylline). The key to preventing asthma attacks, hospitalizations, and death from asthma is reducing and preventing further inflammation.

A *peak flow meter* is a handheld device used to measure the volume of air exhaled and how fast the air is exhaled. Regular measurements can enable a person with asthma to spot trends that signal an impending attack. A peak flow meter permits patients to manage their asthma, similar to the way in which patients with diabetes monitor their blood glucose levels to manage their disease. Low peak flow numbers signal that asthma is not controlled. *Spirometry* is a test that is performed to measure the volume of air that is expired (blown out of the lungs) after taking a deep breath and how rapidly the volume of air is expired.

Drugs Used for the Treatment of Acute Symptoms: Relievers

Rescue medicines, also known as relievers, provide rapid and short-term relief of asthma symptoms. They reverse bronchospasm and open airways. Albuterol (also known as salbutamol) is a short-acting β_2-adrenergic agonist and the most frequently prescribed *bronchodilator*. Other β_2-adrenergic agonists prescribed for the treatment of asthma include levalbuterol, metaproterenol, and terbutaline. β_2-Adrenergic agonists are commonly administered by oral inhalation using a *metered-dose inhaler* (MDI) or *nebulizer*. Ipratropium bromide is also administered by the inhalation route. Ipratropium bromide may be administered in combination with a β_2-adrenergic agonist for the relief of acute symptoms.

> **TECH NOTE!**
> In 2008, manufacturers were required to remove chlorofluorocarbon (CFC) compounds from propellants used in metered-dose inhalers because CFCs deplete the ozone layer.

Mechanism of Action

Bronchial airways are composed of smooth muscle that is innervated by β_2, α_1, α_2, and muscarinic (M1 and M3) receptors. Short-acting β_2-adrenergic agonists relax bronchial smooth muscle, causing airways to dilate and thus reversing bronchospasms. Levalbuterol is an isomer of albuterol and is a moderately selective β_2-adrenergic receptor agonist.

> **TECH NOTE!**
> To determine whether the contents of some metered-dose inhalers are low, patients should check the counter mechanism on the inhaler. The counter shows the number of doses that are left.

Pharmacokinetics

Short-acting β_2-adrenergic agonists have a rapid onset and short duration of action. The onset of action for albuterol is within 15 minutes and the peak effect occurs within 30 minutes to 2 hours.

The duration of action of albuterol is 2 to 6 hours compared with its isomer, levalbuterol, which has a duration of action of approximately 3 to 6 hours.

The bioavailability of ipratropium bromide is low, which accounts for the low incidence of adverse reactions.

Adverse Reactions

Drugs such as albuterol can produce nervousness, difficulty sleeping, dry mouth, mild headache, and throat irritation (inhalants only). Beta receptors are also located on heart and skeletal muscle, so the use of β_2-adrenergic agonists can increase the heart rate and can lead to arrhythmias, hypertension, palpitations, tachycardia, and tremors. β_2-adrenergic stimulation may also produce hyperglycemia, hypokalemia, and increased insulin secretion. Ipratropium bromide can cause difficulty urinating and blurred vision.

> **TECH NOTE!**
> Excessive use of reliever medication is a sign that the asthma is not well controlled.

Precautions

Store the canister at room temperature, because exposure to excessive heat can cause the canister to explode. Excessive cold can reduce the effectiveness of albuterol. Keep the albuterol nebulizer solution in its foil package until time of use; protect from light.

Maintenance Therapy to Prevent Asthma Flare-Ups

Drugs that are intended for long-term use and taken daily to prevent asthma symptoms are called controllers. The five classes of drugs used for asthma prophylaxis are long-acting β_2-adrenergic agonists, inhaled corticosteroids, leukotriene modifiers, mast cell stabilizers, and xanthine derivatives.

Long-Acting β_2-Adrenergic Agonists

The US Food and Drug Administration (FDA) and Health Canada updated the indications for the use of long-acting beta agonists (LABAs) in the treatment of asthma because of safety concerns. To ensure the safe use of these products, the following guidelines are recommended:

- LABAs are contraindicated without the use of an inhaled corticosteroid. Single-ingredient LABAs should not be used alone.
- LABA use should be limited to the shortest duration of time required to achieve control of asthma symptoms and then discontinued.

Long-term use of LABAs should be restricted to patients whose asthma cannot be adequately controlled with controller medications:

- Combination inhaled corticosteroid and a LABA are recommended for pediatric and adolescent patients when the addition of an LABA is required.

> **❶ TECH ALERT!**
> The following drugs have look-alike and sound-alike issues:
> Foradil and Toradol
> salmeterol and salbutamol

Short-Acting β₂-Adrenergic Agonists

Generic Name	US Brand Names Canadian Brand Names	Dosage Forms and Strengths
albuterol[a] (salbutamol)	AccuNeb, Proair HFA, Proair Respiclick, Proventil HFA, Ventolin HFA, VoSpire ER Airomir, Ventolin Diskus, Ventolin HFA, Ventolin Nebules	**Inhaler, metered-dose (Proventil, Proair, Ventolin):** 90 mcg/actuation, 100 mcg/actuation (Airomir) **Solution, for inhalation:** 0.021%,[b] 0.42%,[b] 0.05%,[c] 0.083%,[b] 0.1%,[c] 0.2%,[c] 0.5%[c] **Powder, for inhalation (Proair Respiclick, Ventolin Diskus):** 90 mcg/dose, 200 mcg/dose **Solution, for IV use:** 1 mg/mL[c] **Syrup:** 2 mg/5 mL[b] **Tablet, immediate-release:** 2 mg, 4 mg **Tablet, extended-release (VoSpire ER):**[b] 4 mg
levalbuterol[a]	Xopenex, Xopenex HFA Not available	**Inhaler (Xopenex HFA):** 45 mcg/actuation **Inhalant solution (Xopenex):** 0.31 mg/3 mL (0.0103%), 0.63 mg/3 mL (0.021%), 1.25 mg/3 mL (0.042%), 1.25 mg/0.5 mL (0.25%)
metaproterenol[a]	Generics Not available	**Solution, oral:** 10 mg/5 mL **Tablet:** 10 mg, 20 mg
terbutaline[a]	Generics Bricanyl inhaler	**Inhaler (Canada only):** 0.5 mg/actuation[c] **Tablet:** 2.5 mg,[b] 5 mg[b] **Solution, for injection:** 1 mg/mL[b]
Combinations		
albuterol + ipratropium bromide[a] (salbutamol + ipratropium bromide in Canada)	Combivent, Combivent Respimat Combivent, Combivent Respimat	**Inhaler MDI:** albuterol 100 mcg + ipratropium bromide 20 mcg/actuation **Inhalant solution:** salbutamol 1 mg + ipratropium bromide 0.5 mg per 2.5 mL unit dose vial[c]; albuterol 3 mcg + ipratropium bromide 0.5 mg per 3 mL unit dose vial[b]

[a]Generic available.
[b]Available in the United States only.
[c]Available in Canada only.

TECH NOTE!

The FDA reports that long-acting β₂-adrenergic agonists, such as salmeterol (Serevent Diskus), may increase the risk for severe asthma exacerbations and asthma-related death; therefore a warning label advising patients not to exceed the prescribed dose is typically applied to dispensed prescriptions.

Glucocorticosteroids

Glucocorticosteroids are antiinflammatory drugs. They reduce the inflammatory response in airway cells, decreasing the mucus and swelling that make breathing difficult (see Fig. 23.1).

Mechanism of Action and Pharmacokinetics

Glucocorticoids decrease the synthesis of proinflammatory substances (e.g., prostaglandins, leukotrienes, cytokines, arachidonic acid, and macrophages) that are released as part of the inflammatory response. Further details about the mechanism of action and pharmacokinetics of glucocorticosteroids are discussed in detail in Chapter 13. The primary route of administration for corticosteroids used for the treatment of asthma is inhalation; however, they may be administered orally for more severe symptoms. Inhaled corticosteroids include beclomethasone, budesonide, ciclesonide, fluticasone, and mometasone.

Adverse Reactions

Adverse reactions to inhaled corticosteroids are primarily local and include coughing, hoarseness, throat irritation, dry mouth, flushing, loss of taste, or unpleasant taste. Some patients may develop an infection in the mouth or throat called thrush; however, the risk can be minimized by gargling or rinsing the mouth after administering each dose of medicine. Systemic effects are dose-dependent and more likely to occur at higher doses. Flovent HFA is contraindicated in children younger than 4 years of age and budesonide, beclomethasone, and triamcinolone inhalers are contraindicated in children younger than 6 years of age. Symbicort and Advair HFA are contraindicated in children younger than 12 years.

TECH ALERT!

Arnuity Ellipta (fluticasone furoate), and Flovent Diskus (fluticasone propionate) are not substitutable.

Leukotriene Modifiers

Leukotrienes are proinflammatory substances that are released as part of the inflammatory response. Leukotriene modifiers are administered to patients with mild asthma to reduce inflammation.

Anticholinergics

Generic Name	US Brand Names / Canadian Brand Names	Dosage Forms and Strengths
aclidinium bromide	Tudorza Pressair	**Powder, for inhalation:** 400 mcg/inhalation
	Tudorza Genuair	
glycopyrrolate (United States) glycopyrronium (Canada)	Seebri Neohaler, Lonhala Magnair, Cuvposa	**Powder, for inhalation:** 15.6 mcg/inhalation[a] 50 mcg/inhalation[b]
	Seebri Breezhaler	**Solution, for inhalation (Lonhala Magnair):** 25 mcg/mL **Solution, oral (Cuvposa):** 1 mg/5 mL
ipratropium bromide	Atrovent HFA	**Inhaler (MDI):** 20 mcg/spray,[b] 21 mcg/spray[a]
	Atrovent HFA	**Solution, for inhalation:** 125 mcg/mL,[b] 200 mcg/mL,[a] 250 mcg/mL[b]
tiotropium bromide	Spiriva, Spiriva Respimat	**Inhaler:** 1.25 mcg/inhalation,[a] 2.5 mcg/inhalation
	Spiriva, Spiriva Respimat	**Powder, for inhalation:** 18 mcg/inhalation[a]
umeclidinium	Incruse Ellipta	**Powder for inhalation:** 62.5 mcg inhalation
	Incruse Ellipta	

Anticholinergic + Long-Acting β_2-Adrenergic Agonists Combinations

aclidinium + formoterol	Not available	**Inhaler:** 400 mcg + 12 mcg/actuation
	Duaklir Genuair	
glycopyrrolate + formoterol	Bevespi Aerosphere	**Inhaler:** 9 mcg glycopyrrolate + 4.8 mcg fomoterol/inhalation
	Not available	
glycopyrronium + indacaterol	Utibron	**Powder, for inhalation:** 50 mcg glycopyrronium + 110 mcg indacaterol[b]
	Ultibro Breezehaler	15.6 mcg glycopyrrolate + 27.5 mcg indacaterol[a]
tiotropium + olodaterol	Stiolto Respimat	**Inhaler:** 2.5 mcg tiotropium +2.5 mcg olodaterol/actuation
	Inspiolto Respimat, Spiolto Respimat	**Inhalation solution:** 2.5 mcg tiotropium +2.5 mcg olodaterol
umeclidinium bromide+ vilanterol	Anoro Ellipta	**Powder for inhalation:** 62.5 mcg umeclidinium + 25 mcg vilanterol
	Anoro Ellipta	

[a]Available in the United States only.
[b]Available in Canada only.

Long-Acting β_2-Adrenergic Agonists

Generic Name	US Brand Names / Canadian Brand Names	Dosage Forms and Strengths
arformoterol	Brovana	**Solution, for inhalation:** 15 mcg/2 mL
	Not available	
formoterol	Foradil, Perforomist	**Powder, for inhalation:** 6 mcg (Oxeze); 12 mcg/actuation (Foradil)
	Foradil, Oxeze Turbuhaler	**Solution, for inhalation (Perforomist):** 20 mcg/2 mL
olodaterol	Striverdi Respimat	**Inhaler:** 2.5 mcg/actuation
	Not Available	
salmeterol	Serevent Diskus	**Inhalation, powder:** 50 mcg/actuation
	Serevent Diskus	

Inhaled Corticosteroids

Generic Name	US Brand Names / Canadian Brand Names	Dosage Forms and Strengths
beclomethasone	Qvar Redihaler / Qvar	**Inhaler:** 40 mcg/actuation,[a] 50 mcg/actuation,[b] 80 mcg/actuation,[a] and 100 mcg/actuation[b]
budesonide	Pulmicort Flexhaler, Pulmicort Respules / Pulmicort Nebuamp, Pulmicort Turbuhaler	**Inhalant powder (Pulmicort Flexhaler)**[a]**:** 80 mcg, 160 mcg/actuation; **Inhaler, metered-dose (Pulmicort Turbuhaler)**[b]**:** 200 mcg, 400 mcg/actuation **Inhalant suspension (Pulmicort Nebuamp, Pulmicort Respules):** 0.25 mg/2 mL, 0.5 mg/2 mL, 1 mg/2 mL
ciclesonide	Alvesco Omnaris*, Zetonna* / Alvesco Omnaris*	**Inhalation, nasal:** 50 mcg/actuation **Inhalation solution:** 80 mcg/actuation,[a] 100 mcg/actuation,[b] 160 mcg/actuation,[a] and 200 mcg/actuation[b]
fluticasone	Armonair Respiclick, Arnuity Ellipta, Flovent Diskus, Flovent HFA / Arnuity Ellipta, Flovent Diskus, Flovent HFA	**Inhaler, MDI (Flovent HFA):** 44 mcg/actuation,[a] 50 mcg/actuation,[b] 110 mcg/actuation,[a] 125 mcg/actuation,[b] 220 mcg/actuation,[a] 250 mcg/actuation[b] **Powder, for inhalation (Armonair Respiclick, Arnuity, Flovent Diskus):** 50 mcg, 55 mcg,[a] 100 mcg, 113 mcg,[a] 200 mcg, 232 mcg,[a] 250 mcg, 500 mcg[b]/actuation
mometasone	Asmanex HFA, Asmanex Twisthaler / Asmanex Twisthaler	**Metered dose inhaler (Asmanex HFA):** 100 mcg, 200 mcg **Powder, for inhalation (Asmanex Twisthaler):** 100 mcg,[b] 110 mcg,[a] 200, mcg,[b] 220 mcg,[a] 400 mcg[b]

Long-Acting β₂-Adrenergic Agonist + Corticosteroid

Generic Name	US Brand Names / Canadian Brand Names	Dosage Forms and Strengths
formoterol + mometasone	Dulera / Zenhale	**Inhalation powder:** 5 mcg formoterol + 100 mcg mometasone, 5 mcg formoterol + 200 mcg mometasone per actuation
formoterol + budesonide	Symbicort / Symbicort	**Inhaler, MDI:** 4.5 mcg formoterol + 80 mcg budesonide/actuation[a]; 4.5 mcg formoterol + 160 mcg budesonide/actuation[a]; 6 mcg formoterol + 100 mcg budesonide/actuation,[b] 6 mcg formoterol + 200 mcg budesonide/actuation[b]
salmeterol + fluticasone	Advair Diskus, Advair HFA, Airduo Respiclick / Advair, Advair Diskus	**Inhalant, powder (Advair Diskus):** 50 mcg salmeterol + 100 mcg fluticasone, 50 mcg salmeterol + 250 mcg fluticasone, 50 mcg salmeterol + 500 mcg fluticasone **Inhalant, powder (Airduo Respiclick):** 14 mcg salmeterol + 55 mcg fluticasone; 14 mcg salmeterol + 113 mcg fluticasone; 14 mcg salmeterol + 232 mcg fluticasone **Inhaler (Advair, Advair HFA):** 21 mcg salmeterol + 45 mcg fluticasone,[a] 21 mcg salmeterol + 115 mcg fluticasone,[a] 21 mcg salmeterol + 230 mcg fluticasone[a]; 25 mcg salmeterol + 125 mcg fluticasone,[b] 25 mcg salmeterol + 250 mcg fluticasone[b]

[a]Available in the United States only.
[b]Available in Canada only.
*Nasal spray (see chapter 24).

TECH NOTE!
A common ending for leukotriene modifiers is -lukast.

Mechanism of Action

Zileuton inhibits the action of the enzyme responsible for converting arachidonic acid to leukotriene A4. This is the first step in the leukotriene pathway.

Montelukast and zafirlukast interfere with the binding of leukotrienes on airway smooth muscle, reducing allergen-induced airway inflammation, airway relaxation, and edema.

Pharmacokinetics

Montelukast is readily absorbed when administered orally. The maximum concentration of oral tablets is reached within 3 to 4 hours. Chewable tablets work faster, reaching a maximum concentration within approximately 2.5 hours. Food does not decrease the bioavailability of montelukast, unlike zafirlukast, which must be taken on an empty stomach. Montelukast, zafirlukast, and zileuton are metabolized in the liver by cytochrome P-450 (CYP450) isozymes and can interfere with the metabolism of other drugs using the same metabolic pathway.

Leukotriene Modifiers

Generic Name	US Brand Names / Canadian Brand Names	Dosage Forms and Strengths
montelukast[a]	Singulair	**Oral granules:** 4 mg/pack
	Singulair	**Tablet:** 10 mg
		Tablet, chewable: 4 mg, 5 mg
zafirlukast[a,b]	Accolate	**Tablet:** 10 mg,[b] 20 mg
	Accolate	
zileuton[a]	Zyflo, Zyflo CR	**Tablet (Zyflo):** 600 mg
	Not available	**Tablet, controlled-release (Zyflo CR):** 600 mg

[a]Generic available.
[b]Available in the United States only.

① TECH ALERT!

The following drugs have look-alike and sound-alike issues:
Singulair and SINEquan

Adverse Reactions

Montelukast and zafirlukast may produce cough, hoarseness or sore throat, headache, indigestion, heartburn or stomach upset, and runny nose. Montelukast may also produce difficulty sleeping, dizziness, drowsiness, muscle aches or cramps, or unusual dreams. Zileuton extended-release tablets may produce abdominal pain in addition to the adverse reactions listed for montelukast and zafirlukast.

Precautions

The packet of montelukast granules should not be opened until ready for use. Once opened, packet contents (with or without mixing with food) must be administered within 15 minutes. Zileuton may cause abnormal liver function and jaundice, so liver function tests should be conducted every 2 to 3 months.

Mast Cell Stabilizers

Mast cells are released as part of the immune system's response to allergens. Mast cell degranulation leads to the release of histamine and mediators of inflammation (e.g., leukotrienes, eosinophils, basophils, cytokines, and prostaglandins). Cromolyn sodium is an example of a mast cell stabilizer. Cromolyn is administered for prophylaxis and does not control acute symptoms.

Mechanism of Action

Cromolyn sodium reduces the release of inflammatory substances responsible for producing the symptoms of asthma by making mast cells less reactive to antigens. It inhibits the degranulation of mast cells and prevents the release of histamine and the slow-reacting substance of anaphylaxis (SRS-A). Cromolyn sodium improves exercise tolerance and reaction to cold air and environmental pollutants by reducing hyperactivity of the bronchi.

Pharmacokinetics

Cromolyn sodium is not used to treat acute symptoms. Several weeks of therapy are required before maximum response to the drug is achieved. Cromolyn produces a local effect on cell membranes. Only 1% of the drug is absorbed systemically.

Adverse Reactions

Cromolyn sodium may be administered using a MDI or nebulizer. Systemic absorption of cromolyn sodium is minimal, so side effects are generally localized. The most common adverse reactions are a bad taste in the mouth, irritated dry throat, and coughing or wheezing.

Mast Cell Stabilizers

Generic Name	US Brand Names / Canadian Brand Names	Dosage Forms and Strengths
cromolyn sodium[a]	Generics	**Solution, for inhalation:** 1%
	Generics	
tiotropium	Spiriva, Spiriva Respimat	**Metered dose inhaler:** 1.25 mcg,[b] 2.5 mcg
	Spiriva, Spiriva Respimat	**Powder, for inhalation:** 18 mcg

[a]Generic available.
[b]Available in the United States only.

Xanthine Derivatives

The xanthines are one of the oldest classes of drug used for the treatment of asthma. Theophylline occurs naturally in tea and is chemically similar to caffeine.

① TECH ALERT!

A common ending for xanthine derivatives is -phylline.

Mechanism of Action

Xanthines have bronchodilator and antiinflammatory properties. The exact mechanism of action of xanthines is unknown however, the drugs are known to inhibit the release of inflammatory substances and act on bronchial smooth muscle to reduce bronchospasms.

• BOX 23.4 Modifiers of Serum Blood Levels of Theophylline

Drugs and Foods That Increase Levels
- Oral contraceptives
- Erythromycin
- Calcium channel blockers
- Cimetidine
- Caffeine
- Chocolate

Drugs That Decrease Levels
- Phenobarbital
- Phenytoin
- Carbamazepine

Pharmacokinetics

The half-life ($t_{1/2}$) of theophylline and aminophylline varies with the patient's age, liver function, smoking status, and use of concurrent drugs. Smoking decreases $t_{1/2}$ by nearly 50%. In children 1 to 9 years of age, $t_{1/2}$ can be as much as 50% shorter than that in adults. Liver disease and pulmonary edema can prolong $t_{1/2}$ up to 24 hours. Theophylline is extensively metabolized by the CYP450 enzyme system and is involved in numerous drug interactions (Box 23.4). The bioavailability of theophylline varies by manufacturer. It is recommended that patients receive the same manufacturer's product each time that their prescriptions are refilled.

Adverse Reactions

Xanthine derivatives (e.g., theophylline) may produce insomnia, dizziness, headache, irritability, decreased appetite, stomach cramps, and urinary retention.

Xanthine Derivatives

Generic Name	US Brand Names / Canadian Brand Names	Dosage Forms and Strengths
aminophylline[a]	Generics / Generics	**Solution, for injection:** 25 mg/mL, 50 mg/mL[b]
theophylline[a]	Elixophyllin, Theo-24, Theochron / Theo ER, Theolair, Uniphyl	**Capsule, extended-release (Theo-24)[c]:** 100 mg, 200 mg, 300 mg, 400 mg **Elixir (Elixophyllin, Theolair):** 80 mg/15 mL **Solution, for injection (dextrose 5% 100 mL)[c]:** 40 mg, 80 mg, 160 mg, 200 mg, 320 mg, 400 mg **Tablet, extended–release (Theochron, Uniphyl):** 100 mg, 200 mg, 300 mg, 400 mg, 600 mg

[a]Generic available.
[b]Available in Canada only.
[c]Available in the United States only.

Monoclonal Antibodies

Omalizumab is a monoclonal antibody (anti-IgE) that is indicated for the treatment of moderate to severe *allergic asthma*. It decreases the body's response to asthma triggers. Asthma triggers and environmental allergens can cause a hypersensitivity reaction that produces overexpression of immunoglobulin E (IgE) antibodies that cause asthma symptoms. Omalizumab is indicated as add-on therapy for patients whose asthma is not controlled with inhaled corticosteroids and β_2-adrenergic agonists.

> **• TECH NOTE!**
> A common ending for monoclonal antibody drugs is *-mab.*

Mechanism of Action and Pharmacokinetics

The action of omalizumab is specifically directed toward IgE. It prevents early- and late-stage allergic responses as well as the release of inflammatory mediators (e.g., cytokines). Reslizumab (Cinqair) is an interleukin-5 inhibitor that inhibits the inflammatory process.

Omalizumab is administered once or twice a month by subcutaneous injection and reslizumab is given by intravenous infusion once monthly. The maximum serum concentration is reached within 7 to 8 hours of the administered dose; however, maximum effects from omalizumab are not achieved for several weeks after administration.

Adverse Reactions

The most common adverse reactions are mild redness, itching, swelling, or bruising at the injection site, headache, and nausea. More serious adverse effects that may be a prelude to anaphylaxis are difficulty breathing, hives, and skin rash.

Precautions

The package inserts for omalizumab and reslizumab carry a boxed warning indicating that patients should be instructed to watch for signs and symptoms of anaphylaxis and patients should be provided with instructions for self-treatment in the event of an emergency.

Monoclonal Antibodies

Generic Name	US Brand Names / Canadian Brand Names	Dosage Forms and Strengths
omalizumab	Xolair / Xolair	**Solution, for injection (prefilled syringes)[a]:** 75 mg/0.5 mL, 150 mg/mL **Powder, for injection:** 75 mg, 150 mg
reslizumab	Cinqair / Cinqair	**Solution, for IV infusion:** 10 mg/mL

[a]Available in Canada only.

Chronic Obstructive Pulmonary Disease

Overview

Chronic obstructive pulmonary disease (COPD) is a progressive disease of the airways that produces a gradual loss of pulmonary function. Emphysema, chronic bronchitis, and chronic obstructive bronchitis are all classified under the heading of COPD. The lungs and airways of patients with COPD are chronically inflamed and air sacs are destroyed. Inflammatory cells (e.g., CD8[+] T lymphocytes and interleukin-6) infiltrate the airways.

Risk Factors

Various lifestyle and environmental factors contribute to the risk for developing COPD. Cigarette smoking (or exposure to second-hand smoke) is the leading cause of COPD; 75% of people with COPD are current or former smokers. Occupational irritants to the lungs such as asbestos, industrial chemicals, dust, and air pollution may all contribute to or worsen existing COPD. Viral infections also aggravate COPD—in particular, respiratory syncytial virus (RSV) and adenovirus.

Symptoms

Airflow obstruction produces SOB. Persons with COPD may also exhibit a chronic persistent cough and wheezing. Airways become clogged with mucus, making breathing more difficult.

Treatment

The aim of COPD management is to (1) relieve symptoms and airway obstruction, (2) increase oxygen, and (3) treat any precipitating factors and/or comorbidities. Pharmacologic treatment of COPD involves the administration of bronchodilators, glucocorticosteroids, and—when infections are present—antibiotics. Nonpharmacologic treatments include oxygen therapy and mechanical ventilation.

Pharmacologic Treatment

The use of bronchodilators and glucocorticosteroids to reduce inflammation and open airways was described earlier (see "Maintenance Therapy to Prevent Asthma Flare-Ups"). Usual doses administered for the treatment of COPD are listed in the drug table at the end of this chapter. Additional drugs specifically indicated for the treatment of COPD are the anticholinergics (tiotropium) and antimucolytics (acetylcysteine). Inhaled anticholinergics are first-line maintenance therapy for COPD in patients with persistent symptoms.

Mechanism of Action

Tiotropium bromide and ipratropium bromide are antimuscarinic anticholinergic bronchodilators. Tiotropium is dosed once daily and is indicated for the treatment of COPD. Ipratropium bromide prescribed for short-term relief of asthma symptoms must be given three or four times daily. Anticholinergics bind to muscarinic receptors and block the effects of acetylcholine (released by the vagus nerve), resulting in the relaxation of bronchial smooth muscle. Antagonism of cholinergic receptors relaxes bronchial smooth muscle, producing bronchodilation. Recall that parasympathetic nervous system stimulation produces increased mucus and bronchoconstriction so antagonism decreases mucus and bronchoconstriction. Review the Unit II opener.

Adverse Reactions

Dry mouth is the most common side effect of tiotropium use. Diarrhea, nausea, hoarseness, dizziness, headache, and cardiac arrhythmias have also been reported.

Drug Delivery Devices for Use With Asthma and Chronic Obstructive Pulmonary Disease Medicines

Delivery of the prescribed dose of medication using an MDI is fast but may be challenging for some individuals and is inappropriate for small children. It is not uncommon for a substantial amount of the drug to be delivered to the back of the throat rather than into the lungs when an MDI is used. A dry powder inhaler (DPI) is similar to an MDI, but the medication is in powder form rather than in liquid form. A puff of the powder is inhaled rather than a mist of liquid. A nebulizer is a device that converts a liquid dose of medicine into an aerosolized mist that can be inhaled by normal breathing when used with a mask (Fig. 23.2). A mouthpiece may also be attached to the end of the nebulizer and the mist inhaled using slow deep breaths.

A *spacer* is a device that is attached to the end of the MDI (Fig. 23.3). The drug is sprayed into the device's chamber and then slowly inhaled into the lungs. Some devices produce a whistling sound to alert the patient when inhalation is too rapid or is not controlled.

• **Fig. 23.2** Nebulizer. (From Hopper T: *Mosby's pharmacy technician*, ed 2, St. Louis, 2007, WB Saunders.)

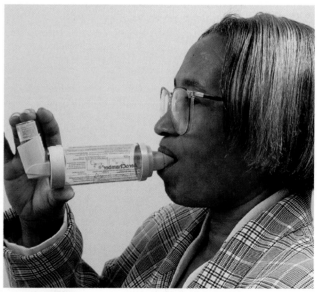

• **Fig. 23.3** Spacer. (From Potter PA, et al: *Fundamentals of nursing*, ed 9, St. Louis, 2017, Elsevier.)

Summary of Drugs Used for the Treatment of Asthma and Chronic Obstructive Pulmonary Disease

Generic Name	US Brand Name	Usual Adult Oral Dose and Dosing Schedule[a]	Warning Labels
Short-Acting β$_2$-Adrenergic Agonists			
albuterol (salbutamol)	Ventolin HFA	**Asthma** **Inhaler:** 1–2 puffs q 4–6 h as needed **Inhalant solution:** 2.5 mg q 6–8 h prn delivered over 5–15 min, *or* **AccuNeb:** 0.63–1.25 mg tid or qid; deliver over 5–15 min as needed **Solution or tablet, immediate-release:** 2–4 mg q 6–8 h (max, 32 mg/day) **Tablet, extended-release:** 4–8 mg q 12 h (max, 32 mg/day)	SHAKE WELL (INHALER).
levalbuterol	Xopenex	**Asthma** **Inhalant solution:** 0.63–1.25 mg q 6–8 h **Inhaler:** 2 puffs q 4–6 h	DO NOT EXCEED RECOMMENDED DOSE.
metaproterenol	Generics	**COPD** **Inhaler:** 100–200 mcg 3–4 times a day **Asthma and COPD** **Syrup or tablets:** 20 mg 3– times a day **Inhaler:** 2–3 puffs every 3–4 h (max, 12 puffs/day) **Inhalant solution:** 0.2–0.3 mL of 5% solution, diluted in 2.5–3 mL normal saline, 3–4 times a day	
terbutaline	Generics	**Asthma and COPD** **Injection:** 0.25 mg SC; repeat in 15–30 min if needed **Tablet:** 2.5–5 mg 3 times a day **Asthma Inhaler:** 2 puffs q 4 h	
Long-Acting β$_2$-Adrenergic Agonists			
formoterol	Foradil	**Asthma and COPD:** Inhale contents of 1 capsule q 12 h	DO NOT SWALLOW CAPSULES (FOR INHALATION DEVICE USE ONLY).
salmeterol	Serevent Diskus	**Asthma and COPD:** 1 inhalation q 12 h	
β$_2$-Adrenergic Agonists + Anticholinergics			
albuterol + ipratropium bromide	Combivent, DuoNeb	**COPD:** Inhale 1 puffs 4 times daily (Combivent) or 3 mL qid (DuoNeb)	SHAKE WELL (INHALER).
fenoterol hydrobromide + ipratropium bromide	DuoVent	**COPD:** Inhale 4 mL q 4–6 h	
Anticholinergics			
aclidinium bromide	Tudorza	**COPD:** Inhale 1 puff twice daily	DISCARD 45 DAYS AFTER OPENING POUCH.
ipratropium bromide	Atrovent HFA	**COPD:** Inhale 2 sprays 3–4 times a day (MDI) or inhale 1 vial of nebulizer solution (500 mcg) q 6–8 h	SHAKE WELL.
tiotropium	Spiriva	**COPD:** Inhale contents of 1 capsule once daily	DO NOT SWALLOW CAPSULES (FOR INHALATION DEVICE USE ONLY).
umeclidinium	Incruse Ellipta	**COPD:** inhale powder once daily	DISCARD 6 WEEKS AFTER OPENING OR WHEN COUNTER IS AT ZERO.
Inhaled Corticosteroids			
beclomethasone	QVar	**Asthma:** 1–4 puffs twice daily (max, 320 mcg/day)	SHAKE WELL (INHALER).
budesonide	Pulmicort	**Asthma:** 1–2 puffs twice daily	

Continued

	Generic Name	US Brand Name	Usual Adult Oral Dose and Dosing Schedule[a]	Warning Labels
	ciclesonide	Alvesco	**Asthma:** 1–2 puffs once daily (800 mcg dose may be given as 400 mcg twice daily)	
	fluticasone	Flovent HFA	**Asthma:** 2 sprays up to twice daily (Maximum dose varies for Armonair Respiclick, Flovent HFA and Flovent Diskus)	
	mometasone	Asmanex	**Asthma:** 1–2 sprays once or twice daily (max, 440 mcg/day	
β₂-Adrenergic Agonists + Inhaled Corticosteroids				
	formoterol + budesonide	Symbicort	**Asthma:** 2 puffs twice daily	SHAKE WELL (INHALER).
	formoterol + mometasone	Dulera (Zenhale)	**Asthma:** 2 puffs twice daily	
	salmeterol + fluticasone	Advair HFA Advair Diskus	**Asthma and COPD:** 1 puff q 12 h (Maximum fluticasone 500 mcg/salmeterol 50 mcg) (Maximum dose varies for Advair Diskus, Advair HFA and Airduo Respiclick)	
Leukotriene Modifiers				
	montelukast	Singulair	**Asthma:** 10 mg once daily in the evening	TAKE WITH A LARGE GLASS OF WATER (CHEWABLE TABLETS). DISCARD UNUSED PORTION OF GRANULES WITHIN 15 MIN.
	zafirlukast	Accolate	**Asthma:** 20 mg (1–2 tablets) twice daily	TAKE ON AN EMPTY STOMACH (1–2 H AFTER EATING).
	zileuton	Zyflo	**Asthma:** 600 mg 4 times a day (immediate-release tabs) 1200 mg bid (extended-release tabs)	TAKE WITH FOOD (within 1 hour after morning and evening meals). SWALLOW WHOLE; DO NOT CRUSH OR CHEW.
Mast Cell Stabilizers				
	cromolyn sodium	Generics	**Asthma** **Inhaler:** 2 sprays 4 times a day **Nebulizer:** 20 mg (2 mL) 4 times a day	SHAKE WELL (INHALER).
Xanthine Derivatives				
	aminophylline[b]	Generics	**Asthma and COPD:** 5 mg/kg/day PO or IV in divided doses q 6–8 h (max, 800 mg/day)	SWALLOW WHOLE; DON'T CRUSH OR CHEW (EXTENDED-RELEASE).
	theophylline	Theolair Theo-24	**Asthma and COPD:** **Immediate-release:** 5 mg/kg/day (max, 300–600 mg/day) PO or IV in divided doses every 6–8 h **Extended-release:** 300–800 mg/day in divided doses q 12–24 h (Theo-24)	TAKE 30–60 MIN BEFORE MEALS WITH A FULL GLASS OF WATER.
Monoclonal Antibody				
	omalizumab	Xolair	**Asthma:** 150–375 mg SC q 2 or 4 weeks (based on baseline IgE levels)	REFRIGERATE POWDER AND RECONSTITUTED SOLUTION BETWEEN 2° AND 8°C (36°–46°F). DISCARD RECONSTITUTED SOLUTION AFTER 24 H.
	reslizumab	Cinqair	3 mg/kg IV once every 4 weeks	DO NOT SHAKE DISCARD IF SOLUTION IS DISCOLORED.

[a]Adult dose for asthma and COPD unless specified.
[b]Aminophylline dose expressed as theophylline.

TECHNICIAN'S CORNER

1. Can lung damage be reversed when a smoker stops smoking?
2. What are some lifestyle modifications that can be implemented to manage asthma?

Key Points

- Asthma is a chronic disease that affects the airways, producing irritation, inflammation, coughing, wheezing, shortness of breath, and chest tightness.
- Asthma is classified according to the frequency and severity of symptoms. The three classifications for asthma are mild, moderate, and severe.
- Family history of asthma, smoking, including exposure to secondhand smoke, chronic exposure to air pollution, exposure to some allergens, and infections early in life are risk factors for developing asthma.
- Symptoms of asthma are caused by airway irritation that results in bronchial constriction and impedes the passage of air. Airways also become inflamed, which produces swelling and restricts the flow of air. Mucus production is increased, which further obstructs breathing passages.
- Asthma "triggers" can precipitate an asthma attack. Examples are animal dander, cockroach droppings, environmental pollutants, cleaning fluids, mold, tobacco smoke, air pollution, upper respiratory infection, vigorous exercise, and even cold air.
- Asthma symptoms can be managed with a combination of medication, lifestyle modification, and home monitoring of breathing using a peak flow meter and medication.
- COPD is a progressive disease of the airways that produces gradual loss of pulmonary function, shortness of breath, chronic persistent cough, wheezing, and increased sputum production.
- Cigarette smoking or exposure to secondhand smoke, occupational irritants, industrial chemicals, or dust can increase the risk of developing COPD.
- Air pollution and viral infections may contribute to and worsen existing COPD.
- A peak flow meter permits self-management of asthma, similar to the way in which the monitoring of blood glucose levels enables self-management of diabetes.
- Low peak flow numbers signal that asthma is not controlled.
- Pharmacologic treatment of COPD involves the administration of bronchodilators, glucocorticosteroids, and antibiotics when infection is present.
- Nonpharmacologic treatments include oxygen therapy and mechanical ventilation.
- Drugs used for the treatment and management of asthma are divided into two classes. Drugs for the treatment of acute symptoms are classified as rescue or reliever medicines. Drugs administered to prevent asthma episodes are classified as maintenance therapies.
- Short-acting β_2-adrenergic agonists provide short-term relief of acute symptoms. Reliever medicines currently prescribed for the treatment of asthma include albuterol, levalbuterol, metaproterenol, and terbutaline.

- The inhaled anticholinergic ipratropium bromide is administered for the relief of acute asthma symptoms; tiotropium is used to treat COPD.
- Drugs such as albuterol can produce nervousness, difficulty sleeping, dry mouth, mild headache, and throat irritation (by inhalants).
- Long-acting β_2-adrenergic agonists (e.g., salmeterol and formoterol) are not recommended as primary therapy because they are associated with an increased risk of severe asthma attacks and asthma-related death.
- Glucocorticosteroids decrease inflammation and mucus in the airways.
- Inhaled corticosteroids include fluticasone (Flovent), budesonide (Pulmicort), mometasone (Asmanex), and beclomethasone (Qvar).
- Adverse reactions to inhaled corticosteroids are primarily local and include coughing, hoarseness, throat irritation, dry mouth, thrush, loss of taste, and/or unpleasant taste.
- Risks for thrush can be minimized by gargling or rinsing the mouth after administering the prescribed dose of glucocorticosteroid.
- Leukotriene modifiers are administered to patients with mild asthma to reduce inflammation.
- Leukotriene modifiers inhibit the release of proinflammatory leukotrienes, substances that are released as part of the inflammatory response.
- The packet of montelukast granules should not be opened until ready for use. Once opened, packet contents (with or without mixing with food) must be administered within 15 minutes.
- Cromolyn sodium is an example of a mast cell stabilizer; it makes mast cells less reactive to antigens and reduces the release of inflammatory substances responsible for producing the symptoms of asthma.
- Xanthines have bronchodilator and antiinflammatory properties.
- Smoking cigarettes decreases the $t_{1/2}$ of theophylline by almost 50%.
- It is recommended that patients receive the same manufacturer's product each time their prescriptions for theophylline are refilled.
- Omalizumab and reslizumab are monoclonal antibodies that are used for the treatment of moderate to severe allergic asthma as add-on therapy for patients whose asthma is not controlled with inhaled corticosteroids and β_2-adrenergic agonists.
- Omalizumab carries a boxed warning that patients should be instructed to watch for signs and symptoms of anaphylaxis.
- A nebulizer is a device that converts a liquid dose of medicine into an aerosolized mist.
- A spacer is a device attached to the end of the metered-dose inhaler that is used to control the delivery of an inhaled medicine.

Review Questions

1. A drug that relaxes tightened airway muscles and improves airflow through the airways is known as a _____.
   a. Bronchodilator
   b. Bronchoconstrictor

2. You receive a prescription for Advair Diskus 1 to 2 puffs every 4 to 6 hours. You consult with the pharmacist because _____.
   a. Advair is not marketed as a "Diskus"
   b. Advair is dosed once daily
   c. Advair is dosed twice a day
   d. Advair has been discontinued and is no longer marketed

3. All of the following are asthma triggers *except*_____.
   a. Family history
   b. Exposure to cigarette smoke
   c. Vigorous exercise
   d. Exposure to environmental pollutants

4. A peak flow meter is a device _____.
   a. That is attached to the end of the metered-dose inhaler
   b. That aids in self-management of asthma
   c. That is used to administer asthma medication
   d. That is used to diagnose and treat COPD

5. Which of the following drugs used for the treatment of allergic asthma is administered by injection?
   a. Xolair
   b. Theolair
   c. Singulair
   d. Advair

6. Persons with _____ may also exhibit a chronic persistent cough, wheezing, and increased mucus production.
   a. Smoking habit
   b. COPD
   c. Bronchitis
   d. None of the above

7. Nonpharmacologic treatments for COPD include which of the following?
   a. Oxygen therapy
   b. Mechanical ventilation
   c. Inhalers
   d. a and b

8. All of the following drugs are marketed as an inhalant solution *except*:
   a albuterol
   b ipratropium
   c metaproterenol
   d tiotropium

9. Tiotropium bromide is administered by the _____ route.
   a. Oral
   b. Inhalation
   c. Transdermal
   d. Intravenous

10. A _____ is a device that converts a liquid dose of medicine into an aerosolized mist that can be inhaled by normal breathing when used with a mask.
    a. Aerosolizer
    b. Nebulizer
    c. Spacer
    d. Inhaler

Bibliography

Centers for Disease Control and Prevention: National Center for Health Statistics-Asthma, 2015. Retrieved September 18, 2017, from http://www.cdc.gov/nchs/fastats/asthma.htm.

FDA, nd. Drugs@FDA: FDA Approved Drug Products. Retrieved August 28, 2018, from http://www.accessdata.fda.gov/scripts/cder/daf/.

Global Initiative for Asthma, 2017. Pocket Guide for Asthma Management and Treatment. From www.ginasthma.org.

Health Canada, 2018. Drug Product Database. Retrieved August 28, 2018, from https://health-products.canada.ca/dpd-bdpp/index-eng.jsp.

National Heart Lung and Blood Institute, 2014. Asthma. Retrieved September 12, 2017, from https://www.nhlbi.nih.gov/book/export/html/4896.

National Heart, Lung, and Blood Institute: What is National Heart Lung and Blood Institute. COPD. Retrieved September 14, 2017, from https://www.nhlbi.nih.gov/book/export/html/4972.

National Institute of Environmental Health Sciences: Asthma and its environmental triggers, 2012. Retrieved September 14, 2017, from http://www.niehs.nih.gov/health/materials/asthma_and_its_environmental_triggers.pdf.

Page C, Curtis M, Sutter M, et al: *Integrated pharmacology*, Philadelphia, 2005, Mosby, pp 415–423.

Papi A, Contoli M, Gaetano C, et al: Models of infection and exacerbations in COPD, *Curr Opin Pharmacol* 7:259–265, 2007.

Shigemitsu H, Afshar K: Nocturnal asthma, *Curr Opin Pulm Med* 13:49–55, 2007.

Statistics Canada, 2014. Asthma, 2014. Retrieved September 14, 2017, from http://www.statcan.gc.ca/pub/82-625-x/2015001/article/14179-eng.htm.

Web MD: Secondhand smoke may harm fetus like smoking, 2012. http://www.webmd.com/baby/news/20050727/secondhand-smoke-may-harm-fetus-like-smoking.

24

Treatment of Allergies

LEARNING OBJECTIVES

1. Learn the terminology associated with allergies.
2. Describe the causes and list the symptoms of allergic reactions.
3. List and categorize medications used for the treatment of allergies.
4. Describe the mechanism of action for drugs used to treat allergies.
5. Identify significant drug look-alike and sound-alike issues.
6. Identify warning labels and precautionary messages associated with medications used for the treatment of allergies.

KEY TERMS

Allergen Substance that produces an allergic reaction.
Allergic conjunctivitis condition characterized by red, watering, itchy, or burning eyes.
Allergic rhinitis Seasonal condition characterized by inflammation and swelling of the nasal passageways (rhinitis) accompanied by runny nose (rhinorrhea).
Allergy Hypersensitivity reaction by the immune system on exposure to an allergen.
Anaphylaxis Life-threatening allergic reaction.
Angioedema Allergic skin disease characterized by patches of circumscribed swelling involving the skin and its subcutaneous layers, the mucous membranes, and sometimes the viscera.

Histamine An organic nitrogen compound involved in local immune responses, as well as regulating physiologic function in the gut and acting as a neurotransmitter.
Immunoglobulin E An antibody associated with allergies.
Leukotriene A proinflammatory mediator released as part of the allergic response. Leukotrienes also trigger contractions in the smooth muscles of airways.
Mast cells Granule-containing cells found in connective tissue. Histamine containing granules are released during allergic reactions.
Urticaria Hives.
Wheal Raised blister-like area on the skin.

Overview

An *allergy* is a hypersensitivity reaction caused by exposure to an allergen. An *allergen* is any substance that produces an allergic reaction.

Occupational Allergens

Pharmacy technicians are at risk for developing latex allergy. Allergic reactions occur when latex-sensitive individuals breathe in or come into physical contact with latex proteins. Latex proteins in disposable gloves may form a complex with the lubricant powder used in some gloves. When the pharmacy technician changes gloves, the protein–powder particle complex may become airborne and then inhaled.

Latex allergy may produce mild reactions such as skin redness, rash, hives, or itching. Respiratory symptoms such as runny nose, sneezing, itchy eyes, and scratchy throat may occur. More severe reactions involve asthma (difficult breathing, coughing spells, and wheezing) and, rarely, *anaphylaxis*, which is life threatening.

The National Institute for Occupational Safety and Health recommends taking the following steps to protect oneself from latex exposure and allergy in the workplace.

1. Avoid contact with latex gloves and products. Select nonlatex gloves when possible to provide barrier protection when handling infectious materials.
2. If you choose latex gloves, use powder-free gloves with reduced protein content.
3. Use appropriate work practices to reduce the chance of reactions to latex.
4. Do not use oil-based hand creams or lotions when wearing latex gloves, because they can cause glove deterioration.
5. After removing latex gloves, wash hands with a mild soap and dry thoroughly.
6. Practice good housekeeping by frequently cleaning areas and equipment contaminated with latex-containing dust.
7. Avoid areas where you might inhale the powder from latex gloves worn by other workers.
8. Tell your employer and health care providers (e.g., physician, nurse, dentist) that you have latex allergy.

Pharmacy technicians may come into contact with additional products containing latex in the workplace. Box 24.1 provides examples of products that may contain latex.

> **TECH NOTE!**
> Symptoms of allergy and a cold are similar; however, cold symptoms rarely last longer than 1 to 2 weeks.

• BOX 24.1 **Products Containing Latex**

- Disposable gloves
- Intravenous tubing
- Intravenous bag ports
- Syringes
- Catheters
- Injection ports
- Rubber tops of multidose vials

• BOX 24.2 **Common Allergy Symptoms**

Dermal
- Redness
- Swelling
- Urticaria
- Wheal

Respiratory
- Itchy eyes, nose, and throat
- Runny nose
- Stuffy nose
- Sneezing
- Coughing and postnasal drip
- Watery eyes
- Conjunctivitis
- Allergic shiners
- Allergic salute

What Triggers an Allergic Response?

The immune system functions to defend the body against invading germs and other substances that it believes are harmful. When a person with allergies first comes into contact with an allergen, the immune system treats the allergen as an invader and produces antibodies to the substance. The allergic reaction sequence is a cascade of events that begins with the ingestion or inhalation of allergen. Exposure to the allergen triggers an immune system reaction and the production of specialized antibodies (immunoglobulin E [IgE]). Antibodies attach to *mast cells* containing *histamine*, which when released produces allergic reaction symptoms such as itching, runny nose, hives, and wheezing.

The production of allergen-specific *immunoglobulin E* antibodies develops within the first few years of life. Exposure to high levels of multiple endotoxins early in life, such as when children live with multiple pets, may reduce the risks for development of asthma and allergies. The degree of IgE antibody response varies, and allergens from some sources (e.g., dust mites, cat) are more potent than others.

Allergic Conditions

Allergic conditions affect between 40 and 50 million people in the United States and are a public health issue because they affect the quality of life, productivity, and performance of sensitive individuals. Seasonal allergic rhinitis (SAR) occurs on exposure to seasonal pollens. Symptoms associated with an allergic reaction may be localized to a specific area of contact, as with contact dermatitis, or may be more generalized. Persons with chronic airborne allergies may develop allergic shiners (dark circles under the eyes caused by increased blood flow near the sinuses) and an allergic salute (a crease across the bridge of the nose caused by persistent upward rubbing of the nose). Common allergy symptoms are listed in Box 24.2. *Urticaria* (also known as hives) is a condition characterized by itching and *angioedema* (swelling). Redness, swelling, and *wheals* (blister-like vesicles) appear on the skin. Urticaria may be caused by an insect bite, drug or food allergy, or injection of allergen extracts (allergy shots). The condition usually subsides within a few days but, if severe, may need to be managed by the administration of antihistamines and glucocorticosteroids. Acute pharyngeal or laryngeal angioedema must be managed by the administration of drugs that rapidly reduce swelling in the throat and restore breathing (e.g., short-acting beta$_2$-adrenergic agonists).

Allergic Rhinitis

Allergic rhinitis is a condition characterized by nasal itching (rhinitis), runny nose (rhinorrhea), nasal congestion (stuffiness), and sneezing. Allergic rhinitis is typically self-limiting and will resolve without treatment with antiinfective agents. Symptoms are caused by inflammation and swelling of the nasal passageways and may occur throughout the year or seasonally. With SAR, allergy symptoms appear seasonally upon re-exposure to allergens after a period of absence. The recurrence of allergic symptoms seasonally is believed to be caused by the presence of memory CD4$^+$ T cells. Memory CD4$^+$ T cells are allergen specific (e.g., tree, grass, weed pollen).

Allergic Conjunctivitis

Allergic conjunctivitis produces red, watering, itchy, or burning eyes. Sufferers may also have ocular puffiness and a stringy discharge from the eyes. Symptoms occur on exposure to an allergen. Seasonal allergic conjunctivitis may worsen during allergy and hay fever season. Overuse of decongestants to treat red eyes may result in *conjunctivitis medicamentosa* or rebound eye redness and congestion. More information about conjunctivitis is found in Chapter 15.

Pharmaceuticals Used in the Management of Allergies and Allergic Conditions

The pharmacologic treatment of allergies is aimed at reducing swelling and inflammation; suppressing the release of cells that mediate immune system and inflammatory responses; and blocking receptor sites of the mediators. Drugs used to treat allergic symptoms include antihistamines, inhaled corticosteroids, mast cell stabilizers, and *leukotriene* receptor antagonists.

> **TECH NOTE!**
>
> Health Canada, the US Food and Drug Administration (FDA) nonprescription Drug Advisory Committee, and FDA Pediatric Advisory Committee recommend that cold and cough products be avoided in children younger than 6 years.

Antihistamines

Antihistamines reduce allergic reactions. Some antihistamines (e.g., meclizine, cyclizine, phenothiazines) also decrease nausea and vomiting or are used for the treatment of schizophrenia (phenothiazines). There are several classes of antihistamines—ethylenediamines, ethanolamines, alkylamines, piperazines, phenothiazines, phthalazinones, and piperidines. Most are available without prescription.

Mechanism of Action and Pharmacokinetics

Administration of antihistamines prevents histamine binding to H1 receptor sites. The drugs compete with free histamine for binding at receptor sites. All H1 receptor antagonists have good oral absorption and reach maximum serum levels within 1 to 2 hours. The half-life ($t^{1/2}$) of the antihistamines varies, ranging from as short as 4 to 6 hours (e.g., diphenhydramine) to 24 hours (fexofenadine). Hydroxyzine is metabolized to the active metabolite cetirizine (Zyrtec). Desloratadine and loratadine are formulated as disintegrating tablets for rapid dissolution and onset of action.

Adverse Reactions

Antihistamines that cross the blood-brain barrier decrease alertness and/or produce sedation. Sedation, dizziness, decreased alertness, dry mouth, blurred vision, lack of coordination, and urinary retention are the most common adverse reactions of antihistamines. Antihistamines that are classified as ethanolamines (e.g., diphenhydramine) and phenothiazines (e.g., promethazine) produce the most sedation and have the greatest anticholinergic effects. Ethylenediamines (e.g., pyrilamine) and piperazines (e.g., cetirizine) produce fewer sedative effects, and newer agents produce the least sedation. Piperidines (e.g., loratadine, fexofenadine) are relatively nonsedating.

● TECH NOTE!

Because of its sedating effects, diphenhydramine is also administered for the treatment of insomnia.

Precautions

Antihistamines should be used cautiously in men with prostate disease, persons with asthma, and women who are breastfeeding. Antihistamine use in children younger than 2 years is not recommended. These drugs can decrease urination, thicken bronchial secretions, and decrease milk production.

⊘ TECH ALERT!

The following drugs have look-alike and sound-alike issues:
diphenhydramine and dimenhydrinate;
Allegra and Viagra;
ZyrTEC, ZyrTEC-D, Zantac, Zocor, ZyPREXA;
Claritin, Claritin-D, and Clarinex

Over-the-Counter Antihistamines

Generic Name	US Brand Name(s) / Canadian Brand Name(s)	Dosage Forms and Strengths
cetirizine[a]	Zyrtec Allergy, Zyrtec Hives	**Capsule:** 5 mg,[b] 10 mg **Syrup:** 1 mg/mL **Tablet, chewable:** 5 mg, 10 mg **Tablet:** 5 mg, 10 mg, 20 mg[c] (RX only) **Tablet, ODT:** 10 mg
	Reactine	
chlorpheniramine[a]	Chlor-Trimeton	**Tablet:** 4 mg[c] **Tablet, extended-release:** 12 mg[b]
	Chlor-Tripolon	
clemastine[a]	Tavist-1	**Tablet:** 1.34 mg
	Not available	
diphenhydramine[a] (Selected products)	Benadryl Allergy, Benadryl Children's Allergy, Benadryl Itch Stopping Extra Strength	**Capsule:** 25 mg, 50 mg **Capsule, liquid-filled:** 25 mg **Cream (Benadryl):** 1%, 2% **Elixir:** 12.5 mg/5 mL **Gel:** 2% **Liquid:** 6.25 mg/5 mL, 12.5 mg/5 mL **Solution, for injection:** 50 mg/mL **Spray:** 2% **Tablet:** 12.5 mg,[c] 25 mg, 50 mg
	Benadryl, Benadryl Allergy Liquigel, Extra Strength Benedryl Allergy Nighttime, Benylin Night for Children	
fexofenadine[a]	Allegra Allergy, Allegra Hives; Children's Allegra Allergy, Children's Allergy Hives	**Suspension:** 30 mg/5 mL **Tablet:** 30 mg,[b] 60 mg, 120 mg,[c] 180 mg[b] **Tablet, oral disintegrating:** 30 mg
	Allegra 12 Hour, Allegra 24 H	
loratadine[a]	Alavert, Claritin, Children's Claritin, Claritin Hives Relief, Claritin RediTab, Claritin Liqui-gel	**Capsule, liquid-filled:** 10 mg **Suspension:** 1 mg/mL **Syrup:** 1 mg/mL **Tablet:** 10 mg **Tablet, chewable:** 5 mg **Tablet, oral disintegrating:** 5 mg, 10 mg
	Claritin, Claritin Kids, Claritin Rapid Dissolve	

[a]Generic available.
[b]Available in the United States only.
[c]Available in Canada only.

Prescription Antihistamines

Generic Name	US Brand Name(s) Canadian Brand Name(s)	Dosage Forms and Strengths
azelastine[a]	Astelin, Astepro Not available	**Nasal spray solution:** 125 mcg (Astelin); 187.6 mcg (Astepro)/actuation **Ophthalmic solution:** 0.05%
bilastine	Not available Blexten	**Tablet:** 20 mg
desloratadine[a] (Prescription in United States and OTC in Canada)	Clarinex Aerius, Aerius Kids (OTC)	**Liquid:** 0.5 mg/mL **Tablet:** 5 mg **Tablet, oral disintegrating (Clarinex RediTab):** 2.5 mg, 5 mg
dexchlorpheniramine[a]	Generics Not available	**Syrup:** 2 mg/5 mL
ketotifen[a] (Prescription and OTC)	Alaway (OTC), Claritin Eye (OTC), Zyrtec Itchy Eye (OTC) Zaditor	**Solution, ophthalmic:** 0.025%, 0.035%[b]
levocetirizine[a] (Prescription and OTC)	Xyzal, Xyzal Allergy 24HR (OTC) Not available	**Solution, oral:** 2.5 mg/5 mL **Tablet:** 5 mg
olopatadine[a]	Pataday, Patanase, Patanol, Pazeo Pataday, Patanol	**Solution, ophthalmic:** 0.1% (Patanol); 0.2% (Pataday); 0.7% (Pazeo) **Spray, Nasal (Patanase):** 0.6%
Antihistamine + Glucocorticoid Combination		
azelastine + fluticasone	Dymista Dymista	Nasal spray solution: 137 mcg azelastine + 50 mcg fluticasone/actuation

[a]Generic available.
[b]Available in the United States only.
OTC, Over-the-counter.

Glucocorticosteroids

Glucocorticosteroids are antiinflammatory drugs that are administered intranasally to control symptoms of allergic rhinitis. When administered intranasally, they inhibit the onset of the inflammatory response by reducing the permeability of the nasal mucosa cells to T-lymphocytes and eosinophils, thereby decreasing the release of mediators of the inflammatory response (e.g., cytokines). They also reduce the number of inflammatory cells. The result is the reduction of the mucus and swelling that make breathing difficult. Additional mechanisms of action and pharmacokinetics of glucocorticosteroids are discussed in detail in Chapters 13 and 23. Fluticasone (Flonase®), budesonide (Rhinocort®), triamcinolone (Nasacort AQ®), mometasone (Nasonex®), and beclomethasone (Beconase AQ®) are examples of glucocorticoids that are marketed for use in the nose.

⚠ TECH ALERT!

The following drugs have look-alike and sound-alike issues:
Flonase and Flovent

Adverse Reactions

Side effects of glucocorticoids, when applied intranasally, are primarily local and include nasal irritation, throat irritation, and nosebleed. Some patients may develop a *Candida* infection in their nose that may present as burning or stinging in the nostril(s).

Mast Cell Stabilizers

Cromolyn sodium and nedocromil are classified as mast cell stabilizers. The drugs make cells less reactive to allergens, decreasing the release of inflammatory substances. Cromolyn is approved for intranasal and ophthalmic use, but nedocromil is manufactured for ophthalmic use only. Cromolyn sodium and nedocromil are not used to treat acute symptoms. Therapy should begin before coming into contact with allergens and continue for the duration of allergen exposure. For more details about the mechanisms of action, pharmacokinetics, and adverse reactions for mast cell stabilizers, read Chapter 23. Adverse effects include bad taste in the mouth, cough, dry throat, difficulty breathing, headache, nosebleeds, runny nose, sneezing, and stinging, burning, or irritation inside the nose. Nasalcrom and Opticrom do not require a prescription; however, nedocromil is a prescription drug.

Leukotriene Receptor Antagonists

The leukotriene receptor antagonist montelukast is used to control allergic rhinitis symptoms. Montelukast is a selective antagonist of the cysteinyl leukotriene D_4 receptor found in the human airway. Montelukast may produce cough, hoarseness, sore throat, headache, indigestion, heartburn, stomach upset, or runny nose. Montelukast may also produce difficulty sleeping, dizziness, drowsiness, muscle aches or cramps, or unusual dreams.

Immunotherapy

Allergy shots represent a form of immunotherapy. They may be administered to persons with perennial (symptoms all year round) or seasonal allergies. The rationale for immunotherapy is to reduce the level of IgE antibodies in the blood while at the same time stimulating the production of IgG, a protective antibody. Allergy shots are administered by subcutaneous injection as a series of shots; each injection has an increased concentration of the allergen that produces sensitivity. Allergy shots can reduce allergy symptoms over a longer period of time than all other treatments.

TECHNICIAN'S CORNER

1. What is the best way to identify what is causing an allergy?
2. Should all antihistamines be available as OTC drugs?

Corticosteroids Used for Allergic Rhinitis or Allergic Conjunctivitis

Generic Name	US Brand Name(s) / Canadian Brand Name(s)	Dosage Forms and Strengths	Prescription Status
beclomethasone	Beconase AQ, QNASL / generics	Pump nasal spray: 40 mcg,[b] 42 mcg,[b] 50 mcg,[a] 80 mcg/actuation[b]	Prescription only
budesonide[c]	Rhinocort Aqua, Rhinocort Allergy (OTC) / Rhinocort Aqua	Pump nasal spray (suspension): 32 mcg/actuation,[b] 64 mcg/actuation,[a] 100 mcg/actuation[a]	Prescription and OTC in the United States
ciclesonide[ca]	Omnaris, Zetonna / Omnaris	50 mcg/actuation	Prescription
flunisolide[c]	Generics / Not available	Pump nasal spray: 25 mcg/actuation	Prescription only
fluticasone[c]	Flonase, Flonase Allergy Relief (OTC), Flonase Sensimist (OTC), Xhance / Avamys, Flonase Allergy Relief (OTC)	Pump nasal spray, as furoate (Avamys, Flonase Sensimist): 27.5 mcg/actuation Pump nasal spray, as propionate (Flonase Allergy Relief): 50 mcg/actuation, 93 mcg/actuation (Xhance)	Prescription and OTC
loteprednol	Alrex, Lotemax / Alrex, Lotemax	Gel, ophthalmic: 0.5% Ointment, Ophthalmic: 0.5% Suspension, Ophthalmic: 0.2% (Alrex), 0.5% (Lotemax)	Prescription only
mometasone[c]	Nasonex / Nasonex, Mosaspray	Pump nasal spray: 50 mcg/actuation	Prescription and OTC in Canada
triamcinolone[a]	Nasacort Allergy 24H (OTC) / Nasacort Allergy 24H (OTC), Nasacort AQ	Pump nasal spray: 55 mcg/actuation	Prescription and OTC

[a]Available in Canada only.
[b]Available in the United States only.
[c]Generic available.
[ca]Generic available in Canada only.
OTC, Over-the-counter.

Mast Cell Stabilizers

Generic Name	US Brand Name(s) / Canadian Brand Name(s)	Dosage Forms and Strengths	Prescription Status
cromolyn sodium[a]	Crolom, Opticrom (OTC) / Opticrom (OTC), Rhinaris-CS Anti-Allergic Nasal Mist (OTC)	Nasal Spray: 2%[b], 4%[c] (5.2 mcg/actuation) Ophthalmic solution: 2% (Opticrom), 4% (Crolom)	Prescription and OTC
nedocromil	Alocril / Alocril	Ophthalmic solution: 2%,	Prescription only

[a]Generic available.
[b]Available in Canada only.
[c]Available in the United States only.
OTC, Over-the-counter.

Leukotriene Receptor Antagonist for Allergic Rhinitis

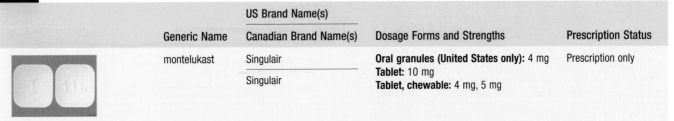

Generic Name	US Brand Name(s) / Canadian Brand Name(s)	Dosage Forms and Strengths	Prescription Status
montelukast	Singulair / Singulair	Oral granules (United States only): 4 mg Tablet: 10 mg Tablet, chewable: 4 mg, 5 mg	Prescription only

Summary of Drugs Used in the Treatment of Allergic Conditions

	Generic Name	US Brand Name(s)	Usual Adult Oral Dose and Dosing Schedule	Warning Labels
Antihistamine				
	azelastine	Astelin, Optivar	**Allergic conjunctivitis:** 1 drop in affected eye(s) twice daily **Allergic rhinitis:** 1–2 sprays each nostril twice daily	DISCARD 30 AFTER REMOVING FROM FOIL POUCH—Astelin PRIME INHALER BEFORE USE. MAY CAUSE SEDATION; DO NOT DRIVE OR OPERATE MACHINERY.
	chlorpheniramine	Chlor-Trimeton	**Allergic rhinitis** **Immediate-release:** 4 mg every 4–6 h up to 24 mg/day **Extended-release:** 8 mg–12 mg 2–3 times a day	MAY CAUSE DIZZINESS OR DROWSINESS; ALCOHOL MAY INCREASE THIS EFFECT: chlorpheniramine, diphenhydramine, clemastine, cetirizine, desloratadine, loratadine, levocetirizine.
	diphenhydramine	Benadryl	**Allergic rhinitis, pruritus, and urticaria:** 25–50 mg 3–4 times a day	SWALLOW WHOLE; DON'T CRUSH OR CHEW—EXTENDED-RELEASE.
	clemastine	Tavist	**Allergic rhinitis and urticaria:** 1.34–2.68 mg 1–3 times daily **Pruritus and angioedema:** 2.68 mg 1–3 times daily	PROTECT FROM MOISTURE; LEAVE IN FOIL PACKET UNTIL READY FOR USE—DISINTEGRATING TABLETS.
	cetirizine	Zyrtec	**Allergic rhinitis and urticaria:** 5–10 mg once daily	DISSOLVE REDITAB UNDER THE TONGUE—DISINTEGRATING TABLETS.
	desloratadine	Clarinex	**Allergic rhinitis, pruritus, and urticaria:** 5 mg once daily	WAIT 10 MIN BEFORE APPLYING ANY OTHER EYE DROPS OR CONTACT LENSES—ketotifen
	fexofenadine	Allegra	**Allergic rhinitis and urticaria:** 60 mg bid or 180 mg once daily	MAY CAUSE DIZZINESS OR DROWSINESS, AVOID ORANGE, GRAPEFRUIT, AND APPLE JUICE—fexofenadine.
	ketotifen	Alaway, Zaditor	**Allergic conjunctivitis:** Instill 1 drop twice daily, every 8–12 h in each affected eye.	
	levocetirizine	Xyzal	**Allergic rhinitis and urticaria:** 5 mg once daily in the evening	
	loratadine	Alavert, Claritin	**Allergic rhinitis and urticaria:** 10 mg once daily	
Glucocorticoids				
	beclomethasone	Beconase AQ	**Allergic rhinitis:** 1–2 sprays each nostril twice daily	SHAKE WELL. RINSE AND DRY TIP AFTER EACH USE (All nasal inhalers).
	budesonide	Rhinocort Aqua	**Allergic rhinitis:** 1–2 sprays each nostril once daily	
	flunisolide	Generic	**Allergic rhinitis:** 2 sprays each nostril 2–3 times daily	
	fluticasone propionate	Flonase	**Allergic rhinitis:** 1 spray each nostril twice daily or 2 sprays in each nostril once daily	
	fluticasone furoate	Flonase Allergy Relief, Avamys	**Allergic rhinitis:** 1–2 sprays each nostril once daily	
	mometasone	Nasonex	**Allergic rhinitis:** 2 sprays each nostril once daily	
	triamcinolone	Nasacort Allergy 24 h	**Allergic rhinitis:** 1–2 sprays each nostril once daily	

Summary of Drugs Used in the Treatment of Allergic Conditions—cont'd

	Generic Name	US Brand Name(s)	Usual Adult Oral Dose and Dosing Schedule	Warning Labels
Mast Cell Stabilizer				
	cromolyn sodium	Rhinaris-CS Anti-Allergic Nasal Mist Opticrom	**Allergic rhinitis:** 1 spray each nostril tid or qid (up to 6 times daily) **Allergic conjunctivitis:** 1–2 drops in affected eye(s) 4–6 times a day	RINSE AND DRY TIP AFTER EACH USE (Rhinaris-CS Anti-Allergic Nasal Mist). REMOVE SOFT CONTACT LENSES DURING TREATMENT (Opticrom)
Leukotriene Receptor Antagonist				
	montelukast	Singulair	**Allergic rhinitis:** 10 mg PO once daily **Adults, chewable tablets:** Chew 1 tablet (4 or 5 mg) once daily. **Children and infants, 6 months to 2 years:** 4 mg PO once daily **Children, 2–5 years, oral granules:** dissolve and consume 1 packet once daily	TAKE WITH A LARGE GLASS OF WATER (CHEWABLE TABLET). DISCARD UNUSED PORTION OF SOLUTION WITHIN 15 MIN.
Antihistamine + Decongestant				
	naphazoline + pheniramine[a]	Visine-A,[b] Naphcon-A,[b] Opcon-A[b]	**Allergic conjunctivitis:** 1–2 drops in affected eye(s) up to qid	OVERUSE CAN LEAD TO CONJUNCTIVITIS MEDICAMENTOSA

Key Points

- An allergy is a hypersensitivity reaction by the immune system on exposure to an allergen.
- Allergic conditions affect the quality of life, productivity, and performance of sensitive individuals.
- When a person with allergies first comes into contact with an allergen, the immune system treats the allergen as an invader and produces antibodies to the substance.
- Allergic rhinitis is a condition characterized by nasal itching (rhinitis), runny nose (rhinorrhea), nasal congestion (stuffiness), and sneezing. Allergic conjunctivitis produces itchy and watering eyes.
- Urticaria (also known as hives) is condition characterized by itching and angioedema (swelling).
- Pharmacy technicians are at risk for developing latex allergy. Allergic reactions occur when latex-sensitive individuals breathe in or come into physical contact with latex proteins.
- Latex allergy may produce mild reactions such as skin redness, rash, hives, or itching. Respiratory symptoms such as runny nose, sneezing, itchy eyes, and scratchy throat may occur.
- Pharmacologic treatment of allergies is aimed at reducing swelling and inflammation and suppressing the release of cells that mediate immune system and inflammatory responses, as well as blocking receptor sites of the mediators.
- Drugs used to treat allergic symptoms include antihistamines, inhaled corticosteroids mast cell stabilizers, and leukotriene modifiers.
- Sedation, dizziness, decreased alertness, dry mouth, blurred vision, lack of coordination, and urinary retention are the most common adverse reactions of antihistamines.
- Antihistamines should be used cautiously in men with prostate disease, persons with asthma, and women who are breastfeeding. They are not recommended for use in children younger than 2 years.
- Glucocorticosteroids are administered intranasally to control symptoms of allergic rhinitis.
- Glucocorticosteroids for intranasal use include fluticasone (Flonase), budesonide (Rhinocort), triamcinolone (Nasacort), flunisolide, mometasone (Nasonex), and beclomethasone (Beconase AQ).
- Adverse reactions to corticosteroids administered intranasally are primarily local and include nasal irritation, throat irritation, and nose bleed.
- Cromolyn sodium is a mast cell stabilizer available for intranasal and ophthalmic use. Nedocromil is manufactured for ophthalmic use only.
- Therapy with cromolyn sodium should be initiated 1 week before coming into contact with allergens and continued for the duration of allergen exposure.
- Montelukast is a leukotriene receptor antagonist used to treat allergic rhinitis.
- Allergy shots are a form of immunotherapy that are administered as a series of subcutaneous injections; they can reduce allergy symptoms over a longer period of time than all other treatments.

Review Questions

1. Which of the following is a life-threatening allergic reaction?
   a. Urticaria
   b. Pruritus
   c. Anaphylaxis
   d. Wheal

2. All of the following drugs are nasal sprays for the treatment of allergic rhinitis EXCEPT_____.
   a. Astelin
   b. Rhinocort
   c. Opticrom
   d. Beconase AQ

3. A condition characterized by nasal itching, runny nose, nasal congestion (stuffiness), and sneezing is called _____.
   a. urticaria
   b. allergic rhinitis
   c. wheals
   d. angioedema

4. Select the drug which may only be purchased by prescription.
   a. Rhinaris-CS
   b. Flonase Allergy Relief
   c. Beconase AQ
   d. Nasacort Allergy 24H

5. All of the following drugs used to treat allergic conjunctivitis require a prescription EXCEPT_____.
   a. Pataday
   b. Alocril
   c. Alrex
   d. Opticrom

6. Glucocorticosteroids are administered orally to control symptoms of rhinitis.
   a. True
   b. False

7. Cromolyn sodium is a (an) _____ available for intranasal use.
   a. mast cell stabilizer
   b. glucocorticoid
   c. antihistamine
   d. leukotriene

8. Diphenhydramine has a side effect of _____.
   a. insomnia
   b. sedation
   c. burning
   d. none of the above

9. Loratadine is the generic name for Clarinex (Aerius).
   a. True
   b. False

10. Cetirizine is available in which of the following dosage forms?
    a. Tablet
    b. Chewable tablet
    c. Syrup
    d. All of the above

Bibliography

Center for Disease Control and Prevention: Allergies, 2017. Retrieved September 25, 2017, from: https://www.cdc.gov/healthcommunication/toolstemplates/entertainmented/tips/allergieshtml.

Centers for Disease Control and Prevention: Occupational latex allergies (NIOSH Alert No. 97–135), 2016. http://www.cdc.gov/niosh/docs/97-135.

Centers for Disease Control and Prevention: Latex allergy: A prevention guide (NIOSH Publ. No. 98–113), 2014. http://www.cdc.gov/niosh/docs/98-113/.

FDA, nd. Drugs@FDA: FDA Approved Drug Products, Retrieved August 27, 2018, from: http://www.accessdata.fda.gov/scripts/cder/daf/.

Health Canada: Drug Product Database, 2018. Retrieved August 27, 2018, from: https://health-products.canada.ca/dpd-bdpp/index-eng.jsp.

Institute for Safe Medication Practices: FDA and ISMP Lists of Look-Alike Drug Names with Recommended Tall Man Letters, 2016.

Institute for Safe Medication Practices: List of Confused Drugs, 2015. Retrieved September 9, 2017, from: https://www.ismp.org/tools/confuseddrugnames.pdf.

Kaiser H, Naclerio R, Given J, et al: Fluticasone furoate nasal spray: a single treatment option for the symptoms of seasonal allergic rhinitis, *J Allergy Clin Immunol* 119:1430–1437, 2007.

Kalant H, Grant D, Mitchell J: *Principles of medical pharmacology*, ed 7, Toronto, 2007, Elsevier Canada, pp 22–27, 397–400, 451, 453–454.

National Institute of Allergy and Infectious Disease: Airborne allergens: Something in the air (NIH Publ. No. 03-7045), 2003. http://www.allergywatch.org/basic/airborne_allergens.pdf.

Page C, Curtis M, Sutter M, et al: *Integrated pharmacology*, Philadelphia, 2005, Mosby, pp 330–336, 428–430.

Woodfolk J: T-cell responses to allergens, molecular mechanisms in allergy and clinical immunology, *J Allergy Clin Immunol* 119:280–294, 2007.

UNIT VIII

Drugs Affecting the Endocrine System

The endocrine system and nervous system both function to maintain the stability of the internal environment. In the endocrine system, regulatory function is performed by chemical messengers called hormones that diffuse into the blood to be carried to almost every point in the body. Their effects appear more slowly and last longer the effects produced by neurotransmitters released by the nervous system. Endocrine glands are known as ductless glands because they secrete hormones directly into the blood.

Hormones are classified by their target site, their chemical composition (steroid or nonsteroid), whether they are hydrophilic or hydrophobic, and the mechanism by which they signal hormonal action. The effects of a particular hormone may be limited to specific tissues in the body (e.g., thyroid releasing hormone) or produce effects throughout the body (e.g., thyroid hormone). Endocrine regulation of body processes first begins during early development in the womb continues throughout life, although the secretion of some hormones declines late in life (such as reproductive hormones). Through the secretion of hormones and autonomic nervous system regulation, almost every process in the human organism is kept in balance.

In Unit IX, the pharmacotherapy for diseases of the endocrine system are described that include hypothyroidism, hyperthyroidism and diabetes. A brief description of each disorder is provided, followed by a description of the drugs indicated for treatment, mechanisms of action, adverse reactions, strength(s) and dosage forms.

25

Treatment of Thyroid Disorders

LEARNING OBJECTIVES

1. Learn the terminology associated with thyroid disorders.
2. Describe the pathophysiology of hyperthyroidism and hypothyroidism.
3. List symptoms of hyperthyroidism and hypothyroidism.
4. List and categorize medications used to treat hyperthyroidism and hypothyroidism.
5. Describe mechanism of action for each class of drugs used to treat hyperthyroidism and hypothyroidism.
6. Identify significant drug look-alike and sound-alike issues.
7. Identify warning labels and precautionary messages associated with medications used to treat hyperthyroidism and hypothyroidism.

KEY TERMS

Graves' disease An autoimmune disorder that causes hyperthyroidism.

Hashimoto's disease An autoimmune disorder that causes hypothyroidism.

Hyperthyroidism A condition in which there is an excessive production of thyroid hormones.

Hypothyroidism A condition in which there is insufficient production of thyroid hormones.

Thyroid-releasing factor A hormone released by the hypothalamus that stimulates the pituitary gland to release thyroid-stimulating hormone.

Thyroid-stimulating hormone A hormone released by the pituitary gland that stimulates the thyroid gland to produce and release thyroid hormones.

Tetraiodothyronine The most abundant thyroid hormone. It contains four atoms of iodine and is also known as thyroxine.

Triiodothyronine A hormone secreted by the thyroid gland containing three atoms of iodine.

Overview

More than 20 million Americans and 3 million Canadians have a thyroid disorder and up to 50% of cases are undiagnosed. The disease affects more than 200 million persons worldwide. Thyroid disorders result in overactivity or underactivity of the thyroid gland, causing hypersecretion or hyposecretion of thyroid hormones, respectively. Thyroid disease is up to eight times more common in women than in men. Hyperthyroidism is most common in women between the ages of 20 and 40 years. Diabetes is a risk factor for thyroid disease; a family history of type 1 diabetes further increases the risk. The incidence of hypothyroidism increases with age and, by age 60 years, up to 17% of women and 9% of men will have an underactive thyroid. Cigarette smoking increases the risk for developing thyroid-related eye disease. Smokers with Graves' disease are five times more likely than nonsmokers to develop thyroid-associated ophthalmopathy.

The thyroid gland secretes hormones that have an effect on almost all cells in the body. The thyroid hormones *tetraiodothyronine* (T_4) and *triiodothyronine* (T_3) regulate growth and metabolism. The physiologic actions of thyroid hormone are listed in Box 25.1. Calcitonin, another hormone secreted by the thyroid gland, helps maintain calcium homeostasis.

Thyroid Hormone Control

Thyroid levels are tightly controlled by a negative feedback loop. When the need for thyroid hormones increases, the hypothalamus secretes *thyroid-releasing factor* (TRF), a hormone that signals the pituitary to release *thyroid-stimulating hormone* (TSH). The target site of TSH is the thyroid gland, which produces and secretes T_4 and T_3. Once desired levels are achieved, TSH release is turned off (Fig. 25.1).

Synthesis of Thyroid Hormones

The thyroid gland is one of the few glands that produces and stores its hormones. Thyroid hormones (T_4, T_3) are synthesized by a coupling process in which atoms of iodine are bound to the thyroid protein thyroglobulin. T_3 is formed by three atoms of iodide bound to thyroglobulin. T_4 is formed by four atoms of iodine bound to thyroglobulin. In the body, T_4 (tetraiodothyronine) is converted to T_3.

Diagnosis of Thyroid Disorders

The TSH test measures the level of TSH in the blood. A low TSH level signals hyperthyroidism. This is to be expected because TSH

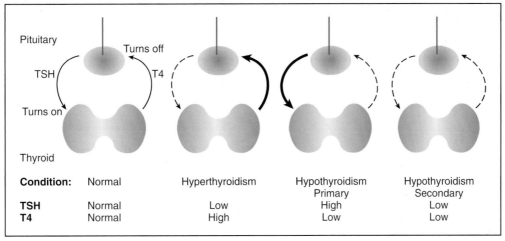

• **Fig. 25.1** Comparison of **thyroid-stimulating hormone** *(TSH)* and **tetraiodothyronine** *(T₄)* levels for normal function, hyperthyroidism, and hypothyroidism. (Courtesy American Thyroid Association, https://www.thyroid.org/thyroid-function-tests/.)

• BOX 25.1   Physiologic Actions of Thyroid Hormones

- Growth of skeletal tissues
- Fetal growth and development (cognitive and physical)
- Growth and development of the central nervous system
- Regulation of protein, lipid, and carbohydrate metabolism
- Regulation of hepatic metabolic enzymes
- Regulation of body temperature
- Cardiac function (heart rate and contractility)
- Circulatory volume
- Respiratory functions
- Peripheral vasodilation
- Bone turnover

Thyroxine (T₄)

Triiodothyronine (T₃)

Dimethyl-isopropyl-thyronine (DIMIT)

• **Fig. 25.2** Structural formula of thyroid hormones. (From Kalant H, Grant DM, Mitchell J: *Principles of medical pharmacology*, ed 7, Philadelphia, 2007, WB Saunders.)

release is turned off when the body recognizes that T_4 levels are high; the body therefore attempts to stop its further production and release. A high TSH level is a signal for hypothyroidism. A tetraiodothyronine test measures free T_4 (FT_4) and the FT_4 index (FT_4I). FT_4 and FT_4I tests measure circulating thyroid hormone. In hyperthyroidism, FT_4 levels are elevated and TSH levels are depressed. The reverse is true in the case of hypothyroidism. The presence of thyroid-stimulating antibodies can be measured by a thyroid antibody test. When thyroid antibodies are present, autoimmune thyroid disease is diagnosed. A radioactive iodine uptake (RAIU) test may also be conducted to test for thyroid disease. Iodine is selectively taken up by the thyroid gland in the process of synthesizing T_4 and T_3 (Fig. 25.2); thus, when a low dose of radioactive iodine (^{131}I) is administered, the amount of radioactivity in the thyroid gland can be measured. The RAIU is high when a person has hyperthyroidism and low when a person has hypothyroidism.

Types of Thyroid Disorders

Hyperthyroidism

Hyperthyroidism is a condition in which the thyroid gland secretes excessive amounts of thyroid hormones. The following conditions are known to cause hyperthyroidism: (1) thyroid nodules (lumps on the thyroid gland that secrete thyroid hormone) and (2) inflammation of the thyroid gland (e.g., subacute thyroiditis, postpartum thyroiditis, lymphatic thyroiditis). *Graves' disease* is an autoimmune disease and a primary cause of thyroid hyperactivity. In Graves' disease, thyroid-stimulating antibodies mimic TSH and cause the thyroid gland to release its hormones (see Fig. 25.1). Graves' disease is the primary cause of hyperthyroidism. When it is left untreated, the severe hyperthyroidism that results may lead to cardiovascular disease and death.

• TECH NOTE!

Potassium iodide can protect the thyroid gland against exposure to radioactive iodine.

• BOX 25.2   Symptoms of Hyperthyroidism

- Rapid heart rate and palpitations
- Muscle weakness
- Muscle wasting
- Tremor
- Weight loss
- Shortness of breath
- Nervousness or irritability
- Restlessness
- Sleeplessness
- Enlarged thyroid (goiter)
- Amenorrhea
- Diarrhea
- Breast enlargement
- Bulging eyes
- Rapid speech
- Sweating
- Heat intolerance, warm skin, facial flushing

Symptoms of Hyperthyroidism

Given that thyroid hormones have an effect on numerous cells throughout the body, it is not surprising that symptoms of thyroid disease are widespread. These are listed in Box 25.2.

Treatment of Hyperthyroidism

Treatment of hyperthyroidism involves the administration of either antithyroid drugs or radioactive iodine; it can also be treated with surgery.

Radioactive Iodine

Low-dose radioactive iodine is used for diagnosis and higher-dose radioactive iodine is administered for the treatment of hyperthyroidism. It is selectively taken up by the thyroid gland, where it causes glandular destruction while minimizing damage to other tissues. The rate of cure is 61% to 86% depending on the dose administered. Pretreatment with an antithyroid drug is recommended for approximately 2 weeks to block the synthesis of thyroid hormone prior to the administration of ^{131}I. The full effects of ^{131}I therapy are achieved after 2 to 3 months in most people, but sometimes a second or third course of therapy is required. Beta blockers (see Chapter 18) may be administered concurrently with ^{131}I until tachycardia and tremors, symptoms of hyperthyroidism, subside. Radioactive iodine that is not retained by the thyroid is eliminated in the urine within 2 or 3 days.

> **TECH NOTE!**
>
> Radioactive iodine ^{131}I is made in nuclear pharmacies and is regulated by the Nuclear Regulatory Commission (NRC).

Adverse Reactions. Treatment with ^{131}I produces few adverse effects. The most common side effect is temporary inflammation of the salivary glands. Most patients also develop an underactive thyroid gland after treatment, requiring lifelong therapy for hypothyroidism.

Precautions. Radioactive iodide therapy is contraindicated in pregnant women because the drug can cross the placenta and cause thyroid damage in the developing fetus. Nursing mothers should also avoid breast-feeding until radioactive iodine can no longer be detected in the breast milk. Nonpregnant women and men treated with radioactive iodide should avoid close physical contact with pregnant women and young children for a few days after the dose is administered.

Radioactive Iodine (^{131}I)

Generic Name	US Brand Names	Dosage Forms and Strengths
	Canadian Brand Names	
radioactive iodine (^{131}I)[a]	No commercial preparations	Individualized
	No commercial preparations	

[a]Generic available.

Thioamides (Thionamides)

Propylthiouracil (PTU) and thiamazole (Canada) or methimazole (United States) are antithyroid drugs. They are used for the primary treatment of hyperthyroidism or to reduce excess thyroid hormone levels in patients awaiting treatment with radioactive iodine or thyroid surgery.

> **! TECH ALERT!**
>
> The following drugs have look-alike and sound-alike issues:
> methimazole and metolazone
> propylthiouracil and Purinethol

Mechanism of Action and Pharmacokinetics. PTU and thiamazole (methimazole) block the synthesis of T_4 and T_3 by blocking the enzyme that catalyzes the coupling of iodinated tyrosine (MIT and DIT). PTU is also capable of blocking the conversion of T_4 to T_3. The maximal benefit of PTU therapy is not achieved until all to the thyroid hormone that is stored in the thyroid gland's follicles is depleted. This can take 2 to 4 months of therapy.

> **! TECH ALERT!**
>
> The abbreviation PTU (propylthiouracil) has been misread as 6-MP (6-mercaptopurine).

Adverse Reactions. Methimazole and PTU may cause nausea or vomiting, muscle aches and pains, and/or minor rash or itching. Side effects requiring medical attention include fever accompanied by sore throat and hoarseness, goiter, severe redness or itching, hepatitis, arthritis, unusual bleeding, bruising, and red spots. Methimazole and PTU may also produce a dangerous decrease in the number of white blood cells (agranulocytosis), which increases the risk for serious infections. Dosages higher than 40 mg/day of methimazole may increase the risk for agranulocytosis.

Like radioactive thyroid therapy, treatment with antithyroid drugs typically induces hypothyroidism. Hypothyroidism may appear as soon as 6 months after the onset of therapy or as long as 25 years after disease remission and discontinuation of drug therapy.

Hypothyroidism

Hypothyroidism is a condition in which the thyroid gland secretes deficient amounts of thyroid hormones. The following conditions are known to cause hypothyroidism: (1) treatment for hyperthyroidism

• BOX 25.3 Symptoms of Hypothyroidism

- Slowed heart rate, slowed pulse
- Extreme fatigue
- Weight gain
- Dry skin and dry coarse hair
- Poor memory, slowed mental processes
- Constipation
- Deep coarse voice, slow speech, thick tongue
- Enlarged heart
- Enlarged thyroid (goiter)
- Cold intolerance
- Depression

• BOX 25.4 Medications That Interact With Thyroid Hormones

- Ferrous products (iron supplements)
- Calcium supplements and dairy products
- Proton pump inhibitors (e.g., omeprazole)
- Raloxifene
- Cholestyramine
- Colestipol
- Oral contraceptives
- Phenytoin
- Carbamazepine

Thioamides

| Generic Name | US Brand Names | | Dosage Forms and Strengths |
	Canadian Brand Names	
methimazole[a] (thiamazole in Canada)	Tapazole		**Tablet:** 5 mg, 10 mg
	Tapazole		
propylthiouracil[a]	Generics		**Tablet:** 50 mg, 100 mg[b]
	Propyl-Thyracil		

[a]Generic available.
[b]Available in Canada only.

with radioactive iodine and antithyroid drugs; (2) treatment with medications for non–thyroid-related conditions (e.g., lithium, amiodarone); (3) thyroidectomy (removal of all or a portion of the thyroid gland); (4) pituitary gland damage that affects TSH secretion; (5) congenital conditions (birth defects); and (6) thyroiditis. *Hashimoto's disease* is an autoimmune disorder in which the body produces antibodies to its own thyroid cells. The antibodies and white blood cells attack and damage the thyroid. Hashimoto's disease is the most common cause of non–iodine-deficiency hypothyroidism.

Symptoms

The effects of insufficient thyroid hormones can be felt throughout the body. Symptoms of hypothyroidism are listed in Box 25.3.

> **TECH NOTE!**
> Levothyroxine is the replacement for naturally occurring thyroxine.

Treatment of Hypothyroidism

Thyroid replacement therapy is the principal treatment for hypothyroidism. Replacement can be achieved by the administration of desiccated (dried, powdered) whole-gland animal thyroid or synthetic T_4, synthetic T_3, or a combination of the two hormones. The most widely prescribed treatment for hypothyroidism is synthetic T_4, which is converted in the body to T_3.

Mechanism of Action

Exogenously administered thyroid hormones, animal gland and synthetic, bind to the same receptor sites and produce the same actions as thyroid hormones made by the body. Synthetic T_4,

known as levothyroxine (L-thyroxine), is generally the only thyroid hormone prescribed for the treatment of hypothyroidism. Additional administration of liothyronine is typically unnecessary because levothyroxine is converted to liothyronine in the body, just as naturally occurring T_4 is metabolized to T_3.

> **! TECH ALERT!**
> The following drugs have look-alike and sound-alike issues: levothyroxine and liothyronine

Pharmacokinetics

Liothyronine (T_3) and levothyroxine are dissimilar in their onset and duration of action. They also differ in potency and dosing frequency.

Bioavailability issues exist between different manufacturers' formulations of synthetic and naturally occurring thyroid preparations. Numerous medications interact with thyroid hormones (Box 25.4). Ferrous products, calcium supplements, cholesterol-lowering agents (e.g., colestipol, cholestyramine), and didanosine interfere with the absorption of thyroid hormones. Food delays absorption. Antiseizure medicines such as phenytoin and carbamazepine accelerate the rate of metabolism of thyroid hormones. Soy isoflavones, oral contraceptives, and raloxifene reduce the clinical response to administered thyroid hormone by altering TSH, thyroglobulin, T_4, and T_3 levels. Thyroid hormones may increase the response to warfarin and decrease the response to oral antidiabetic agents, requiring close monitoring of the international normalized ratio (INR) and blood glucose levels.

> **TECH NOTE!**
> Pharmacy technicians should attempt to dispense the same manufacturer's product each time a patient's prescription is refilled.

Adverse Reactions. Given that thyroid replacement therapy is achieved by administering naturally occurring or synthetic thyroid hormone, adverse effects produced are the same as symptoms of hypothyroidism (subtherapeutic doses) or symptoms of hyperthyroidism (taking too much thyroid hormone).

Precautions. Diabetic patients may require an adjustment in their dose of diabetes medicine once thyroid replacement therapy is initiated. Thyroid hormones can affect blood sugar levels.

> **TECH NOTE!**
> The various strengths of levothyroxine are color-coded to help avoid dispensing errors.

Thyroid Replacements

	Generic Name	US Brand Names	Dosage Forms and Strengths
		Canadian Brand Names	
	levothyroxine[a] (T$_4$)	Levoxyl, Levo-T, Synthroid, Tirosint, Unithroid	**Capsule (Tirosint)**[b]:13 mcg, 25 mcg, 50 mcg, 75 mcg, 88 mcg, 100 mcg, 112 mcg, 125 mcg, 137 mcg, 150 mcg, 175 mcg, 200 mcg
		Eltroxin[c], Synthroid	**Powder, for injection:** 100 mcg,[b] 200 mcg,[b] 500 mcg per vial
			Tablet: 25 mcg, 50 mcg, 75 mcg, 88 mcg, 100 mcg, 112 mcg, 125 mcg, 137 mcg, 150 mcg, 175 mcg, 200 mcg, 300 mcg
	liothyronine[ab] (T$_3$)	Cytomel, Triostat	**Solution, injection (Triostat)**[b]: 10 mcg/mL
		Cytomel	**Tablet (Cytomel):** 5 mcg, 25 mcg, 50 mcg[b]
	liotrix[a] (T$_4$:T$_3$)	Thyrolar-$\frac{1}{4}$, Thyrolar-$\frac{1}{2}$, Thyrolar-1, Thyrolar-2, Thyrolar-3	**Tablet:** levothyroxine 12.5 mcg + liothyronine 3.1 mcg (Thyrolar-$\frac{1}{4}$),
		Not available	levothyroxine 25 mcg + liothyronine 6.25 mcg (Thyrolar-$\frac{1}{2}$), levothyroxine 50 mcg + liothyronine 12.5 mcg (Thyrolar-1), levothyroxine 100 mcg + liothyronine 25 mcg (Thyrolar-2), levothyroxine 150 mcg + liothyronine 37.5 mcg (Thyrolar-3)
	desiccated thyroid[a]	Not available	**Tablet:** 30 mg, 60 mg, 125 mg
		Generics	

[a]Generic available.
[b]Available in the United States only.
[c]Eltroxin is only marketed in 4 strengths (75 mcg, 100 mcg, 150 mcg and 200 mcg).
[c]Generic available in the United States only.

Congenital Hypothyroidism

Congenital hypothyroidism is a condition that occurs when the neonatal thyroid gland fails to develop or function properly. It may also occur if a woman has a iodine deficiency during pregnancy. If untreated, the condition causes severely stunted growth or dwarfism and intellectual disability. In the United States and Canada, all newborns are routinely tested for congenital hypothyroidism. Newborns diagnosed with the condition are treated with thyroid hormones.

Summary of Drugs Used in the Treatment of Thyroid Disorders

	Generic Name	Brand Name	Usual Dose and Dosing Schedule	Warning Labels
Hyperthyroidism				
	methimazole	Tapazole	Begin: 15–60 mg in three divided doses/day Maintenance: 5–15 mg daily	AVOID PREGNANCY.
	propylthiouracil	Generics	Begin 50 to 150 mg 3 times daily. Maintenance dose is 50 mg 2-3 times a day.	
	radioactive iodine,[131]I	Manufactured in pharmacy	6–15 µCi as a single dose	
Hypothyroidism				
	levothyroxine	Synthroid, Eltroxin	25–150 mcg once daily	AVOID ANTACIDS, DAIRY, CALCIUM, AND IRON PILLS WITHIN 4 H OF DOSE. TAKE ON AN EMPTY STOMACH. TAKE WITH A FULL GLASS OF WATER. DO NOT SKIP DOSES.
	liothyronine	Cytomel	25–75 mcg once daily	
	liotrix	Thyrolar	50–100 mcg T$_4$ + 12.5–25 mcg T$_3$ once daily	
	desiccated thyroid	Generics	Initial: 30–300 mg daily; Maintenance: 30–125 mg once daily	

TECHNICIAN'S CORNER

1. What is an autoimmune disease, and what are the effects of an autoimmune disease such as Graves' disease?
2. What types of food provide iodine?

Key Points

- Thyroid disorders result in either overactivity or underactivity of the thyroid gland.
- Hyperthyroidism is a condition in which the thyroid gland secretes excessive amounts of thyroid hormones.
- Graves' disease is an autoimmune disease that causes hyperthyroidism.
- Hypothyroidism is a condition in which the thyroid gland secretes deficient amounts of thyroid hormones.
- Hashimoto's disease is an autoimmune disorder that causes hypothyroidism.
- Hyperthyroidism and hypothyroidism are more prevalent in women than in men.
- The incidence of hypothyroidism increases with age.
- Patients with an autoimmune disease (e.g., type 1 diabetes) are at increased risk for developing thyroid disease.
- Cigarette smoking increases the risk for developing thyroid-related eye disease.
- The thyroid gland secretes hormones that affect almost all cells in the body. Thyroid hormones regulate growth and metabolism.
- The thyroid gland is one of the few glands that produces and stores its hormones.
- Treatment of hyperthyroidism involves the use of antithyroid drugs or high-dose radioactive iodine (^{131}I); it may also be treated with surgery.
- Radioactive iodine is selectively taken up by the thyroid gland, where it causes glandular destruction without producing damage to other tissues.
- Most patients treated with ^{131}I develop an underactive thyroid gland after treatment, requiring lifelong therapy for hypothyroidism.
- Radioactive iodide therapy is contraindicated in pregnant women because it can cause thyroid damage in the developing fetus.
- Radioactive iodine ^{131}I is made in nuclear pharmacies and is regulated by the Nuclear Regulatory Commission.
- Propylthiouracil and methimazole block the synthesis of T_4 and T_3. Propylthiouracil is capable of blocking the process that converts T_4 to T_3.
- Thyroid replacement therapy is the principal treatment for hypothyroidism. Synthetic T_4, known as levothyroxine (L-thyroxine), is the most commonly prescribed drug for the treatment of hypothyroidism.
- Levothyroxine is converted to liothyronine in the body, just as naturally occurring T_4 is metabolized to T_3.
- Liothyronine (T_3) and levothyroxine differ in their onset of action, duration of action, potency, and dosing frequency.
- Pharmacy technicians should attempt to dispense the same manufacturer's product each time a patient's prescription for levothyroxine is refilled.
- Ferrous products, calcium supplements, and food can decrease the absorption of thyroid hormones.
- The various strengths of levothyroxine are color-coded to help avoid dispensing errors.

Review Questions

1. Tetraiodothyronine is the most abundant thyroid hormone. It contains _____ atom(s) of iodine and is also known as thyroxine.
   a. Three
   b. Four
   c. Two
   d. One
2. Hyperthyroidism and hypothyroidism are more prevalent in women than in men.
   a. True
   b. False
3. _____ is an autoimmune disease that is the primary cause of thyroid hyperactivity.
   a. Hashimoto's disease
   b. TSH disease
   c. Graves' disease
   d. All of the above
4. Treatment of hyperthyroidism involves the administration of _____.
   a. Antithyroid drugs
   b. Radioactive iodine
   c. Surgery
   d. All of the above
5. Select the drug that is used to treat hypothyroidism.
   a. Propylthiouracil
   b. Tapazole
   c. Synthroid
   d. Iodine^{131}
6. Select the drug that is used to treat hyperthyroidism.
   a. Cytomel
   b. Synthroid
   c. Eltroxin
   d. Tapazole

7. A brand name for levothyroxine is _____.
    a. Cytomel
    b. Thyrolar
    c. Proloid
    d. Synthroid

8. Select the warning label might be placed on a prescription filled for Synthroid.
    a. Take with food.
    b. Avoid antacids, dairy, and iron pills.
    c. May cause drowsiness.
    d. Avoid prolonged exposure to sunlight.

9. Hashimoto's disease is an autoimmune disorder that causes _____.
    a. Hypothyroidism
    b. Hyperthyroidism

10. Diabetes is not a risk factor for thyroid disease.
    a. True
    b. False

Bibliography

Alexander EK, Pearce EN, Brent GA, et al: 2017 Guidelines of the American Thyroid Association for the Diagnosis and Management of Thyroid Disease During Pregnancy and the Postpartum, *Thyroid* 27(3):2017. doi:10.1089/thy.2016.0457.

American Thyroid Association: 2017. General Information/Press Room: Prevalence and Impact of Thyroid Disease. Retrieved October 30, 2017, from https://www.thyroid.org/media-main/about-hypothyroidism/.

Becker D, Hurley J, Detres R: Thyroid Foundation of Canada: Radioactive iodine treatment of hyperthyroidism. 1992 (http://www.thyroid.ca/thyrotoxicosis.php).

Burch HB, Wartofsky L: 2017a. Graves' Disease. Retrieved October 31, 2017, from https://www.niddk.nih.gov/health-information/endocrine-diseases/graves-disease.

Burch HB, Wartofsky L: 2017b. Hashimoto's Disease. Retrieved October 31, 2017, from https://www.niddk.nih.gov/health-information/endocrine-diseases/hashimotos-disease.

Cawood T, Moriarty P, O'Farrelly C, et al: Smoking and thyroid-associated ophthalmopathy: a novel explanation of the biological link, *J Clin Endocrinol Metab* 92:59–64, 2007.

De Moraes A, Pedro A, Romaldini J: Spontaneous hypothyroidism in the follow-up of Graves' hyperthyroid patients treated with antithyroid drugs, *South Med J* 99:1068–1072, 2006.

FDA: nd. Drugs@FDA: FDA Approved Drug Products. Retrieved August 29, 2018, from http://www.accessdata.fda.gov/scripts/cder/daf/.

Genovese BM, Noureldine SI, Gleeson EM, et al: What is the best definitive treatment for Graves' disease? A systematic review of the existing literature, *Annals or Surgical Oncology* 20:660–667, 2013. doi:10.1245/s10434-012-2606-x.

Health Canada: 2018. Drug Product Database. Retrieved August 29, 2018, from https://health-products.canada.ca/dpd-bdpp/index-eng.jsp.

Institute for Safe Medication Practices: 2015. List of Confused Drugs. Retrieved September 9, 2017, from https://www.ismp.org/tools/confuseddrugnames.pdf.

Kalant H, Grant D, Mitchell J: *Principles of medical pharmacology*, ed 7, Toronto, 2007, Elsevier Canada, pp 613–619.

National Institute of Diabetes and Digestive and Kidney Diseases: 2017 Hashimoto's disease. Retrieved November 8, 2017 from https://www.niddk.nih.gov/health-information/endocrine-diseases/hashimotos-disease.

Okosieme OE, Lazarus JH: Current trends in antithyroid drug treatment of Graves' disease, *Expert Opin Pharmacother* 17(15):2005–2017, 2016. doi:10.1080/14656566.2016.1232388.

Page C, Curtis M, Sutter M, et al: *Integrated pharmacology*, Philadelphia, 2005, Mosby, pp 288–291.

Raffa R, Rawls S, Beyzarov E: *Netter's illustrated pharmacology*, Philadelphia, 2005, Saunders Elsevier, pp 10–11, 136–142.

Ross DS, Burch HB, Cooper DS, et al: 2016 American Thyroid Association Guidelines for Diagnosis and Management of Hyperthyroidism and Other Causes of Thyrotoxicosis, *Thyroid* 26(10):2016.

Schellack N, Schellack G: A review of drugs acting on the thyroid gland, *South African Pharmaceutical Journal* 80(2):12–17, 2013.

Wang S, Baker J Jr: Targeting B cells in Graves' disease, *Endocrinology* 147:4559–4560, 2006.

26

Treatment of Diabetes Mellitus

LEARNING OBJECTIVES

1 Learn the terminology associated with diabetes mellitus.
2 Identify risk factors for diabetes mellitus.
3 Describe the causes of diabetes mellitus.
4 List the symptoms of diabetes mellitus.
5 List and categorize medications used to treat diabetes mellitus.
6 Describe mechanism of action for each class of drugs used to treat diabetes mellitus.
7 Identify significant drug look-alike and sound-alike issues.
8 List common endings for drug classes used in the treatment of diabetes mellitus.
9 Identify warning labels and precautionary messages associated with medications used to treat diabetes mellitus.

KEY TERMS

Diabetes mellitus Chronic condition in which the body is unable to use glucose (sugar) as energy properly.
Diabetic neuropathy Damage to peripheral nerves by diabetes causes numbness in the lower limbs.
Fasting blood glucose Blood glucose level that is taken after a person has not eaten for 8 to 12 hours (usually overnight).
Gestational diabetes Diabetes that may be caused by the hormones of pregnancy or a shortage of insulin.
Hemoglobin A1c Blood test that measures a person's average blood glucose level over a period of 2 to 3 months.
Hyperglycemia Elevated blood glucose levels.
Hypoglycemia Low blood glucose levels.

Insulin resistance Condition in which the body does not respond to insulin; contributes to the development of type 2 diabetes.
Postprandial After a meal.
Prediabetes Condition of impaired fasting glucose and impaired glucose tolerance in which the body consistently has elevated glucose levels.
Type 1 diabetes An autoimmune disease that results in high blood glucose levels. Pancreatic beta cells are destroyed and insufficient amounts of insulin are produced.
Type 2 diabetes A condition that results in high blood glucose levels. People with type 2 diabetes have insulin resistance.

Overview

Diabetes mellitus is a disorder of metabolism that involves glucose use. It is a chronic condition in which the body cannot properly use glucose as energy. Glucose is the body's primary energy source. Under normal conditions, as glucose levels in the blood rise, hormones are released that move the glucose out of the bloodstream and into cells, where it is needed for growth and energy. In diabetes, glucose accumulates in the blood. Much like a person with sticky hands walking through a room, glucose in the bloodstream leaves a sticky residue over all the body's organs and cells and causes damage.

Diabetes affects approximately 422 million people globally. In the United States, more than 30 million adults have the disease, according to the Centers for Disease Control and Prevention, *National Diabetes Statistics Report (2017)*. In Canada, more than 3 million people are living with diabetes, and it is estimated the 2.1 million additional cases will be diagnosed by 2020. Approximately 84 million adults in the United States and 5.7 million Canadians have prediabetes. Diabetes mellitus is one of the leading causes of disability in the United States. It is the leading cause of non–war-related amputations.

The global cost for treating diabetes is $825 billion annually! In the United States, one of every eight federal health care dollars is spent treating people with diabetes. NIDDK National Statistics has estimated the direct cost of diabetes in the United States is $105 billion. The costs in Canada were estimated to be $15.3 billion, approximately $6,741 per person with diabetes.

Hormone Regulation of Blood Glucose Level

The control of glucose levels occurs by a second-messenger reaction. Insulin, a hormone that is essential for the regulation of carbohydrates, fat, and protein metabolism, is secreted by the beta cells in the islets of Langerhans when the blood glucose level rises. Insulin binds to receptors on the cell membrane. This stimulates the docking of intracellular glucose transporters that carry glucose out of the bloodstream and into cells where it is needed. Insulin, along with glucagon, is released by the pancreas in response to the rise and fall of blood glucose, amino acid, and gut-derived hormone levels (Fig. 26.1).

Excess glucose that is not needed for energy immediately, is stored in the liver as glycogen, a reservoir for future energy needs (Fig. 26.2). When glucose levels drop, glucagon is secreted by

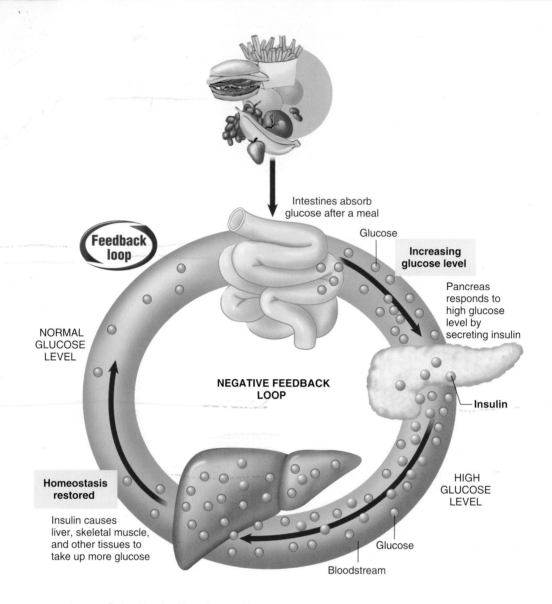

• **Fig. 26.1** Role of insulin. (From Patton KT, Thibodeau GA: *The human body in health and disease*, ed 7, St. Louis, 2018, Elsevier.)

alpha cells in the islets of Langerhans. Glucagon stimulates the release of the stored energy. The physiologic effects of insulin are listed in Box 26.1.

Types of Diabetes Mellitus

Prediabetes, type 1 diabetes, type 2 diabetes, and gestational diabetes all produce elevated blood glucose levels *(hyperglycemia)*. A normal *fasting blood glucose* level is 70 to 99 mg/dL, or less than 4 to 6 mmol/L. Symptoms of *hyperglycemia* are listed in Box 26.2.

Prediabetes

Prediabetes causes impaired fasting glucose (IFG) and impaired glucose tolerance (IGT). When blood glucose levels range between 100 and 125 mg/dL (6.1 to 6.9 mmol/L) after an overnight fast, glucose levels are said to be impaired. After a 2-hour oral glucose tolerance test (OGTT), blood glucose levels are high and range from 140 to 199 mg/dL (7.8 to 11.0 mmol/L) in individuals with IGT. Prediabetes increases the risk of cardiovascular disease (CVD).

Type 1 Diabetes

Type 1 diabetes is an autoimmune disease. The immune system attacks and destroys the insulin-producing beta cells in the pancreas. Only 5% to 10% of all persons with diabetes have type 1 diabetes. People who have type 1 diabetes must inject insulin daily because their body no longer produces sufficient amounts of the hormone insulin. The onset of type 1 diabetes is typically in childhood; hence the condition was formerly called juvenile-onset diabetes mellitus. However, it can occur at any age.

Type 2 Diabetes

Type 2 diabetes is most common, accounting for 90% to 95% of all cases of diabetes. In type 2 diabetes, the pancreas initially produces sufficient amounts of insulin, but the body is unable to use the insulin effectively. This condition is called *insulin resistance*. Insulin production eventually decreases; however, this may not occur for several years. Risk factors of type 2 diabetes are obesity, lack of physical activity, family history of diabetes, prior gestational

• **Fig. 26.2** Algorithm for management of diabetes (or equivalent). (From Garber AJ, Abrahamson MJ, Barzilay JI, et al: Consensus statement by the American Association of Clinical Endocrinologists and American College of Endocrinology on the comprehensive type 2 diabetes management algorithm—2017 executive summary, *Endocr Pract* 23(2):207–238, 2017.)

TABLE 26.1   Risk Factors for Diabetes Mellitus

Type of Risk Factor	Description
Nonmodifiable	Age (≥40 year), family history of diabetes
Modifiable	Obesity (body mass index ≥25 kg/m²) Physical inactivity Smoking
Disease	Hypertension, angina, myocardial infarction, stroke, metabolic syndrome, insulin resistance, hyperlipidemia, schizophrenia, polycystic ovary syndrome

• BOX 26.2   Symptoms of Hyperglycemia

Hyperglycemia
- Blurred vision
- Breath that smells fruity
- Decreased consciousness
- Dry mouth
- Elevated blood glucose level
- Extreme hunger
- Extreme thirst
- Frequent urination
- Shortness of breath
- Upset stomach and vomiting
- Weakness

• BOX 26.1   Physiologic Effects of Insulin

Carbohydrate Metabolism
- Increased glycogen synthesis (liver)
- Decreased gluconeogenesis (liver)
- Increased glucose transport (muscle and fat cells)

Lipid Metabolism
- Sets the level of triglyceride production from free fatty acids
- Decreased lipolysis

Protein Metabolism
- Increased amino acid synthesis
- Increased amino acid transport (precursors for protein synthesis)

diabetes, and increasing age (Table 26.1). Approximately 80% of persons diagnosed with type 2 diabetes are overweight. Type 2 diabetes was formerly called non–insulin-dependent diabetes (NIDDM) or adult-onset diabetes; however, these terms have been replaced, because people with type 2 diabetes may sometimes be required to manage their condition with insulin and childhood

obesity has caused children to become the fastest growing population with diabetes.

In Canada, the prevalence of type 2 diabetes is greater in Canadians of South Asian descent and First Nations and Métis Peoples. In the United States, African Americans and Latino and First Nations Peoples have the highest prevalence. It is believed that internalized racism, chronic stress, and consumption of a "diabetes" diet that is high in fat and carbohydrates may contribute to the higher level of diabetes in these groups.

Gestational Diabetes

Gestational diabetes occurs in approximately 3% to 8% of all pregnant women. It typically occurs late in pregnancy and may be caused by the hormones of pregnancy or by a shortage of insulin. Pregnant women are routinely tested for gestational diabetes. An elevated blood glucose level is an early sign of gestational diabetes. Symptoms often disappear after delivery; however, women who have had gestational diabetes have a 20% to 50% increased risk for the development of type 2 diabetes within 5 to 10 years.

• BOX 26.3 **Symptoms of Diabetes Mellitus**

Type 1
- Blurred vision
- Constant hunger (polyphagia)
- Diabetic ketoacidosis
- Extreme fatigue
- Frequent urination (polyuria)
- Hyperglycemia
- Increased thirst (polydipsia)
- Weight loss

Type 2
- Blurred vision
- Fatigue
- Frequent urination
- Hunger
- Hyperglycemia
- Increased thirst
- Slow healing of wounds or sores
- Weight loss

• BOX 26.4 **Diabetes Complications**

- Amputation
- Angina
- Blindness
- Blurred vision
- Heart attack
- Hyperlipidemia
- Hypertension
- Increased birth defects
- Infections
- Ketoacidosis
- Nephropathy
- Peripheral neuropathy
- Pregnancy complications
- Retinopathy
- Stroke

Insulin Resistance as a Cause of Diabetes

Insulin resistance is a condition in which the body does not respond to insulin. It is a precursor to type 2 diabetes. Insulin resistance is a syndrome that increases the risk for CVD, hypertension, dyslipidemia, elevated triglyceride and low-density lipoprotein (LDL) levels, decreased high-density lipoprotein (HDL) levels, microalbuminuria, and diabetes. It may also increase risk for obesity, a risk factor for type 2 diabetes, because insulin signals the body to increase food intake.

Symptoms and Diagnosis of Diabetes Mellitus

Symptoms

Symptoms of diabetes mellitus are listed in Box 26.3.

Diagnostic Tests

The *hemoglobin A1c* (Hb$_{A1c}$) test is the principal method used to diagnose diabetes. It is the only test that provides information about blood glucose levels over a 2- to 3-month period. Additional test are blood glucose levels measured after fasting or after the consumption of a dose of glucose (OGTT)
- Fasting blood glucose test: Blood glucose level 126 mg/dL or higher (≥7 mmol/L) or more after an 8-hour fast.
- OGTT: Blood glucose level 200 mg/dL or higher (≥11 mmol/L) 2 hours after drinking a beverage containing 75 g of glucose dissolved in water.
- Random blood glucose: Blood glucose level 200 mg/dL or higher (≥11 mmol/L), along with the presence of diabetes symptoms.

Diabetes Complications

Untreated or poorly controlled diabetes mellitus produces damage throughout the body (Box 26.4). It may cause microvascular and macrovascular damage. Microvascular damage weakens blood vessels in the eye, and retinopathy can lead to blurred vision and blindness. Nephropathy (kidney damage) and *diabetic neuropathy* also occur. Diabetic neuropathy causes numbness in the lower limbs. Patients

with diabetes must frequently inspect their feet because if they develop a foot injury, they might not feel it. Diabetes causes poor wound healing, so foot infections sometimes become serious enough to require limb amputation. Macrovascular changes can lead to hypertension, angina, and myocardial infarction. Diabetes can also cause hyperlipidemia. Individuals with untreated or poorly controlled type 1 diabetes may develop ketoacidosis, a condition in which the body breaks down fats to obtain its energy needs. Ketones are a by-product of lipid metabolism, and their accumulation can lead to coma and death.

> ● **TECH NOTE!**
>
> Alcohol, aspirin, and decongestants can alter blood glucose levels. A list of drugs that increase and decrease blood glucose levels is provided in Box 26.2.

> ● **TECH NOTE!**
>
> It is recommended that alcohol consumption be limited in a patient with diabetes to no more than one or two drinks/day (maximum, 14 drinks/week for men and 9 drinks/week for women).

Management of Diabetes

Nonpharmacologic Management

Diabetes mellitus is sometimes classified as a disease of lifestyle because lifestyle factors can increase the risk for type 2 diabetes. All types of diabetes can be improved by weight loss, engaging in physical activity, consuming foods with a low glycemic index, quitting smoking, reducing alcohol consumption, and other lifestyle changes. Physical activity lowers the risk of type 2 diabetes by up to 30%. For those with diabetes, increased physical activity decreases risks of mortality from the disease. A minimum of 150 minutes of exercise weekly is recommended to maintain glycemic control, of which at least 90 minutes should be vigorous aerobic exercise. Loss of 5% to 7% of body weight through diet and increased physical activity can lower the risks of diabetes (Fig. 26.2).

• **Fig. 26.3** (A) Blood glucose monitor. (B) Blood glucose testing using a blood glucose meter. ([A], From Bonewit-West K: *Clinical procedures for medical assistants*, ed 7, St. Louis, 2008, Saunders. [B], From MedlinePlus: *Diabetes*. http://www.nlm.nih.gov/medlineplus/diabetes.html. 2017.)

Blood Glucose Monitoring

Blood glucose monitoring is an essential component of diabetes management (Fig. 26.3A). Measurement of blood glucose levels may be recommended 1 to 4 times daily, depending on the type of diabetes (type 1, type 2, or gestational) and on the antihyperglycemic drug regimen that the patient is prescribed. Blood glucose monitoring enables individuals with diabetes to take control of their disease by adjusting their level of diet, exercise, and insulin (see Fig. 26.3B).

Keeping the blood glucose level within a normal range has been shown to minimize the risk of diabetic complications. According to the Diabetes Control and Complications Trial (DCCT), a 10-year study sponsored by the NIDDK and the United Kingdom Prospective Diabetes Study, intensive control of blood glucose and blood pressure reduces complications in types 1 and 2 diabetes.

● TECH NOTE!

Pharmacy technicians knowledgeable about the various blood glucose monitors can help patients select the monitor that best suits their needs.

Pharmacologic Management

At present, type 1 diabetes is primarily managed with insulin. Type 2 diabetes may be managed with oral antidiabetic agents or insulin (Fig. 26.4). Pramlintide (Symlin) is a synthetic analogue of the hormone amylin that is also used for the treatment of type 1 diabetes. Type 2 diabetes may be treated with oral agents and/or insulin. Oral antidiabetic agents are indicated only as an adjunct to diet and exercise in the treatment of type 2 diabetes mellitus.

Insulin

Insulin is administered for the management of all types of diabetes. It helps the body metabolize carbohydrates, fats, and proteins from the diet. It may be the sole drug administered, as in type 1 diabetes, or may be added to oral therapy or replace oral therapy in type 2 diabetes. Insulin was originally manufactured from animal sources (pig and cow); however, genetically engineered insulin using recombinant DNA technology (see Chapter 1) to match human insulin has replaced animal source insulin. Pork and bovine insulins are no longer marketed in the United States but are still available in Canada and other parts of the world.

• **Fig. 26.4** Algorithm for glycemic control. (From Garber AJ, Abrahamson MJ, Barzilay JI, et al: Consensus statement by the American Association of Clinical Endocrinologists and American College of Endocrinology on the comprehensive type 2 diabetes management algorithm—2017 executive summary, *Endocr Pract* 23(2):207–238, 2017.)

● TECH NOTE!

Remember, when mixing insulin, that if one is cloudy, it gets drawn up second. Lantus or Levemir should not be mixed together in a syringe with any other form of insulin.

● TECH NOTE!

Rapid-acting insulin (aspart, glulisine, lispro), regular insulin, and long-acting insulin (detemir, glargine) are clear solutions that should be discarded if they appear cloudy.

Mechanism of Action and Pharmacokinetics

Insulin facilitates the transport of glucose that is in the blood stream into the body's cells where the glucose provides energy (Fig. 26.5). Insulin is administered parenterally. Solutions, such as regular insulin may be administered intravenously; all other insulins are injected subcutaneously. Insulin is formulated in rapid-acting, short-acting, intermediate-acting, and long-acting form. The onset of action for rapid-acting insulin (aspart, glulisine, lispro insulin) begins within 15 minutes, whereas the onset of action for long-acting insulin (detemir, glargine insulin) is 90 minutes (Table 26.2). Rapid-acting

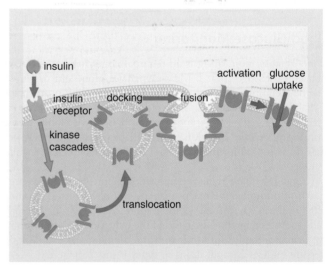

• **Fig. 26.5** Insulin Mechanism of Action. (From Page C, Curtis M, Sutter M, et al: *Integrated pharmacology*, ed 3, Philadelphia, 2006, Mosby.)

A

B

C

• **Fig. 26.6** Dosage Delivery Systems for the Administration of Insulin. (A) Standard insulin syringe. (B) Insulin pen. (C) Insulin pump. ([A and B], From Fulcher EM, Fulcher RM, Soto CD: *Pharmacology principles and applications*, ed 3, St. Louis, 2012, Elsevier. [C], Courtesy of MiniMed, Sylmar, California. In Fulcher EM, Fulcher RM, Soto CD: *Pharmacology principles and applications*, ed 3, St Louis, 2012, Saunders.)

TABLE 26.2	Onset, Peak, and Duration of Action of Insulin		
Insulin	Onset of Action	Peak Action	Duration of Action
Ultra-Rapid Acting (Prandial)			
insulin lispro	10–15 min	1–1.5 h	6–8 h
insulin aspart	10–15 min	1–2 h	3–5 h
insulin glulisine	10–15 min	1–1.5 h	5–6 h
Short Acting (Prandial)			
insulin regular	15 min (IV)	—	30–60 min (IV)
	30 min (SC)	2–3 h	8–12 h (SC)
Intermediate Acting (Basal)			
Neutral protamine Hagedorn (NPH), recombinant	1–3 h	5–8	Up to 18 h
Long Acting (Basal)			
insulin glargine - Lantus	1.5 h	—	Up to 24 h
- Basaglar	—	12 h	Up to 24 h
- Toujeo	6 h	12-16	Up to 24 hours (blood glucose lowering effect increases over time - up to 5 days)
insulin detemir	1.5 h	6–8 h	Up to 24 h

insulin is injected 5 to 15 minutes before eating, or even after a meal for some individuals. Long-acting basal insulin, administered at bedtime, has the advantage of lower risk for nighttime *hypoglycemia* (low blood sugar) when compared with NPH insulin, which is also used for basal insulin needs. Basal bolus insulin administration is recommended by the Canadian Diabetes Association Clinical Guidelines for people with type 1 diabetes. Intermediate- or long-acting basal insulin is typically administered once or twice daily, and rapid-acting prandial insulin is injected at mealtime.

Dosage delivery systems used for the administration of insulin are the insulin pump, vial and syringe, inhaler, and insulin pen (Fig. 26.6).

> **TECH NOTE!**
> Individuals with diabetes must eat scheduled meals. Basal bolus insulin administration mimics normal fluctuations of insulin levels throughout the day in response to preprandial and *postprandial* glucose levels.

> **TECH NOTE!**
> Insulin is the most effective agent for glycemic control and reduces the Hb$_{A1c}$ level by more than 2%.

Adverse Reactions

Insulin replacement therapy produces symptoms similar to effects produced by the naturally secreted hormone at its target site. In addition to hypoglycemia, insulin therapy may cause weight gain, pain, or irritation at the injection site and lipohypertrophy or lipoatrophy. Signs of lipohypertrophy are fat accumulation around the injection site. Signs of lipoatrophy are depressions around the site of injection caused by fat loss. Patients should be advised to rotate the site of injection to minimize these adverse reactions. Symptoms of hypoglycemia are listed in Box 26.5.

• BOX 26.5 Symptoms of Hypoglycemia

Hypoglycemia

- Anxiety, nervousness, irritability
- Blurred vision
- Cold sensations
- Confusion
- Difficulty concentrating
- Fatigue, uncontrolled yawning
- Headache
- Hunger
- Loss of consciousness
- Low blood glucose level
- Muscle weakness
- Nausea
- Numbness of the mouth
- Pale skin
- Palpitations, rapid heartbeat
- Shallow breathing
- Sweating
- Tingling in the fingers
- Tremors

• BOX 26.6 Drugs That Increase or Decrease Blood Glucose Levels

Drugs Associated With Hyperglycemia

- Atypical antipsychotics
- Beta blockers
- Diuretics, thiazides (>25 mg hydrochlorothiazide)
- Glucocorticoids
- Growth hormone
- Nicotinic acid
- Pentamidine
- Phenytoin
- Protease inhibitors
- Sympathomimetics

Drugs Associated With Hypoglycemia

- Acetylsalicylic acid (ASA; salicylates)
- Alcohol
- Angiotensin-converting enzyme inhibitors; angiotensin II receptor blockers
- Beta blockers

> **■ TECH NOTE!**
>
> Insulin must be protected from extremes in heat and cold. Refrigerate unopened vials; do not freeze. Opened vials of insulin may be stored at room temperature, but this will shorten the expiry date for most insulin. Check the manufacturer's insert (Table 26.3).

> **■ TECH NOTE!**
>
> Many drugs may produce hyperglycemia or hypoglycemia (Box 26.6).

Sulfonylureas

Sulfonylureas are sometimes categorized as oral hypoglycemic agents. They are effective only for the treatment of type 2 diabetes. They are very effective in producing glycemic control and can reduce the Hb$_{A1c}$ level by 1% to 2%.

> **❶ TECH ALERT!**
>
> The following drugs have look-alike and sound-alike issues:
> TOLAZamide and TOLBUTamide;
> glyBURIDE, glipiZIDE, and glicazide;
> Diabeta and Zebeta;
> Micronase and Microzide;
> Glucotrol and Glucotrol XL;
> Amaryl and Reminyl

Mechanism of Action and Pharmacokinetics

Sulfonylureas primarily stimulate insulin release from pancreatic beta cells. Sulfonylureas also decrease the breakdown of glycogen to glucose (glycogenolysis). Glycogen is the storage form of glucose.

Sulfonylureas are classified as first- or second-generation agents. First-generation agents—chlorpropamide, tolbutamide, and tolazamide—are still marketed but are rarely prescribed. Sulfonylureas differ in pharmacokinetics, pharmacodynamics, and incidence of hypoglycemic reactions. The second-generation agents, glyburide and glicazide, have the highest risk for hypoglycemia and glimepiride

TABLE 26.3 Recommended Storage for Opened Vials and Cartridges of Insulin

Type of Insulin	Storage
insulin aspart and insulin glulisine	Vials: Room temperature or refrigerated—discard after 28 days. Cartridges: Store at room temperature; discard after 28 days.
insulin detemir	Vials: Room temperature or refrigerated—discard after 42 days. Cartridges: Store at room temperature; discard after 42 days.
insulin glargine	Vials and cartridges: Refrigerated—discard after 28 days (5 and 10 mL).
insulin lispro	Vial, cartridges, and pens: Room temperature or refrigerated—once opened, discard after 28 days. Insulin pump: Discard after 7 days.
NPH insulin	Vial: Room temperature or refrigerated—discard after 42 days. Cartridges: Room temperature or refrigerated—once opened, store at room temperature; discard after 14 days.

NPH, Neutral protamine Hagedorn.

has the lowest risk. Glyburide has active metabolites that can accumulate in patients with kidney disease.

Adverse Reactions

Sulfonylureas can produce hypoglycemia, a serious side effect. Other common side effects are weight gain, abdominal pain, diarrhea, dyspepsia, nausea and vomiting, headache, and dizziness.

> **■ TECH NOTE!**
>
> Conventional and micronized dosage forms of glyburide are not substitutable.

Insulin

Generic Name	US Brand Name(s) / Canadian Brand Name(s)	Dosage Forms and Strengths
insulin aspart	Fiasp, Fiasp FlexTouch Novolog, Novolog FlexPen, Novolog Penfill	**Suspension, for injection (vial, pen, cartridge):** 100 units/mL
	Fiasp, Novorapid	
insulin degludec	Tresiba	**Solution:** 100 units/mL, 200 units/mL
	Tresiba	
insulin detemir	Levemir, Levemir FlexTouch	**Solution, for injection (vial, pen, cartridge):** 100 units/mL
	Levemir Penfill, Levemir FlexTouch	
insulin glargine	Basaglar, Lantus, Lantus SoloStar, Toujeo	**Solution, for injection (vial, pen, cartridge):** 100 units/mL 300 units/mL (Toujeo)
	Basaglar, Lantus, Lantus SoloStar, Toujeo	
insulin glulisine	Apidra, Apidra SoloStar	**Injection, solution (vial, pen, cartridge):** 100 units/mL
	Apidra, Apidra SoloStar, Apidra cartridge	
insulin lispro	Admelog, Admelog Solostar, Humalog, Humalog cartridge, Humalog KwikPen	**Solution, for IV or subcutaneous injection (Admelog):** 100 units/mL **Suspension, for injection (vial, pen, cartridge):** 100 units/mL, 200 units/mL
	Humalog, Humalog cartridge, Humalog KwikPen	
insulin, recombinant human	Afrezza	**Powder, for inhalation:** 4 units/inhalation, 8 units/inhalation, 12 units/inhalation
	Not Available	
insulin regular recombinant human	Humulin R, Humulin R KwikPen, Novolin R	**Injection, solution (vial, pen, cartridge):** 100 units/mL, 500 units/mL
	Humulin R, Humulin R cartridge, Humulin R KwikPen	
insulin isophane recombinant human	Humulin N, Humulin N KwikPen, Novolin N	**Suspension, for injection (vial, pen, cartridge):** 100 units/mL
	Humulin N, Humulin N KwikPen, Humulin N cartridge, Novolin GE NPH, Novolin GE NPH pen, Novolin GE Toronto[a]	
insulin isophane pork	Not available	**Suspension:** 100 units/mL
	Hypurin NPH	
Insulin regular pork	Not available	**Solution:** 100 units/mL
	Hypurin R	

Insulin Mixtures

Generic Name	US Brand Name(s) / Canadian Brand Name(s)	Dosage Forms and Strengths
insulin regular + insulin isophane	Humulin 70/30, Novolin 70/30	**Suspension, for injection (vial, pen, cartridge):** 30 units/mL insulin + 70 units/mL insulin isophane 50 units/mL insulin + 50 units/mL insulin isophane 40 units/mL insulin + 60 units/mL insulin isophane[a]
	Humulin 30/70, Humulin 30/70 cartridge Novolin GE Penfill 30/70 Novolin GE Penfill 40/60 Novolin GE Penfill 50/50	
lispro insulin + lispro protamine suspension	Humalog Mix 50/50, Humalog Pen 50/50, Humalog KwikPen 50/50, Humalog Mix 75/25, Humalog Mix Pen 75/25, Humalog Mix KwikPen 75/25	**Suspension, for injection (cartridge, pen):** 75 units lispro protamine suspension + 25 units lispro insulin 50 units lispro insulin + 50 units lispro protamine suspension
	Humalog Mix 25 (Cartridge), Humalog Mix 25 KwikPen, Humalog Mix 50 (Cartridge), Humalog Mix 50 KwikPen	
insulin aspart + insulin aspart protamine	Novolog Mix 50/50, Novolog Mix 70/30, Novolog Mix Flexpen 70/30, Novomix Penfill 70/30	**Suspension, for injection (vial, pen, cartridge):** 30 units insulin aspart + 70 units insulin aspart protamine, 50 units insulin aspart + 50 units insulin aspart protamine
	Novomix-30 penfill	
insulin aspart + insulin degludec	Ryzodeg 70/30	**Solution:** 30 units insulin aspart/mL + 70 units insulin degludec/mL
	Not Available	
insulin degludec + liraglutide	Xultophy 100/3.6	**Solution:** 100 units insulin degludec + 3.6 mcg liraglutide/mL
	Xultophy	
insulin glargine + lixisenatide	Soliqua 100/33	**Solution:** 100 units insulin glargine/mL + 33 mcg lixisenatide/mL
	Not Available	

[a]Strength available in Canada only.

Sulfonylureas

	US Brand Name(s)	
Generic Name	Canadian Brand Name(s)	Dosage Forms and Strengths
glyburide[a]	Diabeta, Glynase Diabeta	**Tablet (Diabeta):** 1.25 mg[b], 2.5 mg, 5 mg **Tablet, micronized (Glynase):** 1.5 mg, 3 mg, 6 mg
gliclazide[a]	Not available Diamicron, Diamicron MR	**Tablet, immediate-release (Diamicron):** 80 mg **Tablet, extended-release (Diamicron MR):** 30 mg, 60 mg
glipizide[a]	Glucotrol, Glucotrol XL Not available	**Tablet, immediate-release (Glucotrol):** 5 mg, 10 mg **Tablet, extended-release (Glucotrol XL):** 2.5 mg, 5 mg, 10 mg
glimepiride[a]	Amaryl Generic	**Tablet:** 1 mg, 2 mg, 4 mg

[a]Generic available.
[b]Available in the United States only.

Biguanides

Metformin is classified as a biguanide antidiabetic agent. Metformin acts to control fasting blood glucose. It is effective in producing glycemic control and reduces Hb_{A1c} levels by 1% to 2% without producing hypoglycemia. This makes metformin a first-line drug for the treatment of type 2 diabetes. Unlike most other antihyperglycemic agents, metformin does not cause weight gain, which is a benefit when treating obese patients with type 2 diabetes.

Mechanism of Action and Pharmacokinetics

Metformin improves glucose tolerance and insulin resistance by increasing peripheral glucose uptake into skeletal muscles and adipose tissue. It increases glucose transport across cell membranes. Metformin also lowers postprandial plasma glucose levels, decreases hepatic gluconeogenesis (new glucose) production, and decreases intestinal absorption of glucose.

Metformin may be administered in immediate-release (tablets and solution) and extended-release dosage forms. Peak blood levels are achieved in 2.5 hours for immediate-release tablets, 2.2 hours for oral solution, and 7 hours for extended-release tablets. Food decreases the absorption of immediate-release tablets but increases the absorption of metformin solution and extended-release tablets. Glumetza, Glucophage XR, and Fortamet are all extended-release dosage forms of metformin; however, they are not substitutable, because different processes are used to make the drug into an extended-release formulation. Glumetza is designed to remain in the stomach and deliver metformin to the upper gastrointestinal tract, where absorption is enhanced.

Adverse Reactions

Gastrointestinal adverse reactions are common. They include gas, heartburn, metallic taste in the mouth, mild stomachache, nausea, and weight loss. Metformin may produce lactic acidosis, a rare but potentially fatal condition. Metformin may stimulate ovulation in infertile women who have polycystic ovary syndrome.

❶ TECH ALERT!

Metformin immediate-release and extended-release forms are available in some of the same strengths. Check strength carefully to avoid dispensing errors.

❶ TECH ALERT!

Glucophage and Glucotrol have look-alike and sound-alike issues.

● TECH NOTE!

Extended-release dosage forms of metformin are not substitutable.

α-Glucosidase Inhibitors

α-Glucosidase inhibitors prolong the digestion of carbohydrates and delay their absorption in the small intestine. They reduce peak plasma glucose levels. α-Glucosidase inhibitors do not promote insulin secretion like many other antidiabetic agents, nor do they cause hypoglycemia. They produce a minimal effect on reducing Hb_{A1c} levels (<1%) and therefore are not used as monotherapy.

Mechanism of Action and Pharmacokinetics

Acarbose and miglitol inhibit α-glucosidases, enzymes that break down carbohydrates. They must be administered with the first bite of each meal. The drugs compete for binding sites with oligosaccharides and disaccharides in foods. It is important to eat a diet rich in complex carbohydrates while taking acarbose and miglitol.

Adverse Reactions

α-Glucosidase inhibitors most commonly produce gastrointestinal side effects. Adverse reactions include a bloated feeling, diarrhea, stomach or intestinal gas, or rumbling stomach and stomach pain or discomfort.

O Zempic

Biguanides

Generic Name	US Brand Name(s) Canadian Brand Name(s)	Dosage Forms and Strengths
metformin[a]	Fortamet, Glucophage, Glucophage XR, Glumetza, Riomet Glucophage, Glumetza	**Solution, oral (Riomet):** 100 mg/mL **Tablet, immediate-release:** 500 mg, 850 mg, 1000 mg[b] **Tablet, extended-release: (Glumetza):** 500 mg, 1000 mg **(Fortamet):** 500 mg, 1000 mg **(Glucophage XR):** 500 mg, 750 mg

Combination Biguanide + Sulfonylureas

metformin + glyburide[a]	Generic Not available	**Tablet:** 250 mg metformin + 1.25 mg glyburide 500 mg metformin + 2.5 mg glyburide 500 mg metformin + 5 mg glyburide
metformin + glipizide[a]	Generic Not available	**Tablet:** 250 mg metformin + 2.5 mg glipizide 500 mg metformin + 2.5 mg glipizide 500 mg metformin + 5 mg glipizide

[a]Generic available.
[b]Available in the United States only.

α-Glucosidase Inhibitors

Generic Name	US Brand Name(s) Canadian Brand Name(s)	Dosage Forms and Strengths
acarbose	Precose Glucobay	**Tablet:** 25 mg,[a] 50 mg, 100 mg
miglitol	Glyset Not available	**Tablet:** 25 mg, 50 mg, 100 mg

[a]Strength available in the United States only.

Meglitinides

Meglitinides are oral antidiabetic agents used in the treatment of type 2 diabetes. Meglitinides, like the sulfonylureas, are effective only in individuals who have functioning pancreatic beta cells. Repaglinide is more effective in producing glycemic control than nateglinide. Repaglinide reduces Hb_{A1c} levels by 1% to 2%, whereas nateglinide reduces Hb_{A1c} levels only by less than 1%.

> **TECH NOTE!**
>
> A common ending for meglitinides is *-glinide*.

Mechanism of Action and Pharmacokinetics

Repaglinide and nateglinide lower postprandial blood glucose levels by stimulating insulin secretion from pancreatic beta cells. Repaglinide is rapidly and completely absorbed from the intestinal tract. The onset of action is within 15 to 30 minutes. Peak effects of repaglinide and nateglinide are achieved in approximately 1 to 1.5 hours, and elimination is equally as rapid. The drugs must be taken only with meals to avoid hypoglycemia. Their short half-life accounts for the multiple daily dosing required. Both drugs are metabolized via the cytochrome P-450 (CYP450) system and are subject to many drug-drug interactions.

Adverse Reactions

Meglitinides may cause hypoglycemia; however, the risk is lower than with sulfonylureas if they are taken appropriately with meals. Other side effects are headache, nausea, and vomiting. Nateglinide and repaglinide should be used with caution in patients with liver dysfunction.

Meglitinides

Generic Name	US Brand Name(s) Canadian Brand Name(s)	Dosage Forms and Strengths
nateglinide[a]	Starlix Not available	**Tablet:** 60 mg, 120 mg
repaglinide[a]	Prandin Gluconorm	**Tablet:** 0.5 mg, 1 mg, 2 mg

[a]Generic available.

Thiazolidinediones

Thiazolidinediones are insulin sensitizers; they are used for the treatment of type 2 diabetes. They treat insulin resistance. Two agents are currently marketed in the United States and Canada, pioglitazone and rosiglitazone. Both drugs reduce fasting plasma glucose (FPG) and Hb_{A1c} levels by approximately 1% to 2%.

> **TECH NOTE!**
>
> A common ending for thiazolidinediones is *-glitazone*.

> **❶ TECH ALERT!**
>
> The following drugs have look-alike and sound-alike issues:
> Avandia, Avandamet, Coumadin, and Prandin;
> Actos and Actonel

Thiazolidinediones

Generic Name	US Brand Name(s) Canadian Brand Name(s)	Dosage Forms and Strengths
pioglitazone[a]	Actos	**Tablet:** 15 mg, 30 mg, 45 mg
	Generics	
rosiglitazone[a]	Avandia	**Tablet:** 2 mg, 4 mg, 8 mg
	Avandia	

Thiazolidinediones + Biguanides

pioglitazone + metformin[a]	Actosplus Met, Actosplus Met XR	**Tablet:** pioglitazone 15 mg + metformin 500 mg pioglitazone 15 mg + metformin 850 mg

	Not available	**Tablet, biphasic extended-release (Actosplus Met XR):**
		    pioglitazone 15 mg + metformin 1000 mg
		    pioglitazone 30 mg + metformin 1000 mg

Thiazolidinediones + Sulfonylureas

pioglitazone + glimepiride[a]	Duetact	**Tablet:** pioglitazone 30 mg + glimepiride 2 mg pioglitazone 30 mg + glimepiride 4 mg
	Not available	

[a]Generic available.

Mechanism of Action and Pharmacokinetics

Thiazolidinediones increase tissue sensitivity to insulin. They do not increase insulin secretion, so they do not produce hypoglycemia when used as monotherapy. Insulin receptor sensitivity is greatest in adipose tissue, skeletal muscle, and the liver. Pioglitazone and rosiglitazone increase the uptake of glucose in the liver and muscles. Pioglitazone also lowers free fatty acid and triglyceride levels, plasma glucose, insulin, and Hb_{A1c}. Pioglitazone and rosiglitazone are both administered orally. The time to reach peak plasma concentration is 1 hour for rosiglitazone and 2 hours for pioglitazone. Food doubles the time needed to reach the maximum concentration for pioglitazone but has no effect on rosiglitazone. Food does not reduce the bioavailability of either drug.

Adverse Reactions

The most common adverse reactions of therapy with pioglitazone and rosiglitazone are headache, weight gain, diarrhea, nausea, and vomiting. Serious side effects linked to pioglitazone and rosiglitazone are heart failure, heart attack, and liver failure. Patients should be instructed to report signs of muscle pain, jaundice, blurred vision, and signs of hypoglycemia or hyperglycemia.

Dipeptidyl Peptidase-4 Inhibitors

Alogliptin, linagliptin, saxagliptin, and sitagliptin are oral antidiabetic agents known as dipeptidyl peptidase-4 (DPP-4) inhibitors. They are indicated for the treatment of type 2 diabetes. They increase insulin release and decrease glucagon levels by potentiating the activity of peptide hormones released in response to eating a meal. They decrease FPG, postprandial glucose, and Hb_{A1c} levels. The decrease in Hb_{A1c} levels is 0.5% to 1%, less than that produced by sulfonylureas and biguanides.

> **● TECH NOTE!**
>
> A common ending for DPP-4 inhibitors is *-gliptin*.

Mechanism of Action and Pharmacokinetics

DPP-4 is the enzyme responsible for the degradation of circulating glucagon-like peptide-1 (GLP-1) and glucose-dependent insulinotropic peptide (GIP). These peptide hormones are key agents in glucose homeostasis. The action of the hormones is prolonged by DPP-4 inhibitors. DPP-4 inhibitors also increase beta-cell responsiveness to glucose in the islets of Langerhans.

Oral absorption and bioavailability of DPP-4 inhibitors are good, and peak effects are reached 1 to 4 hours after administration. Sitagliptin and saxagliptin are primarily eliminated in the urine, so dosage adjustments may be required in those with kidney disease.

Adverse Reactions

The most common adverse reactions are intestinal upset, gas, heartburn, stomach pain, decreased appetite, metallic taste, and stuffy or runny nose. Pancreatitis is a rare but serious adverse reaction associated with the use of sitagliptin. The drug may also cause hypoglycemia when used in combination with sulfonylureas.

Sodium-Glucose Cotransporter-2 Inhibitors

Canagliflozin, dapagliflozin, empagliflozin, and ertugliflozin are sodium-glucose cotransporter-2 (SGLT2) inhibitors that are used to treat type 2 diabetes. They increase urinary elimination of glucose,

Dipeptidyl Peptidase-4 Inhibitor

Generic Name	US Brand Name(s) / Canadian Brand Name(s)	Dosage Forms and Strengths
alogliptin	Nesina / Nesina	**Tablet:** 6.25 mg, 12.5 mg, 25 mg
linagliptin	Tradjenta / Trajenta	**Tablet:** 5 mg
saxagliptin	Onglyza / Onglyza	**Tablet:** 2.5 mg, 5 mg
sitagliptin	Januvia / Januvia	**Tablet:** 25 mg, 50 mg, 100 mg

Combination Dipeptidyl Peptidase-4 Inhibitors

Generic Name	US Brand Name(s) / Canadian Brand Name(s)	Dosage Forms and Strengths
alogliptin + metformin	Kazano / Kazano	**Tablet:** alogliptin 12.5 mg + metformin 500 mg, alogliptin 12.5 mg + metformin 850 mg,[a] alogliptin 12.5 mg + metformin 1000 mg
linagliptin + metformin	Jentadueto, Jentadueto XR / Jentadueto	**Tablet:** linagliptin 2.5 mg + metformin 500 mg, linagliptin 2.5 mg + metformin 850 mg, linagliptin 2.5 mg + metformin 1000 mg **Tablet, extended release (Jentadueto XR):** linagliptin 2.5 mg + metformin 1000 mg, linagliptin 5 mg+ metformin 1000 mg
saxagliptin + metformin	Kombiglyze XR / Komboglyze	**Tablet (Komboglyze)[a]:** saxagliptin 2.5 mg + metformin 500 mg, saxagliptin 2.5 mg + metformin 850 mg, saxagliptin 2.5 mg + metformin 1000 mg **Tablet, extended release (Kombiglyze XR):** saxagliptin 2.5 mg + metformin 1000 mg, saxagliptin 5 mg + metformin 500 mg, saxagliptin 5 mg + metformin 1000 mg
sitagliptin + metformin	Janumet, Janumet XR / Janumet, Janumet XR	**Tablet:** sitagliptin 50 mg + metformin 500 mg sitagliptin 50 mg + metformin 850 mg[a] sitagliptin 50 mg + metformin 1000 mg **Tablet, extended release:** sitagliptin 50 mg + metformin 500 mg sitagliptin 50 mg + metformin 1000 mg sitagliptin 100 mg + metformin 1000 mg
alogliptin + pioglitazone	Oseni / Not available	**Tablet:** alogliptin 12.5 mg + pioglitazone 15 mg, alogliptin 12.5 + pioglitazone 30 mg, alogliptin 12.5 mg + pioglitazone 45 mg, alogliptin 25 mg + pioglitazone 15 mg, alogliptin 25 mg + pioglitazone 30 mg, alogliptin 25 mg + pioglitazone 45 mg

[a]Strength available in Canada only.

thereby reducing plasma glucose. They may be prescribed as monotherapy or in combination with other antidiabetic agents for adults with type 2 diabetes that is not well controlled. They lower Hb_{A1c} by approximately 0.5% to 1%

Mechanism of Action and Pharmacokinetics

Glucose in the bloodstream is filtered by the kidney and then reabsorbed to be used by the body's cells. Sodium-glucose cotransporter inhibitors work by blocking the transporter proteins that are responsible for reabsorbing glucose (SGLT1 and SGLT2). SGLT2 is responsible for reabsorbing 90% of the glucose that is filtered by the kidneys. The SGLT2 inhibitors differ in selectivity for SGLT receptors. Empagliflozin has the greatest selectivity, and canagliflozin has the lowest selectivity. The drugs work best in patients who have normal kidney function.

Adverse Effects

Canagliflozin, dapagliflozin, or empagliflozin may increase urinary tract and genital infections. They promote weight loss, which is a beneficial side effect for treating obese patients. They may increase the risk for hypoglycemia if prescribed in combination with sulfonylureas (e.g., gliclazide and glyburide). They may also increase potassium levels.

> **● TECH NOTE!**
> "gliflozin" is a common ending for sodium-glucose cotransporter-2 (SGLT2) Inhibitors.

Sodium-Glucose Cotransporter-2 Inhibitors

Generic Name	US Brand Name(s) Canadian Brand Name(s)	Dosage Forms and Strengths
canagliflozin	Invokana Invokana	**Tablet:** 100 mg, 300 mg
dapagliflozin	Farxiga Forxiga	**Tablet:** 5 mg, 10 mg
empagliflozin	Jardiance Jardiance	**Tablet:** 10 mg, 25 mg
ertugliflozin	Steglatro Steglatro	**Tablet:** 5 mg, 15 mg
Combination SGLT2 Inhibitors		
canagliflozin + metformin	Invokamet, Invokamet XR Invokamet	**Tablet:** canagliflozin 50 mg + metformin 500 mg, canagliflozin 50 mg + metformin 850 mg,[a] canagliflozin 50 mg + metformin 1000 mg, canagliflozin 150 mg + metformin 500 mg, canagliflozin 150 mg + metformin 850 mg,[a] canagliflozin 150 mg + metformin 1000 mg **Tablet, extended release:** canagliflozin 50 mg + metformin 500 mg, canagliflozin 50 mg + metformin 1000 mg, canagliflozin 150 mg + metformin 500 mg, canagliflozin 150 mg + metformin 1000 mg
dapagliflozin + metformin	Xigduo XR Xigduo	**Tablet (Xigduo):** dapagliflozin 5 mg + metformin 850 mg, dapagliflozin 5 mg + metformin 1000 mg **Tablet, extended release (Xigduo XR):** dapagliflozin 2.5 mg + metformin 1000 mg, dapagliflozin 5 mg + metformin 500 mg, dapagliflozin 5 mg + metformin 1000 mg, dapagliflozin 10 mg + metformin 500 mg, dapagliflozin 10 mg + metformin 1000 mg
empagliflozin + metformin	Synjardy, Synjardy XR Synjardy	**Tablet:** empagliflozin 5 mg + metformin 500 mg, empagliflozin 5 mg + metformin 850 mg[a] empagliflozin 5 mg + metformin 1000 mg empagliflozin 12.5 mg + metformin 500 mg, empagliflozin 12.5 mg + metformin 850 mg[a] empagliflozin 12.5 mg + metformin 1000 mg **Tablet, extended release:** empagliflozin 5 mg + metformin 1000 mg, empagliflozin 10 mg + metformin 1000 mg, empagliflozin 12.5 mg + metformin 1000 mg, empagliflozin 25 mg + metformin 1000 mg
ertugliflozin + metformin	Segluromet Segluromet	**Tablet:** 2.5 mg ertugliflozin + 500 mg metformin 2.5 mg ertugliflozin + 1000 mg metformin 7.5 mg ertugliflozin + 500 mg metformin 7.5 mg ertugliflozin + 1000 mg metformin
dapagliflozin + saxagliptin	Qtern Qtern	**Tablet:** dapagliflozin 10 mg + saxagliptin 5 mg
empagliflozin + linagliptin	Glyxambi Glyxambi	**Tablet:** empagliflozin 10 mg + linagliptin 5 mg empagliflozin 25 mg + linagliptin 5 mg
ertugliflozin + sitagliptin	Steglujan Steglujan	**Tablet:** 5 mg ertugliflozin + 100 mg sitagliptin 15 mg ertugliflozin + 100 mg sitagliptin

[a]Available in Canada only.

Parentaly admin.

Glucagon-Like Peptide Receptor Agonists (Incretin Mimetics)

Dulaglutide (Trulicity), exenatide (Byetta), lixisenatide (Adlyxin, Adlyxine), liraglutide (Victoza), and semaglutide (Ozempic) are parenterally administered agents. Glucagon-like peptide (GLP-1) receptor agonist drugs are administered as adjuncts to diet and exercise and may be administered only for type 2 diabetes mellitus. Exenatide is approved as monotherapy or in combination with other antidiabetic agents. Liraglutide is not approved as monotherapy. Exenatide is approved for use with insulin glargine but not prandial insulin.

Mechanism of Action and Pharmacokinetics

Dulaglutide, exenatide, lixisenatide, simaglutide, and liraglutide stimulate GLP-1 receptors in the pancreatic alpha and beta cells, stimulating insulin secretion when glucose levels are elevated. Alpha-cell stimulation suppresses glucagon release. GLP-1 receptor agonists also delay gastric emptying, slowing the rise of blood glucose levels after eating, and decreasing appetite. Exenatide is administered subcutaneously within 60 minutes before the morning and evening meals. It is rapidly absorbed and has a half-life ($t_{1/2}$) of 2.5 hours. Exenatide powder for injection is a long-acting formulation that is administered once per week. Liraglutide is administered subcutaneously once daily. It is absorbed slowly, and the $t_{1/2}$ is 11 to 14 hours. Exenatide reduces Hb_{A1c} levels by 0.5% to 1%. Liraglutide reduces Hb_{A1c} levels by 0.8% to 1.5%.

Glucagon-Like Peptide Receptor Agonists

Generic Name	US Brand Name(s) / Canadian Brand Name(s)	Dosage Forms and Strengths
dulaglutide	Trulicity / Trulicity	Solution, for subcutaneous injection: 0.75 mg/0.5 mL, 1.5 mg/0.5 mL
exenatide	Byetta, Bydureon / Byetta, Bydureon	Solution, for injection (Byetta): 250 mcg/mL Suspension, for subcutaneous injection (extended release): 2 mg/vial Powder, for subcutaneous injection (extended release): 2 mg/vial
liraglutide	Saxenda, Victoza / Saxenda, Victoza	Solution, for injection: 18 mg/3 mL (6 mg/mL)
lixisenatide	Adlyxin / Adlyxin	Solution: 0.05 mg/mL, 0.1 mg/mL
semaglutide	Ozempic / Ozempic	Solution, for injection: 2 mg/1.5 mL (1.34 mg/mL)

Adverse Effects

Nausea is the most common side effect with exenatide and liraglutide, affecting up to 50% of patients. Gastrointestinal side effects are most common in the first month of therapy. Nausea associated with both drugs may be minimized by increasing the dose gradually. Other side effects include hypoglycemia; heartburn; itching, burning, swelling, or rash at the injection site; diarrhea or constipation; reduced appetite; and a slight weight loss. Exenatide may cause mild dizziness, weakness, headaches, or nausea. Pancreatitis is a rare but serious side effect of liraglutide.

Amylin Analogue

Pramlintide (Symlin) is a synthetic analogue of the hormone amylin. Amylin levels are absent in type 1 diabetes and decreased in type 2 diabetes. Pramlintide is used with mealtime insulin to control blood sugar levels in people who have type 1 or 2 diabetes mellitus.

> **TECH NOTE!**
> Pramlintide may cause hypoglycemia. The risk is greater during the first 3 hours after pramlintide is injected.

Mechanism of Action and Pharmacokinetics

Like amylin, pramlintide slows gastric emptying, reduces postprandial glucagon secretion, and reduces appetite. It should be injected subcutaneously immediately prior to each meal. The maximum concentration of pramlintide is reached within 20 minutes of administration, and the therapeutic effects last approximately 3 hours.

Adverse Reactions

Adverse reactions associated with pramlintide include hypoglycemia; redness, swelling, bruising, itching at the injection site; loss of appetite; stomach pain; indigestion; upset stomach; excessive tiredness; dizziness; coughing; sore throat; and joint pain. Nausea and vomiting are dose dependent and may be reduced by gradually titrating the dose. This side effect decreases over time. To avoid lipodystrophy, patients should be advised to rotate the site of injection.

> **TECH NOTE!**
> Rotate the site of injection to minimize risk of developing an increase or a decrease in fatty tissue under the skin at the injection site.

> **TECH NOTE!**
> Do not mix pramlintide with any other injection, including insulin.

Amylin Analogue

Generic Name	US Brand Name(s) / Canadian Brand Name(s)	Dosage Forms and Strengths
pramlintide	Symlin / Not available	Solution, for injection (pen cartridge): 1.5 mg/1.5 mL 2.7 mg/2.7 mL

Miscellaneous Agents

Colesevelam (Welchol) is a cholesterol-lowering agent that is FDA approved for the management of type 2 diabetes. The mechanism of action for reducing FPG and Hb_{A1c} levels is unknown. Bromocriptine (Cycloset) is a dopamine agonist that improves glycemic control; the mechanism of its effect on postprandial glucose levels is unknown. Both drugs are approved as an adjunct to diet and exercise. The most common side effects of colesevelam are heartburn and upset stomach. Nausea, drowsiness, and headache are side effects of bromocriptine.

Dopamine Agonist

Generic Name	US Brand Name(s)	Dosage Forms and Strengths
	Canadian Brand Name(s)	
bromocriptine	Cycloset	**Tablet:** 0.8 mg
	Not available	

Management of hypoglycemia

Some medicines used to treat diabetes cause hypoglycemia, especially when individuals increase exercise, do not eat regularly, or take other medicines that can also decrease blood sugar. Individuals experiencing symptoms of hypoglycemia may raise their blood sugar by consuming: 3-4 glucose tablets or a tube of glucose gel, 1 tablespoon of sugar, honey, or corn syrup, 4 ounces (1/2 cups) of juice or regular soda (not diet) or 8 ounces of nonfat or 1% milk, eat several hard candies, jellybeans, or gumdrops. Severe hypoglycemia is treated by administering the hormone glucagon. It is administered by intravenous or intramuscular injection. Glucagon kits are available by prescription. The kit contains one vial with 1 mg glucagon powder and a vial of diluent.

Complementary and Alternative Medicines and Diabetes

Six dietary supplements have been of particular interest in recent years as adjunct therapy for people with diabetes. They are alpha-lipoic acid (ALA), chromium, coenzyme Q10, garlic, magnesium, and omega-3 fatty acids. None has been extensively studied using randomized, double-blind studies. Of the six dietary supplements, ALA, magnesium, and omega-3 fatty acids have shown the most evidence of possible usefulness.

Alpha-Lipoic Acid

ALA is an antioxidant. Antioxidants prevent cell damage caused by oxidative stress from substances called free radicals. Elevated blood glucose levels can cause oxidative stress. ALA might lower the blood sugar level too much, so blood glucose levels must be monitored closely when it is used.

Magnesium

Magnesium is a mineral found in green leafy vegetables, nuts, seeds, and some whole grains. Magnesium levels are depressed in people with diabetes. Low magnesium levels may worsen glucose control in type 2 diabetes by interrupting insulin secretion and increasing insulin resistance.

Omega-3 Fatty Acids

Omega-3 fatty acids are naturally found in fish, fish oil, canola and soybean oils, walnuts, and wheat germ. Studies have shown that supplementation with omega-3 fatty acids can reduce the incidence of CVD and slow the progression of atherosclerosis. Omega-3 fatty acids have been of interest because diabetes increases the risk for developing CVD.

Garlic

Evidence about the value of garlic is mixed. It is believed that garlic may be involved in some biologic activities associated with type 2 diabetes. The mechanism is not known.

TECHNICIAN'S CORNER

1. If your family has a history of type 2 diabetes, which lifestyle precautions should you take to reduce your risk for developing the disease?
2. What are some basic changes in diet that can be implemented to avoid developing type 2 diabetes?

Summary of Drugs Used in the Treatment of Diabetes

	Generic Name	Brand Name	Usual Dose and Dosing Schedule	Warning Labels
Insulin				
	insulin	Afrezza, Apidra, Basaglar, Detemir, Fiasp, Humulin, Humalog, Lantus, Levemir, Novolin, Novolog, Novolin GE Toronto, Ryzodeg, Tresiba	Individualized	STORE IN THE REFRIGERATOR; DO NOT FREEZE.—All except Afrezza USE AFREZZA CARTRIDGES ONLY WITH THE AFREZA INHALER DISCARD 14–15 DAYS AFTER FIRST USE— Afrezza cartridge, Soliqua
	insulin/non-insulin combination	Soliqua, Xultophy		

	Generic Name	Brand Name	Usual Dose and Dosing Schedule	Warning Labels
Sulfonylureas				
	gliclazide	Diamicron, Diamicron MR 30 and MR 60	Immediate release tabs: 80–160 mg twice daily (max, 320 mg/day); extended release tabs: 30-120 mg once daily (max, 120 mg/day)	AVOID PROLONGED EXPOSURE TO SUNLIGHT (GLIPIZIDE, GLIMEPIRIDE). LIMIT OR AVOID ALCOHOL (ALL). TAKE 30 MIN BEFORE BREAKFAST (GLIPIZIDE, GLYBURIDE). SWALLOW WHOLE; DON'T CRUSH OR CHEW (SUSTAINED RELEASE). TAKE WITH A MEAL (GLICLAZIDE, GLIMEPIRIDE).
	glipizide	Glucotrol	5–40 mg daily in divided doses	
		Glucotrol XL	5–20 mg once daily	
	glyburide	Diabeta, Micronase	1.25–20 mg/day given in single or 2 divided doses	
		Glynase	0.75–12 mg/day, given in single or 2 divided doses	
	glimepiride	Amaryl	1–4 mg once daily, (max, 8 mg/day)	
Biguanides	metformin	Glucophage	Maintence: 500–1000 mg twice daily or 850 mg PO 3 times daily (max, 2,000 mg/day)	TAKE WITH MEALS. SWALLOW WHOLE; DON'T CRUSH OR CHEW (SUSTAINED-RELEASE).
		Glumetza	1000 mg once or twice daily	
		Fortamet	500–1000 mg once daily	
Combination Biguanide + Sulfonylureas				
	metformin + glyburide	Generic	1 tablet (500 mg/2.5 mg or 500 mg/5 mg) twice daily	TAKE WITH MEALS.
	metformin + glipizide	Generic	1 tablet (500 mg/2.5 mg or 500/5 mg) twice daily	TAKE WITH MEALS.
α-Glucosidase Inhibitors				
	acarbose	Precose	25–100 mg 3 times a day	TAKE WITH THE FIRST BITE OF A MEAL.
	miglitol	Glyset	25–100 mg 3 times a day	
Dipeptidyl Peptidase-4 Inhibitors				
	alogliptin	Nesina	25 mg once daily	TAKE AT THE SAME TIME EACH DAY, WITH OR WITHOUT FOOD.
	linagliptin	Tradjenta	5 mg once daily	
	saxagliptin	Onglyza	2.5–5 mg once daily	
	sitagliptin	Januvia	100 mg once daily	
Combination Dipeptidyl Peptidase-4 Inhibitors				
	alogliptin + metformin	Kazano	1 tablet twice daily	TAKE WITH FOOD—All SWALLOW WHOLE; DON'T CRUSH OR CHEW— Extended release tabs
	linagliptin + metformin	Jentadueto, Jentadueto XR	1 tablet twice daily 1 tablet once daily (XR tab)	
	saxagliptin + metformin	Kombiglyze XR, Komboglyze	1 tablet twice daily tablet once daily (XR tab)	
	sitagliptin + metformin	Janumet, Janumet XR	1 tablet twice daily 1 tablet once daily (XR tab)	
Meglitinides				
	nateglinide	Starlix	60–120 mg 3 times a day	TAKE IMMEDIATELY PRIOR TO MEALS (SKIP DOSE IF THE MEAL IS MISSED). TAKE WITH A FULL GLASS OF WATER.
	repaglinide	Prandin	1–4 mg prior to each meal, up to 4 times a day	

Continued

	Generic Name	Brand Name	Usual Dose and Dosing Schedule	Warning Labels
Thiazolidinediones				
	pioglitazone	Actos	15–45 mg once daily	LIMIT OR AVOID ALCOHOL. TAKE WITH A FULL GLASS OF WATER.
	rosiglitazone	Avandia	4–8 mg daily in single or divided doses	
Combination Thiazolidinediones				
	alogliptin + pioglitazine	Oseni	1 tablet once daily	TAKE WITH MEALS (ALL). LIMIT OR AVOID ALCOHOL (ALL). AVOID PROLONGED EXPOSURE TO SUNLIGHT (METAGLIP, GLUCOVANCE). SWALLOW WHOLE; DON'T CRUSH OR CHEW (ACTOPLUS MET XR, SUSTAINED-RELEASE).
	metformin + pioglitazone	Actoplus Met Actoplus Met XR	1 tablet once or twice daily (max, 2250 mg metformin + 45 mg pioglitazone/day)	
	pioglitazone + glimepiride	Duetact	1 tablet daily with the first meal of the day	
Glucagon-Like Peptide Receptor Agonist				
	dulaglutide	Trulicity	Inject 0.75 mg–1.5 mg subcutaneously once weekly	REFRIGERATE; DO NOT FREEZE. DISCARD PEN UNIT 30 DAYS AFTER OPENING. -Victoza, Byetta. INJECT 60 MIN PRIOR TO MORNING AND EVENING MEAL- Byetta. USE IMMEDIATELY AFTER RECONSTITUTION- Bydureon. DO NOT USE DILUENT IF CLOUDY- Bydureon. INJECT 1 H BEFORE THE FIRST MEAL OF THE DAY—Adlyxin
	liraglutide	Victoza	Inject 0.6 mg subcutaneously once daily for 1 week; then increase to 1.2–1.8 mg subcutaneously once daily	
	exenatide	Byetta	Initiate with 5 mcg subcutaneously twice daily, may increase to 10 mcg after 1 month	
		Bydureon	Inject 2 mg subcutaneously once every 7 days	
	lixisenatide	Adlyxin	Inject 10–20 mcg once daily 1 hour prior to the first meal of the day	
	semaglutide	Ozempic	Inject 0.25–1 mg subcutaneously once weekly	
Sodium-Glucose Cotransporter-2 (SGLT2) Inhibitors				
	canagliflozin	Invokana	100–300 mg once daily	TAKE 1 H BEFORE THE FIRST MEAL OF THE DAY—Invokana AVOID ALCOHOL TAKE WITH FOOD— Invokamet, Invokamet XR, Xigduo, Xigduo XR, Synjardy, Synjardy XR, Segluromet
	dapagliflozin	Farxiga, Forxiga	5–10 mg once daily in the morning	
	empagliflozin	Jardiance	10–25 mg once daily in the morning	
	ertugliflozin	Steglatro	5–15 mg once daily	
	canagliflozin + metformin	Invokamet, Invokamet XR	1 tablet twice daily 1 tablet once daily (XR)	
	dapagliflozin + metformin	Xigduo, Xigduo XR	1 tablet twice daily 1 tablet once daily (XR)	
	empagliflozin + metformin	Synjardy, Synjardy XR	1 tablet twice daily 1 tablet once daily (XR)	
	ertugliflozin + metformin	Segluromet	1 tablet twice daily (maximum 15 mg ertugliflozin + 2000 mg metformin daily)	
	dapagliflozin + saxagliptin	Qtern	1 tablet once daily in the morning	
	empagliflozin + linagliptin	Glyxambi	1 tablet once daily in the morning	
	ertugliflozin + sitagliptin	Steglujan	1 tablet once daily in the morning (maximum 15 mg ertugliflozin + 100 mg sitagliptin daily)	

Summary of Drugs Used in the Treatment of Diabetes—cont'd

	Generic Name	Brand Name	Usual Dose and Dosing Schedule	Warning Labels
	ertugliflozin + metformin	Segluromet	1 tablet twice daily	
Amylin Analogue				
	pramlintide	Symlin	Inject 15–60 mcg before meals (Type 1 diabetes) Inject 60–120 mcg before meals (Type 2 diabetes)	REFRIGERATE; DON'T FREEZE
Dopamine Agonist				
	bromocriptine	Cycloset	1.6–4.8 mg once daily within 2 h after waking in the morning	TAKE WITH FOOD.

SGLT2, Sodium-glucose cotransporter-2.

Key Points

- Diabetes mellitus is a disorder in which glucose accumulates in the blood.
- Insulin is released by the beta cells in the islets of Langerhans of the pancreas in response to the rise of blood glucose, amino acid, and gut-derived hormone levels.
- When glucose levels drop, glucagon is secreted by alpha cells in the islets of Langerhans.
- Prediabetes causes impaired fasting glucose and impaired glucose tolerance.
- Type 1 diabetes is an autoimmune disease. The immune system attacks and destroys the insulin-producing beta cells in the pancreas.
- In type 1 diabetes, the body can no longer produce sufficient amounts of the hormone insulin.
- Type 2 diabetes is most common, accounting for 90% to 95% of all cases of diabetes.
- In type 2 diabetes, the pancreas usually produces sufficient amounts of insulin early in the disease, but the body is unable to use the insulin effectively.
- Gestational diabetes may be caused by the hormones of pregnancy or a shortage of insulin.
- Insulin resistance is a condition in which the body does not respond to insulin. It is a precursor to type 2 diabetes.
- The hemoglobin A1c (Hb$_{A1c}$) test is the only test that provides information about blood glucose levels over a 2- to 3-month period.
- Blood glucose testing is the principal method used to diagnose diabetes.
- Individuals with type 1 or 2 diabetes will reduce risks for complications by weight loss, engaging in physical activity, consuming foods with a low glycemic index, quitting smoking, and other lifestyle changes.
- Insulin may be administered for the management of all types of diabetes. It is available in dosage forms to be administered by intravenous infusion, insulin pump, powder for inhalation, and subcutaneous injection.

- Insulin is formulated in rapid-acting, short-acting, intermediate-acting, and long-acting forms.
- Rapid-acting insulins are typically injected 5 to 15 minutes before eating.
- Rapid-acting insulin (aspart, glulisine, lispro), regular insulin, and long-acting insulin (detemir, glargine) are clear solutions that should be discarded if they appear cloudy.
- Sulfonylureas are also known as oral hypoglycemic agents. They are only effective for the treatment of type 2 diabetes because they stimulate insulin release from pancreatic beta cells.
- Metformin improves glucose tolerance and insulin resistance, lowers postprandial plasma glucose levels, decreases hepatic gluconeogenesis, and decreases the intestinal absorption of glucose.
- α-Glucosidase inhibitors (acarbose, miglitol) prolong the digestion of carbohydrates, delay their absorption in the small intestine, and are administered with the first bite of each meal.
- Meglitinides (nateglinide and repaglinide) stimulate insulin secretion from pancreatic beta cells, similar to sulfonylureas.
- Pioglitazone and rosiglitazone are insulin sensitizers that are used in the treatment of type 2 diabetes.
- Sitagliptin, saxagliptin, alogliptin, and linagliptin are dipeptidyl peptidase-4 inhibitors. They decrease fasting plasma glucose, postprandial glucose, and Hb$_{A1c}$ levels.
- Exenatide, dulaglutide, lixisenatide, semaglutide, and liraglutide are glucagon-like peptide receptor agonists.
- Colesevelam is a cholesterol-lowering agent that, along with diet and exercise, is approved for the treatment of type 2 diabetes.
- Bromocriptine is a dopamine agonist that, along with diet and exercise, is approved for the treatment type 2 diabetes.
- Alpha-lipoic acid, magnesium, omega-3 fatty acids, and garlic are nutritional supplements that show some evidence of effectiveness for the treatment of diabetes mellitus.

Review Questions

1. The condition of elevated blood glucose levels is termed _____.
   a. Hypoglycemia
   b. Hyperglycemia

2. An autoimmune disease in which beta cells are destroyed and insufficient amounts of insulin are produced is _____.
   a. Type 1 diabetes
   b. Type 2 diabetes
   c. Gestational diabetes
   d. All of the above

3. In diabetes, _____ accumulates in the blood.
   a. Calcium
   b. Glucose
   c. Magnesium
   d. Insulin

4. A hormone that is essential for the regulation of carbohydrate, fat, and protein metabolism is _____.
   a. Aldosterone
   b. Serotonin
   c. Dopamine
   d. Insulin

5. Type 2 diabetes is most common, accounting for 90% to 95% of all cases of diabetes.
   a. True
   b. False

6. Which insulin product is administered by inhalation?
   a. Afrezza
   b. Humulin N
   c. Humalog
   d. Soliqua

7. All of the following are recommendations for lifestyle changes to reduce the risk for diabetes mellitus EXCEPT_____.
   a. Exercise 150 minutes week
   b. Stop smoking
   c. Limit alcohol
   d. Eat carbohydrates

8. Insulin is only administered for the management of type 1 diabetes.
   a. True
   b. False

9. Januvia and Onglyza are examples of _____.
   a. Sulfonylureas
   b. Dipeptidyl peptidase-4 inhibitors
   c. Thiazolidinediones
   d. Nutritional supplements

10. Which of the following antidiabetic agents is administered by subcutaneous injection?
    a. Jardiance
    b. Glumetza
    c. Trulicity
    d. Januvia

Bibliography

AACE/ACE: Consensus Statement by the American Association of Clinical Endocrinologists and American College of Endocrinology on the Comprehensive Type 2 Diabetes Management Algorithm-2017 Executive Summary, *Endocr Pract* 23(2):2017.

Bilandzic A, Rosella L: The cost of diabetes in Canada over 10 years: applying attributable health care costs to a diabetes incidence prediction model, *Health Promot Chronic Dis Prev Can* 37(2):2017.

Bosi E, Camisasca R, Collober C, et al: Effects of vildagliptin on glucose control over 24 weeks in patients with type 2 diabetes inadequately controlled with metformin, *Diabetes Care* 30:890–895, 2007.

Canadian Institute for Health Information: *International comparisons: a focus on diabetes*, Ottawa, ON, 2015, CIHI.

Chatterjee S, Davies MJ, Tarigopula G: Pharmacological control of blood sugar, *Anaesthesia and Intensive Care Medicine* 18(10):532–534, 2017.

FDA: nd. Drugs@FDA: FDA Approved Drug Products. (Retrieved August 30, 2018). From: http://www.accessdata.fda.gov/scripts/cder/daf/.

Gangji A, Cukierman T, Gerstein H, et al: A systemic review and meta-analysis of hypoglycemia and cardiovascular events, *Diabetes Care* 30:389–394, 2007.

Health Canada: 2018. Drug Product Database. (Retrieved August 30, 2018). From: https://health-products.canada.ca/dpd-bdpp/index-eng.jsp.

Kalant H, Grant D, Mitchell J: *Principles of medical pharmacology*, ed 7, Toronto, 2007, Elsevier Canada, pp 635–642.

Kalra S: Sodium Glucose Co-Transporter-2 (SGLT2) inhibitors: a review of their basic and clinical pharmacology, *Diabetes Ther* 5:355–366, 2014.

Morrato E, Hill J, Wyatt H, et al: Physical activity in U.S. adults with diabetes and at risk for developing diabetes, 2003, *Diabetes Care* 30:203–209, 2007.

National Institute of Diabetes and Digestive and Kidney Diseases: 2016. Diabetes. (Retrieved 4 November 2017). From: https://www.niddk.nih.gov/health-information/diabetes.

National Institute of Diabetes and Digestive and Kidney Diseases: 2017. National Diabetes Statistics Report, 2017. (Retrieved 4 November 2017). From: https://www.niddk.nih.gov/health-information/health-statistics.

National Center for Complementary and Integrative Health: 2017. Type 2 Diabetes and Dietary Supplements. (Retrieved 4 November 2017). From: https://nccih.nih.gov/health/providers/digest/diabetes.

NCD Risk Factor Collaboration (NCD-RisC): Worldwide trends in diabetes since 1980: a pooled analysis of 751 population-based studies with 4·4 million participants, *Lancet* 387(10027):1513–1530, 2016. doi: http://dx.doi.org/10.1016/S0140-6736(16)00618-8.

Page C, Curtis M, Sutter M, et al: *Integrated pharmacology*, ed 3, Philadelphia, 2006, Mosby, pp 293–299.

Public Health Agency Canada. 2016. *Health Status of Canadians 2016*. (Cat: 978-0-660-05480-3). Retrieved from: https://www.canada.ca/content/dam/hc-sc/healthy-canadians/migration/publications/department-ministere/state-public-health-status-2016-etat-sante-publique-statut/alt/pdf-eng.pdf.

Whalen K, Miller S, St.Onge E: The role of sodium-glucose co-transporter 2 inhibitors in the treatment of type 2 diabetes, *Clin Ther* 37(6):2015.

Overview of the Reproductive System

The human reproductive system undergoes change throughout its lifecycle. During puberty the male and female reproductive hormones surge, producing changes necessary for reproduction. The hypothalamus produces the hormones that signal the gonads (the testes in males and the ovaries in females) to produce the hormones testosterone, estrogen, and progesterone. These hormones stimulate sperm production, menstruation, ovulation, and secondary sexual characteristics such as facial hair, pubic hair, breast enlargement, and vaginal and uterine growth. Reproductive hormones decline with the onset of menopause in women signaling changes that produce the symptoms of menopause (e.g., "hot flashes"), the cessation of ovarian function, and the end of reproduction capacity.

In Unit IX, diseases of the reproductive system that include amenorrhea, infertility, endometriosis, premenstrual syndrome, abnormal uterine bleeding, prostate disease, and erectile dysfunction covered. This unit also provides information about contraception and emergency contraception. A description of the drugs indicated for the treatment, including mechanisms of action, adverse reactions, strength(s), and dosage forms is provided. It is important for pharmacy technicians to know about prescription and OTC agents that affect the reproductive system.

27

Drugs That Affect the Reproductive System

LEARNING OBJECTIVES

1. Learn the terminology associated with the reproductive system.
2. Describe the pathophysiology of reproductive system disorders.
3. Describe the physiology of pregnancy and methods of pregnancy prevention.
4. List and categorize medications that affect the reproductive system.
5. Describe the mechanism of action for each class of drugs that affects the reproductive system.
6. Identify significant drug look-alike and sound-alike issues.
7. List common endings for drug classes that affect the reproductive system.
8. Identify warning labels and precautionary messages associated with medications that affect the reproductive system.
9. Identify over-the-counter contraceptive methods.

KEY TERMS

Abnormal uterine bleeding Irregular or excessive uterine bleeding that results from a structural problem or hormonal imbalance.

Amenorrhea Absence of normal menstruation.

Atrophic vaginitis Postmenopausal thinning and dryness of the vaginal epithelium related to decreased estrogen levels.

Dysmenorrhea Difficult or painful menstruation.

Endometriosis Presence of functioning endometrial tissue outside the uterus.

Hypogonadism Inadequate production of sex hormones.

Hysterectomy Surgical removal of the uterus.

Infertility Inability to achieve pregnancy during 1 year or more of unprotected intercourse.

Menopause Termination of menstrual cycles; an event usually marked by the passage of at least 1 full year without menstruation.

Menorrhagia Excessive menstrual bleeding.

Pelvic inflammatory disease Infection of the uterus, fallopian tubes, and adjacent pelvic structures that is not associated with pregnancy or surgery.

Polycystic ovary disease Condition characterized by ovaries twice the normal size that contain fluid-filled cysts.

Premenstrual dysphoric disorder Disorder characterized by symptoms such as depression, anxiety, hopelessness, sad feelings, and self-deprecation.

Premenstrual syndrome Condition involving a set of symptoms (headache, irritability, depression, fatigue, sleep changes, weight gain) that occur before the start of the menstrual cycle.

Supraovulation Simultaneous rupture of multiple mature follicles.

Toxic shock syndrome Rare disorder caused by certain *Staphylococcus aureus* strains that occurs in women using tampons.

Overview

Sixty-one million U.S. women are of reproductive age (15–44 years) and approximately 70% are at risk for unintended pregnancy. A significant portion of Canadian women are also at risk. To prevent unintended pregnancy, nearly 60% of all women of reproductive age in the United States and Canada are using some contraceptive method. The use of effective contraceptive methods is underutilized, however, according to the 2015 Canadian Contraception Consensus.

Contraception: Prevention of Pregnancy

A variety of methods exist to prevent pregnancy. They are mechanical or barrier methods, hormonal methods, intrauterine devices (IUDs), abstinence, and emergency contraception (EC).

Mechanical and Barrier Methods of Contraception

Condoms, diaphragm, cervical cap, vaginal sponge, and spermicide (e.g., foams, jellies, creams) are mechanical barrier methods for contraception. They act to kill sperm or to block sperm from entering the uterus.

A condom is a device, usually made of latex or polyurethane, which is placed on a man's erect penis prior to sexual intercourse to block ejaculated semen from physically entering the body of the sexual partner. Female condoms are placed in the vagina. Condoms are used to prevent pregnancy and transmission of sexually transmitted infections (STIs) such as gonorrhea, syphilis, and human immunodeficiency virus (HIV). Condoms are used with a spermicide to provide greater protection.

■ *TECH NOTE!*

Lambskin condoms made from lamb intestines are the oldest form of condom available. They are ineffective in preventing the transmission of STIs.

Diaphragms

The diaphragm is a dome-shaped cup made of latex or silicone. The spring-molded rim creates a seal against the wall of the vagina. The rim of the diaphragm is squeezed into an arc shape for insertion. A water-based lubricant (usually spermicide) may be applied to the rim of the diaphragm to aid insertion. One teaspoonful (5 mL) of spermicide is placed in the dome of the diaphragm before insertion or with an applicator after insertion. The diaphragm must be inserted some time before sexual intercourse and remain in the vagina for 6 to 8 hours after a male's last ejaculation. The diaphragm must be removed for cleaning with warm soapy water at least once every 24 hours. Diaphragms should be refitted after a weight change of 4.5 kg (10 lb) or more or after any pregnancy. In the United States and Canada, diaphragms are available by prescription only. Many European countries do not require prescriptions.

Adverse Reactions. Diaphragms are associated with an increased risk of urinary tract infection. *Toxic shock syndrome* (TSS) occurs at a rate of 2.4 cases/100,000 women using diaphragms, almost exclusively when the device is left in place longer than 24 hours.

Types of Diaphragms

Generic Name	US Brand Name(s) Canadian Brand Name(s)	OTC/Prescription
diaphragm	Arcing spring, Omniflex (50–105 mm)	Prescription OTC (Caya)
	Caya Contoured Diaphragm (One size)	

OTC, Over the counter.

Cervical Cap, Contraceptive Sponge, and Vaginal Contraceptive Film

The cervical cap is placed over the cervix opening and is the size of a thimble. It is used with spermicide and has a 9% to 16% failure rate in women who have not previously been pregnant and is even less effective in women who have given birth. The cervical cap is a reusable silicone cup placed over the cervix and held in place by a one-way suction valve. It is also used with spermicide. It comes in one size and does not need to be specifically fitted to each woman. It is available by prescription in the United States, although it is obtainable over the counter in Europe and Canada. The contraceptive sponge (Today Sponge) is used with spermicide and has a 9% to 28% failure rate. It provides protection immediately after insertion and should remain inserted for 6 hours after intercourse. The vaginal contraceptive film (VCF) is a thin film that is impregnated with the spermicide nonoxynol-9. It is placed over the cervix 15 minutes prior to intercourse. The failure rate for VCF is approximately 6%.

Cervical Contraceptive Devices

Generic Name	US Brand Name(s) Canadian Brand Name(s)	OTC/Prescription
cervical cap	FemCap, Pro-Ception	Prescription (US) OTC (Canada)
	FemCap	
cervical sponge	Today Sponge	OTC
	Today Sponge	
contraceptive film	VCF	OTC
	VCF	

OTC, Over the counter; *VCF*, vaginal contraceptive film.

Intrauterine Device

An IUD is a contraceptive device that is placed in the uterus and is the most widely used long-acting reversible birth control method, globally. The device has to be inserted or removed from the uterus by a physician or qualified medical practitioner. Depending on the type, a single IUD is approved for 5 to 10 years use. The IUD is more than 99% effective. There are two broad categories, copper-releasing and hormone-releasing IUDs. Levonorgestrel, a progestin is released from hormone-releasing IUDs. In addition to contraception, levonorgestrel reduces menstrual bleeding, making it useful for the treatment of *menorrhagia* (heavy periods).

Mechanism of Action. The presence of an object in the uterus prompts the release of leukocytes and prostaglandins by the endometrium. These substances are hostile to sperm and eggs; the presence of the copper prevents the sperm from reaching the egg and the egg from attaching to the uterus. Progestin-releasing IUDs prevent ovulation and thicken cervical mucus, thus preventing the sperm from reaching the egg. IUDs do not protect against STIs, and their use is contraindicated in women with *pelvic inflammatory disease* (PID) or who are pregnant.

Adverse Reaction. Insertion of an IUD may introduce bacteria into the uterus. The insertion carries a small transient risk of PID in the first 20 days after insertion. If pregnancy does occur, presence of the IUD increases the risk of miscarriage, particularly during the second trimester.

Hormonal Methods of Contraception

Oral contraceptives (OCs), hormone-impregnated vaginal inserts, hormone injections, skin patches, surgical implants, and some IUDs are hormone dosage delivery systems marketed for contraception.

Oral Contraceptives

OCs have been collectively called the pill. Numerous OC products are available containing estrogen and progestins combinations, as well as progestin-only pills (Table 27.1). The pill can be used to regulate menstruation and prevent pregnancy. If used correctly and consistently, the pill is an extremely effective contraceptive, with an unintended pregnancy rate estimated at between 0.1% and 3%. In real life, the pill is approximately 91% effective.

Mechanism of Action. Hormonal contraceptives prevent pregnancy by initiating negative feedback inhibition of follicle-stimulating hormone (FSH) and luteinizing hormone (LH) secretion. As a result, mature follicles do not develop, and LH does not reach the level

Intrauterine Devices

Generic Name	US Brand Name(s) / Canadian Brand Name(s)	Strength
Copper releasing T shaped	Paraguard	
	Flex-T 300, Flex-T 380, Nova T	
levonorgestrel releasing	Liletta, Kyleena, Mirena, Skyla	**Levonorgestrel-releasing IUD:** 13.5 mg (Jaydess, Skyla), 19.5 mg (Kyleena), 52 mg (Liletta, Mirena)
	Jaydess, Kyleena, Mirena	

TABLE 27.1 Oral Contraceptives

Estrogen-Progestin Combination	Description
Monophasic	Provides a fixed dose of estrogen and progestin throughout cycle of 21- or 28-day package
Biphasic	Amount of estrogen remains the same throughout cycle; less progestin in first half of cycle, increased progestin in second half of cycle
Triphasic	Amount of estrogen is the same or varies throughout cycle; progestin amount varies

required to initiate ovulation. Menses takes place during the week with nondrug-containing pills (28-day cycle) or when the pill is stopped (21-day cycle). When the progestin and estrogen levels fall, as they normally do near the end of the cycle, menstruation occurs.

Adverse Reactions. Common side effects are breast tenderness and changes in menstrual pattern. Smoking increases the risk of adverse reactions, including increased risk of thromboembolic events and heart attacks. Loss of appetite and constipation can also occur. Women taking OCs should immediately report pain, muscle soreness, heat, or redness in calves; shortness of breath; sudden loss of vision; unresolved leg or foot swelling; weight gain (>5 lb [2.3 kg]); breast tenderness that does not go away; acute abdominal cramping; signs of vaginal infection; or changes in mood.

Other Hormone-Releasing Contraceptive Dosage Forms

Etonogestrel (Nexplanon) and medroxyprogesterone (Depo-Provera) are progestins. They prevent pregnancy by preventing ovulation, thickening cervical mucus to inhibit the passage of sperm, and maintaining the endometrium. Depo-Provera is administered by injection, once every 3 months. Etonogestrel (Nexplanon) is formulated as a micro-size rod, the size of a match stick, that is surgically implanted. The birth control injection is 94% effective, and the birth control implant is 99% effective at preventing pregnancy. Once inserted, Nexplanon prevents pregnancy for up to 4 years. Evra and Xulane are transdermal patches containing a combination of estrogen and progestin. A single patch is applied each week for 3 weeks, followed by 1 patch-free week. Each patch should be applied on the same day each week and only one patch should be worn at a time. No more than 7 days should pass during the patch-free interval. An advantage over other methods of contraception is that it is a weekly dose, noninvasive, and easy to use. The contraceptive patch is 91% effective in preventing pregnancy. Disadvantages are that the patch can become partially or completely detached and can irritate the skin.

Oral Contraceptives

Generic Name	US Brand Name(s) / Canadian Brand Name(s)	Dosage Forms and Strengths
Estrogen and Progestin Combinations		
ethinyl estradiol + desogestrel[a]	Bekyree, Cyclessa, Desogen, Emoquette, Enskyce, Isibloom, Kalliga, Kariva, Kimidess, Pimtrea, Velivet, Viorele, Volnea	**Tablet, monophasic (Apri, Desogen, Freya, Marvelon, Mirvala):** 21 days ethinyl estradiol 0.03 mg + desogestrel 0.15 mg **Tablet, biphasic (Kariva):** 21 days ethinyl estradiol 0.02 mg + desogestrel 0.15 mg; 5 days ethinyl estradiol 0.01 mg **Tablet, triphasic (Cyclessa, Linessa, Velivet):** 7 days ethinyl estradiol 0.025 mg + desogestrel 0.125 mg; 7 days ethinyl estradiol 0.025 mg + desogestrel 0.15 mg; 7 days ethinyl estradiol 0.025 mg + desogestrel 0.1 mg
	Apri, Freya, Linessa, Marvelon, Mirvala	
ethinyl estradiol + drospirenone[a]	Angeliq, Loryna, Lo-Zumandimine, Melamisa, Nikki, Syeda, Yaela, Yasmin, Yaz, Zumandimine	**Tablet, monophasic:** ethinyl estradiol 0.02 mg + drospirenone 3 mg, ethinyl estradiol 0.03 mg + drospirenone 3 mg (Zamine, Zarah)
	Mya, Yasmin, Yaz, Zamine, Zarah	
ethinyl estradiol + drospirenone + levomefolate[a]	Beyaz, Safyral Tydemy	**Tablet, monophasic:** 24 days ethinyl estradiol 0.02 mg + drospirenone 3 mg + levomefolate 0.451 mg; 4 days levomefolate 0.451 mg
	Yaz Plus	
ethinyl estradiol + ethynodiol[a]	Kelnor, Zovia 1+ 35, Zovia 1+ 50 E	**Tablet, monophasic:** ethinyl estradiol 0.035 mg + ethynodiol 1 mg (Zovia 1 + 35); ethinyl estradiol 0.05 mg + ethynodiol 1 mg (Zovia 1 + 50); ethinyl estradiol 0.03 mg + ethynodiol 2 mg (Demulen 30)
	Demulen 30	

Oral Contraceptives—cont'd

Generic Name	US Brand Name(s) Canadian Brand Name(s)	Dosage Forms and Strengths
ethinyl estradiol + levonorgestrel[a]	Afirmelle, Altavera, Ashlyna, Aviane, Ayuna, Balcoltra, Daysee, Elifemme, Enpresse, Falmina, Fayosim, Iclevia, Introvale, Jaimiess, Kurvelo, Lessina, Levonest, Levora, Lo-Seasonique, Lo-Simpesse, Marlissa, Myzilra, Portia, Quartette, Quasense, Seasonale, Seasonique, Setlakin, Trivora, Vienva Alesse, Alysena, Aviane, Indayo, Min-Ovral, Ovima, Portia, Seasonale, Seasonique, Triquilar	**Tablet, monophasic:** ethinyl estradiol 0.03 mg + levonorgestrel 0.15 mg (Altavera, Ayuna, Indayo, Kurvelo, Levora, Min-Ovral, Nordette, Ovima, Portia); ethinyl estradiol 0.02 mg + levonorgestrel 0.1 mg (Afirmelle, Alesse, Alysena, Aviane, Balcoltra, Esme, Lessina) **Tablet, triphasic:** 6 days ethinyl estradiol 0.03 mg + levonorgestrel 0.05 mg; 10 days ethinyl estradiol 0.03 mg + levonorgestrel 0.125 mg; 5 days ethinyl estradiol 0.04 mg + levonorgestrel 0.75 mg (Elifemme, Enpresse, Triquilar, Trivora) **Tablet, 84-day extended cycle (Introvale, Seasonale):** 84 days each—ethinyl estradiol 0.03 mg + levonorgestrel 0.15 mg **Tablet, 84-day biphasic cycle (Lo-Seasonique, Seasonique):** 7 days ethinyl estradiol 0.01 mg; 84 days ethinyl estradiol 0.02 mg + levonorgestrel 0.1 mg
ethinyl estradiol + norethindrone[a] More than 80 products...	Alyacen, Aranelle, Aurovela, Balziva, Briellyn, Brevicon, Cyclafem, Dasetta, Junel 1/20, Larin 1/20, Loestrin 1/20, Loestrin 1.5/30, Microgestin 1.5/30, Norinyl 1 + 35, Nortrel 7/7/7, Ortho-Novum 1/35, Ortho-Novum 7/7/7, Tri-Norinyl Brevicon 0.5/35, Brevicon 1/35, Loestrin 1.5/30, Lolo, Minestrin 1/20, Select 1/35, Synphasic	**Tablet, chewable:** ethinyl estradiol 0.035 mg + norethindrone 0.4 mg (Femcon FE, Nexesta FE); ethinyl estradiol 0.025 mg + norethindrone 0.8 mg (Kaitlib) **Tablet, monophasic:** ethinyl estradiol 0.035 mg + norethindrone 0.4 mg (Balziva, Briellyn, Ovcon 35); ethinyl estradiol 0.035 mg + norethindrone 0.5 mg (Brevicon, Cyclafem, Ortho 0.5/35); ethinyl estradiol 0.035 mg + norethindrone 1 mg (Norinyl 1 + 35 and 1 + 50, Ortho 1/35); ethinyl estradiol 0.05 mg + norethindrone 1 mg (Ovcon 50); ethinyl estradiol 0.03 mg + norethindrone 1.5 mg (Aurovela 1.5/30, Loestrin 1.5/30); ethinyl estradiol 0.02 mg + norethindrone 1 mg (Aurovela 1/20, Loestrin 1/20, Minestrin 1/20) **Tablet, biphasic:** 12 days ethinyl estradiol 0.035 + norethindrone, 0.5 mg; 9 days ethinyl estradiol 0.035 mg + norethindrone 1 mg Aranelle, Synphasic, Tri-Norinyl; 10 days ethinyl estradiol 0.035 + norethindrone, 0.5 mg; 11 days ethinyl estradiol 0.035 mg + norethindrone 1 mg (generic) **Tablet, triphasic (Cyclafem 7/7/7, Ortho Novum 7/7/7):** 7 days each—ethinyl estradiol 0.035 + norethindrone, 0.5 mg; 7 days each—ethinyl estradiol 0.035 mg + norethindrone 0.75 mg, 7 days each—ethinyl estradiol 0.035 mg + norethindrone 1 mg
ethinyl estradiol + norgestimate[a]	Estarylla, Mili, Mono-Linyah, Ortho-Cyclen, Ortho Tri-Cyclen, Ortho Tri-Cyclen Lo, Previfem, Sprintec, Tri-Estarylla, Tri-Lo Estarylla, TriNessa, Tri-Prevofem, Tri-Lo-Mili, Tri-Mili, Tri-Sprintec, Tri-Lo-Sprintec, Tri-Linyah Cyclen, Tri-Cyclen, Tri-Cyclen Lo, Tricira Lo	**Tablet, monophasic (Cyclen, Ortho-Cyclen, Previfem, Sprintec):** ethinyl estradiol 0.035 mg + norgestimate 0.25 mg **Triphasic formulation:** 7 days each—ethinyl estradiol 0.035 mg + norgestimate 0.18 mg, 7 days each—ethinyl estradiol 0.035 mg + norgestimate 0.215 mg, 7 days each—ethinyl estradiol 0.035 mg + norgestimate 0.25 mg (Ortho Tri-Cyclen, Tri-Cyclen, TriNessa, Tri-Sprintec); 7 days each—ethinyl estradiol 0.025 mg + norgestimate 0.18 mg, 7 days each—ethinyl estradiol 0.025 mg + norgestimate 0.215 mg, 7 days each—ethinyl estradiol 0.025 mg + norgestimate 0.25 mg (Ortho Tri-Cyclen Lo, Tri-Cyclen Lo, Tri-Lo-Sprintec)
Progestins		
norethindrone[a] norethindrone acetate[a]	Camila, Errin, Heather, Incassia, Jencycla, Micronor, Nor QD Jencycla, Micronor, Movisse, Norlutate	**Tablet:** 0.35 mg, 5 mg[b] (Norlutate)

[a]Generic available.
[b]Strength not used for contraception; used for amenorrhea, abnormal uterine bleeding, and endometriosis.

NuvaRing is a hormonal vaginal ring inserted for 3 weeks and then removed for 1 week. A new ring is inserted 7 days after the last one was removed and should be inserted the same time as the insertion of the previous ring. Advantages are that it is easy to use and is a once-monthly dosing. Although rare, it is possible for the ring to slip outside the vagina; if this occurs, it must be replaced within 3 hours. The contraceptive ring is 91% effective in preventing pregnancy.

Adverse Reactions. Depo-Provera and Nexplanon may cause irritation, redness, or pain at the site of administration. Patients may also experience dizziness, weight gain, leg cramps or joint pain, lower sex drive, hot flashes, increased body hair (reversible when drug is discontinued), and loss of bone mineral density (prolonged use). Rarely, the Nexplanon is rejected by the body. The most common side effects for the birth control patches (Evra, Xulane) and birth control ring (NuvaRing) are breast tenderness, weight gain, changes in appetite, or vaginal infection. Smoking increases the risk of thromboembolic events, stroke, and heart attacks.

Emergency Contraception

Emergency contraceptives reduce the risk of pregnancy after unprotected intercourse. Levonorgestrel (Plan B) is approximately 75% to 85% effective when taken as soon as possible after unprotected intercourse. It is most effective if taken within the first 72 hours after unprotected sexual intercourse. Plan B 1.5 mg is taken as a single dose or 0.75 mg followed by a second (0.75 mg) tablet 12 hours later. Ulipristal (Ella) is effective if taken within 5 days of unprotected intercourse. Ulipristal is a selective progesterone receptor modulator (SPRM) that delays ovulation and prevents implantation of a fertilized egg. Emergency contraception (EC) may be used at any time during the menstrual cycle. If conception has already occurred, EC will not terminate pregnancy. EC use is contraindicated in pregnancy or suspected pregnancy. The most common side effects are nausea, headache, and abdominal pain.

The emergency insertion of a copper IUD also is highly effective, reducing the risk of pregnancy by as much as 99%.

> ### ◗ TECH NOTE!
>
> In Canada, Plan B is listed as a schedule II nonprescription drug (requires pharmacist intervention) and a schedule III nonprescription drug (may be sold without pharmacist intervention). For schedule II, the manufacturer's labeled dosing is one (0.75 mg) tablet followed by a second tablet 12 hours later. For schedule III, the manufacturer's labeled dosing is two tablets as a single dose.

Miscellaneous Contraceptive Dosage Forms

Generic Name	US Brand Name(s) / Canadian Brand Name(s)	Dosage Forms and Strengths
ethinyl estradiol + etonogestrel	NuvaRing / NuvaRing	**Intravaginal ring:** ethinyl estradiol 15 mcg/24 h + etonogestrel 120 mcg/24 h
ethinyl estradiol + norelgestromin	Xulane / Evra	**Patch, weekly:** ethinyl estradiol 35 mcg/24 h + norelgestromin 200 mcg/24 h (Evra), ethinyl estradiol 35 mcg/24 h + norelgestromin 150 mcg/24 h (Xulane)
ethinyl estradiol + segesterone acetate	Annovera / Not available	**Intravaginal ring:** ethinyl estradiol 13 mcg/24 h + segesterone acetate 150 mcg/24 h
etonogestrel	Nexplanon / Not available	**Implantable rod:** etonogestrel 68 mg
medroxyprogesterone[a]	Depo-Provera, Depo-subQ Provera 104 / Depo-Provera	**Injection:** 50 mg/mL,[b] 104 mg/0.65 mL (Depo-SubQ Provera 104),[c] 150 mg/mL, 400 mg/mL[c]

[a]Generic available.
[b]Available in Canada only.
[c]Available in the United States only.

Emergency Contraceptives

Generic Name	US Brand Name(s) / Canadian Brand Name(s)	Dosage Forms and Strengths	OTC/Prescription Status
levonorgestrel[a]	Fallback Solo, Her Style, Opcicon One Step, Plan B, Plan B One-Step / Backup Plan Onestep, Contingency Plan, Next Choice, Option 2, Plan B	**Tablet:** 0.75 mg, 1.5 mg	OTC
ulipristal	Ella, Logilia / Ella, Fibristal	Tablet: 5 mg,[b] 30 mg	Prescription

[a]Generic available.
[b]Indicated to treatment of fibroids.

Surgical Methods of Contraception

Surgical methods such as tubal ligation and male vasectomy result in permanent sterility. Behavioral methods involve abstaining from sexual intercourse for a specified number of days before, during, and after ovulation. The rhythm method is a natural method based on calculating the fertile period by the use of a calendar, on which the supposed infertile days are marked. The ovulation method includes keeping a temperature chart to detect a minute change in temperature at the time of ovulation or determining the time of ovulation by observing changes in cervical mucus.

Menopause and Atrophic Vaginitis

Menopause is the termination of the menstrual cycle and is usually marked by the passage of at least 1 full year without menstruation. Natural menopause will occur in 25% of women by age 47, 50% by age 50, 75% by age 52, and 95% by age 55 years. Menopause caused by surgical removal of the ovaries *(hysterectomy)* occurs in almost 30% of US women who are 50 years or older.

Symptoms of menopause may last from a few months to years and vary from hardly noticeable to severe. Symptoms include mood changes, hot flashes (flushes), chills, fatigue, insomnia, palpitation, vertigo, headache, myalgia, urinary disturbances (e.g., incontinence), atrophic vaginitis, and various disorders of the gastrointestinal system. The long-range effects of lower estrogen levels are osteoporosis and atherosclerosis.

Atrophic vaginitis is the postmenopausal thinning and dryness of the vaginal epithelium related to decreased estrogen levels. Symptoms include burning and pain during intercourse. Hormone replacement therapy (HRT) or application of topical estrogen restores the integrity of the vaginal epithelium and relieves symptoms.

Hormone Replacement Therapy

HRT is prescribed to treat symptoms of menopause, such as hot flashes, vaginal dryness, mood swings, sleep disorders, and decreased sexual desire. HRT contains one or more female hormones, commonly estrogen plus progestin. Estrogen-only therapy is usually reserved for women who have had their uterus removed. It typically involves the administration of oral or vaginal estrogens, with or without progestins. The medication may be taken in the form of a pill, patch, or vaginal cream. The dosage form may vary according to the symptoms to be treated. For example, a vaginal cream can ease vaginal dryness but does not relieve hot flashes. Treatment protocols vary according to whether or not the woman has a uterus or has had a hysterectomy.

The Women's Health Initiative (WHI) HRT study (2002) showed that HRT increased the risk of developing breast cancer, heart attacks, strokes, and blood clots. The estrogen-progestin study showed that there was a 26% increase in the incidence of breast cancer, and the estrogen-only therapy study in women who no longer had a uterus showed that stroke risk was increased.

> **❶ TECH ALERT!**
>
> The following drugs have look-alike and sound-alike issues:
> Ortho Tri-Cyclen and Ortho TriCyclen Lo;
> FemHRT and Femara;
> Alora and Aldara;
> Premphase and Prempro

Adverse Reactions

HRT may increase the risk of heart disease, pulmonary embolism, and breast and endometrial cancers. Other adverse effects are nausea, vomiting, bloating, cramping, breast tenderness, return of menstruation or spotting, migraine headaches, and weight gain.

Selective Serotonin Reuptake Inhibitors (SSRIs)

Paroxetine is a SSRI that is used to treat the some symtoms of menopause, in addition to depression. Brisdelle is a low-dose paroxetine formulation that is approved for the treatment of moderate to severe vasomotor symptoms ("hot flashes").

Menstrual Disorders

Premenstrual Syndrome

Premenstrual syndrome (PMS) is a condition that involves a collection of symptoms that regularly occur in women prior to menstruation. Symptoms include headache, mood changes, fatigue, weight gain, sleep changes, and other problems that are distressing enough to limit activity and affect personal relationships. Because the causes of PMS are still unclear, current treatments focus on relieving the symptoms. A more severe form of PMS is *premenstrual dysphoric disorder* (PMDD). It is characterized by more pronounced features of PMS and occurs during the last week of the luteal phase in most menstrual cycles during the year preceding diagnosis. These symptoms disappear a few days after the onset of the menses. Symptoms may be accompanied by suicidal thoughts. Women commonly report that their symptoms worsen with age but go away with the onset of menopause. PMDD is treated with antidepressants such as SSRIs such as fluoxetine, paroxetine, and sertraline. SSRIs and other antidepressants are described in Chapter 6. Dosage forms specifically marketed for the treatment of PMDD are shown in the following table.

> **❶ TECH ALERT!**
>
> The following drugs have look-alike and sound-alike issues:
> FLUoxetine and DULoxetine;
> PROzac, PriLOSEC, Prograf, and Provera;
> Sarafem and Serophene;
> PARoxetine, FLUoxetine, and piroxicam;
> Paxil and Taxol;
> Sertraline and cetirizine

Dysmenorrhea

Dysmenorrhea, or painful menstruation, is the term used to describe menstrual cramps. Up to 85% of all women will have painful periods sometime during their reproductive years. Severe lower abdominal cramping and back pain accompanied by headache, nausea, and vomiting will disrupt their education, work, athletic, or other activities. Primary dysmenorrhea is the most common type, occurring primarily in adolescents and young women. Symptoms, which can last from hours to days vary in severity from cycle to cycle, are caused by an abnormally increased concentration of certain prostaglandins produced by the uterine lining. High concentrations of prostaglandin E2 (PGE2) and prostaglandin F2 (PGF2) cause painful spasms by decreasing blood flow and oxygen to the uterine muscle.

Primary dysmenorrhea can generally be treated effectively with over-the-counter (OTC) drugs such as nonsteroidal antiinflammatory drugs (NSAIDs) such as ibuprofen (Advil, Motrin, Midol), naproxen (Aleve, Pamprin), and prescription drugs ketoprofen and meclofenamate. Antiinflammatory drugs are listed and described in Chapter 10.

Hormone Replacement Therapy

Generic Name	US Brand Name(s) / Canadian Brand Name(s)	Dosage Forms and Strengths
Estrogen		
conjugated estrogens	Premarin Premarin	**Vaginal cream:** 0.625 mg/g **Powder, for injection:** 25 mg/vial **Tablet:** 0.3 mg, 0.45 mg,[a] 0.625 mg, 0.9 mg,[a] 1.25 mg
estradiol[b]	Alora, Climara, Depo-Estradiol, Delestrogen, Divigel, Elestrin, Estrace, Estrogel, Evamist, Femring, Imvexxy, Menostar, Minivelle, Vagifem, Vivelle, Vivelle Dot Climara, Divigel, Estrace, Estraderm, Estra Dot, Estring, Estrogel, Oesclim, Vagifem	**Gel, topical:** 0.1% (Divigel), 0.06% (Elestrin, Estrogel) **Solution, for injection, as cypionate (Depo-Estradiol):** 5 mg/mL **Solution, for injection, as valerate (Delestrogen):** 10 mg/mL, 20 mg/mL, 40 mg/mL **Spray, topical (Evamist):** 1.53 mg/spray **Tablet (Estrace):** 0.5 mg, 1 mg, 2 mg **Transdermal patch, biweekly (Alora, Estraderm, Estradot, Minivelle, Oesclim, Vivelle dot):** 0.025 mg/24 h, 0.0375 mg/24 h, 0.5 mg/24 h, 0.075 mg/24 h, 0.1 mcg/24 h **Transdermal patch, weekly (Climara, Menostar):** 0.014 mg/24 h, 0.025 mg/24 h, 0.0375 mg/24 h, 0.05 mg/24 h, 0.06 mg/24 h, 0.075 mg/24 h; 0.1 mg/24 h, **Vaginal cream (Estrace)[a]:** 0.01% **Vaginal ring:** 0.5 mg/24 h, 0.1 mg/24 h (Femring); 2 mg (Estring) **Vaginal insert (Imvexxy):** 4 mcg, 10 mcg **Vaginal tablet (Vagifem):** 10 mcg/tablet
estrogen (esterified)	Menest Not available	**Tablet:** 0.3 mg, 0.625 mg, 1.25 mg, 2.5 mg
estropipate[b]	Ogen 5 Not available	**Tablet:** 6 mg
Estrogen and Progestin Combinations		
estradiol + levonorgestrel	Climara Pro Not available	**Transdermal patch, weekly:** 0.45 mg/24 h estradiol + 0.15 mg/24 h levonorgestrel
estradiol + norethindrone[b]	Activella, Combipatch Activelle, Activelle LD, Estalis	**Tablet:** 0.5 mg estradiol + 0.1 mg norethindrone (Activelle LD); 1 mg estradiol + 0.5 mg estradiol (Activella, Activelle) **Transdermal patch, biweekly:** 0.05 mg/24 h estradiol + 0.14 mg/h norethindrone (Combipatch 50/140, Estalis 50/140); 0.05 mg/h estradiol + 0.25 mg/h norethindrone (Combipatch 50/250, Estalis 50/250)
estradiol + norgestimate	Generic Not available	**Tablet:** estradiol 1 mg + norgestimate 0.09 mg
conjugated estrogens + medroxyprogesterone	Prempro, Premphase 14/14, Prempro/Premphase Not Available	**Tablet (Premphase 14/14):** conjugated estrogens 0.625 mg + medroxyprogesterone 5 mg (Premphase) **Tablet (Prempro):** conjugated estrogens 0.3 mg + medroxyprogesterone 1.5 mg; conjugated estrogens 0.45 mg + medroxyprogesterone 1.5 mg; conjugated estrogens 0.625 mg + medroxyprogesterone 2.5 mg; conjugated estrogens 0.625 mg + medroxyprogesterone 5 mg
ethinyl estradiol + norethindrone	FemHRT Not Available	**Tablet:** 2.5 mcg ethinyl estradiol + 0.5 mg norethindrone
Estrogen agonist-antagonist		
Conjugated estrogen + bazedoxifene	Duavee Duavive	**Tablet:** 0.45 mg conjugated estrogens + 20 mg bazedoxifene

[a]Available in the United States only.
[b]Generic available.

Selective Serotonin Reuptake Inhibitors for Treatment of Premenstrual Dysphoric Disorder or Menopause

	Generic Name	US Brand Name(s) / Canadian Brand Name(s)	Dosage Forms and Strengths
	fluoxetine[a]	Sarafem, Selfemra / Prozac	**Capsule (Prozac):** 10 mg, 20 mg / **Tablet, as HCl (Sarafem, Selfemra):** 10 mg, 15 mg, 20 mg
	paroxetine	Brisdelle* / Not available	**Capsule:** 7.5 mg[b]

[a]Generic available.
[b]Available in the United States only.
*For vasomotor symptoms.

Amenorrhea

Amenorrhea is the absence of normal menstruation. Primary amenorrhea is the failure of the menstrual cycles to begin, and it may be caused by various factors, such as hormone imbalances, genetic disorders, or structural deformities of the reproductive organs. Secondary amenorrhea occurs when a woman who has previously menstruated slows to three or fewer cycles per year. Amenorrhea may be a symptom of excessive weight loss, pregnancy, lactation, menopause, or disease of the reproductive system. Amenorrhea is treated with bromocriptine, a dopamine receptor agonist that restores normal ovulatory menstrual cycles. Bromocriptine's mechanism of action and adverse effects are described in detail in Chapter 8. OCs may also be prescribed to establish a normal menstrual cycle.

Pharmaceutical Treatment of Amenorrhea

Generic Name	US Brand Name(s) / Canadian Brand Name(s)	Dosage Forms and Strengths
bromocriptine[a,b]	Parlodel / Generics	**Tablet:** 2.5 mg **Capsule:** 5 mg
oral contraceptives	See earlier, "Oral Contraceptives"	See earlier, "Oral Contraceptives"

[a]Generic available.
[b]Also available as Cycloset (used to treat diabetes).

Abnormal Uterine Bleeding

Abnormal uterine bleeding (AUB), a condition that causes heavy menstrual bleeding, affects up to $\frac{1}{3}$ of all reproductive-age women. AUB may occur in women who have fibroids, but the exact association is unknown. In severe cases, excessive uterine bleeding from any cause can result in life-threatening anemia. In addition to excessive bleeding, women may experience cramping for an abnormal period of time beyond the normal menstrual cycle.

Treatment with NSAIDs and hormonal manipulation using low-dose birth control pills may be prescribed. If conservative treatment fails to stop the endometrial lining from hemorrhaging, hysterectomy remains one of the most curative options.

Reproductive Disorders

Infertility

Conception is a normal biologic process that results in pregnancy; however, for infertile women and men, conception may be aided by pharmacotherapy. *Infertility* is often defined as a failure to conceive after 1 year of regular unprotected intercourse. It is caused by a wide variety of biologic, environmental, and even lifestyle factors, such as smoking or alcohol abuse. Infertility affects men and women. *Polycystic ovary disease*, characterized by enlarged ovaries that contain fluid-filled cysts, and *hypogonadism*, a condition in which the sex glands produce little or no hormones, are examples of medical conditions that can cause infertility. In men, gonads are the testes; in women, they are the ovaries.

Infertility may be treated with fertility drugs, alone or in combination with other assisted reproductive procedures, such as artificial insemination. Pharmaceutical treatment of infertility may involve the administration of selective estrogen receptor modulators (SERMs; e.g., clomiphene), menotropins (Menopur), gonadotropin-releasing hormone (GnRH) antagonists (e.g., Ganirelix), and recombinant human FSH (follitropin alfa). FSH and LH stimulate normal follicular growth, maturation, and subsequent ovulation.

Selective Estrogen Receptor Modulator

Clomiphene is a SERM that stimulates ovulation. It is taken for 5 days, starting on day 3 to 5 of the menstrual cycle. If treatment is successful, ovulation begins 6 to 12 days after a course of the drug.

Mechanism of Action and Pharmacokinetics

Clomiphene competes with estrogen for estrogen-receptor binding sites. It works by effectively tricking the pituitary gland into producing FSH and LH, necessary for ovulation.

Adverse Reactions

Clomiphene may cause visual disturbances, dizziness, and headache. It should not be used during pregnancy. The incidence of multiple births when clomiphene is administered is approximately 5% to 7% (mostly twins). This percentage is much lower than that observed following direct administration (injection) of FSH and LH, in which the intent is to produce multiple follicles before inducing ovulation.

❗ TECH ALERT!

The following drugs have look-alike and sound-alike issues: clomiphene and clomipramine

Pharmacotherapy for Infertility

Generic Name	US Brand Name(s)	Dosage Forms and Strengths
	Canadian Brand Name(s)	
clomiphene	Generic	**Tablet:** 50 mg
	Not available	

Gonadotropins

Menotropins, human chorionic gonadotropin (hCG), choriogonadotropin alfa, and follitropin are gonadotropins that are administered to promote ovulation. Menotropins are purified combination preparations of FSH and LH that are derived from the urine of postmenopausal women. Urofollitropin is purified human follitropin derived from urine. Follitropin alfa and follitropin beta are recombinant version of human FSH (rFSH). Choriogonadotropin alfa (rhCG) is a synthetic recombinant formulation of hCG

Gonadotropins stimulate *supraovulation*, or simultaneous rupture of multiple mature follicles, which is an infertility treatment option that may be used if clomiphene proves ineffective or if multiple ova are considered to be useful for assisted reproductive procedures, such as in vitro fertilization.

Mechanism of Action and Pharmacokinetics

Gonadotropins promote follicular growth, maturation, and ovulation. Menotropins, hCG, rhCG, and follitropin are peptides that are quickly destroyed in the gastrointestinal tract; therefore they must be administered parenterally as an intramuscular injection or, for select products, as an subcutaneous injection. Urine-derived hCG is administered IM, and recombinant hCG is administered subcutaneously.

Adverse Reactions

Side effects of gonadotropin administration include headache, lightheadedness, nausea, abdominal discomfort, flushing, and local inflammation at the injection site.

Gonadotropin-Releasing Hormone

GnRH analogues may be agonists or antagonists. GnRH antagonists are approved for the treatment of infertility. GnRH agonists are indicated for the treatment hypogonadism, endometriosis, AUB, and various other conditions.

Gonadotropin-Releasing Hormone Antagonists

Cetrorelix (Cetrotide) and ganirelix (Ganirelix) and GnRH antagonists that are approved for treating infertility. They are

Gonadotropins

Generic Name	US Brand Name(s)	Dosage Forms and Strengths
	Canadian Brand Name(s)	
follitropin-alpha/beta	Follistim AQ, Gonal-f, Gonal-f RFF	**Powder, for injection:** 75 units/vial (Gonal RFF),[a] 300 units/vial,[a] 450 units/vial (Gonal-F), 900 units/vial[a] 1050 units/vial (Gonal-F)
	Gonal-f, Gonal-f pen, Puregon	**Solution, for injection (Follistim AQ):** 300 units/0.36 mL, 600 units/0.72 mL, 900 units/1.08 mL
follitropin-beta Puregon		**Solution, for injection (Puregon):** 50 units/0.5 mL, 100 units/0.5 mL, 833 units/1 mL
urofollitropin	Bravelle	**Powder, for injection:** 75 units/vial
	Not available	
choriogonadotropin	Ovidrel	**Solution, prefilled syringe, for injection (Ovidrel):** 0.25 mg/0.5 mL, 0.25 mg/vial
	Ovidrel	
menotropins	Menopur	**Powder, for injection:** 75 units/vial
	Menopur, Repronex	

[a]Available in Canada only.

administered to prevent premature LH surges in women undergoing controlled ovarian hyperstimulation stimulation. GnRH antagonists decrease the production and release of LH by competitively binding GnRH receptor sites.

Gonadotropin-Releasing Hormone Agonists

Gonadotropin-releasing hormone agonist analogues are used to treat endometriosis, endometrial thinning, and AUB (Lupaneta Pak, Lupron Depot, Zoladex), hypogonadism (Luveris, Pergoveris), precocious puberty (Suprellin LA, Synarel), prostate cancer (Eligard, Zoladex), and advanced breast cancer (Zoladex).

Mechanism of Action

GnRH agonists produce initial stimulation followed by inhibition the body's release of naturally occurring gonadotropins (LH and FSH). Antagonists competitively bind to GnRH receptor sites to block the action of GnRH. Continuous administration of agonist and antagonist suppresses ovulation and decreases testosterone levels.

Gonadotropin-Releasing Hormone Antagonists

Generic Name	US Brand Name(s) / Canadian Brand Name(s)	Dosage Forms and Strengths
cetrorelix	Cetrotide	Powder, for injection: 0.25 mg/mL
	Cetrotide	
ganirelix	Ganirelix	Solution, for injection (prefilled syringe): 250 mcg/0.5 mL
	Orgalutran	

Adverse Reactions

Side effects of GnRH analogues include pain, redness, or swelling around the injection or implant site. Additional adverse reactions include headache, breast swelling and tenderness, postmenopausal symptoms, vaginal spotting, breakthrough bleeding, decreased libido, impotence, and bone loss. rhLH may additionally produce abdominal bloating, diarrhea, and gas.

> **⊘ TECH ALERT!**
>
> The following drugs have look-alike and sound-alike issues: Lupron Depot-3 Month and Lupron Depot-Ped

Endometriosis

Endometriosis is a benign but painful condition that is characterized by the presence of functioning endometrial tissue outside the uterus. The displaced endometrial tissue is usually attached to an ovary or to the pelvic or abdominal organs; it is occasionally found in other areas of the body. Endometriosis often causes infertility, dysmenorrhea, and severe pain. Symptoms reflect the fact that displaced endometrial tissue reacts to ovarian hormones in the same way as the normal endometrium—exhibiting a cycle of growth and sloughing off. The disorder affects approximately 10% of women; most are aged 30 to 45 years.

Danazol

Danazol is an androgenic steroid that is used to treat endometriosis and fibrocystic breast disease. It reduces breast pain, tenderness, and nodules.

Mechanism of Action

Danazol works by suppressing the pituitary output of FSH and LH, resulting in anovulation and associated amenorrhea. It interrupts the progression and pain of endometriosis by shrinking normal and ectopic endometrial tissue.

Adverse Reactions

Adverse reactions include masculinity effects, gastrointestinal distress, diarrhea, or jaundice, and menstrual irregularities.

Gonadotropin-Releasing Hormone Agonists

Generic Name	US Brand Name(s) / Canadian Brand Name(s)	Dosage Forms and Strengths
buserelin	Not available	Implant (Suprefact Depot): 6.3 mg (2-months), 9.45 mg (3-months) Solution, injection: 1 mg/mL
	Suprefact, Suprefact Depot	
goserelin	Zoladex, Zoladex LA	Injection (Zoladex), 1-month implant: 3.6 mg Injection (Zoladex LA), 3-month implant: 10.8 mg
	Zoledex, Zoladex LA	
leuprolide[a]	Eligard, Lupron, Lupron Depot	Solution, for injection: 5 mg/mL Suspension, for injection: 7.5 mg (1 month); 22.5 mg (3 months); 30 mg (4 months), 45 mgb (6 months)/syringe [Eligard]; 3.75 mg, 11.25 mg, 15 mg, 22.5 mg, 30 mg/vial (Lupron, Lupron Depot)
	Eligard, Lupron, Lupron Depot	
leuprolide + norethindrone	Lupaneta Pak	Suspension, for injection + tablets: leuprolide 3.75 mg/vial + norethindrone 5-mg tablets; leuprolide 11.25 mg/vial + norethindrone 5- mg tablets
	Not Available	
lutropin alfa	Not Available	Powder, for Injection: 75 units
	Luveris	
lutropin alfa + follitropin alfa	Not Available	Powder, for Injection: 75 units lutropin alfa + 150 units follitropin alfa
	Pergoveris	
nafarelin	Synarel	Solution, nasal spray: 2 mg/mL, 60 metered doses
	Synarel	
histrelin	Supprelin LA, Vantas	Implant: 50 mg
	Not available	

[a]Generic available.

Treatment of Endometriosis

Generic Name	US Brand Name(s) / Canadian Brand Name(s)	Dosage Forms and Strengths
danazol[a]	Generics / Cyclomen	**Capsule:** 50 mg, 100 mg, 200 mg

[a]Generic available.

Androgen Deficiency in Men

The male hormone testosterone and its derivatives are collectively called androgens. They are secreted by the anterior pituitary gland and are responsible for masculinization (development of male secondary sexual characteristics). Small amounts are produced by the adrenal gland.

Androgens and Anabolic Steroids

Anabolic steroids are synthetic drugs that closely resemble the androgen testosterone. They promote the tissue-building process and, in normal dosages, can have a minimal effect on accessory sex organs and secondary sex characteristics. Androgen therapy is used as replacement therapy for testosterone deficiency such as hypogonadism, select cases of delayed puberty, and postpuberty testosterone deficiency.

> **⊘ TECH ALERT!**
>
> Testosterone patches are not substitutable.

Mechanism of Action and Pharmacokinetics

Androgens aid in the development and maintenance of secondary sexual characteristics, such as facial hair, deepening of voice, growth of body hair, fat distribution, and muscle development, in adolescent boys. Testosterone also stimulates the growth of accessory sex organs (penis, testes, vas deferens, prostate). Androgens also promote tissue-building processes (anabolism) and tissue-depleting processes (catabolism).

They are available in different dosage forms as patches, gels, tablets, capsules, injections, transdermal patches, and pellets. The mucoadhesive form produces twice the androgen activity of oral tablets, the transdermal patch is applied daily to the scrotum or other parts of the body, and the gel is applied to the shoulder, upper arm, and abdomen (it should not be applied to the genitals).

Adverse Reactions

Androgens may produce gynecomastia (breast enlargement), testicular atrophy, impotence, decreased testicular function, penis enlargement, nausea, jaundice, headache, anxiety, male pattern baldness, acne, and depression. Fluid electrolyte imbalances (e.g., sodium, chloride, potassium, calcium, phosphate, water retention) may also occur. Prolonged use of anabolic steroids can cause many of the same serious adverse effects as androgens, as well as testicular atrophy, blood-filled cysts in the liver or spleen, malignant and benign liver tumors, increased risk of atherosclerosis, and mental changes (e.g., rage). These adverse effects are why androgens (anabolic steroids) are regulated as controlled substances.

> **⊘ TECH ALERT!**
>
> The following drugs have look-alike and sound-alike issues: Testoderm (scrotal patch) and Testoderm TTS (transdermal patch)

> **⊘ TECH ALERT!**
>
> Testosterone and other anabolic steroids are schedule C-III controlled substances in the United States and C3 controlled substances in Canada.

Androgen Agonists

Generic Name	US Brand Name(s) / Canadian Brand Name(s)	Dosage Forms and Strengths
fluoxymesterone	Generics / Not available	**Tablet:** 10 mg
methyltestosterone[a]	Android 25, Testred / Not available	**Capsule (Testred):** 10 mg **Tablet (Android):** 25 mg
testosterone[a]	Androderm, Androgel, Aveed, Fortesta, Natesto, Striant, Testim, Testopel, Vogelxo / Androderm, Androgel, Axiron, Delatestryl, Nastesto, Testim	**Capsule, as undecanoate:** 40 mg **Gel, topical (Androgel, Testim, Vogelxo):** 1% **Implant (Testopel):** 75 mg **Nasal spray (Natesto):** 5.5 mg/actuation (4.5%) **Spray, transdermal solution (Axiron):** 2% **Spray, transdermal gel:** 10 mg/actuation (Fortesta), 12.5 mg/actuation (Androgel) **Solution, injection:** 100 mg/mL,[b] 200 mg/mL, 250 mg/mL (Aveed) **Oil, as enanthate injection (Delestryl):** 200 mg/mL **Tablet, extended release; buccal (Striant):** 30 mg **Transdermal Patch (Androderm):** 2 mg/24 h,[c] 2.5 mg/24 h,[b] 4 mg/24 h,[c] 5 mg/24 h[b]

[a]Generic available.
[b]Available in Canada only.
[c]Available in the United States only.

Summary of Drugs That Affect the Reproductive System

	Generic Name	Brand Name	Usual Dose and Dosing Schedule	Warning Labels
Selective Serotonin Reuptake Inhibitors				
	fluoxetine	Prozac, Sarafem	**PMDD:** 20 mg/day dosed continuously or intermittently (starting 14 days prior to menstruation through the onset of menses)	MAY CAUSE DIZZINESS. MAY IMPAIR ABILITY TO DRIVE. SWALLOW WHOLE; DON'T CRUSH OR CHEW (DELAYED-RELEASE).
	sertraline	Zoloft	**PMDD:** 50–150 mg/day dosed continuously or intermittently (starting 14 days prior to menstruation through the onset of menses)	
	paroxetine	Brisdelle	**Menopause vasomotor symptoms:** 7.5 mg daily at bedtime	
Dopamine Receptor Agonist				
	bromocriptine	Parlodel	**Female infertility – In vitro fertilization:** 1.25 mg/day on days 4 to 6 of follicular phase, then 2.5 mg/day until 3 days after onset of menstruation.	TAKE WITH FOOD OR MILK. MAY CAUSE DROWSINESS. LIMIT ALCOHOL USE.
Oral Contraceptives				
Estrogen and Progestin Combinations				
	ethinyl estradiol + desogestrel	Numerous (See OC table in chapter)	Take 1 tablet daily at same time every day for 21 days; off 7 days (21-day cycle), or take 1 tablet daily at same time every day (28-day cycle)	MAY TAKE WITH FOOD. TAKE AT THE SAME TIME EACH DAY. AVOID PROLONGED EXPOSURE TO SUNLIGHT USE EXACTLY AS PRESCRIBED. AVOID SMOKING.
	ethinyl estradiol + drospirenone	Yasmin, Yaz		
	ethinyl estradiol + etonogestrel	NuvaRing	Insert ring vaginally and leave in place for 3 weeks. Remove for 1 week. Insert new ring 7 days after last one was removed.	
	ethinyl estradiol + levonorgestrel	Numerous (See OC table in chapter)	Take 1 tablet at same time every day for 21 days; off 7 days (21-day cycle), or take 1 tablet daily at same time every day (28-day cycle)	
	ethinyl estradiol + norethindrone	Numerous (See OC table in chapter)		
	ethinyl estradiol + norgestimate	Numerous (See OC table in chapter)		
Intrauterine Devices				
	copper-releasing	ParaGard	**Intrauterine device:** Insert IUD into uterine cavity; replace 10 years after insertion.	CALL YOUR HEALTH CARE PROVIDER IF YOU CANNOT FEEL THE IUD THREADS OR HAVE PELVIC PAIN OR PAIN DURING SEXUAL INTERCOURSE.
	levonorgestrel	Kyleena, Mirena	**Intrauterine device:** Insert IUD into uterine cavity; replace 5 years after insertion.	
Contraceptive Implant				
	etonogestrel	Implanon	Insert 1 rod under the skin in upper arm; replace 3 years after insertion.	CALL YOUR DOCTOR IF YOU CANNOT FEEL THE IMPLANT.
Emergency Contraceptives				
	levonorgestrel	Plan B, Plan B One Step	Take 1 tablet within 72 h of unprotected sexual intercourse; take another tablet 12 h later or take 2 tablets as a single dose.	TAKE WITH FOOD AVOID SMOKING

Continued

Summary of Drugs That Affect the Reproductive System—cont'd

	Generic Name	Brand Name	Usual Dose and Dosing Schedule	Warning Labels
Hormone Replacement Therapy				
Estrogen				
	estradiol	Numerous (See estrogen table in chapter)	**Moderate to Severe symptoms of Menopause (vasomotor symptoms or atrophic vulva) Vaginal cream:** Insert 2 to 4 g/day intravaginally for 2 weeks; then reduce to half the initial dose for 2 weeks, followed by maintenance dose of 1 g two or three times/week **Tablet, oral:** 1–2 mg orally once daily in a cyclical pattern (3 weeks on, 1 week off) **Topical emulsion:** Apply 3.84 g once daily in the morning. **Topical gel:** 1.25 g/day applied at same time daily **Transdermal spray (Evamist):** Apply 1 spray once daily to forearm; increase to 2 or 3 sprays daily based on clinical response. **Patch:** Apply once weekly (Climara, Menostar) or twice weekly (Vivelle-Dot). **Vaginal ring:** Insert ring intravaginally: leave in for 3 months. **Vaginal tablet:** Insert 1 tablet daily for 2 weeks; maintenance, insert 1 tablet twice weekly.	ROTATE SITE OF APPLICATION (TRANSDERMAL PATCH). AVOID SMOKING. TAKE WITH FOOD (TABLET) INSERT PRESCRIBED DOSE VAGINALLY AS DIRECTED—vaginal cream, vaginal tablet
	estrogens (conjugated)	Premarin	**Moderate to Severe symptoms of Menopause (vasomotor symptoms or atrophic vulva) Vaginal cream:** Insert 0.5–2 g/day intravaginally for 3 weeks, then 1 week off (cyclically) **Tablet:** 0.3 mg/day cyclically or daily	
	estrogen (esterified)	Menest	0.3–1.25 mg/day tablet cyclically	
	estropipate	Ogen 5	1 tablet daily; administer cyclically	
Estrogen and Progesterone Combinations				
	estradiol + levonoregestrel	ClimaraPro	**Transdermal:** apply 1 patch weekly	ROTATE SITE OF APPLICATION. AVOID PROLONGED EXPOSURE TO SUNLIGHT.
	estradiol + norethindrone	Activella, CombiPatch, Estalis	**Transdermal patch:** apply new patch twice weekly during 28-day cycle	
	estradiol + norgestimate	Prefest	**Tablet:** 1 mg pink tablet daily for 3 days followed by 0.09 mg white tablet for 3 days: repeat sequence	
	estrogens + medroxyprogesterone acetates (MPA)	Premphase, Premplus, Prempro	**Premphase:** 1 maroon tablet days 1–14 followed by 1 light blue tablet days 15–28 **Prempro:** 1 tablet daily	
Selective Estrogen Receptor Modulator				
	clomiphene	Generic	**Female infertility:** 50 mg once daily for 5 days starting on the 5th day of cycle. May repeat cycle in 30 days increasing dose to 100 mg if ovulation has not occurred. **Male hypogonadism:** 25 mg once daily or 25–50 mg every other day.	TAKE EXACTLY AS DIRECTED; DON'T SKIP DOSES.

Summary of Drugs That Affect the Reproductive System—cont'd

	Generic Name	Brand Name	Usual Dose and Dosing Schedule	Warning Labels
Gonadotropins				
	choriogonadotropin (recombinant)	Ovidrel	**Infertility:** Inject 250 mcg subcutaneously 1 day after the last dose of the follicle stimulating agent (Ovidrel) **Hypogonadism (males):** Inject 500–4000 units 3 times a weekly for 3 weeks to 6 months depending on protocol.	DISCARD ANY UNUSED RECONSTITUTED SOLUTION.
	follitropin-alpha	Gonal-f	**Ovulation Induction:** 75 IU/day SC; if no response in 5–7 days, may increase by 37.5 IU weekly until max 300 IU **Hypogonadism (men):** 150 IU SC 3 times/week following hCG pretreatment, 1000 units	USE IMMEDIATELY AFTER RECONSTITUTION
	menotropins	Menopur	On day 2 of cycle inject 225–450 IU daily for up to 20 days based on ovarian response	REFRIGERATE DILUTED POWDER; DO NOT FREEZE. PROTECT FROM LIGHT.
	urofollitropin	Bravelle	**Ovulation induction:** 150 units once daily SC or IM for 5 days according to protocol	USE IMMEDIATELY AFTER RECONSTITUTION
Gonadotropin-Releasing Hormone Antagonists				
	cetrorelix	Cetrotide	**Ovulation Induction:** Inject 0.25 mg SC once daily beginning on morning of stimulation day 5 or 6 and continue until hCG administration according to protocols	REFRIGERATE; DON'T FREEZE—(0.25 mg) STORE AT ROOM TEMPERATURE (3 mg cetrorelix, ganirelix) PROTECT FROM LIGHT— ganirelix
	ganirelix	Ganirelix, Orgalutran Orgalutran	Inject 250 mg SC once daily during mid- to late-follicular phase	
Gonadotropin-Releasing Hormone Agonists				
	buserelin	Suprefact	**Endometriosis:** 2 sprays in each nostril 3 times daily for 6–9 months	DISCARD 5 WEEKS AFTER FIRST OPENING
	goserelin	Zoladex	**Endometriosis:** Inject 3.6 mg SC every 28 days	STORE AT ROOM TEMPERATURE UNTIL READY FOR USE. DO NOT FREEZE.
	histrelin	Suprellin LA	**Precocious puberty:** Insert 1 implant SC annually	REFRIGERATE; DON'T FREEZE
	leuprolide	Eligard, Lupron, Lupron Depot,	**Endometriosis:** 11.25 mg IM every 3-months for 1–2 doses. Max course of treatment is 12 months **Precocious puberty:** Dose varies by weight. 7.5–15 mg IM monthly or 11.25–30 mg IM depot once every 3 months **Anemia caused by uterine fibroids (Lupron Depot):** 3.5 mg monthly or 11.25 mg Max: 3 months	SHAKE IF SETTLING OCCURS (Suspension) DISCARD ANY UNUSED PORTION. STORE AT ROOM TEMPERATURE (Solution). ROTATE INJECTION SITE.
	lutropin alfa	Luveris	**Stimulate Follicle development:** 75 IU SC once daily	DISCARD ANY UNUSED PORTION OF VIAL.
	nafarelin	Synarel	**Endometriosis:** 1 spray in one nostril in the morning and 1 spray in the other nostril in the evening **Precocious puberty:** 2 sprays in each nostril every morning and evening	DO NOT USE NASAL DECONGESTANTS FOR 30 MIN AFTER USING NAFARELIN SPRAY.

Continued

Summary of Drugs That Affect the Reproductive System—cont'd

	Generic Name	Brand Name	Usual Dose and Dosing Schedule	Warning Labels
	leuprolide + norethindrone	Lupaneta Pak	**Endometriosis:** Inject 3.75 mg monthly + take 1 norethindrone tablet once daily	STORE AT ROOM TEMPERATURE
	lutropin alfa + follitropin alfa	Pergoveris	**Varies**	STORE AT ROOM TEMPERATURE PROTECT FROM LIGHT
Androgen Agonists				
	fluoxymesterone	Generics	**Hypogonadism:** 5–20 mg/day	TAKE AS DIRECTED.—All
	methyltestosterone	Android	**Hypogonadism:** 10–50 mg/day	TAKE WITH FOOD.—All ROTATE SITE OF APPLICATION (PATCH, INJECTION).
	testosterone	Androderm, Delatestryl, Striant, Testoderm	**Hypogonadism** **Pellet:** SC implantation, 150–450 mg every 3–6 months **Scrotal patch (Testoderm):** 6 mg daily to scrotum **Transdermal patch (Androderm, Testoderm TTS):** Apply daily to back, abdomen, thigh, or arm **Injection:** 50–400 mg every 2–4 weeks **Gel:** 5 g daily **Oral, buccal (Striant):** 30 mg every 12 h **Nasal gel:** 2 pump actuations 3 times a day (max 33 mg/day)	APPLY TO THE UPPER GUM ABOVE THE INCISOR TOOTH (BUCCAL TABLET). APPLY TO ARM, ABDOMEN, BACK, OR THIGH (ANDRODERM). APPLY TO SCROTUM (TESTODERM).
Miscellaneous				
	danazol	Generics	**Endometriosis:** 200–800 mg daily in 2 divided doses	PROTECT FROM LIGHT AND MOISTURE

OC, oral contraceptive; *IUD*, intrauterine device; *IU*, international unit; *SC*, subcutaneously; *PMDD*, Premenstrual Dysphoric Disorder.

TECHNICIAN'S CORNER

1. Since the WHI study, many women have turned to herbal preparations to combat menopausal symptoms. How effective are these preparations in improving these symptoms?
2. Many athletes have been using anabolic steroids to gain an edge in their sport. What are some long-term effects of these steroids on the body and mind?

Key Points

- Infertility may be caused by a wide variety of medical, environmental, and even lifestyle factors, such as smoking or alcohol abuse.
- Symptoms of premenstrual syndrome include headache, mood changes, fatigue, weight gain, sleep changes, and other problems that are distressing enough to limit activity and affect personal relationships.
- Amenorrhea may be a symptom of weight loss, pregnancy, lactation, menopause, or disease of the reproductive system.
- Abnormal uterine bleeding is irregular or excessive uterine bleeding.
- Sexually transmitted infections are caused by communicable pathogens such as viruses, bacteria, fungi, and protozoa.
- Menopause is the termination of menstrual cycles and is usually marked by the passage of at least 1 full year without menstruation.

- Endometriosis is a benign but painful condition that is characterized by the presence of functioning endometrial tissue outside the uterus.
- Condoms are used to prevent pregnancy and transmission of sexually transmitted infections such as gonorrhea, syphilis, and HIV.
- Most hormonal contraceptives were developed to prevent pregnancy by initiating negative feedback inhibition of follicle-stimulating hormone and luteinizing hormone secretion.
- The diaphragm must be inserted sometime before sexual intercourse and remain in the vagina for 6 to 8 hours after a male's last ejaculation.
- The presence of an intrauterine device in the uterus prompts the release of leukocytes and prostaglandins by the endometrium interfering with fertilization and implantation.

- If used correctly and consistently, the pill is an extremely effective contraceptive, with an unintended pregnancy rate estimated at between 0.1% and 3%.
- Emergency contraceptive pills must be taken within 3 days (Plan B) or 5 days (Ella) after unprotected intercourse.
- Hormone replacement therapy may be prescribed to treat symptoms of menopause such as hot flashes, vaginal dryness, mood swings, sleep disorders, and decreased sexual desire.
- Gonadotropin-releasing hormone analogues are used to treat prostate cancer, endometriosis, advanced breast cancer, and endometrial thinning.
- The male hormone testosterone and its derivatives are called androgens. Androgens are responsible for masculinization (development of male secondary sexual characteristics).

Review Questions

1. Hormonal contraceptives are manufactured in all of the following dosage forms EXCEPT _____.
   a. tablet
   b. transdermal patch
   c. vaginal cream
   d. implant
2. Select the contraceptive that is marketed as an over-the-counter (OTC) product.
   a. Contraceptive sponge
   b. Diaphragm
   c. Intrauterine device (IUD)
   d. Transdermal patch
3. Testoderm is applied to _____.
   a. back
   b. thigh
   c. abdomen
   d. scrotum
4. Select the emergency contraceptive that must be dispensed by prescription.
   a. Plan B One Step
   b. Next Choice
   c. Fallback Solo
   d. Ella
5. Menopause is the termination of menstrual cycles that is usually marked by the passage of at least 2 full years without menstruation.
   a. True
   b. False

6. Oral contraceptives (the pill) are 100% effective in preventing pregnancy.
   a. True
   b. False
7. The WHI study on hormonal replacement therapy concluded that hormonal replacement therapy may increase the risk for _____.
   a. heart disease and breast cancer
   b. heart attack and blood clots
   c. strokes
   d. all of the above
8. Clomiphene is a drug used to treat _____.
   a. contraception
   b. infertility
   c. hypogonadism
   d. amenorrhea
9. Gonadotropin-releasing hormone agonist, Synarel is a(n) _____.
   a. transdermal patch
   b. nasal spray
   c. injection
   d. capsule
10. Testosterone and anabolic steroids are _____ controlled substances in the United States and _____ in Canada.
    a. schedule I, C1
    b. schedule II, C2
    c. schedule III, C3
    d. schedule IV, C4

Bibliography

Barnes MN, Wiemer D: Therapeutic Management of Infertility: A Pharmacist's Perspective, 2015. https://www.uspharmacist.com/ce/therapeutic-management-of-infertility-a.

Borgelt L: Emergency Contraception: An Update for Pharmacists, 2016. http://www.powerpak.com/course/preamble/113221.

Borgelt L: Emergency Contraception: Key Concepts for the Pharmacy Technician, 2016. http://www.powerpak.com/course/preamble/115023.

Centers for Disease Control and Prevention, Workowski KA, Berman SM: Sexually transmitted diseases treatment guidelines, *MMWR Recomm Rep* 64(3):2015.

FDA: Drugs@FDA: FDA Approved Drug Products, nd. Retrieved September 7, 2018, from http://www.accessdata.fda.gov/scripts/cder/daf/.

Health Canada: Drug Product Database, 2018. Retrieved September 7, 2018, from https://health-products.canada.ca/dpd-bdpp/index-eng.jsp.

Hutten-Czapski P, Goertzen J: The occasional intrauterine contraceptive device insertion, *Can J Rural Med* 13:31–35, 2008.

Institute for Safe Medication Practices: List of Confused Drugs, 2015. Retrieved September 9, 2017, from https://www.ismp.org/tools/confuseddrugnames.pdf.

Kallmann's syndrome, tabers medical dictionary, ed 20, Philadelphia, 2005, FA. Davis, p 1163.

Kumar P, Sharma A: Gonadotropin-releasing hormone analogs: Understanding advantages and limitations, *J Hum Reprod Sci* 7(3):170–174, 2014. doi:10.4103/0974-1208.142476.

National Heart Lung and Blood Institute: NHLBI Stops Trial of Estrogen Plus Progestin Due to Increased Breast Cancer Risk, Lack of Overall Benefit, 2002. Retrieved June 13, 2012, from http://www.nhlbi.nih.gov/news/press-releases/2002/nhlbi-stops-trial-of-estrogen-plus-progestin-due-to-increased-breast-cancer-risk-lack-of-overall-benefit.html.

National Heart Lung and Blood Institute: NIH Asks Participants in Women's Health Initiative Estrogen-Alone Study to Stop Study Pills, Begin Follow-up Phase, 2004. Retrieved June 13, 2012, from http://www.nhlbi.nih.gov/news/press-releases/2004/nih-asks-participants-in-womens-health-initiative-estrogen-alone-study-to-stop-study-pills-begin-follow-up-phase.html.

National Heart, Lung and Blood Institute: Facts about menopausal hormone therapy (NIH Publ. No. 05-5200), 2005 (http://www.nhlbi.nih.gov/health/women/pht_facts.pdf).

Roach S: *Pharmacology for health professionals*, Baltimore, 2005, Lippincott, Williams & Wilkins.

Shannon M, Wilson B, Stang C: *Health professionals drug guide, 2005–2006*, Upper Saddle River, NJ, 2006, Prentice-Hall.

Thibodeau G, Patton K: *Anatomy and physiology*, ed 6, St. Louis, 2007, Mosby.

U.S. Department of Health and Human Services Office on Women's Health: Birth Control Methods, 2017. Retrieved November 12, 2017, from https://www.womenshealth.gov/a-z-topics/birth-control-methods.

Whitaker L, Critchley H: Abnormal uterine bleeding, *Best Pract Res Clin Obstet Gynaecol* 34:54–65, 2016. doi:10.1016/j.bpobgyn.2015.11.012.

28

Treatment of Prostate Disease and Erectile Dysfunction

LEARNING OBJECTIVES

1. Learn the terminology associated with prostate disease and erectile dysfunction.
2. List symptoms of prostate disease and erectile dysfunction.
3. List and categorize medications used for the treatment of prostate disease and erectile dysfunction.
4. Describe mechanism of action for drugs used for the treatment of prostate disease and erectile dysfunction.

5. List common endings for drug classes used in the treatment of prostate disease and erectile dysfunction.
6. Identify significant drug look-alike and sound-alike issues.
7. Identify warning labels and precautionary messages associated with medications used for the treatment of prostate disease and erectile dysfunction.

KEY TERMS

Benign prostatic hyperplasia Noncancerous, abnormal increase in the growth of the prostate gland.
Erectile dysfunction Persistent inability to achieve and/or maintain an erection sufficient for satisfactory sexual intercourse.
Incontinence Loss of bladder or bowel control.
Prostate gland Gland in the male reproductive system just below the bladder surrounding the urethra.
Prostate-specific antigen Protein produced by the prostate gland. Levels are elevated in men with conditions ranging from prostate infection to prostate cancer.

Prostate-specific antigen test Blood test to measure the percentage of prostate-specific antigen that is unbound. Free prostate-specific antigen is linked to benign prostate hyperplasia but not to cancer.
Prostatitis Inflammation of the prostate gland.
Urinary frequency Need to urinate more often than is normal.

Benign Prostatic Hyperplasia

The *prostate gland* is a part of the male reproductive system located just below the bladder that surrounds the urethra. The gland produces semen, the fluid that contains sperm. *Prostatitis* is an inflamed or infected prostate gland. Symptoms may be burning on urination, fever, body ache, groin, rectal, or low back pain, difficulty urinating, urge *incontinence*, painful ejaculation, and decreased libido. Although some of the symptoms are similar, prostatitis is usually an acute condition, unlike *benign prostatic hyperplasia* (BPH). BPH is a condition in which noncancerous cells in the prostate grow and increase the size of the prostate gland (Fig. 28.1). It is a condition associated with bladder obstruction and lower urinary tract symptoms (LUTS), because as the gland grows, it begins to obstruct the flow of urine through the urethra. The urethra is a small tube that carries urine and semen through the penis.

The risk for developing BPH increases with age. By age 60, more than 50% of men will have the condition; 90% or more men will develop BPH/LUTS by 80 years old, and nearly all men will have an enlarged prostate.

Diagnosis

Several tests are available to check the health of the prostate. A digital rectal examination involves the insertion of a gloved finger into the rectum and palpating the prostate to determine whether it is enlarged. A *prostate-specific antigen* (PSA) *test* may be performed to determine whether levels of the PSA protein are elevated. A higher than normal level is a sign of BPH, infection, inflammation, or prostate cancer. A free PSA test, the percentage of PSA that is not attached to another chemical, may be conducted to differentiate between BPH and cancer. Free PSA is linked to

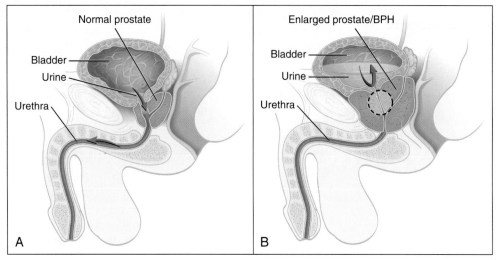

• **Fig. 28.1** (A) Normal prostate. (B) Enlarged prostate. *BPH,* Benign prostatic hyperplasia. (Courtesy National Institutes of Health, Bethesda, MD.)

• **BOX 28.1** **Symptoms of Benign Prostatic Hyperplasia**

- Weak or slow stream of urine
- Delay in starting urination
- Urinary stream that starts and stops
- Frequent urination
- Urinary urgency
- Nighttime awakening to urinate
- Need to strain to urinate

BPH but not to cancer. Urinalysis and a biopsy of prostate tissue may also be taken.

Symptoms of Benign Prostatic Hyperplasia

The first symptom of an enlarged prostate gland is a weak or slow stream of urine (Box 28.1). There may also be a delayed start in the flow of urine or straining to urinate. As the disease progresses, the bladder becomes hypersensitive and the need to urinate becomes more frequent *(urinary frequency)*. Some men may develop urinary infection(s) from the condition. BPH may also produce bladder stones, sudden inability to urinate, or kidney damage.

Treatment of Benign Prostatic Hyperplasia

Pharmacotherapy for BPH is initiated when symptoms are uncomfortable enough to warrant treatment (Fig. 28.2). Watchful waiting is recommended when patients are asymptomatic or symptoms do not produce much discomfort. Alpha blockers and 5α-reductase inhibitors may be administered to manage symptoms.

α₁-Adrenergic Antagonists

α_1-adrenergic antagonists relax prostate and bladder smooth muscle, which reduces urethral resistance and improves the flow of urine. Some alpha blockers are also prescribed for the treatment of hypertension (see Chapter 18).

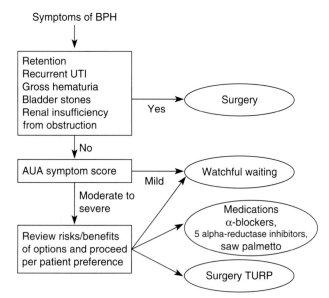

• **Fig. 28.2** Summary of treatment options for benign prostatic hyperplasia *(BPH).* *TURP,* Transurethral resection of the prostate. (From Page C, Hoffman B, Curtis M, et al: *Integrated pharmacology,* ed 3, Philadelphia, 2006, Mosby.)

⬛ *TECH NOTE!*

A common ending for 5α-reductase inhibitors is *-steride.*

---

❶ *TECH ALERT!*

The following drugs have look-alike and sound-alike issues: Cardura and Coumadin

---

Mechanism of Action and Pharmacokinetics

Alfuzosin, doxazosin, silodosin, tamsulosin, and terazosin bind to α_1-adrenergic receptor sites. Binding to α_1-adrenergic receptors blocks adrenergic-mediated vasoconstriction in the prostate.

Alfuzosin, doxazosin, and tamsulosin are available in extended-release dosage forms and are dosed once daily. The half-life ($t^{1/2}$)

α₁-Adrenergic Antagonists

Generic Name	US Brand Name(s) / Canadian Brand Names(s)	Dosage Forms and Strengths
alfuzosin[a]	Uroxatral	Tablet, extended-release: 10 mg
	Xatral	
doxazosin[a]	Cardura, Cardura XL	Tablet: 1 mg, 2 mg, 4 mg, 8 mg[b]
	Cardura	Tablet, extended release (Cardura XL)[b]: 4 mg, 8 mg
silodosin[a]	Rapaflo	Capsule: 4 mg, 8 mg
	Rapaflo	
tamsulosin[a]	Flomax	Capsule, controlled release: 0.4 mg
	Flomax CR	Tablet, controlled release[c]: 0.4 mg
terazosin[a]	Generics	Capsule[b]: 1 mg, 2 mg, 5 mg, 10 mg
	Generics	Tablet[c]: 1 mg, 2 mg, 5 mg, 10 mg

[a]Generic available.
[b]Available in the United States only.
[c]Available in Canada only.

for all agents ranges between 10 and 22 hours. Absorption of tamsulosin is increased if the drug is taken with high fat content meal, increasing the effects and side effects. Rapaflo (silodosin) should be taken with food. Urine flow rates are usually improved within the first 2 weeks of therapy.

Adverse Reactions

Adverse drug effects linked to the administration of α-adrenergic antagonists are postural hypotension, dizziness, reflex tachycardia, headache, stuffy nose, weakness, and fatigue.

5α-Reductase Inhibitors

High testosterone levels can stimulate growth of prostate tissue, whereas deprivation results in a reduction in glandular size. Finasteride and dutasteride are 5α-reductase inhibitors that reduce testosterone levels.

Mechanism of Action and Pharmacokinetics

Finasteride and dutasteride inhibit 5α-reductase, an enzyme that controls the production of dihydrotestosterone (DHT) from testosterone. Drug effects accumulate over time, and it may take 6 to 12 months for full therapeutic effects to be achieved.

> **● TECH NOTE!**
>
> Finasteride, 1 mg, is prescribed for the treatment of male pattern baldness.

Adverse Reactions

Dutasteride and finasteride may decrease desire for sex, cause *erectile dysfunction* (ED), and/or reduce semen volume. Both drugs are harmful to the developing fetus; therefore pregnant women and women of childbearing age should be advised to avoid contact with broken or crushed tablets. The use of a barrier contraceptive, such as condoms, is also recommended.

5α-Reductase Inhibitors

Generic Name	US Brand Name(s) / Canadian Brand Names(s)	Dosage Forms and Strengths
dutasteride[a]	Avodart	Capsule: 0.5 mg
	Avodart	
finasteride[a]	Proscar, Propecia	Tablet (Proscar): 5 mg
	Proscar, Propecia	Tablet (Propecia)[b]: 1 mg
Combination: 5α-Reductase Inhibitor and Alpha Blocker		
dutasteride + tamsulosin[a]	Jalyn	Capsule: 0.5 mg dutasteride + 0.4 mg tamsulosin
	Jalyn	

[a]Generic available.
[b]Propecia is used for hair loss.

> **❶ TECH ALERT!**
>
> Proscar and Provera have look-alike and sound-alike issues.

Nonpharmacologic Treatment Options

When symptoms of BPH are severe, surgery is indicated. There are several surgical options. Some procedures are more invasive

Summary of Drugs Used in the Treatment of Benign Prostatic Hyperplasia

Generic Name	US Brand Name	Usual Adult Oral Dose and Dosing Schedule	Warning Labels
α₁-Adrenergic Antagonist			
alfuzosin	Uroxatral	10 mg once daily	DO NOT DISCONTINUE WITHOUT MEDICAL SUPERVISION. MAY CAUSE DIZZINESS OR LIGHTHEADEDNESS. AVOID DRIVING OR OPERATING HAZARDOUS MACHINERY. SWALLOW WHOLE; DO NOT CRUSH OR CHEW (Flomax, Cardura XL, Uroxatral). TAKE WITH MEAL (alfuzosin silodosin).
doxazosin	Cardura	1–8 mg once daily	
	Cardura XL	4–8 mg once daily	
terazosin	Generics	1–10 mg at bedtime	
silodosin	Rapaflo	8 mg daily	
tamsulosin	Flomax	0.4–0.8 mg once daily	
5α-Reductase Inhibitors			
dutasteride	Avodart	0.5 mg once daily	SWALLOW CAPSULES WHOLE; DO NOT CHEW (dutasteride). SWALLOW THE TABLETS WITH A DRINK OF WATER (finasteride). PREGNANT WOMEN SHOULD AVOID CONTACT WITH BROKEN OR CRUSHED TABLETS.
finasteride	Proscar	5 mg once daily	
Combination: 5α-Reductase Inhibitor and Alpha Blocker			
dutasteride + tamsulosin	Jalyn	1 capsule daily	MAY CAUSE DIZZINESS. SWALLOW CAPSULES WHOLE; DO NOT CHEW. PREGNANT WOMEN SHOULD AVOID CONTACT WITH BROKEN OR CRUSHED TABLETS.

than others. Following are brief definitions of surgical procedures for BPH:

Prostatic stent: A stent (scaffolding) is inserted into the urethra to open a passage and improve urine flow.

TUIP (transurethral incision of the prostate): One or two slits are made in the prostate to relieve the pressure and improve urine flow.

TUMT (transurethral microwave thermal therapy of the prostate): Computer-regulated microwaves are sent through a catheter to heat portions of the prostate.

TUNA (transurethral needle ablation): Delivers a low-level radiofrequency signal directly into the prostate and destroys the prostate tissue, improving the symptoms of BPH.

TURP (transurethral resection of the prostate): Excess prostate tissue is trimmed away.

TUVP: Excess prostate tissue is vaporized using an electrical current.

Erectile Dysfunction

An erection occurs when the arteries and sinusoids in the corpus cavernosum fill with blood (Fig. 28.3). Intracorporal blood pressure increases while at the same time venous outflow decreases, resulting in penile rigidity that enables effective intercourse. ED is defined as the total inability to achieve erection, an inconsistent ability to achieve erection, or difficulty maintaining erection long enough to sustain sexual intercourse. It is also known as impotence. Up to 30 million American men have reported symptoms of ED. ED appears to increase with age; however, it is not an inevitable part of the aging process. By age 40 years, approximately 5% of men experience ED. By age 65, approximately 15% to 25% of men have ED.

What Causes Erectile Dysfunction?

ED may have physiologic, psychological, neurologic, or endocrinologic causes. Physiologic causes include age-related changes and chronic disease (e.g., hypertension, hyperlipidemia, or multiple sclerosis). Neurologic and endocrinologic causes may be the result of diabetes, a disease of the endocrine system that can cause vascular and nerve changes that affect erectile function. ED may also be caused by depression. ED may also be caused by lifestyle factors such as smoking, obesity, and alcoholism.

Drugs Used for the Treatment of Erectile Dysfunction

ED is managed by the administration of drugs that promote penile engorgement and slow loss of erection. Neurotransmitters are involved in producing an erection, listed in Box 28.2.

Nitric oxide (NO) is a mediator of smooth muscle relaxation that is released in response to sexual stimulation. It activates several intracellular enzymes such as phosphodiesterase type 5 (PDE5), an enzyme involved in the reversal of an erection. PDE5 inhibitors and prostaglandin E analogues are drugs that are used in the treatment of ED.

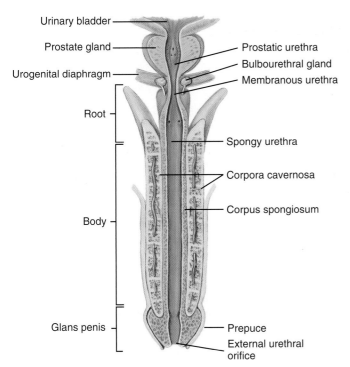

• **Fig. 28.3** Structure of the penis. (From Page C, Hoffman B, Curtis M, et al: *Integrated pharmacology*, ed 3, Philadelphia, 2006, Mosby.)

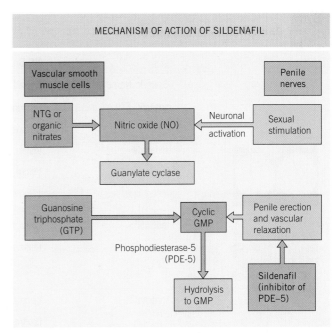

• **Fig. 28.4** Mechanism of action for sildenafil. Sildenafil binds to receptors that block the degradation of cGMP and increase the effects of nitric oxide *(NO)* on the corpus cavernosum (relaxation and increased erectile response). *NTG,* Nitroglycerine; *GMP,* guanosine monophosphate. (From Page C, Hoffman B, Curtis M, et al: *Integrated pharmacology*, ed 3, Philadelphia, 2006, Mosby.)

• **BOX 28.2** **Neurotransmitters That Relax Smooth Muscle in the Penis**

- Acetylcholine (ACh)
- Nitric oxide (NO)
- Prostaglandin E1 (PGE1)
- Vasoactive intestinal polypeptide (VIP)
- Calcitonin gene-related peptide (CGRP)

Phosphodiesterase Inhibitors

Sildenafil, tadalafil, and vardenafil are the most commonly prescribed drugs for the treatment of ED. They are taken prior to intercourse to produce an erection. Sildenafil and tadalafil are taken 30 minutes prior to intercourse. Vardenafil is taken up to 60 minutes before sexual activity.

Mechanism of Action

Avanafil, sildenafil, tadalafil, and vardenafil relax smooth muscle and blood vessels that supply the corpus cavernosum and control penile engorgement (Fig. 28.4). At the cellular level, the drugs increase levels of Nitric oxide (NO) in the corpus cavernosum, which blocks the opening of calcium voltage-gated channels and reduces calcium-mediated vascular contractions.

Pharmacokinetics

The oral absorption of sildenafil, vardenafil, and tadalafil is good, and maximum concentration (C_{max}) and onset of action of vardenafil are reached between 30 minutes and 2 hours after a dose of drug is administered. C_{max} for tadalafil and sildenafil is similar, averaging approximately 2 hours. The bioavailability of the drugs may be reduced by up to 50% when they are taken with a meal that is high in fat. Protein binding is approximately 94% to 95% for all PDE5s.

Adverse Reactions

Many of the adverse reactions associated with the use of phosphodiesterase inhibitors are a result of vasodilation. These side effects include dizziness, flushing, headache, and nasal congestion. Diarrhea and indigestion are gastrointestinal side effects. Sildenafil, tadalafil, and vardenafil may also produce sudden hearing loss or visual effects that range from light sensitivity and difficulty distinguishing between green and blue to loss of vision. The incidence of visual disturbances is greater with sildenafil than with vardenafil and tadalafil.

Precautions

PDE5 inhibitors are involved in numerous drug interactions. A life-threatening drop in blood pressure has occurred in men who have taken nitrates such as nitroglycerin (for angina), so the use of nitrates, in all dosage forms, is contraindicated while taking PDE5 inhibitors. Concurrent administration of α-adrenergic agonists (e.g., alfuzosin, terazosin, doxazosin), used for the treatment of BPH, requires caution, and it is recommended that alpha blockers should not be taken within 4 hours of PDE5 inhibitors. Patients taking PDE5 inhibitors should avoid antifungals *(-azoles),* cimetidine, grapefruit juice, and macrolide antiinfectives (e.g., erythromycin, clarithromycin) and excessive alcohol consumption (more than five glasses of wine or five shots of whiskey). Drug interactions also occur with the coadministration of selective serotonin reuptake inhibitor and monoamine oxidase inhibitor (MAOI) antidepressants.

Phosphodiesterase Inhibitors

Generic Name	US Brand Name(s) Canadian Brand Names(s)	Dosage Forms and Strengths
avanafil	Stendra	**Tablet:** 50 mg, 100 mg, 200 mg
	Not available	
sildenafil[a]	Viagra, Revatio[b]	**Solution, oral (Revatio)**[c]: 10 mg/mL
	Viagra, Revatio[b]	**Solution, IV (Revatio):** 0.8 mg/mL **Tablet (Viagra):** 25 mg, 50 mg, 100 mg **Tablet (Revatio):** 20 mg
tadalafil[a]	Cialis, Adcirca[b]	**Tablet:** 2.5 mg, 5 mg, 10 mg, 20 mg
	Cialis, Adcirca[b]	
vardenafil[a]	Levitra, Staxyn	**Tablet:** 2.5 mg,[c] 5 mg, 10 mg, 20 mg **Tablet, oral disintegrating (Staxyn):** 10 mg
	Levitra, Staxyn	

[a]Generic available.
[b]Indicated for pulmonary arterial hypertension (20 mg tablet only).
[c]Available in the United States only.

Prostaglandins

Alprostadil is naturally occurring prostaglandin E1 (PGE1) present in the seminal vesicles and cavernous tissues of males. It can also be found in the placenta of the fetus. PGE1 mediates the relaxation of penile smooth muscle.

Mechanism of Action and Pharmacokinetics

PGE1 mobilizes intracellular calcium in the corpus cavernosum, resulting in smooth muscle contraction; however, in the endothelium, PGE1 mediates the release of NO, which relaxes cavernosal smooth muscle, causing an erection.

The oral absorption of alprostadil is poor; therefore the drug is formulated for intraurethral insertion and intracavernosal injection. The intracavernosal route of administration is more effective than is the intraurethral route. Instructions for inserting alprostadilintraurethral inserts are provided in Box 28.3. Instructions for using the alprostadilintracavernosal injection are provided in Box 28.4.

Adverse Reactions

Adverse reactions are specific to the route of administration. Hypotension, dizziness, bleeding, bruising, or pain at the site of injection and painful erection are associated with intracavernosal administration. Itching in the penis, testicles, legs, and perineum, redness of the penis, warmth or burning sensation in the urethra, and leg swelling are adverse effects associated with intraurethral administration of alprostadil. Urethral bleeding or spotting may occur when the drug is administered improperly. Both dosage forms may produce prolonged erection (lasting >4 hours).

• BOX 28.3 Instructions for Administration of Intraurethral Pellets

1. Gently and slowly stretch the penis upward to its full length.
2. Slowly insert the stem of the applicator into the urethra up to the collar; then gently and completely push down the button at the top of the applicator until it stops (and medicated pellet is released).
3. Hold the applicator in this position for 5 seconds; then remove applicator while keeping the penis upright. Roll the penis firmly between the hands for at least 10 seconds to ensure that the medication is adequately distributed along the walls of the urethra.
4. An erection should begin to form within 10 minutes of application.

• BOX 28.4 Instructions for Administration of Intracavernosal Injection

1. Gently and slowly stretch the penis upward to its full length.
2. Insert the needle into the corpus cavernosum at 90 degrees until the metal portion of the needle is almost completely into the penis. Avoid visible veins, urethra, and corpus spongiosum.
3. Slowly inject the contents of the syringe over 5 to 10 seconds.
4. Withdraw syringe and apply pressure to injection site for 5 minutes or until bleeding stops.

Nonpharmacologic Management of Erectile Dysfunction

ED may also be treated by attaching a mechanical vacuum device to the penis, which uses suction to produce engorgement. An alternative approach is to surgically implant a device with inflatable tubes that can cause the penis to become erect. Vascular surgery

Prostaglandins

Generic Name	US Brand Name(s) / Canadian Brand Names(s)	Dosage Forms and Strengths
alprostadil[a]	Caverject, Caverject Impulse, Edex cartridge, Muse, Prostin VR[b]	**Powder, for injection, (Caverject):** 5 mcg,[c] 10 mcg,[c] 20 mcg, 40 mcg[c]
	Caverject, Muse, Prostin VR[b]	**Urethral insert (Muse):** 125 mcg,[c] 250 mcg, 500 mcg, 1000 mcg
		Injection, solution (Prostin VR): 500 mcg/mL

[a]Generic available.
[b]Prostin VR is administered as a continuous infusion to neonates with congenital heart disease such as ductus arteriosus, pulmonary stenosis, or interruption of the aortic arch until corrective surgery can be performed.
[c]Available in the United States only.
[d]Available in Canada only.

Summary of Drugs Used in the Treatment of Erectile Dysfunction

	Generic Name	US Brand Name	Usual Adult Oral Dose and Dosing Schedule	Warning Labels
Phosphodiesterase Inhibitors (PDE5)				
	avanafil	Stendra	50–200 mg 15 minutes prior to sexual activity	MAY CAUSE DIZZINESS. AVOID GRAPEFRUIT JUICE (avanafil, tadalafil, vardenafil). DISSOLVE ORAL DISINTEGRATING TABLETS UNDER TONGUE.
	sildenafil	Viagra	25–100 mg ½–4 h prior to sexual intercourse; not more than once daily	
	tadalafil	Cialis	10–20 mg prior to sexual intercourse; not more than once daily or 2.5–5 mg once daily	
	vardenafil	Levitra	5–20 mg up to 60 min prior up to sexual intercourse; not more than once daily	
Prostaglandins				
	alprostadil	Muse	Insert 1 pellet 30–60 min prior to sexual intercourse; not more than once daily	REFRIGERATE (MAY BE STORED AT ROOM TEMPERATURE FOR 14 DAYS).
		Caverject	Inject individualized dose not more than once in 24 h or >3 times/weeks	ROTATE SITE OF INJECTION. MAY STORE AT ROOM TEMPERATURE FOR UP TO 3 MONTHS. AVOID DRUG EXPOSURE TO EXTREMES IN HEAT OR COLD.

may be performed to reconstruct arteries that supply the penis and to block off veins that allow blood to leak from penile tissue.

Herbal Remedies for Benign Prostatic Hyperplasia and Erectile Dysfunction

The ripened fruit of saw palmetto contains fatty acids and plant sterols that inhibit 5α-reductase and cystolic androgen binding, producing antiinflammatory and antiestrogenic effects. Saw palmetto may reduce urinary symptoms of BPH. Prostate cancer should be ruled out prior to taking saw palmetto. Yohimbe is an evergreen tree found in West Africa. Its bark contains an α_2-adrenergic blocker related to reserpine that may improve ED. Clinical trials have not been conducted and evidence to support yohimbe's effectiveness is lacking. Adverse effects include increased blood pressure and heart rate, headache, insomnia, anxiety, nausea, and vomiting. Drug interactions may occur if yohimbe is taken concurrently with MAOIs, tricyclic antidepressants (TCAs), and phenothiazines.

TECHNICIAN'S CORNER

1. How are complementary and alternative medicines (e.g., herbs) used in managing BPH?
2. How might lifestyle changes reduce the risks erectile dysfunction?

Key Points

- The prostate gland is part of the male reproductive system.
- Prostatitis is an inflamed or infected prostate gland.
- Benign prostatic hyperplasia (BPH) is a condition in which noncancerous cells in the prostate grow and increase the size of the prostate gland.
- The risk for developing BPH increases with age; by 80 years old, nearly all men will have an enlarged prostate.
- Higher than normal prostate-specific antigen levels are a sign of BPH, infection, inflammation, or prostate cancer.
- Two classes of drugs are administered to manage symptoms of BPH. They are alpha blockers and 5α-reductase inhibitors.
- Alfuzosin, doxazosin, silodosin, terazosin, and tamsulosin are $α_1$-adrenergic blockers.
- Alfuzosin, doxazosin, and tamsulosin are available in extended-release dosage forms.
- Adverse drug effects linked to the administration of α-adrenergic antagonists are postural hypotension, dizziness, reflex tachycardia, headache, stuffy nose, weakness, and fatigue.
- Finasteride and dutasteride are 5α-reductase inhibitors that decrease testosterone levels. It may take 6 to 12 months to achieve maximum effects.
- Dutasteride and finasteride are harmful to the developing fetus. Pregnant women and women of childbearing age should be advised to avoid contact with broken or crushed tablets. The use of barrier contraceptive is also recommended.
- Erectile dysfunction (ED) is defined as a total inability to achieve erection, an inconsistent ability to achieve erection, or difficulty maintaining erection long enough to sustain sexual intercourse.
- Drugs currently marketed for the treatment of ED are phosphodiesterase inhibitors and prostaglandin E analogues.
- Avanafil, sildenafil, tadalafil, and vardenafil are selective inhibitors of cyclic guanosine monophosphate–specific PDE5.
- PDE5 inhibitors relax smooth muscle and blood vessels that supply the corpus cavernosum and control penile engorgement by increasing levels of nitric oxide.
- Side effects of PDE5 inhibitors are dizziness, flushing, headache, nasal congestion, diarrhea, indigestion, and visual disturbances.
- The administration of nitrates, such as nitroglycerin, in all dosage forms, is contraindicated in patients taking PDE5 inhibitors.
- Patients taking avanfil, tadalafil, and vardenafil should avoid consuming grapefruit juice with the drugs.
- Alprostadil is a naturally occurring prostaglandin E1 present in male seminal vesicles and cavernous tissues.
- Prostaglandin E1 mediates the relaxation of penile smooth muscle.
- Oral absorption of alprostadil is poor; therefore the drug is formulated for intraurethral insertion and intracavernosal injection.
- Both dosage forms may produce prolonged erection (lasting >4 hours).

Review Questions

1. Benign prostatic hyperplasia is a condition that is cancerous.
   a. True
   b. False
2. The first symptom(s) of an enlarged prostate gland is(are) _____.
   a. A weak or slow urine stream
   b. A delayed start in the flow of urine
   c. Straining to urinate
   d. All of the above
3. Class(es) of drugs administered to manage the symptoms of benign prostatic hyperplasia are _____.
   a. Alpha blockers and beta blockers
   b. α-Reductase inhibitors and beta blockers
   c. Alpha blockers and α-reductase inhibitors
   d. All of the above
4. Which warning label is NOT typically placed on prescription vials for avanafil, tadalafil, and vardenafil?
   a. Avoid grapefruit juice
   b. Avoid nitrates
   c. Report sudden hearing loss or vision disturbances
   d. Report signs of bleeding
5. The generic name for Flomax is _____.
   a. doxazosin
   b. tamsulosin
   c. alfuzosin
   d. terazosin

6. Which of the following is NOT an adverse effect of dutasteride and finasteride?
   a. Decreased desire for sex
   b. Erectile dysfunction
   c. Increased desire for sex
   d. Reduced semen
7. Which of the following drugs is not used for erectile dysfunction?
   a. sildenafil
   b. penadafil
   c. tadalafil
   d. vardenafil
8. Higher than normal levels of PSA may be a sign of _____.
   a. BPH
   b. Infection and inflammation
   c. Prostate cancer
   d. All of the above
9. Finasteride and dutasteride work by reduce testosterone levels.
   a. True
   b. False
10. _____ are currently marketed for the treatment of erectile dysfunction.
    a. Phosphodiesterase inhibitors
    b. Prostaglandin E analogues
    c. Testosterone therapy
    d. All of the above

Bibliography

Agency for Health Research and Quality: Treating Localized Prostate Cancer: A review of the research for adults, 2016. (Pub. No. 15(16)-EHC004-A, pp. 1-16): AHRQ.

FDA: Drugs@FDA: FDA Approved Drug Products, nd. September 12, 2018, from http://www.accessdata.fda.gov/scripts/cder/daf/.

Health Canada: Drug Product Database, 2017. Retrieved September 12, 2018, from https://health-products.canada.ca/dpd-bdpp/index-eng.jsp.

Kapoor A: Benign prost hyper (BPH) management in the primary care setting, *Can J Urol* 19(Suppl 1):10–17, 2012. www.canjurol.com.

Knapp-Dlugosz C: OTC advisor: Popular herbal and dietary supplements, Washington, DC, 2010, American Pharmacists Association.

National Cancer Institute: Understanding Prostate Changes: A Health Guide for Men (NIH Publication No. 11-4303 ed.), 2011. U.S. Department of Health and Human Services, National Institutes of Health. Retrieved from http://www.cancer.gov/cancertopics/screening/understanding-prostate-changes/prostate_booklet.pdf.

National Center for Complementary and Integrative Health: Yohimbe (NCCIH Publication No. D356), 2016. Bethesda: U.S. Department of Health & Human Services, National Institutes of Health. https://nccih.nih.gov/health/herbsataglance.htm.

National Center for Complementary and Integrative Health: Saw Palmetto (NCCIH Publication No. D275), 2016. Bethesda: U.S. Department of Health & Human Services, National Institutes of Health. https://nccih.nih.gov/health/herbsataglance.htm.

National Kidney and Urologic Diseases Information Clearinghouse: Prostatitis: Inflammation of the Prostate (NIH Publication No. 14–4553 ed.), 2014. Bethesda: National Institute of Diabetes and Digestive and Kidney Diseases.

National Kidney and Urologic Diseases Information Clearinghouse: Prostate Enlargement: Benign Prostatic Hyperplasia (NIH Publication No. 14–3012), 2014. Bethesda: The National Institute of Diabetes and Digestive and Kidney Diseases.

National Kidney and Urologic Diseases Information Clearinghouse: Erectile Dysfunction (NIH Publication No. 14–3923), 2015. Bethesda: National Institute of Diabetes and Digestive and Kidney Diseases. https://www.niddk.nih.gov/-/media/Files/Urologic-Diseases/Erectile_Dysfunction_Section_508.

Page C, Curtis M, Sutter M, et al: *Integrated pharmacology*, Philadelphia, 2005, Mosby, pp 495–500.

U.S. Food and Drug Administration: Questions and answers about Viagra, Levitra, Cialis, and Revatio: Possible sudden hearing loss, 2013 http://www.fda.gov/Drugs/DrugSafety/PostmarketDrugSafetyInformationforPatientsandProviders/ucm106525.htm.

USP Center for Advancement of Patient Safety: Use caution–avoid confusion (USP Quality Review No. 79), Rockville, MD, 2004, USP Center for Advancement of Patient Safety.

Drugs Affecting the Immune System

The immune system, along with the nervous and endocrine systems, maintains the relative constancy of the body's internal environment. The immune system is made up of antibodies, proteins (immunoglobulins), on the surface of B cells that mount an immune response and fight disease by recognizing and attacking antigens (foreign or abnormal substances). The immune system is continually patrolling the body for harmful or internal enemies. Our own cells have unique cell markers (antigens) that identify our cells as self. Foreign cells or particles have nonself molecules that serve as recognition markers for our immune system. Autoimmune disorders such as diabetes type 1 are a result of a hyperactive immune response. The body destroys beta cells in the pancreas that the body perceives as harmful invaders.

Cells that trigger immune responses are epithelial barrier cells, phagocytic cells (neutrophils, macrophages), natural killer (NK) cells and cytokines, chemicals released from cells to (e.g., interleukins, leukotrienes, and interferons) are involved in innate immunity. Adaptive immunity involves mechanisms that recognize specific threatening agents and then adapts, or responds, by targeting their activity only against these agents. Lymphocytes (T-cells and B-cells) are the primary leukocytes (white blood cells) involved in adaptive immunity. The densest populations of lymphocytes occur in the bone marrow, thymus gland, lymph nodes, and spleen. Antibodies are proteins called immunoglobulins (Ig). There are five classes of antibodies, identified by letter names as immunoglobulins M, G, A, E, and D. The function of antibody molecules is to produce antibody-mediated immunity. They fight disease first by recognizing substances that are foreign or abnormal.

In Unit X, the treatment of bacterial infections, viral infections, common types of cancers as well as vaccines, immunomodulators, and immunosuppressants are covered. A brief description of each disorder is provided, followed by a description of the drugs and antivirals indicated for treatment, including mechanisms of action, adverse reactions, strength(s), and dosage forms.

29

Treatment of Bacterial Infection

LEARNING OBJECTIVES

1 Learn the terminology associated with treatments for infection.
2 Compare bacteriostatic with bactericidal.
3 Describe the morphology of bacterial cells.
4 Explain microbial resistance and list several reasons for its development.
5 List and categorize antiinfective agents.

6 Describe the mechanism of action for antiinfective agents.
7 List common beginnings and endings for antiinfective agents.
8 Identify significant drug look-alike and sound-alike issues.
9 Identify warning labels and precautionary messages associated with antiinfective agents.

KEY TERMS

Antibiotic A substance produced by or derived from a microorganism that is capable of destroying or inhibiting the growth of another microorganism (e.g., penicillin mold).
Antimicrobial A substance capable of destroying or inhibiting the growth of a microorganism.
Bactericidal Able to destroy bacteria.

Bacteriostatic Able to inhibit bacterial proliferation; host defense mechanisms destroy the bacteria.
Broad-spectrum antibiotic Antimicrobial that is capable of destroying a wide range of bacteria.
Microbial resistance Ability of bacteria to overcome the bactericidal or bacteriostatic effects of an antiinfective. Resistance traits are encoded on bacterial genes and can be transferred to other bacteria.

Overview

Although chronic noninfectious disease is a leading cause of disability and death in developed and industrialized countries, infectious disease is still one of the leading causes of morbidity and mortality globally. In developing countries, infectious diarrhea is a major cause of infant mortality. New infections of malaria and tuberculosis continue to grow. Poverty, malnutrition, the lack of clean water, poor sanitation, and inadequate housing increase the risk for infectious disease and decrease the likelihood for adequate treatment.

Antimicrobial agents, also called antibiotics or antiinfectives, play a key role in improving the survival of individuals with bacterial infections but do not treat viral infections. Technically, an *antibiotic* is a naturally occurring substance that is produced by or derived from a microorganism and is able to destroy or inhibit the growth of another microorganism. Bacteria that cause infection may be sensitive to the effects of one antiinfective but not another; therefore a culture and sensitivity test may also be performed. A small disk with antibiotic is placed in a culture from the infected patient and incubated in a Petri dish. The larger the zone of inhibition (area of no bacterial growth) around the disk, the more effective the antibiotic will be in treating the bacterial infection. Effective treatment of bacterial infections is dependent on host factors, bacterial factors, and drug factors (Fig. 29.1). A drug factor that can influence how quickly a patient begins to "feel better" after starting pharmacotherapy is whether the antiinfective is bactericidal

or bacteriostatic. *Bactericidal* agents (e.g., penicillins) are able to destroy rapidly proliferating bacteria. Patients may begin to "feel better" within the first 24 hours. *Bacteriostatic* agents (e.g., tetracyclines) slow the growth of bacteria enough for the host's (our body's) defense mechanism to destroy the invading bacteria. It may take up to 3 days before patient start to "feel better."

Mechanisms of Antimicrobial Action

Antiinfective agents work by a variety of mechanisms of action such as (1) inhibiting bacterial wall synthesis, (2) inhibiting cell wall function, (3) inhibiting protein synthesis, (4) inhibiting bacterial deoxyribonucleic acid (DNA) or ribonucleic acid (RNA), and (5) inhibiting folic acid. Fortunately, the anatomy of bacteria differs enough from humans that it is possible to destroy some bacteria without harming host cells.

Inhibition of Bacterial Cell Wall Synthesis

Many bacteria have a cell wall that is the target of some antibacterial agents. Because human cells lack cell walls, antibacterial agents that target the cell wall harm the bacteria without damaging the human host. Penicillins, cephalosporins, carbapenems, and monobactams are β-lactam antibiotics that inhibit cell wall synthesis (Fig. 29.2). The β-lactam ring is highlighted in pink. The β-lactam ring can be broken by some bacteria, which inactivates the antibiotics effects.

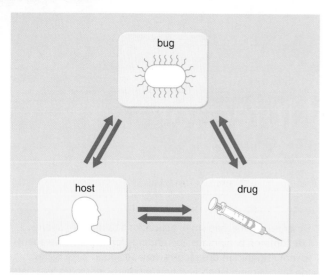

• **Fig. 29.1** Factors that influence successful antimicrobial therapy. (From Page C, Curtis M, Sutter M, et al: *Integrated pharmacology*, ed 3, Philadelphia, 2006, Mosby.)

Glycopeptides also target the bacterial cell wall. Vancomycin is the only glycopeptide antibiotic available in the United States and Canada.

Inhibition of Bacterial Cell Wall Function

Antibiotics that inhibit the function of the bacterial cell wall work by binding to bacterial membranes, where the antibiotic produces a detergent-like action that increases cell membrane permeability. This causes essential cell contents to leak out of the cell and destroys the bacteria. Polymyxin B is an example of an antibiotic that interferes with cell wall function.

Inhibition of Protein Synthesis

Aminoglycosides, macrolides, tetracyclines, amphenicols, and oxazolidinone are classes of antibacterial agents that inhibit the formation of the proteins bacteria need to replicate. Specifically, they act to disrupt ribonucleic acid (RNA) function in the bacterial replication process (Fig. 29.3).

Inhibition of Bacterial Deoxyribonucleic Acid and Ribonucleic Acid Synthesis

Genetic code is stored in DNA. In the replication process, a strand of RNA forms along a strand of DNA. RNA regulates specific cell functions, such as editing strands of code. Without the ability to transfer the genetic code for the synthesis of bacteria cell constituents, bacteria are unable to replicate and spread. Fluoroquinolones and nitroimidazoles are classes of antibiotics capable of inhibiting DNA synthesis. Fluoroquinolones (e.g., ciprofloxacin) and nitroimidazoles (e.g., metronidazole) are predominantly bactericidal. Rifampin inhibits bacterial RNA synthesis.

Inhibition of Folic Acid

Folic acid is needed for the bacteria to synthesize DNA because unlike humans, they cannot get it from external sources. Bacteria synthesize folic acid from para-aminobenzoic acid (PABA). Antifolate agents and dihydrofolate reductase inhibitors block

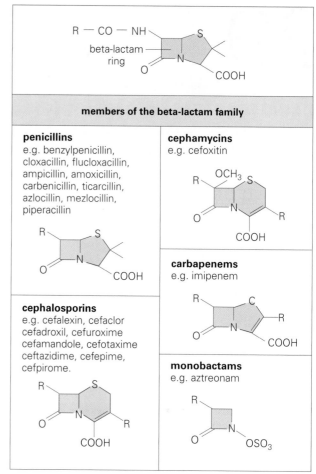

• **Fig. 29.2** Basic structure of β-lactam antibiotics. (From Page C, Curtis M, Sutter M, et al: *Integrated pharmacology*, ed 3, Philadelphia, 2006, Mosby.)

the bacterial synthesis of folic acid. Sulfonamides are antifolate drugs, and trimethoprim is a dihydrofolate reductase inhibitor (Fig. 29.4).

Microbial Resistance

Microbes spread rapidly, mutate frequently, and adapt with relative ease to new environments and hosts. Unfortunately, microbes can learn how to withstand the effects of antibiotics. Superbugs are resistant to currently available antimicrobial agents. Multidrug resistance is a serious problem, and, although previously only a risk for hospitalized patients, multidrug-resistant tuberculosis (MDR-TB), vancomycin-resistant enterococci (VRE), and methicillin-resistant *Staphylococcus aureus* (MRSA) are spreading outside of hospitals. *Microbial resistance* is the ability of bacteria to overcome the bactericidal effects of an antibiotic. Bacteria may overcome the effects of antiinfective agents by secreting an enzyme (e.g., β-lactamase) that inactivates the β-lactam antibiotics like amoxicillin. There are three β-lactamase inhibitors—clavulanic acid (clavulanate), sulbactam, and tazobactam. Macrolide antibiotics are inactivated by bacterial production of enzymes (e.g., erythromycin ribosomal methylase). Bacteria can mutate to modify the site on the ribosome to which the antibiotic normally binds. This is a mechanism for resistance to macrolide antibiotics (e.g., erythromycin). Bacteria that are resistant to macrolides are capable of lowering the concentration of

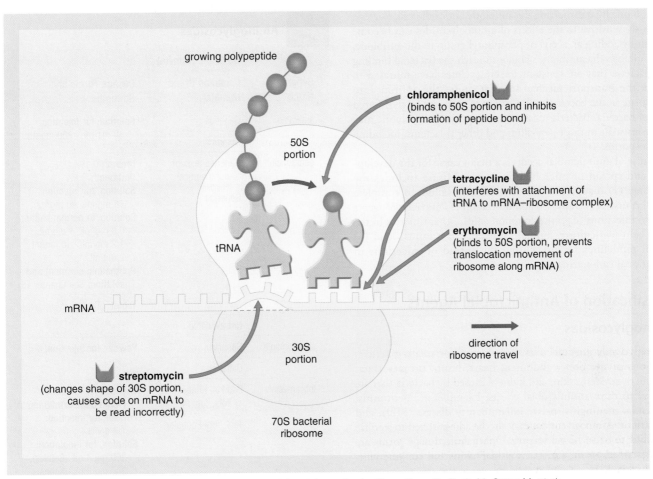

• **Fig. 29.3** Antibiotics that inhibit bacterial protein synthesis. (From Page C, Curtis M, Sutter M, et al: *Integrated pharmacology*, ed 3, Philadelphia, 2006, Mosby.)

• **Fig. 29.4** The folate biosynthetic pathway. *DHFR,* Dihydrofolate reductase; *DHPS,* dihydropteroate synthase; *PABA,* para-aminobenzoic acid. (From Page C, Curtis M, Sutter M, et al: *Integrated pharmacology,* ed 3, Philadelphia, 2006, Mosby.)

the antibiotic by transporting the antibiotic out of the cell. Bacteria previously sensitive to the effects of aminoglycosides can become resistant by adding an acetyl or phosphoryl group to the antibiotic, which inhibits the antibiotic's ability to reach the bacterial binding site. Bacteria that are resistant to tetracyclines have mutated to change the transport mechanism that causes the antibiotic to accumulate in the bacterial cell. Resistance traits can be transferred to other bacteria. Bacteria resistant to one penicillin antibiotic may also be resistant to most penicillins and other β-lactams, including cephalosporins.

Misuse of antimicrobial agents is a major cause for the development and spread of microbial resistance. Misuse includes the following: (1) inappropriate prescribing; (2) failure to complete the full course of therapy; (3) administration of antibacterial agents for viral infections (e.g., the common cold); (4) antibiotics in the food chain (agriculture, animal husbandry, fish farms); and (5) lack of guidelines for preventing the spread of infections in institutional care settings.

Classification of Antimicrobial Agents

Aminoglycosides

Aminoglycoside antiinfectives are effective for treating serious infections of the bone, abdomen, heart, brain, urinary tract, reproductive system, skin, and kidneys caused by bacteria that are sensitive to their antimicrobial effects. Examples are peritonitis, septicemia, meningitis, pelvic inflammatory disease (PID), and endocarditis. Aminoglycosides may also be administered to sterilize the bowel prior to bowel surgery. Ophthalmic dosage forms are also prescribed for the treatment of blepharitis and conjunctivitis (see Chapter 15).

Mechanism of Action and Pharmacokinetics

Aminoglycosides inhibit bacterial protein synthesis. They enter the bacterial cell via an oxygen-dependent transport system, which explains why they are effective against aerobic bacteria and not anaerobic bacteria. They bind to a site on the bacterial ribosome that causes the genetic code carried by messenger RNA (mRNA) to be read incorrectly.

Aminoglycosides are not absorbed systemically when administered by mouth. The only aminoglycoside that is administered orally (neomycin) is used to reduce the bacteria in the bowel prior to colorectal surgery. Other nonparenteral use is topical application for skin, eye, and ear infections. Aminoglycosides for topical use are commonly marketed in combination products that contain additional antiinfectives, local anesthetics, and/or antiinflammatories, such as Lanobiotic and Viaderm KC.

Adverse Reactions

Aminoglycoside may cause hearing loss (ototoxicity) and kidney damage (nephrotoxicity). These effects limit their use to the treatment of serious infections. There is little risk for this side effect when it is applied topically.

Cephalosporins

Cephalosporins have a β-lactam ring structure (Fig. 29.2). Like penicillins, the different side chains added to the basic β-lactam ring structure can affect the antimicrobial spectrum of activity. They are classified as first-, second-, third-, and fourth-generation cephalosporins. First-generation cephalosporins are most effective

Aminoglycosides

Generic Name	US Brand Name(s) Canadian Brand Name(s)	Dosage Forms and Strengths
amikacin[a]	Generics	**Solution, for injection:** 50 mg/mL,[b] 250 mg/mL
	Generics	
gentamicin[a]	Generics (except ophthalmics)	**Cream**[b]: 0.1% **Ointment**[b]: 0.1% **Solution, for injection:** 10 mg/mL, 40 mg/mL
	Generics	**Solution, in normal saline:** 0.8 mg/mL, 1 mg/mL, 1.2 mg/mL, 1.6 mg/mL, 2 mg/mL[b] **Ophthalmic ointment and solution:** See Chapter 15
neomycin[a]	Generics	**Tablet:** 500 mg
	Not available	
streptomycin[a]	Generics	**Powder, for injection:** 1 g/vial
	Generics	
tobramycin[a]	Bethkis, Kitabis Pak, Tobi, Tobi Podhaler	**Capsule, for inhalation (Tobi Podhaler):** 28 mg **Powder, for injection:** 1.2 g/vial
	Tobi, Tobi Podhaler	**Solution, for inhalation:** 300 mg/4 mL (Bethkis),[b] 300 mg/5 mL (Kitabis Pak, Tobi) **Solution, for injection:** 10 mg/mL, 40 mg/mL **Solution, for injection in NS**[b]: 0.8 mg/mL, 1.2 mg/mL, 1.6 mg/mL **Ophthalmic ointment and solution:** See Chapter 15

[a]Generic available.
[b]Available in the United States only.

against staphylococcal infections and streptococcal infections of the skin and soft tissue caused by gram-positive aerobic (require oxygen) bacteria. Gram's Stain is a process used to identifying types of bacteria. A crystal violet stain is applied to a sample taken from the site of the infection. When the stain is washed out, gram-positive bacteria retain a dark purple color. Gram-negative bacteria retain a pink color. Second-generation cephalosporins are effective for treating upper respiratory infections (URIs) such as *Haemophilus influenzae* caused by gram-positive and gram-negative bacteria. Third-generation cephalosporins are used to treat bacterial meningitis, gonorrhea, intraabdominal infections (e.g., peritonitis), and bone and joint infections caused by gram-negative anaerobic bacteria. The fourth-generation cephalosporin cefepime is administered to treat pneumonia (community-acquired and nosocomial) and urinary tract infections (UTIs).

⏺ TECH ALERT!

A common beginning for cephalosporin drugs is *ceph-* or *cef-*.

⏺ TECH ALERT!

The following drugs have look-alike and sound-alike issues:
ceFAZolin and cefTRIAXone

Mechanism of Action

Cephalosporins inhibit the third and final stage of bacterial cell wall synthesis by binding to specific penicillin-binding proteins (PBPs) located inside the bacterial cell wall. Because PBPs vary among different bacterial species, cephalosporin spectrum of activity is dependent on the drug's ability to bind to a specified bacterial PBP.

Pharmacokinetics

Cephalosporins are formulated for oral, intramuscular, and intravenous use. Cefixime is the only third-generation cephalosporin that is administered orally. In contrast, all but two second-generation cephalosporins (cefotetan, cefoxitin) are available for oral use. First-generation cephalosporins do not penetrate the cerebrospinal fluid (CSF) in adequate concentration to treat meningitis, whereas most third-generation agents reach a high-enough level. The fourth-generation agent has a greater ability to penetrate the bacterial cell wall of gram-negative bacteria than third-generation agents and is more resistant to destruction by β-lactamases.

Adverse Reactions

Adverse reactions produced by cephalosporins include diarrhea, headache, dizziness, nausea, vomiting, gas, abdominal pain, dry mouth, and heartburn.

Cephalosporins

Generic Name	US Brand Name(s) Canadian Brand Name(s)	Dosage Forms and Strengths
First-Generation Cephalosporins		
cefazolin[a]	Kefzol	**Powder, for injection:** 0.5 g, 1 g, 10 g, 100 g[c]
	Generics	
cefadroxil[a]	Generics	**Capsule:** 500 mg
		Powder, for oral suspension[b]**:** 250 mg/5 mL, 500 mg/5 mL
	Generics	**Tablet**[b]**:** 1 g
cephalexin[a]	Keflex	**Capsule:** 250 mg, 333 mg[b], 500 mg, 750 mg[b]
		Powder, for oral suspension: 125 mg/5 mL, 250 mg/5 mL
	Generics	**Tablet:** 250 mg, 500 mg
Second-Generation Cephalosporins		
cefaclor[a]	Generics	**Capsule:** 250 mg, 500 mg
		Powder for oral suspension: 125 mg/5 mL, 187 mg/5 mL,[b]
	Not available	250 mg/5 mL, 375 mg/5 mL
		Tablet, extended release: 375 mg, 500 mg
cefotetan[a]	Cefotan	**Powder for injection:** 1 g/vial, 2 g/vial, 10 g/vial
	Not available	
cefoxitin[a]	Mefoxin	**Solution, for injection**[b]**:** 20 mg/mL, 40 mg/mL
		Powder for injection: 1 g/vial, 2 g/vial, 10 g/vial
	Generics	
cefuroxime[a]	Zinacef	**Powder for injection:** 750 mg, 1.5 g, 7.5 g/vial
		Powder for oral suspension[c]**:** 125 mg/5 mL
	Ceftin	**Solution, for injection**[b]**:** 1.5 g/20 mL, 1.5 g/100 mL
		Tablet: 125 mg,[b] 250 mg, 500 mg
Third-Generation Cephalosporins		
cefotaxime	Generics	**Powder for injection:** 500 mg/ vial[b], 1 g/vial, 2 g/vial, 10 g/vial[b]
	Generics	
ceftazidime[a]	Fortaz, Tazicef	**Powder, for injection:** 500 mg/vial[b], 1 g/vial, 2 g/vial, 3 g/vial,[c] 6 g/vial
	Generic	
ceftriaxone[a]	Generics	**Powder for injection:** 250 mg, 500 mg,[b] 1 g, 2 g, 10 g
		Solution, for injection[b]**:** 20 mg/mL, 40 mg/mL
	Generics	

Continued

Cephalosporins—cont'd

Generic Name	US Brand Name(s) / Canadian Brand Name(s)	Dosage Forms and Strengths
cefixime[a]	Suprax	**Capsule**[b]: 400 mg
	Suprax	**Powder, for oral suspension:** 100 mg/5 mL, 200 mg/5 mL[b]
		Tablet: 400 mg
		Tablet, Chewable[b]: 100 mg, 150 mg, 200 mg
cefpodoxime[a]	Generics	**Powder, for oral suspension:** 50 mg/5 mL, 100 mg/5 mL
	Not Available for human use	**Tablet:** 100 mg, 200 mg
Fourth-Generation Cephalosporin		
cefepime[a]	Maxipime	**Powder, for injection:** 500 mg/vial,[b] 1 g/vial, 2 g/vial
	Generics	

[a]Generic available.
[b]Available in the United States only.
[c]Available in Canada only.

Fluoroquinolones

Fluoroquinolones are indicated for the treatment of UTIs, sinusitis, sexually transmitted infections, bacterial conjunctivitis (see Chapter 15), infectious diarrhea, anthrax, and numerous other infections.

> ### ❗ TECH ALERT!
> A common ending of fluoroquinolone is -floxacin.

> ### ❗ TECH ALERT!
> The following drugs have look-alike and sound-alike issues:
> Noroxin and Neurontin

Mechanism of Action and Pharmacokinetics

Fluoroquinolones inhibit the enzyme DNA gyrase that is responsible for blocking one of the processes of DNA replication. This results in the inhibition of bacterial DNA synthesis.

Fluoroquinolones are formulated for oral, ophthalmic, and parenteral use. Oral absorption is good. The half-life ($t^{1/2}$) of the newer agents such as moxifloxacin is long, permitting once-daily dosing, whereas ciprofloxacin ($t^{1/2} \cong 4$ hours) is dosed every 12 hours.

Adverse Reactions and Precautions

Common adverse reactions are diarrhea, crystalluria, photosensitivity, dizziness, drowsiness, headache, nausea, and stomach upset. Cartilage deformities may occur in children and developing fetuses, so quinolones are contraindicated in children and pregnant women. Quinolones can also cause arrhythmias by prolongation of the QT interval, musculoskeletal pain, and, rarely, peripheral neuropathy.

Macrolides

Azithromycin, clarithromycin, and erythromycin are macrolide antibiotics that are primarily used for the treatment of URIs. Other important uses are the treatment of peptic ulcer disease (PUD), eye infections, and acne. Erythromycin, the prototype for the macrolides, is used for the prevention of neonatal eye infections and acne, in addition to treatment of upper respiratory infections. Clarithromycin is one of the ingredients in multidrug treatment regimens for PUD caused by the bacterium *Helicobacter pylori* (see Chapter 21).

Mechanism of Action

Macrolides inhibit bacterial protein synthesis by binding to the 50S ribosomal subunit and blocking the translocation movement along mRNA.

Pharmacokinetics

Macrolides are formulated for oral, parenteral, and ophthalmic use. Erythromycin base is formulated for immediate release and delayed release. Delayed-release tablets have a lower incidence of gastrointestinal (GI) side effects than do immediate-release tablets.

The expiration date of powder for the oral suspension of erythromycin, clarithromycin, and azithromycin is shortened once the drug is reconstituted. Refrigeration is recommended for oral suspensions of erythromycin; storage at room temperature is recommended for clarithromycin and azithromycin.

Adverse Reactions

GI upset is common with the use of macrolides. It occurs in up to 21% of those who take erythromycin. The incidence of GI upset is less with clarithromycin (10%) and azithromycin (5%). Erythromycin and clarithromycin can cause arrhythmias by prolongation of the QT interval. Other adverse reactions include headache and tinnitus. Macrolides may decrease the effectiveness of oral contraceptives.

Oxazolidinones

Linezolid is a newer antimicrobial agent indicated for the treatment of gram-positive bacterial pneumonia and skin structure infections. Its use is limited because of adverse side effects and to limit the development of bacterial resistance.

Fluoroquinolones

Generic Name	US Brand Name(s) / Canadian Brand Name(s)	Dosage Forms and Strengths
ciprofloxacin[a]	Cetraxal, Ciloxan, Cipro, Cipro XR Ciloxan, Cipro, Cipro XL, Otixal	**Powder, for oral suspension (Cipro):** 250 mg/5 mL,[b] 500 mg/5 mL **Tablet (Cipro):** 100 mg,[b] 250 mg, 500 mg, 750 mg **Tablet, extended-release (Cipro XL, Cipro XR):** 500 mg, 1000 mg **Ophthalmic and Otic solution (Ciloxan, Cetraxal, Otixal):** See Chapter 15 **Solution, for injection:** 2 mg/mL,[c] 10 mg/mL[b] **Solution, for injection in 5% dextrose:** 200 mg/100 mL
gatifloxacin[a,b]	Zymar, Zymaxid Zymar	**Ophthalmic solution:** See Chapter 15
gemifloxacin[a]	Factive Not available	**Tablet:** 320 mg
levofloxacin[a]	Generics Levaquin, Quinsair	**Ophthalmic solution:** See Chapter 15 **Solution for injection:** 25 mg/mL[b] **Solution for injection in 5% dextrose:** 5 mg/mL **Solution, oral:** 25 mg/mL[b] **Solution, for inhalation (Quinsair)[c]:** 240 mg/2.4 mL **Tablet:** 250 mg, 500 mg, 750 mg
moxifloxacin[a]	Avelox, Moxeza, Vigamox Avelox, Vigamox	**Ophthalmic solution (Moxeza, Vigamox):** See Chapter 15 **Tablet:** 400 mg **Solution for IV:** 400 mg/250 mL 0.8% NaCl
ofloxacin[a]	Generics (except ophthalmic) Ocuflox	**Ophthalmic and Otic solution (Ocuflox):** See Chapter 15 **Tablet[b]:** 200 mg, 300 mg, 400 mg
norfloxacin[a]	Not Available Generics	**Tablet:** 400 mg

[a]Generic available.
[b]Available in the United States only.
[c]Available in Canada only

Macrolides and Related Antiinfectives

Generic Name	US Brand Name(s) / Canadian Brand Name(s)	Dosage Forms and Strengths
azithromycin[a]	Azasite, Zithromax Zithromax	**Ophthalmic solution (Azasite):** See Chapter 15 **Powder, for injection:** 500 mg/vial **Powder, for oral suspension (Zithromax):** 100 mg/5 mL, 200 mg/5 mL, 1 g (single dose) **Tablet (Zithromax):** 250 mg, 500 mg,[b] 600 mg
clarithromycin[a]	Biaxin, Biaxin XL Biaxin, Biaxin BID, Biaxin XL	**Powder, for suspension:** 125 mg/5 mL, 250 mg/5 mL **Tablet (Biaxin, Biaxin BID):** 250 mg, 500 mg **Tablet, extended-release (Biaxin XL):** 250 mg,[b] 500 mg
erythromycin base[a] (immediate-release)	Ery-gel Generics	**Gel, topical (Ery-gel):** 2% **Ophthalmic ointment:** 0.5% **Tablet (generics):** 250 mg, 500 mg[b] **Solution, topical:** 2% **Swab:** 2%
erythromycin base[a] (delayed-release)	ERYC, PCE ERYC	**Capsule:** 250 mg, 333 mg[c]

Continued

Macrolides and Related Antiinfectives—cont'd

Generic Name	US Brand Name(s) / Canadian Brand Name(s)	Dosage Forms and Strengths
erythromycin stearate[a]	Erythrocin	**Tablet:** 250 mg
	Generic	
erythromycin ethylsuccinate[a]	EES, Eryped	**Granules, for oral suspension:** 200 mg/5 mL, 400 mg/5 mL
	Not available	**Tablet:** 400 mg
erythromycin lactobionate[a]	Erythrocin	**Powder, for injection:** 500 mg, 1 g[c]
	Generic	

[a]Generic available.
[b]Available in the United States only.
[c]Available in Canada only.

Mechanism of Action and Pharmacokinetics

Linezolid inhibits bacterial protein synthesis. Its action on the bacterial ribosome blocks a key step in the translation process, which inhibits bacterial replication. The metabolism of linezolid is not well understood. Linezolid has no effect on cytochrome P-450 (CYP450) isoenzymes so has fewer drug interactions involving drug metabolism.

Adverse Reactions

The most common side effects of linezolid are skin rash, itching, change in taste, headache, mild diarrhea, dizziness, mild stomach upset, nausea, vomiting, and temporary tongue discoloration.

Oxazolidinones

Generic Name	US Brand Name(s) / Canadian Brand Name(s)	Dosage Forms and Strengths
linezolid[a]	Zyvox	**Powder, for suspension:** 100 mg/5 mL
	Zyvoxam	**Solution, for injection:** 2 mg/mL
		Tablet: 600 mg

[a]Generic available.

Penicillins and Carbapenems

Penicillin is one of the first antibiotics discovered. It is a naturally occurring substance originally produced by the mold *Penicillium chrysogenum* (also known as *Penicillium notatum*) and can grow on stale bread and fruit. Oral penicillins are used to treat many infections, including URIs, otitis media, skin infections, strep throat, and to prevent recurrent rheumatic fever. Penicillins may be administered before dental and other medical procedures to prevent bacterial endocarditis in individuals with prosthetic heart valves. Parenteral penicillins are used for the treatment of numerous infections, including bone and joint infections, diabetic foot ulcers, infectious arthritis, sexually transmitted infections, meningitis, and septicemia.

> **⊘ TECH ALERT!**
> A common ending of the penicillin family of drugs is -*cillin*.

> **⊘ TECH ALERT!**
> Persons who are allergic to penicillin may also be allergic to cephalosporins.

> **⊘ TECH ALERT!**
> The following drugs have look-alike and sound-alike issues:
> penicillin and penicillAMINE;
> Augmentin and Augmentin XR

Mechanism of Action

Penicillins are β-lactam antibiotics; they inhibit the synthesis of the cell wall of sensitive microbes. Side chains on this structure alter the antibacterial and pharmacologic properties of the basic penicillin molecule. The side chains can extend the antimicrobial spectrum. For example, amoxicillin and ticarcillin are effective against more types of bacteria than is penicillin. Antistaphylococcal penicillins are penicillinase resistant and are not inactivated by penicillinase (staphylococcal β-lactamase), a substance produced by the bacteria that destroys the antibiotic's β-lactam ring.

Carbapenems have a β-lactam ring fused with a penem ring. Carbapenems inhibit the third step in bacterial cell wall synthesis. Their spectrum of activity is broad, and they resist inactivation by microbial enzymes (e.g., β-lactamase).

Pharmacokinetics

Many penicillins lack stability in gastric acids, which is why most are administered intramuscularly or must be taken on an empty stomach. The exception is penicillin VK, which is relatively acid stable.

Procaine penicillin G and benzathine penicillin G are formulated to delay absorption and achieve prolonged blood levels. Levels of benzathine penicillin G can be detected in the blood up to 1 month after an intramuscular injection of the drug is given.

Penicillins that are formulated as powders for reconstitution have shortened expiration dates once mixed with water. Expiration dates range from 10 to 14 days, depending on the drug. Most suspensions should be refrigerated after they are reconstituted.

⚠ TECH ALERT!

The quantity of clavulanic acid varies widely between products. It is important to read the stock bottle label carefully before making product substitutions.

Adverse Reactions

GI side effects such as diarrhea, loss of appetite, nausea, vomiting, sore mouth, stomach gas, and heartburn are the most common adverse reactions to penicillins. Other adverse effects include superinfection and hypersensitivity and reactions. Penicillins may decrease the effectiveness of oral contraceptives.

Sulfonamides

Sulfonamides are the oldest antimicrobial agents. They were developed in the 1930s, but their use did not spread until the 1940s in World War II. Sulfonamides are commonly called sulfa

Penicillins

Generic Name	US Brand Name(s) / Canadian Brand Name(s)	Dosage Forms and Strengths
Penicillin		
penicillin G potassium[a]	Pfizerpen	**Powder, for injection:** 1 million units, 5 million units, 20 million units
	Not available for human use	
phenoxymethyl penicillin potassium[a] (penicillin VK)	Generics	**Powder for oral suspension**[b]:125 mg/5 mL, 250 mg/5 mL **Tablets:** 250 mg, 300 mg,[c] 500 mg
	Generics	
benzathine penicillin G[a]	Bicillin L-A	**Suspension, for IM injection:** 600,000 units/mL
	Bicillin L-A	
benzylpenicillin (penicillin G sodium)	Generics	**Powder, for injection:** 1,000,000 units/vial,[c] 5,000,000 units/vial, 10,000,000 units/vial[c]
	Generics	
Aminopenicillins: Extended Spectrum		
amoxicillin[a]	Amoxil, Larotid, Moxatag	**Capsule:** 250 mg, 500 mg **Powder for oral suspension:** 50 mg/mL,[b] 125 mg/5 mL, 200 mg/5 mL,[b] 250 mg/5 mL, 400 mg/5 mL[b] **Tablet**[b]**:** 500 mg, 875 mg **Tablet, chewable**[b]**:** 125 mg, 200 mg, 250 mg, 400 mg[b] **Tablet, extended-release (Moxatag):** 775 mg[b]
	Generics	
ampicillin[a]	Generics	**Capsule:** 250 mg, 500 mg **Powder, for injection:** 125 mg,[b] 250 mg, 500 mg, 1 g, 2 g, 10 g[b] **Powder, for oral suspension**[b]**:** 125 mg/5 mL, 250 mg/5 mL
	Generics	
Antistaphylococcal Penicillins: Penicillinase Resistant		
cloxacillin[a]	Not available	**Capsule:** 250 mg, 500 mg **Powder, for oral suspension:** 125 mg/5 mL **Powder, for injection:** 0.5 g, 1 g, 2 g, 10 g
	Generics	
dicloxacillin[a]	Generics	**Capsule:** 125 mg, 250 mg, 500 mg
	Not available	
nafcillin[a]	Nallpen	**Powder, for injection:** 1 g, 2 g, 10 g **Solution, for injection (Nallpen):** 20 mg/mL
	Not available	
oxacillin[a]	Bactocill	**Powder, for injection:** 1 g, 2 g, 10 g **Solution, for injection (Bactocill):** 20 mg/mL, 40 mg/mL
	Not available	
Antipseudomonal Penicillins		
piperacillin[a]	Generic	**Powder for injection:** 2 g,[b] 3 g, 4 g,[b] 40 g[b]
	Generic	

Continued

Penicillins—cont'd

Generic Name	US Brand Name(s) Canadian Brand Name(s)	Dosage Forms and Strengths
Penicillin Combinations		
amoxicillin + clavulanic acid[a]	Augmentin, Augmentin XR Clavulin	**Powder for oral suspension:** amoxicillin 125 mg + clavulanic acid 31.25 mg/5 mL amoxicillin 200 mg + clavulanic acid 28.5 mg/5 mL amoxicillin 250 mg + clavulanic acid 62.5 mg/5 mL amoxicillin 400 mg + clavulanic acid 57 mg/5 mL **Tablet:** amoxicillin 250 mg + clavulanic acid 125 mg amoxicillin 500 mg + clavulanic acid 125 mg amoxicillin 875 mg + clavulanic acid 125 mg **Tablet, chewable (Augmentin):** amoxicillin 200 mg + clavulanic acid 28.5 mg amoxicillin 400 mg + clavulanic acid 57 mg **Tablet, extended-release (Augmentin XR)[b]:** amoxicillin 1000 mg + clavulanic acid 62.5 mg
ampicillin + sulbactam[a]	Unasyn Not available	**Powder, for injection:** ampicillin 1 g + sulbactam 0.5 g ampicillin 2 g + sulbactam 1 g ampicillin 10 g + sulbactam 5 g
piperacillin + tazobactam	Zosyn Tazocin	**Powder, for injection:** piperacillin 2 g + tazobactam 0.25 g/vial piperacillin 3 g + tazobactam 0.375 g/vial piperacillin 4 g + tazobactam 0.5 g/vial piperacillin 12 g + tazobactam 1.5 g[c] piperacillin 36 g + tazobactam 4.5 g/vial

[a]Generic available.
[b]Available in the United States only.
[c]Available in Canada only.

Carbapenems

Generic Name	US Brand Name(s) Canadian Brand Name(s)	Dosage Forms and Strengths
ertapenem[ab]	Invanz Invanz	**Powder, for injection:** 1 g per vial
imipenem + cilastatin[a]	Primaxin Primaxin	**Powder, for injection:** imipenem 250 mg + cilastatin 250 mg/vial imipenem 500 mg + cilastatin 500 mg/vial
meropenem[a]	Merrem Merrem	**Powder, for injection:** 500 mg, 1 g
meropenem + vabobactam	Vabomere Not Available	Powder, for injection: meropenem 1 g + vabobactam 1 g

[a]Generic available.
[ab]Generic available in the United States.

drugs because the generic name of all agents begins with *sulf-*. Sulfonamides and trimethoprim are used in the treatment of various upper respiratory, urinary tract, and skin infections. They are also indicated for the treatment of AIDS-related pneumonia (caused by *Pneumocystis jiroveci*).

> **⊘ TECH ALERT!**
> A common beginning for sulfonamides *sulf-*.

> **⊘ TECH ALERT!**
> The following drugs have look-alike and sound-alike issues:
> sulfADIAZINE, sulfiSOXAZOLE, and sulfaSALAzine;
> sulfamethoxazole + trimethoprim single-strength and sulfamethoxazole + trimethoprim double-strength;

Mechanism of Action and Pharmacokinetics

Sulfonamides and trimethoprim are antifolate drugs. They interfere with the microbial synthesis of folic acid at separate steps in the biosynthetic pathway that ultimately leads to bacterial DNA synthesis (see Fig. 29.4). Food may slightly decrease the absorption of sulfonamides; however, the drug may be taken with small amounts of food to reduce GI upset.

⚠ TECH ALERT!

The warning label "Take with Lots of Water" is put on prescription vials for sulfonamides. This reduces the risk of kidney damage caused by crystalluria.

Adverse Reactions

Common adverse reactions are nausea, vomiting, abdominal pain, headache, drowsiness, dizziness, diarrhea, and photosensitivity. Sulfonamides may promote the formation of crystals in the urine (crystalluria), especially if taken with acidic foods or beverages.

Tetracyclines

Tetracylines are *broad-spectrum antibiotic* (antibacterial) agents. They may be bactericidal or bacteriostatic. They are used for the treatment of acne, sexually transmitted infections such as chlamydia, Lyme disease, and Rocky Mountain spotted fever.

⚠ TECH ALERT!

A common ending for the tetracycline family of drugs is *-cycline*.

Mechanism of Action and Pharmacokinetics

Tetracyclines inhibit bacterial protein synthesis. Doxycycline and minocycline are more stable in the acidic stomach contents than tetracycline. They also have a longer duration of action. They are given once or twice daily compared with tetracycline, which is given four times daily. Tetracycline interacts with dairy products, calcium, aluminum, and ferrous supplements to form a chelated complex. The complex significantly reduces the absorption of tetracycline and should be avoided.

⚠ TECH ALERT!

Apply the following warning label to prescription vials for tetracycline: "Avoid Antacids and Dairy Products within 2 Hr of Dose."

Adverse Reactions

The tetracylines can cause nausea, vomiting, diarrhea, and photosensitivity. Serious but less common side effects include hepatotoxicity, pseudomembranous colitis, and kidney disease. Outdated tetracycline becomes toxic. Patients should be advised to discard old medicines. Tetracyclines may decrease the effectiveness of oral contraceptives.

⚠ TECH ALERT!

Apply the following warning label to prescription vials for tetracycline: "Avoid Tanning and Prolonged Exposure to Sunlight."

⚠ TECH ALERT!

Tetracyclines are contraindicated in pregnancy and small children because they can weaken fetal bone, retard bone growth, weaken tooth enamel, and stain teeth.

Miscellaneous Antibacterials

Isoniazid is used for the treatment of tuberculosis. It inhibits the synthesis of mycolic acid, an important constituent of the highly lipid cell wall of mycobacteria. Isoniazid may cause liver disease and nerve damage. Concurrent administration of vitamin B_6 is recommended to prevent neurotoxicity.

Metronidazole is an amebicide. It destroys the protozoa that cause giardiasis (traveler's diarrhea) and trichomoniasis (a sexually transmitted infection). It is the drug of choice for the treatment of *Clostridium difficile* enteritis, a condition that may cause pseudomembranous colitis. Topical preparations are used for the

Sulfonamides

	Generic Name	US Brand Name(s) / Canadian Brand Name(s)	Dosage Forms and Strengths
Sulfonamides			
	sulfadiazine[a]	Generics	**Tablet:** 500 mg
		Not available	
Combination Sulfonamides			
	sulfamethoxazole + trimethoprim[a] (SMX-TMP; Cotrimox)	Bactrim, Bactrim DS, Septra, Septra DS, Sulfatrim DS	**Solution for injection:** sulfamethoxazole 80 mg/mL + trimethoprim 16 mg/mL
		Septra, Sulfatrim DS	**Tablet:** sulfamethoxazole 100 mg + trimethoprim 20 mg[b] sulfamethoxazole 400 mg + trimethoprim 80 mg sulfamethoxazole 800 mg + trimethoprim 160 mg
			Suspension: sulfamethoxazole 200 mg/5 mL + trimethoprim 40 mg/5 mL

[a]Generic available.
[b]Available in Canada only.

Tetracyclines

	Dosage Forms and Strengths	US Brand Name(s) / Canadian Brand Name(s)	Dosage Forms and Strengths
	demeclocycline[a]	Generics	**Tablet:** 150 mg, 300 mg
		Not available	
	doxycycline anhydrous	Oracea	**Capsule, immediate + delayed release (Oracea):** 40 mg
		Not available	
	doxycycline calcium	Vibramycin	**Powder, for oral suspension:** 25 mg/5 mL, 50 mg/5 mL
		Not available	
	doxycycline hyclate[a]	Acticlate, Atridox, Doryx, Vibramycin	**Capsule:** 20 mg (Periostat),[b] 50 mg,[c] 75 mg (Acticlate), 100 mg
		Atridox, Periostat	**Powder, for injection:** 100 mg/vial, 200 mg/vial **Gingival gel (Atridox):** 10% **Tablet:** 75 mg, 150 mg (Acticlate) **Tablet, delayed release (Doryx):** 50 mg, 75 mg, 120 mg, 100 mg, 150 mg, 200 mg
	doxycycline monohydrate[a]	Monodox	**Capsule (Apprilon):** 40 mg **Tablet:** 50 mg, 75 mg, 100 mg (Monodox)
		Apprilon	
	minocycline[a]	Arestin, Dynacin, Minocin, Minolira, Solodyn, Ximino	**Capsule:** 50 mg, 75 mg,[c] 100 mg **Capsule, extended release (Ximino):** 45 mg, 90 mg, 135 mg **Powder, for injection[c]:** 100 mg/vial **Powder, periodontal-sustained release (Arestin):** 1 mg/4 mg **Tablet:** 50 mg, 75 mg, 100 mg **Tablet, extended-release (Minolira, Solodyn):** 55 mg, 65 mg, 80 mg, 105 mg, 115 mg, 135 mg
		Arestin	
	tetracycline[a]	Achromycin V	**Capsule:** 250 mg, 500 mg[c]
		Generics	
	tigecycline[b]	Tygacil	**Powder, for injection:** 50 mg/vial
		Tygacil	

[a]Generic available.
[b]Available in Canada only.
[c]Available in the United States only.

treatment of acne rosacea. It is formulated for oral, parenteral, vaginal, and topical use. Alcoholic beverages or medicines containing high levels of alcohol may produce nausea, vomiting, stomach pains, headache, and dizziness. The drug may also produce a metallic taste.

Mupirocin is a topically applied antimicrobial used to treat staphylococcal infections of the skin, such as impetigo.

Chloramphenicol is a broad-spectrum antimicrobial agent that inhibits protein synthesis. It is typically prescribed a second line therapy, when other less toxic drugs cannot be used (e.g., for drug allergy). It may be used for the treatment of bacterial meningitis, brain abscess, and Rocky Mountain spotted fever. It is contraindicated in neonates and children.

Clindamycin is an antimicrobial agent used topically for the treatment of acne and vaginosis. Systemic use of clindamycin is associated with the development of *C. difficile*, a bacterium that causes diarrhea and pseudomembranous colitis. Drinking plenty of fluids can lower the risk of the development of this condition.

TECHNICIAN'S CORNER

1. With microbial resistance developing against antibiotics, what steps should be taken by the pharmaceutical and food industries, patients, and health care providers to combat this problem?
2. Can the practice of universal precautions (e.g., handwashing) reduce the incidence of nosocomial infections?

Miscellaneous Antibacterial Agents

Generic Name	US Brand Name(s) / Canadian Brand Name(s)	Dosage Forms and Strengths
dalbavancin	Dalvance Not available	**Powder, for infusion:** 500 mg per vial
oritavancin	Orbactiv Not available	**Powder, for infusion:** 400 mg per vial
isoniazid[a]	Generics Generics	**Solution, for injection:** 100 mg/mL[b] **Syrup, oral:** 50 mg/5 mL **Tablet:** 100 mg, 300 mg
metronidazole[a]	Flagyl, Metrocreme, Metrogel, Metrolotion, Noritate, Nuvessa, Vandazole Flagyl, Metrogel, Nidagel, Noritate	**Capsule (Flagyl):** 375 mg[b], 500 mg[c] **Cream:** 0.75% (Metrocreme), 1% (Noritate) **Cream, vaginal (Flagyl)[c]:** 10% **Gel, topical (Metrogel):** 0.75%, 1% **Gel, vaginal:** 0.75% Metrogel, Nidagel, Vandazole), 1.3% (Nuvessa) **Lotion:** 0.75% (Metrolotion) **Tablet (Flagyl):** 250 mg, 500 mg[b] **Tablet, extended-release:** 750 mg
mupirocin[a]	Centany Bactroban, Bactroban Cream	**Cream:** 2% **Ointment, topical:** 2%
chloramphenicol[a]	Generics Chloromycetin	**Powder, for injection:** 1 g per vial
clindamycin[a]	Cleocin, Cleocin T, Clinda-derm, Clindagel, Clindesse, Clindets, Evoclin Clinda-T, Dalacin C, Dalacin T 1%	**Capsule:** 75 mg,[b] 150 mg, 300 mg **Foam (Evoclin)[b]:** 1% **Swab(Clindets)[b]:** 1% **Solution, for injection:** 150 mg/mL, **Solution, for infusion:** 6 mg/mL,[b] 12 mg/mL, 18 mg/mL **Powder, for oral solution:** 75 mg/5 mL **Topical gel and lotion (Clinda-T, Cleocin T, Clindagel, Clindamax):** 1% **Topical solution (Cleocin T, Dalacin T):** 1% **Vaginal cream (Clindesse, Cleocin, Dalacin):** 2% **Vaginal suppositories (Cleocin)[b]:** 100 mg
telavancin	Vibativ Vibativ	**Powder, for injection:** 250 mg,[b] 750 mg
vancomycin	Firvanq Kit, Vancocin Vancocin	**Capsule:** 125 mg, 250 mg **Powder, for oral solution (Firvanq Kit)[b]:** 25 mg/mL, 50 mg/mL **Powder, for injection:** 500 mg, 750 mg,[b] 1 g, 5 g, 10 g per vial

[a]Generic available.
[b]Available in the United States only.
[c]Available in Canada only.

Summary of Drugs Used for the Treatment of Bacterial Infections

	Generic Name	Brand Name	Usual Dose and Dosing Schedule	Warning Labels
Cephalosporins				
	cefadroxil	Duricef	1 g orally/day given in 1 or 2 daily doses until course of therapy is finished	COMPLETE FULL COURSE OF THERAPY (ALL).
	cephalexin	Keflex	Varies (max, 4 g/day)	TAKE WITH FOOD (CEFADROXIL, DELAYED RELEASE).
	cefaclor	Generics	**Immediate-release:** 250–500 mg orally every 8 h until course of therapy is finished **Extended release:** 375–500 mg every 12 h until course of therapy is finished (max, 1.5 g/day)	REFRIGERATE, SHAKE WELL, AND DISCARD AFTER 14 DAYS (CEFADROXIL, CEPHALEXIN, CEFACLOR ORAL SUSPENSIONS). REFRIGERATE, SHAKE WELL, AND DISCARD AFTER 10 DAYS (CEFUROXIME SUSPENSION). REFRIGERATE OR STORE AT ROOM TEMPERATURE, SHAKE WELL, AND DISCARD AFTER 14 DAYS (CEFIXIME ORAL SUSPENSION).
	cefuroxime	Ceftin	250–500 mg orally every 12 h until course of therapy is finished.	
	cefixime	Suprax	400 mg orally once every 24 h until course of therapy is finished	
Fluoroquinolones				
	ciprofloxacin	Cipro Cipro XR	**Immediate-release:** 500–750 mg orally every 12 h until course of therapy is finished **Extended-release:** 500–1000 mg once daily until course of therapy is finished	COMPLETE FULL COURSE OF THERAPY. TAKE WITH LOTS OF WATER. AVOID PROLONGED EXPOSURE TO SUNLIGHT. MAY CAUSE DIZZINESS OR DROWSINESS. AVOID ANTACIDS AND VITAMINS CONTAINING IRON AND ZINC.
	levofloxacin	Levaquin	250–500 mg every 24 h (max, 750 mg/day) until course of therapy is finished	SHAKE WELL, AND DISCARD AFTER 14 DAYS (CIPRO SUSPENSION).
	moxifloxacin	Avelox	400 mg orally or IV once daily until course of therapy is finished	SWALLOW WHOLE; DON'T CRUSH OR CHEW (EXTENDED-RELEASE). TAKE ON AN EMPTY STOMACH.
	norfloxacin	Noroxin	400 mg orally twice daily until course of therapy is finished	
Macrolides				
	azithromycin	Zithromax	500 mg day 1, followed by 250 mg once daily for 4 days	COMPLETE FULL COURSE OF THERAPY. SHAKE WELL—ALL SUSPENSIONS STORE AT ROOM TEMPERATURE AND DISCARD IN 14 DAYS (CLARITHROMYCIN AND AZITHROMYCIN EXTENDED-RELEASE SUSPENSION).
	clarithromycin	Biaxin, Biaxin XL	**Immediate-release:** 250–500 mg every 12 h up to 1000 mg once daily until course of therapy is finished **Extended-release:** 1000 mg once daily until course of therapy is finished	REFRIGERATE; DISCARD IN 10 DAYS (AZITHROMYCIN SUSPENSION, IMMEDIATE-RELEASE). TAKE ON AN EMPTY STOMACH (AZITHROMYCIN SUSPENSION).
	erythromycin base, delayed-release	ERYC, PCE	250–500 mg every 6–8 h until course of therapy is finished	MAY DECREASE THE EFFECTIVENESS OF ORAL CONTRACEPTIVES.
	erythromycin ethylsuccinate	EES	400–800 mg every 6–8 h until course of therapy is finished (max, 4 g/day)	TAKE WITH FOOD (DELAYED-RELEASE).
Sulfonamides and Sulfonamide Combinations				
	sulfamethoxazole + trimethoprim	Septra, Bactrim	40–160 mg trimethoprim + 200–800 mg sulfamethoxazole every 12 h until course of therapy is finished	COMPLETE FULL COURSE OF THERAPY. TAKE WITH PLENTY OF WATER. AVOID PROLONGED SUNLIGHT. SHAKE WELL (SUSPENSION). STORE AT ROOM TEMPERATURE

Summary of Drugs Used for the Treatment of Bacterial Infections—cont'd

	Generic Name	Brand Name	Usual Dose and Dosing Schedule	Warning Labels
Penicillins				
	ampicillin	Generics	250–1000 mg orally every 6 h until course of therapy is finished	COMPLETE FULL COURSE OF THERAPY. TAKE ON AN EMPTY STOMACH (AMPICILLIN, CLOXACILLIN, DICLOXACILLIN). REFRIGERATE, SHAKE WELL, AND DISCARD AFTER 14 DAYS (SUSPENSION AMPICILLIN, DICLOXACILLIN, PENICILLIN VK). MAY DECREASE EFFECTIVENESS OF ORAL CONTRACEPTIVES. REFRIGERATE, SHAKE WELL, AND DISCARD AFTER 10 DAYS (SUSPENSION, AMOXICILLIN + CLAVULANIC ACID).
	amoxicillin	Amoxil	Varies; 500–875 mg every 12 h or 250–500 mg PO every 8 h until course of therapy is finished	
	dicloxacillin	Generics	125–500 mg orally every 6 h until course of therapy is finished	
	penicillin VK	Generics	125–500 mg orally every 6 h until course of therapy is finished	
	amoxicillin + clavulanic acid	Augmentin	Varies; 250–500 mg every 8 h or 500–875 mg every 12 h until course of therapy is finished	
	penicillin G benzathine	Bicillin L-A	Varies	REFRIGERATE; DO NOT FREEZE.
Tetracyclines				
	doxycycline	Vibramycin, Monodox	Varies; commonly 100 mg bid on day 1 followed by 100 mg daily or 100 mg bid until course of therapy is completed	COMPLETE FULL COURSE OF THERAPY. TAKE WITH LOTS OF WATER. AVOID PROLONGED SUNLIGHT. AVOID ANTACIDS AND VITAMINS CONTAINING IRON AND ZINC. MAY DECREASE EFFECTIVENESS OF ORAL CONTRACEPTIVES. SHAKE WELL (TETRACYCLINE SUSPENSION). TAKE ON AN EMPTY STOMACH (TETRACYCLINE).
	minocycline	Minocin	Varies (max, 350 mg on day 1, then 200 mg/day)	
	tetracycline	Generics	Varies (max, 4 g/day)	
Miscellaneous				
	metronidazole	Metrogel, Metrocreme, Noritate Flagyl	**Acne rosacea:** Apply a thin film once or twice daily. **Bacterial vaginosis:** One applicatorful once daily at bedtime **Other infections:** varies 250–1000 mg 2–3 times daily until course of therapy is completed	COMPLETE FULL COURSE OF THERAPY. TAKE WITH A FULL GLASS OF WATER. AVOID ALCOHOL.
	isoniazid	Generics	**Tuberculosis prophylaxis:** 300 mg orally once daily or 900 mg/day twice weekly with pyridoxine (50 mg once daily or 100 mg twice weekly) for 9 months	COMPLETE FULL COURSE OF THERAPY. AVOID ANTACIDS. AVOID ALCOHOL.
	clindamycin	Cleocin	Varies: Take in 3–4 divided doses daily until course of therapy is completed	COMPLETE FULL COURSE OF THERAPY. TAKE WITH A FULL GLASS OF WATER. SHAKE WELL, STORE AT ROOM TEMPERATURE- SUSPENSION
	mupirocin	Bactroban	Apply tid or bid for intranasal infections.	COMPLETE FULL COURSE OF THERAPY.
	ertapenem	Invanz	Varies: 1 gram IM or IV once daily for up to 14 days	
	dalbavancin	Dalvance	Varies: Administer by IV infusion	
	oritavancin	Orbactiv	Infuse 1200 mg as a single dose over 3 hours	

Key Points

- Chronic noninfectious disease is a leading cause of disability and death in developed, industrialized countries; however, infectious disease is still one the leading causes of morbidity and mortality globally.
- Poverty, malnutrition, the lack of clean water, poor sanitation, and inadequate housing increase the risk for infectious disease and decrease the likelihood for successful treatment.
- Antibiotics have played a key role in improving the survival of those with bacterial infections.
- Microbes can learn how to resist the effects of antibiotics; superbugs are resistant to some currently available antimicrobial agents. Multidrug resistance is a serious problem.
- Microbial resistance occurs because of the following: (1) inappropriate prescribing; (2) failure to complete the full course of therapy; (3) administration of antibacterial agents for viral infections (e.g., the common cold); (4) antibiotics in the food chain (agriculture, animal husbandry, fish farms); and (5) lack of guidelines for preventing the spread of infections in institutional care settings.
- Bactericidal agents are able to destroy rapidly proliferating, pathogenic bacteria.
- Bacteriostatic agents slow the growth of bacteria enough for the host's (our body's) defense mechanism to destroy the invading bacteria.
- β-Lactam antibiotics target the bacterial cell wall. Penicillins, cephalosporins, carbapenems, and monobactams are β-lactam antibiotics that inhibit cell wall synthesis.
- There are five classes of antiinfective agents that act to inhibit bacterial protein synthesis—the aminoglycosides, macrolides, tetracyclines, amphenicols, and oxazolidinones.
- Fluoroquinolones (e.g., ciprofloxacin) and nitroimidazoles (e.g., metronidazole) inhibit bacterial DNA synthesis.
- Rifampin inhibits bacterial RNA synthesis.

- Sulfonamides are antifolate drugs; trimethoprim is a dihydrofolate reductase inhibitor that interferes with bacterial folic acid synthesis.
- Aminoglycosides are not absorbed systemically when administered by mouth but may be given orally to reduce the number of bacteria in the bowel prior to colorectal surgery.
- A common beginning for cephalosporin drugs is *ceph-* or *cef-*.
- Cephalosporins are classified as first-, second-, third-, and fourth-generation agents.
- A common ending of fluoroquinolones is *-floxacin*.
- Clarithromycin is a key component of treatment regimens for peptic ulcer disease caused by the bacterium *H. pylori*.
- Macrolides, penicillins, and tetracyclines may decrease the effectiveness of oral contraceptives.
- Penicillins may be administered before dental and other medical procedures to prevent bacterial endocarditis in individuals with prosthetic heart valves.
- Antistaphylococcal penicillins are penicillinase resistant.
- A common beginning for sulfonamides is *sulf-*.
- Tetracyclines are used for the treatment of acne, sexually transmitted infections such as chlamydia, Lyme disease, and Rocky Mountain spotted fever.
- Tetracyclines are contraindicated in pregnancy and small children because they can weaken fetal bone, retard bone growth, weaken tooth enamel, and stain teeth.
- Isoniazid is used for the treatment of tuberculosis. Vitamin B_6 should be taken with isoniazid to reduce neurotoxicity.
- Individuals taking metronidazole should avoid drinking alcoholic beverages or taking medicines containing alcohol.
- Mupirocin is a topically applied antimicrobial used to treat staphylococcal infections of the skin such as impetigo.

Review Questions

1. Antibiotics are used to treat_____.
   a. Bacterial infections
   b. Viral infections
   c. Fungal infections
   d. None of the above
2. Misuse of antimicrobial agents is a major cause for the development and spread of microbial resistance.
   a. True
   b. False
3. Antibacterial agents may be classified as _____.
   a. Bactericidal
   b. Bacteriolytic
   c. Bacteriostatic
   d. a and c
4. Each of the following antiinfective agents is marketed as a pediatric solution or suspension EXCEPT _____.
   a. amoxicillin
   b. trimethoprim + sulfamethoxazole
   c. vancomycin
   d. clindamycin

5. All of the following antiinfective agents must be refrigerated after reconstitution EXCEPT _____.
   a. Amoxil 250 mg/5 mL
   b. Keflex 250 mg/5 mL
   c. Augmentin 250 mg/5 mL
   d. Ceftin 250 mg/5 mL
6. Fluoroquinolones are formulated for oral, ophthalmic, and parenteral use.
   a. True
   b. False
7. All of the following antiinfective agents must be stored at room temperature EXCEPT: _____.
   a. Augmentin 250 mg/5 mL
   b. Septra 200 mg/40 mg/5 mL
   c. Biaxin 250 mg/5 mL
   d. Cleocin 75 mg/5 mL
8. Oral penicillins are used to treat many infections, including

   _____.
   a. Upper respiratory infections
   b. Otitis media, skin infections
   c. Strep throat
   d. All of the above

9. Outdated tetracycline becomes toxic and should be discarded.
   a. True
   b. False

10. Isoniazid is used for the treatment of _____.
   a. Upper respiratory infections
   b. AIDS
   c. Tuberculosis
   d. Peptic ulcers

Bibliography

Costello J, King E, Patel D: Core elements of antibiotic stewardship, 2017. From http://www.powerpak.com/course/preamble/115367.

FDA: Drugs@FDA: FDA approved drug products, nd. Retrieved September 14, 2018, from http://www.accessdata.fda.gov/scripts/cder/daf/.

Geisler WM, Uniyal A, Lee JY, et al: Azithromycin versus Doxycycline for urogenital chlamydia trachomatis infection, *NEJM* 373:2512–2521, 2015. doi:10.1056/NEJMoa1502599.

Health Canada: Drug product database, 2018. Retrieved September 14, 2018, from https://health-products.canada.ca/dpd-bdpp/index-eng.jsp.

Institute for Safe Medication Practices: List of confused drugs, 2015. Retrieved September 9, 2017, from https://www.ismp.org/tools/confuseddrugnames.pdf.

Kalant H, Grant D, Mitchell J: *Principles of medical pharmacology*, ed 7, Toronto, 2007, Elsevier Canada, pp 671–686, 702–707, 713.

National Institute of Allergy and Infectious Diseases: Understanding Microbes in Sickness and in Health, 2006. (NIH Publication No. 06-4914). National Institutes of Health Retrieved from www.niaid.nih.gov.

Page C, Curtis M, Sutter M, et al: *Integrated pharmacology*, Philadelphia, 2005, Elsevier Mosby, pp 111–134.

30

Treatment of Viral Infections

LEARNING OBJECTIVES

1. Learn the terminology associated with the treatment of viral infections.
2. Describe the mechanism of virus entry into cells.
3. Describe antiviral resistance.
4. List and categorize antiviral agents.

5. Describe mechanism of action for antiviral agents.
6. List common endings for antiviral agents.
7. Identify significant drug look-alike and sound-alike issues.
8. Identify warning labels and precautionary messages associated with antiviral agents.

KEY TERMS

AIDS (acquired immunodeficiency syndrome) The most severe form of human immunodeficiency virus (HIV) infection. HIV-infected patients are diagnosed with AIDS when their CD4 cell count falls below 200 cells/mm^3 or if they develop an AIDS-defining illness (an unusual illness in someone who is not HIV positive).

Antiretroviral Medication that interferes with the replication of a retrovirus (e.g., HIV).

Antiviral Medication that is able to inhibit viral replication.

Antiviral resistance Ability of a virus to overcome the suppressive action of antiviral agents.

CD4 T lymphocyte White blood cells that fight infection.

Cross-resistance Development of resistance to one drug in a particular class that results in resistance to other drugs in that class.

Highly active antiretroviral therapy (HAART) Combination of three or more antiretroviral medications taken in a regimen.

Human immunodeficiency virus (HIV) Virus that causes acquired immunodeficiency syndrome (AIDS).

Oncovirus A virus that is a causative agent in a cancer.

Virion Infectious particles of a virus.

Virustatic Able to suppress viral proliferation.

Virus Intracellular parasite that consists of a DNA and RNA core surrounded by a protein coat and sometimes an outer covering of lipoprotein.

Overview

A *virus* is an intracellular parasite that consists of a deoxyribonucleic acid (DNA) or ribonucleic acid (RNA) core surrounded by a protein coat and sometimes an outer covering of lipoprotein. The infectious particle (*virion*) does not have the cellular components necessary for reproduction, so they use the host's cellular machinery to replicate (Fig. 30.1). The virus attaches itself to susceptible host cells and then releases viral genetic material (RNA and DNA) into the host cell. The viral material takes control of the host cell machinery for replication. The host cell eventually dies because the virus keeps it from performing its normal functions. When it dies, the cell releases replicated viruses that proliferate and attack more and more host cells. The ability of viruses to transfer genetic material between cells is beneficial in the development of bioengineered drugs and vaccines (e.g., *Haemophilus influenzae* type B conjugate vaccine). See Chapter 32.

Viruses may cause minor illnesses, such as the common cold and warts, or serious infections such as *human immunodeficiency virus* (HIV), smallpox, and hepatitis C infection. Some viral infections are linked to cancers. For example, human papillomavirus (HPV) is linked to cervical cancer. Epstein-Barr virus (EBV) is associated with nose and throat cancers, and hepatitis B and C

viruses are associated with liver cancer. Viruses that can cause cancer are called *oncoviruses*.

An *antiviral* is a medication that is able to inhibit viral replication. Antiviral agents work best when the host (the individual with the infection) has a healthy immune system. This is because antivirals do not destroy viruses; they slow the rate of virus proliferation (*virustatic*). Macrophages, immunoglobulins, T cells, interleukins, interferons, and other cells released by the host in response to the virus's attack ultimately are responsible for recovery from the infection. Like bacterial infections, effective treatment of viral infections is dependent on host factors, virus factors, and antiviral agent factors. Fig. 30.1 shows factors that influence successful therapy.

The following factors influence the outcome of antiviral therapy: (1) stage of illness at the time therapy begins; (2) antiviral dose; (3) ability of the virus to penetrate the central nervous system; (4) ability of the virus to remain latent within its host; and (5) development of antiviral resistance. Herpes simplex virus types 1 and 2 (HSV-1, HSV-2) are viruses that demonstrate the importance of timing related to the initiation of antiviral therapy. Antiviral therapy reduces the severity of the infection and symptoms only if it begins within the first 24 to 48 hours of exposure to the virus or the onset of symptoms. Other viral infections improved by early initiation of antiviral therapy are influenza (Box 30.1) and varicella

1. Attachment to host cell
2. Uncoating of virus, and entry of viral nucleic acid into host cell nucleus
3. Control of DNA, RNA, and/or protein production
4. Production of viral subunits
5. Assembly of virions
6. Release of virions

• **Fig. 30.1** Virus invasion of a host cell, viral replication, and release of virions. (Adapted from Brody TM, Larner J, Minneman KP: *Human pharmacology: molecular to clinical*, ed 3, St. Louis, 1998, Mosby.)

• **BOX 30.1** **CDC Recommendations for Antiviral Treatment of Influenza**

- Children < 2 years
- Adults > 65 years
- Persons with chronic pulmonary (including asthma), cardiovascular (except hypertension alone), renal, hepatic, hematological (including sickle cell disease), and metabolic disorders (including diabetes mellitus), or neurologic and neurodevelopment conditions (including disorders of the brain, spinal cord, peripheral nerve, and muscle, such as cerebral palsy, epilepsy [seizure disorders], stroke, intellectual disability [mental retardation], moderate to severe developmental delay, muscular dystrophy, or spinal cord injury)
- Persons with immunosuppression, including that caused by medications or by human immunodeficiency virus infection
- Women who are pregnant or postpartum (within 2 weeks after delivery)
- Persons aged younger than 19 years who are receiving long-term aspirin therapy
- American Indians/Alaska Natives
- Persons who are morbidly obese (i.e., body mass index is equal to or greater than 40)

Residents of nursing homes and other chronic care facilities
Adapted from Centers for Disease Control and Prevention: Antiviral agents for the treatment and chemoprophylaxis of influenza erratum: 2017. MWR Morb Mortal Wkly Rep 66(No. RR-1):707, 2017. doi:http://dx.doi.org/10.15585/mmwr.mm6626a7.

zoster virus (VZV). HSV-1, HSV-2, and VZV are also examples of viruses that lay dormant in host cells and periodically awaken to cause recurrent disease.

Antiviral agents are typically effective against specific viral strains. For example, amantadine acts against influenza A but not influenza B. Oseltamivir (Tamiflu) is indicated for the treatment of influenza but is not effective for the treatment of HIV, HPV, or HSV. Antibiotics are not effective against viral infections.

Antiviral Resistance

The growth of viral colonies involves viral replication. In the process of replication, the virus may mutate. Mutations often result in adaptations that make it easier for the virus to exist in new environments and hosts. *Antiviral resistance* is the ability of a virus to overcome the suppressive action of antiviral agents. It may occur when an individual taking an antiviral drug skips doses or takes them irregularly. Vomiting may cause subtherapeutic levels of antiviral agents resulting in insufficient levels to suppress viral replication, yet sufficient residual exposure to permit antiviral resistance to develop. The virus may accidentally mutate into a form that is resistant to the antiviral drug(s) taken.

Because viruses continually mutate, it is difficult to develop a vaccine to prevent viral infections. For example, each year a new flu vaccine must be developed against the latest virulent strain of influenza. A triple cocktail of drugs is administered for the treatment of HIV and AIDS, known as highly active antiretroviral therapy (HAART), to decrease mutations and improve antiretroviral therapy. There are several strains of human papilloma virus (HPV). Cervarix and Gardasil are effective against HPV types 16 and 18, which cause most cervical cancers. Gardasil is also effective against HPV types 6 and 11.

Mechanisms of Antiviral Action

Antivirals interfere with virus-specific steps in the replication cycle, specifically:
- virus attachment to the host cell receptors, cell penetration, and viral uncoating;
- virus regulatory proteins;
- virus cleavage;
- viral assembly; and
- release of virus.
  Antivirals inhibit:
- reverse transcriptase, transamidase, and other virion-associated enzymes;

- viral transcription; and
- viral messenger RNA (mRNA).

Treatment of Influenza

Two types of antivirals are used to prevent or treat influenza. They are adamantanes (amantadine and rimantadine) and neuraminidase inhibitors (oseltamivir, zanamivir, and peramivir).

> **! TECH ALERT!**
> A common ending for antivirals that inhibit viral uncoating is *-mantidine*.

Adamantanes

Amantadine and rimantadine are classified as adamantane antivirals that are used for the prevention and treatment of influenza A.

> **! TECH ALERT!**
> The following drugs have look-alike and sound-alike issues:
> Amantadine and amiodarone

Amantanes

Mechanism of Action and Pharmacokinetics

Amantadine and rimantadine interfere with the uncoating of the influenza A virus, a necessary step in the viral replication process. More specifically, they inhibit the activity of the influenza virus M2 protein, which forms a channel in the virus membrane and enables replication after the virus enters the host cell. Amantadine is rapidly absorbed, and peak plasma levels are achieved within two to four hours of an oral dose. Peak plasma levels for rimantadine occur in approximately 6 hours. Rimantadine is approximately 40% protein-bound. It is also highly metabolized in the liver and has active metabolites that account for the drug's long half-life of 13 to 65 hours.

Adverse Reactions and Precautions

Amantadine and rimantadine may produce anxiety, irritability, nervousness, drowsiness, confusion, and headache. They can also cause diarrhea or constipation, difficulty sleeping or nightmares, dry mouth, loss of appetite, nausea or vomiting, unusual tiredness, and, rarely, kidney damage. Antiviral resistance limits their effectiveness in treating influenza A and influenza B.

Neuraminidase Inhibitors

Oseltamivir, zanamivir, and peramivir are indicated for the treatment of influenza A and influenza B. Nearly 98% H1N1 and H3N3 strains of influenza A are susceptible to the effects of oseltamivir and zanamivir; however, one strain of H1N1 influenza that is resistant to oseltamivir and zanamivir has been identified.

> **! TECH ALERT!**
> Tamiflu and Theraflu have look-alike and sound-alike issues.

Mechanism of Action and Pharmacokinetics

The surfaces of influenza viruses are dotted with neuraminidase proteins. Neuraminidase inhibitors inhibit viral release by inhibiting the enzyme that breaks the bonds that hold the virus particle to the outside of the infected cell. They inhibit virus spread by blocking virus release from the host cell. Oseltamivir (Tamiflu) is formulated for oral use, zanamivir (Relenza) is a powder that is inhaled by mouth, and peramivir (Rapivab) is formulated for an intravenous infusion.

Adverse Reactions

Side effects common to the use of oseltamivir and zanamivir are nausea and vomiting, coughing, dizziness, and headache. Psychosis and other emotional changes have been reported with the use of neuraminidase inhibitors. Zanamivir is not recommended for patients with pulmonary disease because it has been reported to produce bronchospasm and deterioration of pulmonary function. Allergic reactions include oropharyngeal or facial edema. The most common side effect with Rapivab is diarrhea; however, serious skin and hypersensitivity reactions may occur.

Treatment of Influenza

Generic Name	U.S. Brand Name(s) / Canadian Brand Name(s)	Dosage Forms and Strengths
Amantanes		
amantadine[a]	Gocovri[b]	**Capsule:** 100 mg
	Generics	**Capsule, extended release (Gocovri):** 68.5mg, 137 mg **Oral solution:** 10 mg/mL **Tablet[c]:** 100 mg
rimantadine[a]	Flumadine	**Tablet:** 100 mg
	Not available	
Neuraminidase Inhibitors		
oseltamivir[a]	Tamiflu	**Capsule:** 30 mg, 45 mg, 75 mg
	Tamiflu	**Powder, for suspension:** 6 mg/mL,
peramivir	Rapivab	**IV infusion:** 200 mg/20 mL
	Not available	
zanamivir	Relenza	**Powder, for inhalation:** 5 mg per actuation
	Relenza	

[a]Generic available.
[b]Gocovri is indicated for the treatment Parkinson's disease-related symptoms.
[c]Available in the United States only.

Treatment of Hepatitis B and Hepatitis C

Hepatitis B and hepatitis C are viral infections that attack the liver. The viruses can spread when blood from an infected person enters the bloodstream of an non-infected person, as can occur with unsafe injection practices (e.g., sharing needles). Hepatitis B can also be transmitted in semen and other body fluids. Five percent of the global population is infected with hepatitis B, and 600,000 people die annually from liver damage and other complications of chronic infection. More than 170 million people worldwide are infected with hepatitis C. Interferons, nucleoside analogues, nucleotide analogues, and protease inhibitors (PIs) are used for the treatment of hepatitis B virus (HBV) and/or hepatitis C virus (HCV) infections. Nucleosides, nucleotides, and PIs are also used for the treatment of HIV infections and are described in the next section.

Interferons

Interferons are a family of naturally occurring proteins that are made and secreted by cells of the immune system. There are approximately 2000 interferon receptors on each normal and malignant cell. Interferons may also be produced by recombinant DNA technology. They are not technically antiviral agents. Instead, they protect uninfected cells by promoting resistance to virus infection.

Interferon alfa-2b, interferon alfacon-1, peginterferon alfa-2a, and peginterferon alfa-2b are administered to treat viral infections. Peginterferon alfa-2b is indicated for the treatment of HCV. Interferon alfa-2b and peginterferon alfa-2a may be used for the treatment of HBV and HCV.

> **⊘ TECH ALERT!**
>
> The following drugs have look-alike and sound-alike issues:
> peginterferon alfa-2a and peginterferon alfa-2b

Interferon Alfa and Interferon Alfa N3 Mechanism of Action and Pharmacokinetics

Interferons inhibit viral transcription by activating enzymes that cleave single-stranded viral RNA. Depending on the virus and cell type, they may also inhibit viral uncoating, inhibit the synthesis of mRNA, and interfere with the translation, assembly, and release of viral proteins.

Adverse Reactions and Precautions

The most common adverse reactions associated with interferons are flu-like symptoms—fever, chills, headache, fatigue, muscle aches, and joint pain. They may also cause nausea, vomiting, diarrhea, dizziness, and depression. More serious adverse effects are neutropenia (a drop in the white blood cell count) and thrombocytopenia (a decrease in the platelet count).

Nucleoside/Nucleotide Analogues

Nucleoside/nucleotide analogue antiviral agents that are used for the treatment of HBV are adefovir, lamivudine, entecavir and telbivudine, and tenofovir. Entecavir is effective against lamivudine-resistant HBV. Ribavirin is indicated for the treatment of hepatitis C when combined with peginterferon alfa. Ribavirin is also indicated for the treatment of respiratory syncytial virus (RSV).

Mechanism of Action

Nucleosides/nucleotides analogues inhibit at least one of the three steps of virus replication. Entecavir, lamivudine, ribavirin, and telbivudine are nucleoside analogues. They inhibit HBV reverse transcriptase. Telbivudine inhibits HBV DNA polymerase, resulting in DNA chain termination and inhibition of viral replication. Ribavirin is effective against RNA and DNA viruses. The mechanism of action is not completely understood, but it is believed that the drug increases the mutation rate of the virus, leading to a growing number of viruses unable to replicate. Adefovir and tenofovir are nucleotide analogues that inhibit HBV DNA polymerase, resulting in DNA chain termination and inhibition of viral replication. Sovaldi (sofosbuvir) is a nucleotide analog NS5B polymerase inhibitor that works by blocking a specific protein that the HCV needs to grow.

Adverse Effects and Precautions

The most common adverse effects of entecavir and lamivudine are headache, fatigue, dizziness, and nausea. Headache, abdominal pain, diarrhea, nausea, dyspepsia, flatulence, and asthenia are the most common side effects associated with adefovir. Adefovir, entecavir, and telbivudine have a boxed warning regarding worsening of hepatitis upon discontinuation. Tenofovir may increase the toxicity of adefovir.

> **⊘ TECH ALERT!**
>
> The US Food and Drug Administration (FDA) requires a boxed warning for adefovir, entecavir, telbivudine, and tenofovir, informing prescribers of the following: (1) severe acute exacerbations of hepatitis B have been reported in patients who have discontinued anti-hepatitis B therapy; (2) fatal lactic acidosis; and (3) renal dysfunction (adefovir).

> **⊘ TECH ALERT!**
>
> The FDA requires a boxed warning that entecavir is not recommended for patients coinfected with HIV and HBV unless also receiving HAART, to reduce the risk for the development of drug resistance.

Direct Acting Antivirals

In 2014, direct acting antivirals (DAAs) were approved by the FDA for the treatment of hepatitis C. Most of the direct acting antivirals are marketed as combination products or are taken in combination with ribavirin or interferons to improve effectiveness and/or reduce the development of antiviral resistance.

Mechanism of Actions

DAAs target specific nonstructural proteins of the HCV to disrupt viral replication and the infection. There are four classes of DAAs: (1) nonstructural proteins 3/4A (NS3/4A) protease inhibitors (PIs); (2) NS5B nucleoside polymerase inhibitors (NPIs); (3) NS5B nonnucleoside polymerase inhibitors (NNPIs); and (4) NS5A inhibitors.

NS3/4A PIs include glecaprevir, grazoprevir, paritaprevir, and voxilaprevir. Sofosbuvir is an NS5B NPI. It is approved by the FDA for the treatment of HIV and HCV coinfection.

Daclatasvir, elbasvir, ledipasvir, ombitasvir, pibrentasvir, and velpatasvir are NS5A inhibitors. NS5B NNPIs are in the clinical phase of development.

Adverse Reactions

The most common side effects of DAA medications are headache, fatigue, and nausea. HBV reactivation has been reported upon initiation of therapy in patients coinfected with HCV and HBV leading to the severe and sudden onset of hepatitis, hepatic failure, and death.

Treatment of Herpes Simplex, Herpes Zoster, and Cytomegalovirus

The virus that causes cold sores (HSV-1), the virus that causes genital warts (HSV-2), and the virus that causes chicken pox and shingles (varicella zoster) are treated with acyclovir, famciclovir, penciclovir, and valacyclovir. Acyclovir and valacyclovir are indicated for the treatment of cold sores, herpes genitalis, and shingles, whereas penciclovir is only indicated for the treatment of herpes labialis, commonly known as a cold sore. Trifluridine is used for the treatment of keratoconjunctivitis of the eye caused by HSV-1 and HSV-2 (see Chapter 15). Cytomegalovirus (CMV) may be treated with cidofovir, ganciclovir, or foscarnet. Foscarnet is also indicated for the treatment of acyclovir-resistant HSV-1, HSV-2, and herpes labialis.

Treatment of Hepatitis B and Hepatitis C

Generic Name	US Brand Name(s) / Canadian Brand Name(s)	Dosage Forms and Strengths
Interferons		
interferon alfa-2b	Intron-A	**Powder, for injection:** 10 million international units (mIU)/vial, 18 mIU/vial,[a] 25 mIU/vial[a]
	Intron-A	**Solution for injection, vial:** 6 mIU/mL,[b] 10 mIU/mL,[b] 15 mIU/mL,[b] 25 mIU/mL,[b] 50 mIU/mL[b]
peginterferon alfa-2a	Pegasys	**Solution for injection, vial[a]:** 180 mcg/mL
	Pegasys	**Solution for injection, prefilled syringe:** 180 mcg/0.5 mL
peginterferon alfa-2b	PegIntron, Sylatron	**Powder for injection (Sylatron):** 296 mcg, 444 mcg, 888 mcg per vial
	Not available	**Solution, for injection (vial and pre-filled syringe):** 50 mcg/0.5 mL, 80 mcg/0.5 mL, 120 mcg/0.5 mL, 150 mcg/0.5 mL
Nucleoside/Nucleotide Analogues[d]		
adefovir[c]	Hepsera	**Tablet:** 10 mg
	Hepsera	
entecavir[c]	Baraclude	**Solution, oral:** 0.05 mg/mL[a]
	Baraclude	**Tablet:** 0.5 mg, 1 mg[a]
lamivudine[c]	Epivir HBV	**Solution, oral:** 5 mg/mL
	Heptovir	**Tablet:** 100 mg
ribavirin[c]	Rebetol, Ribasphere	**Capsule (Rebetol, Ribasphere):** 200 mg
	Ibavyr, Moderiba	**Oral solution (Rebetol)[a]:** 40 mg/mL
		Tablet (Copegus, Ibavyr, Moderiba): 200 mg, 400 mg, 500 mg,[a] 600 mg
telbivudine	Not avsailable	**Tablet:** 600 mg
	Sebivo	
tenofovir alafenamide	Vemlidy	**Tablet:** 25 mg
	Vemlidy	
Direct- Acting Antivirals		
daclatasvir	Daklinza	**Tablet:** 30 mg, 60 mg, 90 mg[a]
	Daklinza	
sofosbuvir	Sovaldi	**Tablet:** 400 mg
	Sovaldi	
Combination Direct Acting Antivirals		
glecaprevir + pibrentasvir	Mavyret	**Tablet:** 100 mg glecaprevir + 40 mg pibrentasvir
	Maviret	
ombitasvir + paritaprevir + ritonavir	Technivie	**Tablet:** 12.5 mg ombitasvir + 75 mg paritaprevir + 50 mg ritonavir
	Not available	
dasabuvir + ombitasvir + paritaprevir + ritonavir tablets	Viekira Pak, Viekira XR	**Tablet (Viekira XR):** 200 mg dasabuvir + 8.33 mg ombitasvir + 50 mg paritaprevir + 33.33 mg ritonavir
	Not available	**Tablet (Viekira Pak):** 250 mg dasabuvir + 12.5 mg ombitasvir + 75 mg paritaprevir + 50 mg ritonavir
sofosbuvir + velpatasvir	Epclusa	**Tablet:** 400 mg sofosbuvir + 100 mg velpatasvir
	Epclusa	
sofosbuvir + ledipasvir	Harvoni	**Tablet:** 400 mg sofosbuvir + 90 mg ledipasvir
	Harvoni	

Treatment of Hepatitis B and Hepatitis C—cont'd

Generic Name	US Brand Name(s) Canadian Brand Name(s)	Dosage Forms and Strengths
sofosbuvir + velpatasvir + voxilaprevir	Vosevi / Vosevi	**Tablet:** 400 mg sofosbuvir + 100 mg velpatasvir + 100 mg voxilaprevir
elbasvir + grazoprevir	Zepatier / Zepatier	**Tablet:** 50 mg elbasvir + 100 mg grazoprevir

[a]Available in the United States only.
[b]Available in Canada only.
[c]Generic available.
[d]Only brand names and strength of nucleoside/nucleotide analogues marketed for the treatment of hepatitis are shown in the table. Additional strengths or Brand names may be marketed for the treatment of additional infections.

Treatment of Respiratory Syncytial Virus: Inhibition of Deoxyribonucleic Acid and Ribonucleic Acid Replication

Generic Name	US Brand Name(s) Canadian Brand Name(s)	Dosage Forms and Strengths
palivizumab	Synagis / Synagis	**Powder, for injection solution:** 50 mg/vial, 100 mg/vial **Solution, for injection**[b]: 50 mg/0.5 mL, 100 mg/mL
ribavirin[a]	Virazole / Virazole	**Powder, for inhalation:** 6 g/vial

[a]Generic available.
[b]Available in Canada only.

> ⚠ **TECH ALERT!**
>
> A common ending for antivirals used for the treatment of herpes virus infections is -cyclovir and -ciclovir.

> ⚠ **TECH ALERT!**
>
> The following drugs have look-alike and sound-alike issues:
> Zovirax and Zostrix;
> Denavir and indinavir.

Mechanism of Action and Pharmacokinetics

Acyclovir inhibits viral DNA synthesis which is an essential step in the process of viral replication because genetic code is stored in DNA. Acyclovir is approximately 10 times more potent against HSV-1 and -2 than against VZV. Higher doses are required for the treatment of chickenpox and shingles. Acyclovir may be administered topically, orally, or parenterally. Gastrointestinal (GI) absorption is poor and the bioavailability of orally administered acyclovir is much lower than parenterally administered acyclovir. Systemic effects from topical administration are limited.

Valacyclovir is an ester of acyclovir. It has greater oral absorption. It treats the same conditions as acyclovir but requires less frequent dosing. Cidofovir inhibits viral DNA polymerase, the enzyme responsible for the replication of new viral RNA and DNA.

Foscarnet inhibits the viral-specific DNA polymerases and reverse transcriptases. It also inhibits the replication of the herpes simplex virus, VZV, EBV, human herpesvirus 6, and CMV.

Ganciclovir is used for the treatment of CMV. It is similar in structure to acyclovir. Ganciclovir is a competitive inhibitor of viral DNA polymerases that results in the inhibition of viral DNA synthesis.

Famciclovir is metabolized to penciclovir. It has a similar spectrum of activity to acyclovir and is also indicated for the treatment of HSV-1, HSV-2, and acute herpes zoster infections. It has a longer duration of action than acyclovir.

Penciclovir is an active metabolite of famciclovir. It is administered topically.

Adverse Reactions

Adverse reactions that are common to acyclovir, famciclovir, ganciclovir, penciclovir, valacyclovir, and cidofovir are diarrhea, nausea, vomiting, headache, fatigue, dizziness, and confusion. Penciclovir and acyclovir topical cream or ointment may also cause local irritation. Cidofovir may produce neutropenia, hair loss, tinnitus, renal failure, and hearing loss. Foscarnet has a side effect profile similar to that of cidofovir but can also cause arrhythmias, heart failure, and peripheral neuropathy.

Human Immunodeficiency Virus and Acquired Immunodeficiency Syndrome

HIV/AIDS (*acquired immunodeficiency syndrome*) is a global public health issue. According to the Joint United Nations Programme on HIV/AIDS (UNAIDS), 36.9 million people were living with HIV in 2017, including 2.1 million children. There were 1.8 million new HIV infections worldwide (5000 new cases per day).

HIV/AIDS is worsened by poverty. Poverty creates the following conditions: individuals knowingly engage in risky sexual behaviors such as the sex trade; it increases malnutrition, which can weaken the immune system; it decreases access to health care and HIV medicines, which can increase drug resistance; and many HIV medicines should be taken with food, and access to regular meals may be limited.

Treatment of Herpes Virus and Cytomegalovirus

Generic Name	US Brand Name(s) / Canadian Brand Name(s)	Dosage Forms and Strengths
acyclovir[a]	Sitavig, Zovirax / Zovirax	**Capsule:** 200 mg **Cream:** 5% **Ointment:** 5% **Solution, for injection:** 25 mg/mL,[c] 50 mg/mL **Suspension:** 200 mg/5 mL **Tablet:** 200 mg,[c] 400 mg, 800 mg **Tablet, buccal (Sitavig):** 50 mg
acyclovir + hydrocortisone	Xerese / Xerese	**Cream:** 5% acyclovir + 1% hydrocortisone
cidofovir[a]	Generics / Not available	**Solution, for injection:** 75 mg/mL
famciclovir[a]	Generics / Famvir	**Tablet:** 125 mg, 250 mg, 500 mg
foscarnet[a]	Generics / Not available	**Solution, for injection:** 24 mg/mL
ganciclovir[a]	Cytovene, Zirgan / Cytovene	**Gel, ophthalmic (Zirgan)[b]:** 0.15% **Powder, for injection:** 500 mg/vial
penciclovir	Denavir / Not available	**Cream:** 1%
trifluridine[a]	Viroptic / Viroptic	**Ophthalmic solution:** 1%
valacyclovir[a]	Valtrex / Valtrex	**Tablet:** 500 mg, 1 g
valganciclovir[a]	Valcyte / Valcyte	**Powder, for oral solution:** 50 mg/mL **Tablet:** 450 mg

[a]Generic available.
[b]Available in the United States only.
[c]Available in Canada only.

HIV is the virus that causes AIDS. The virus attacks *CD4 T lymphocytes* and weakens the immune system. As the CD4 count declines below 200 cells/mm³ and the viral load increases, the risk for developing opportunistic infections such as tuberculosis (TB), candidiasis, and cytomegalovirus (CMV) and other AIDS-defining conditions also increases. The viral load is the amount of materials from the virus that are released into the bloodstream when the HIV reproduces.

Human Immunodeficiency Virus Life Cycle

HIV, like other viruses, lacks the cellular machinery to reproduce itself. It incorporates its DNA into the DNA of the host cell; then, when the host cell tries to make new proteins, it accidentally makes new HIV as well. HIV treatments interfere with specific steps in the HIV life cycle briefly described here:

- Step 1: Binding. The HIV binds to CD4 surface receptors.
- Step 2: Fusion. The HIV is activated by proteins on the cell's surface, allowing the HIV envelope to fuse to the outside of the cell.
- Step 3: Uncoating. The virus is uncoated, permitting the contents of the viral capsid (viral RNA and enzymes) to be released into the infected host cell.
- Step 4: Reverse transcription. A viral enzyme called reverse transcriptase makes a DNA copy of the viral RNA.
- Step 5: Integration. Viral DNA is incorporated into the host cellular DNA.
- Step 6: Genome replication. The strands of viral DNA in the nucleus separate and mRNA provides instructions for making new virus (genome). This process is called transcription.
- Step 7: Protein synthesis. The HIV mRNA genome acts as a template for synthesizing viral proteins needed to make a new virus in a process called translation.

Summary of Drugs Used for the Treatment of Influenza, Herpes, Hepatitis, Respiratory Syncytial Virus, and Cytomegalovirus Viral Infections

Generic Name	Brand Name	Usual Dose and Dosing Schedule	Warning Labels
Influenza A or B Treatment			
amantadine	Generics *Symmetrel*	**Influenza A treatment and prophylaxis:** 200 mg/day as one or two divided doses; begin 24–48 h of onset of signs or symptoms and continue for 24–48 h after symptoms resolve or for prophylaxis at least 10 days	MAY CAUSE DIZZINESS OR DROWSINESS. COMPLETE FULL COURSE OF THERAPY
rimantadine	Flumadine	**Influenza A treatment and prophylaxis:** 100 mg twice daily; begin 24–48 h of onset of signs or symptoms, continue for 5–7 days	
oseltamivir	Tamiflu	**Influenza A or B treatment and prophylaxis:** 75 mg twice daily for 5 days for acute infection, once daily for 10 days—prophylaxis	REFRIGERATE; SHAKE WELL; DISCARD AFTER 10 DAYS (oseltamivir suspension). COMPLETE FULL COURSE OF THERAPY.
peramavir	Rapivab	Influenza Treatment—600 mg/100 mL IV infusion over 15–30 min	
zanamivir	Relenza	**Influenza A treatment:** Two doses to start; then two oral inhalations twice daily for 5 days; begin within 48 h of onset of signs or symptoms **Influenza A prophylaxis:** Two oral inhalations daily for 10 or 28 days, as directed	INHALE USING DISKHALER DELIVERY DEVICE (zanamivir)
Hepatitis B			
adefovir[a]	Hepsera	10 mg once daily	TAKE WITH OR WITHOUT FOOD—adefovir, lamivudine, telbivudine, tenofovir. TAKE ON AN EMPTY STOMACH—entecavir. REFRIGERATE; DO NOT FREEZE-interferon alfa-2b, peginterferon alfa-2a
entecavir	Baraclude	0.5–1 mg once daily	
interferon alfa-2b	Intron A	30–35 mIU weekly SC or IM for 16 weeks	
lamivudine	Epivir HBV, Heptovir	HIV negative patients—100 mg once daily for up to 1 year	
peginterferon alfa-2a	Pegasys	180 mcg SC once weekly for 48 weeks *Hep B*	
telbivudine	Sebivo	600 mg once daily	
tenofovir	Vemlidy	25 mg once daily	
Hepatitis C			DO NOT SKIP DOSES—all REFRIGERATE; DO NOT FREEZE-peginterferon alfa-2b. TAKE WITH FOOD—ribavirin, Mavyret, Technivie, Viekira Pak, Vosevi DO NOT CRUSH OR CHEW-ribavirin. TAKE WITH FOOD (NOT LOW FAT)—simiprevir. TAKE WITH OR WITHOUT FOOD-daclatasvir, sofosbuvir, Epclusa, Harvoni, Zepatier SWALLOW WHOLE, DON'T CRUSH OR CHEW—Viekira XR
daclatasvir	Daklinza	60 mg taken orally once daily (Administer in combination with sofosbuvir)	
peginterferon alfa-2b	PEG-Intron	1.5 mcg/kg once weekly for 1 year	
ribavirin	Copegus	**Monoinfection:** 800–1400 mg daily according to body weight with 180 mcg of peginterferon alfa-2a **Coinfection with HIV:** 800 mg PO daily for 48 weeks with 180 mcg of peginterferon alfa-2a	
simiprevir	Olysio	150 mg once daily (with sofosbuvir or pegintron alfa and ribavirin	
sofosbuvir	Sovaldi	400 mg once a day	
glecaprevir + pibrentasvir	Mavyret, Maviret	Take three tablets once daily	
ombitasvir + paritaprevir + ritonavir	Technivie	Take two tablet once daily (Administer in combination with ribavirin)	
dasabuvir + ombitasvir + paritaprevir + ritonavir	Viekira Pak	Take two ombitasvir + paritaprevir + ritonavir tablets and 1 dasabuvir tablet twice daily	

Continued

Summary of Drugs Used for the Treatment of Influenza, Herpes, Hepatitis, Respiratory Syncytial Virus, and Cytomegalovirus Viral Infections—cont'd

Generic Name	Brand Name	Usual Dose and Dosing Schedule	Warning Labels
sofosbuvir + velpatasvir	Epclusa	Take one tablet once daily	
sofosbuvir + ledipasvir	Harvoni	Take one tablet once daily	
sofosbuvir + velpatasvir + voxilaprevir	Vosevi	Take one tablet once daily	
elbasvir + grazoprevir	Zepatier	Take one tablet once daily	PROTECT FROM MOISTURE
Respiratory Syncytial Virus			
palivizumab	Synagis	15 mg/kg IM monthly	STORE AT ROOM TEMPERATURE PROTECT FROM LIGHT AND MOISTURE—virazole DON'T SHAKE- palivizumab
ribavirin	Virazole	**RSV:** 20 mg/mL administered as continuous aerosol administration for 12–18 h/day for 3–7 days	
Herpes Simplex, Herpes Zoster Infections			
acyclovir	Zovirax	Varies according to type of infection (HSV-1, HSV-2, VZV) and acute versus recurrent infection **Dosage range:** **IV:** 5–10 mg/kg every 8 h for 5–10 days **Oral:** 200 mg 5 times/day or 400 mg tid for 5–10 days **Topical:** Apply every 3 h for 7 days	SHAKE WELL (acyclovir suspension). COMPLETE FULL COURSE OF THERAPY; BEGIN THERAPY WITHIN 72 HR OF ONSET OF SYMPTOMS. SWALLOW WHOLE; DON'T CRUSH OR CHEW (ganciclovir). AVOID PREGNANCY (ganciclovir). TAKE WITH FOOD (ganciclovir). WASH YOUR HANDS WITH SOAP AND WATER AFTER USING (penciclovir). DO NOT SKIP DOSES—all SHAKE WELL, STORE IN THE REFRIGERATOR, DISCARD AFTER 28 DAYS—valacyclovir suspension
famciclovir	Famvir	Varies according to type of infection (HSV-1, HSV-2, VZV) and acute versus recurrent infection **Dosage range:** 125–500 mg bid or tid for 5–10 days or 1000–1500 mg bid for 1 day	
ganciclovir	Cytovene	Varies according to acute or recurrent CMV infection **Dosage range:** **IV:** 5 mg/kg IV every 12–24 h for 7–21 days **Oral:** 1000 mg tid or 500 mg six times daily	
penciclovir	Denavir	**Cold sores:** Apply every 2 h while awake for 4 days; start within 1 h of symptom onset	
valacyclovir	Valtrex	Varies according to type of infection (HSV-1, HSV-2, VZV) and acute versus recurrent infection **Dosage range:** 500 mg–2 g 2-3 times a day for 5–10 days	
foscarnet	Foscavir	Varies according to type of infection (HSV-1, HSV-2, VZV, CMV) and acute versus recurrent infection **Dosage range:** 40–90 mg/kg IV every 8–12 h for 2–3 weeks	STORE AT ROOM TEMPERATURE; DISCARD DISCOLORED SOLUTION—foscarnet. REMOVE CONTACT LENSES BEFORE USE—trifluridine
trifluridine	Viroptic	1 drop in affected eye(s) every 2 h while awake (max, 9 drops/day)	
Cytomegalovirus			
cidofovir	Vistide	**CMV retinitis:** 5 mg/kg IV once weekly for 2 weeks with probenecid; prophylaxis 5 mg/kg IV once every other week	USE WITHIN 24 HR OF PREPARATION- cidofovir. STORE BETWEEN 2-8°C (36–46°F)- Cytogam USE WITHIN 6 H OPENING- Cytogam
cytomegalovirus Immune globulin	Cytogam	100–150 mg/kg/dose	

ªGeneric available.

SC, subcutaneously; *IM,* intramuscularly; *PO,* orally; *IV,* intravenously; *RSV,* respiratory syncytial virus.

- Step 8: Protein cleavage and viral assembly. Protease is an enzyme that cuts the long chain of viral protein into smaller individual proteins. Some of the cleaved proteins become structural elements of new HIV and others become enzymes, such as reverse transcriptase. The new particles are assembled into new HIV.
- Step 9: Virus release. New virus buds off from the host cell.

Pharmacological Treatment

UNAIDS 2020 treatment targets are: 90% of people living with HIV know their HIV status; 90% of people who know their HIV-positive status are accessing treatment; and 90% of people on treatment have a suppressed viral load. Global HIV treatment and prevention programs have been credited with the 16% decline in new AIDS infections between 2010 and 2016 worldwide. *Antiretrovirals* are administered to reduce viral load, increase CD4 counts, delay the development of AIDS-related conditions and opportunistic infections, and improve survival. Antiretrovirals fall into six classes:

- Nucleoside/nucleotide reverse transcriptase inhibitors (NRTIs)
- Nonnucleoside reverse transcriptase inhibitors (NNRTIs)
- Protease Inhibitors (PIs)
- Fusion inhibitors
- Chemokine receptor antagonist, type 5 (CCR5)
- HIV integrase strand inhibitors

International treatment guidelines have been established for initiation of antiretroviral therapy based on CD4 counts and whether patients are symptomatic or asymptomatic. Antiretroviral therapy is a lifelong commitment and requires strict adherence to treatment regimens.

To reduce antiviral resistance, *HAART*—a regimen of three or more medications from two or more antiretroviral classes—is prescribed. Combination therapy improves effectiveness and decreases the risk of developing resistance, but may increase adverse reactions. Antiretroviral agent resistance testing is recommended prior to the initiation of therapy with antiretrovirals, and prior to changing therapy.

Nucleoside and Nucleotide Reverse Transcriptase Inhibitors

Many Nucleoside and Nucleotide Reverse Transcriptase Inhibitors (NRTIs) are prodrugs that are activated by host cell enzymes. They competitively inhibit reverse transcriptase, the enzyme that makes a DNA copy of the viral RNA.

Abacavir

Abacavir is an NRTI. It is an ingredient in the triple antiretroviral therapy that combines abacavir with zidovudine and lamivudine. It is also formulated with lamivudine as a dual combination therapy. It is linked to a fatal hypersensitivity reaction that necessitates discontinuation of the drug. Symptoms include fever and chills, muscle and joint pain, fatigue and feeling rundown, nausea and vomiting, skin rash, and shortness of breath.

Didanosine

Didanosine (DDI) is an NRTI. It is metabolized to an active metabolite that has an intracellular half-life ($t_{1/2}$) of 25 to 40 hours; therefore, the drug can be dosed once daily. It is acid-labile, so it must be buffered to prevent inactivation by gastric acids. DDI is formulated for pediatric use as a powder for solution and as delayed-release capsules. Side effects, such as pancreatitis and peripheral neuropathy, limit its use.

Emtricitabine

Emtricitabine (FTC) is an NRTI similar to lamivudine. *Cross-resistance* occurs between lamivudine and emtricitabine.

Cross-resistance refers to the development of resistance to one agent in a particular class that results in resistance to the other agents in that class. Emtricitabine is formulated as an oral capsule and an oral solution. Refrigeration is recommended for the oral solution; however, the solution is stable at room temperature for three months if refrigeration is not available.

Lamivudine

Lamivudine (3TC) is an NRTI that is effective against HIV, including zidovudine-resistant strains of HIV. Lamivudine also inhibits replication of HBV. It is a good choice of therapy for those who have HIV and HBV coinfections. Lamivudine is an ingredient in HIV combination therapies. The drug has good oral absorption, and the relatively long intracellular $t_{1/2}$ (12 hours) permits once-daily dosing.

Stavudine

Stavudine (d4T) is an NRTI. It is similar to zidovudine. Stavudine has a short $t_{1/2}$ and must be administered more frequently than some of the other NRTIs. It is formulated for oral administration and food does not interfere with absorption.

Tenofovir

Tenofovir (TDF) is an NRTI. It is administered orally. Food increases bioavailability of the drug. It has a long intracellular $t_{1/2}$, up to 50 hours. WHO 2017 guidelines for preexposure prevention (PrEP) of HIV infection recommend the use of formulations containing TDF. TDF should not be administered concurrently with adefovir (used to treat hepatitis C) because it increases the risk of toxicity.

Zidovudine

Zidovudine (AZT) was the first available antiretroviral, and was introduced in 1987. It is an NRTI and is formulated for oral and parenteral administration. The drug may be administered orally to pregnant women and intravenously during delivery, and as a suspension to neonates. It has been shown to decrease perinatal mother-to-child transmission (MTCT) of HIV from 25% to 8%. WHO 2015 Prevention of MTCT Guidelines, adopted by many countries, replaces AZT with a triple drug regimen for pregnant women. WHO 2015 guidelines are shown in Table 30.1.

Adverse Reactions

Common side effects associated with almost all NRTIs are headache, stomach upset, fatigue or insomnia, muscle ache, and diarrhea.

TABLE 30.1	World Health Organization Option B+ Prevention of Mother-to-Child Transmission Guidelines (2015)
B+	**Mother:** Lifelong triple antiviral therapy (TDF + 3TC [or FTC] + EFV) for pregnant and breastfeeding women with HIV
	Breastfeeding infants: Daily NVP antiretroviral drug regimen for 6 weeks
	Nonbreastfeeding infants: Daily NVP for 4–6 weeks or twice daily AZT

3TC, Lamivudine; *AXT,* zidovudine; *EFV,* efavirenz; *FTC,* emtricitabine; *HIV,* human immunodeficiency virus; *NVP,* nevirapine; *TDF,* tenofovir.
Adapted from World Health Organization: WHO HIV and AIDS guidelines for PMTCT and breastfeeding, 2010 (http://www.avert.org/pmtct-guidelines.htm) and WHO PMTCT update 2012 (www.who.int/hiv/PMTCT_update.pdf).

Nucleoside Reverse Transcriptase Inhibitors Used for the Treatment of HIV and AIDS[d]

Generic Name	US Brand Name(s) Canadian Brand Name(s)	Dosage Forms and Strengths
abacavir (ABC)	Ziagen	**Tablet:** 300 mg **Solution:** 20 mg/mL
	Ziagen	
didanosine[a] (DDI)	Videx, Videx EC	**Powder, for pediatric solution**[b]**:** 10 mg/mL **Capsule/Tablet, delayed-release (Videx EC):** 125 mg, 200 mg, 250 mg, 400 mg
	Videx EC	
emtricitabine (FTC)	Emtriva	**Capsule:** 200 mg **Solution**[b]**:** 10 mg/mL
	Not available	
lamivudine[a] (3TC)	Epivir	**Solution:** 10 mg/mL **Tablet:** 150 mg, 300 mg
	Epivir	
stavudine[a] (d4T)	Zerit	**Capsule, immediate-release:** 15 mg, 20 mg, 30 mg, 40 mg **Powder, for oral solution:** 1 mg/mL[b]
	Zerit	
tenofovir DF[a] (TDF)	Viread	**Powder, for oral suspension**[b]**:** 40 mg/scoopful **Tablet:** 150 mg,[b] 200 mg,[b] 250 mg,[b] 300 mg
	Viread	
zidovudine[a] (AZT)	Retrovir	**Capsule:** 100 mg **Solution, injection:** 10 mg/mL **Syrup:** 10 mg/1 mL
	Retrovir	
Fixed-Dose Combinations		
abacavir + lamivudine[a]	Epzicom	**Tablet:** 600 mg abacavir + 300 mg lamivudine
	Kivexa	
emtricitabine + tenofovir DF[a]	Truvada	**Tablet:** 200 mg emtricitabine + 300 mg tenofovir DF, 100 mg emtricitabine + 150 mg tenofovir[b], 133 mg emtricitabine + 200 mg tenofovir[b], 167 mg emtricitabine + 250 mg tenofovir[b]
	Truvada	
emtricitabine + tenofovir AF	Descovy	**Tablet:** 200 mg emtricitabine + 25 mg tenofovir AF, 200 mg emtricitabine + 10 mg tenofovir AF[c]
	Descovy	
lamivudine + zidovudine[a]	Combivir	**Tablet:** 150 mg lamivudine + 300 mg zidovudine
	Combivir	
efavirenz + emtricitabine + tenofovir[a]	Atripla	**Tablet:** 600 mg efavirenz + 200 mg emtricitabine + 300 mg tenofovir
	Atripla	
abacavir + lamivudine + zidovudine[a]	Trizivir	**Tablet:** 300 mg abacavir + 150 mg lamivudine + 300 mg zidovudine
	Trizivir	
emtricitabine + rilpivirine + tenofovir DF	Complera	**Tablet:** 200 mg emtricitabine + 25 mg rilpivirine + 300 mg tenofovir
	Complera	
emtricitabine + rilpivirine + tenofovir AF	Odefsey	**Tablet:** 200 mg emtricitabine + 25 mg rilpivirine + 25 mg tenofovir
	Odefsey	
lamivudine + tenofovir + efavirenz	Symfi, Symfi Lo	**Tablet:** 300 mg lamivudine + 300 mg tenofovir + 600 mg efavirenz, 300 mg lamivudine + 300 mg tenofovir + 400 mg efavirenz
	Not Available	

[a]Generic available.
[b]Available in the United States only.
[c]Available in Canada only.
[d]Only Brand names and strength of nucleoside reverse transcriptase inhibitors marketed for the treatment of HIV/AIDS are shown in the table. Additional strengths or Brand names may be marketed for the treatment of additional infections.

AZT may also cause nail discoloration. More severe, less common side effects, are liver problems, muscle inflammation and weakness, diabetes, abnormal fat distribution (lipodystrophy syndrome), high cholesterol, decreased bone density caused by osteonecrosis and osteopenia, skin rash, pancreatitis (inflammation of the pancreas), peripheral neuropathy (especially with DDI and d4T), leukopenia (a drop in the white blood cell count), and increased bleeding in patients with hemophilia.

Nonnucleoside Reverse Transcriptase Inhibitors

NNRTIs bind to viral transcriptase. They differ from NRTIs in three important ways:

1. NNRTIs are noncompetitive inhibitors of reverse transcriptase.
2. They do not need to be activated by host enzymes.
3. They are not effective against HIV-2.

With the exception of nevirapine, NNRTIs are only used in combination therapy with NRTIs and PIs because resistance develops rapidly. All NNRTIs are metabolized by cytochrome P-450 (CYP450) hepatic enzymes and reduce their own $t_{1/2}$ as well as the $t_{1/2}$ of other drugs coadministered with them that are metabolized by the same enzymes. Numerous drug interactions are seen when NNRTIs are administered concurrently with benzodiazepines, HMG-CoA inhibitors (-*statins*), and proton pump inhibitors (-*prazoles*).

Delavirdine

Delavirdine has a short half-life and must be given in multiple daily doses. It is administered three times daily compared with nevirapine and efavirenz, which are dosed once daily. Cross-resistance, frequency of dosing, and the number of tablets per dose (four tablets) have limited the use of delavirdine.

Efavirenz

Efavirenz is an ingredient in several fixed-dose combination medicines used for the treatment of HIV-1 infection. It is also available as a single-ingredient product; however, monotherapy is not recommended because of the rapid development of resistance. The drug is administered by mouth and, because of its long $t_{1/2}$ (40 to 55 hours), it may be given once daily.

Efavirenz is teratogenic. The drug should not be administered in the first trimester of pregnancy, and women taking the drug should be advised to avoid pregnancy.

Nevirapine

Nevirapine is the one NNRTI that may be administered as monotherapy for the prevention of mother-to-child transmission (PMTCT) of HIV. It is administered as a single dose. Controversy exists about the use of single-dose nevirapine therapy because of the risk of developing drug resistance. Treatment of mothers with triple antiretroviral therapy reduces the risk for developing antiretroviral resistance.

Nevirapine is associated with fatal liver toxicity and the FDA has required changes in the package labeling to warn of this adverse effect. Risk for the development of liver toxicity with the use of single doses of nevirapine to the mother and child for the prevention of perinatal HIV infection is minimal.

Adverse Reactions

Rash is a common side effect of all NNRTIs. Nevirapine is associated with fatal hepatotoxicity. The risk is greatest during the first 6 to 18 weeks of therapy and is more common in women than in men. Efavirenz may cause dizziness, drowsiness or insomnia, abnormal dreams, confusion, abnormal thinking, impaired concentration, amnesia, agitation, hallucinations, depersonalization, and euphoria.

Nonnucleoside Reverse Transcriptase Inhibitors Used for the Treatment of Human Immunodeficiency Virus and Acquired Immunodeficiency Syndrome

Generic Name	US Brand Name(s) / Canadian Brand Name(s)	Dosage Forms and Strengths
delavirdine (DLV) Discontinued in the US after available stock depleted in 2020	Rescriptor / Rescriptor	**Tablet:** 100 mg, 200 mg[b]
efavirenz (EFV)[a]	Sustiva / Sustiva	**Capsule:** 50 mg, 200 mg **Tablet:** 600 mg
etravirine (ETV)	Intelence / Intelence	**Tablet:** 25 mg, 100 mg, 200 mg
nevirapine[a] (NVP)	Viramune, Viramune XR / Viramune	**Suspension:** 10 mg/1 mL[b] **Tablet:** 200 mg **Tablet, extended-release (Viramune XR):** 400 mg
rilpivirine (RIL)	Edurant / Edurant	**Tablet:** 25 mg

[a]Generic available.
[b]Available in the United States only.

🛈 TECH ALERT!

A common ending for protease inhibitors is -*navir*.

Protease Inhibitors

PIs interfere with step 8 of the HIV life cycle. They block the cleavage of long-chain viral proteins into individual proteins that are assembled to make a new virus. PIs are administered as combination therapy; most are recommended to be given along with ritonavir.

Fosamprenavir

Fosamprenavir is indicated for the treatment of HIV-1 infection. Fosamprenavir is a prodrug that is metabolized to the active drug amprenavir. The effect of fosamprenavir is boosted with the coadministration of ritonavir.

Atazanavir

Atazanavir is another PI that is effective against HIV-1. Its effectiveness is increased when the drug is coadministered with ritonavir. Concurrent administration with the NNRTI efavirenz can decrease its bioavailability. Atazanavir may be given orally once daily. Administration with a light meal increases bioavailability compared with a heavy meal or fasting.

Darunavir

Darunavir has advantages over other PIs in that cross-resistance is low and it produces a greater reduction in viral load after 24 weeks of treatment. Like other PIs, it must be administered along with ritonavir. Darunavir and atazanavir are also formulated as a combination product with cobicistat and other antiviral agents. Cobicistat (Tybost®) is a CYP3A inhibitor that decreases the metabolism of the drugs, thereby increasing systemic exposure to antiretroviral agents used for the treatment of HIV-1 infection.

Indinavir

Indinavir must be administered in three daily doses. Absorption is affected by food so the drug is taken on an empty stomach. To avoid the formation of kidney stones, indinavir should be taken with at least 1.5 L of water daily. The effects of indinavir are boosted by the coadministration of ritonavir.

Nelfinavir

Nelfinavir is a competitive inhibitor of HIV protease that is typically administered as part of a three-drug regimen that includes indinavir, efavirenz, and/or abacavir. Unlike indinavir and atazanavir, the absorption of nelfinavir is enhanced by a fatty meal. Nelfinavir should be taken with food. Nelfinavir oral powder is stable for six hours, once mixed with food or liquid, if refrigerated.

Ritonavir

Ritonavir is a competitive inhibitor of HIV protease. It differs from other PIs in that it is effective against HIV-1 and HIV-2 proteases. Ritonavir boost the effects of other PIs by inhibiting their metabolism, and resistance appears to occur more slowly than with other PIs. Ritonavir inhibits the metabolic enzyme CYP3A4. It is formulated as single entity and a fixed-dose combination with lopinavir (Kaletra). Lopinavir/ritonavir (LPV/r) is available in multiple formulations. The syrup formulation must be refrigerated thus the cold chain must be maintained until dispensing. It has good oral bioavailability but adverse effects are common and occur in more than 85% of those taking the drug.

Saquinavir

Saquinavir is formulated as a hard gelatin capsule and a film-coated tablet. Bioavailability following oral administration is low for both formulations. Extensive first-pass metabolism further reduces the actions of the drug. Similar to other PIs, saquinavir's effects are boosted by coadministration with ritonavir. Saquinavir should be taken with food.

Tipranavir

Tipranavir is a sulfonamide that selectively binds to HIV-1 protease. It has a lower rate for the development of resistance than some other PIs. Like other PIs, tipranavir is not used for monotherapy but is administered with other antiretrovirals. It should be taken with food to increase absorption.

Adverse Reactions

PIs can elevate triglyceride, cholesterol (see Chapter 19), and blood glucose levels, and can produce insulin resistance (see Chapter 26). They also cause the redistribution of fat, causing its accumulation in the abdomen and loss in the face and limbs. All PIs produce nausea, vomiting, and diarrhea.

Fusion Inhibitors

Fusion inhibitors interfere with step 2 in the HIV life cycle. Fusion (the attachment of the HIV to the host cell membrane) is required for the virus capsid to release its contents (genetic material) into the host cell.

Protease Inhibitors Used for the Treatment of HIV and AIDS

Generic Name	US Brand Name(s) / Canadian Brand Name(s)	Dosage Forms and Strengths
atazanavir (ATV)[a]	Reyataz / Reyataz	**Powder, oral:** 50 mg per packet **Capsule:** 150 mg, 200 mg, 300 mg
darunavir (DRV)	Prezista / Prezista	**Suspension:** 100 mg/mL **Tablet:** 75 mg, 150 mg, 600 mg, 800 mg
fosamprenavir (FPV)[ab]	Lexiva / Telzir	**Suspension:** 50 mg/mL **Tablet:** 700 mg
indinavir (IDV)	Crixivan / Not available	**Capsule:** 200 mg, 400 mg
nelfinavir (NFV)	Viracept / Viracept	**Tablet:** 250 mg, 625 mg
ritonavir (RTV)[ab]	Norvir / Norvir	**Powder, oral**[b]: 100 mg per packet **Solution, Oral:** 80 mg/mL **Tablet:** 100 mg
saquinavir (SQV)	Invirase / Invirase	**Capsule:** 200 mg **Tablet:** 500 mg
tipranavir	Aptivus / Aptivus	**Capsule:** 250 mg **Solution, oral**[b]: 100 mg/mL
Combination		
atazanavir + cobicistat	Evotaz / Not available	**Tablet:** 300 mg atazanavir + 150 mg cobicistat
darunavir + cobicistat	Prezcobix / Prezcobix	**Tablet:** 800 mg darunavir + 150 mg cobicistat
lopinavir + ritonavir[ab]	Kaletra / Kaletra	**Solution, oral:** 80 mg/mL lopinavir + 20 mg/mL ritonavir **Tablet:** 100 mg lopinavir + 25 mg ritonavir; 200 mg lopinavir + 50 mg ritonavir
darunavir + cobicistat + emtricitabine + tenofovir	Symtuza / Symtuza	**Tablet:** 800 mg darunavir + 150 mg cobicistat + 200 mg emtricitabine + 10 mg tenofovir

[ab]Generic available in the United States.
[b]Available in the United States only.

Enfuvirtide must be administered by subcutaneous injection in the thigh, arm, or abdomen. It is formulated as a powder that is reconstituted prior to administration. Once reconstituted, the solution is stable for only 24 hours if refrigerated. Enfuvirtide is intended to be administered in combination with other antiretrovirals.

Adverse Reactions

Irritation, pain, redness, itchiness, and the formation of nodules and cysts at the site of injection are common adverse reactions. Allergic reactions also occur and produce rash, chills, fever, stiffness, hypotension, nausea, and vomiting.

Fusion Inhibitors Used for the Treatment of Human Immunodeficiency Virus and Acquired Immunodeficiency Syndrome

Generic Name	US Brand Name(s) Canadian Brand Name(s)	Dosage Forms and Strengths
enfuvirtide (T-20)	Fuzeon Fuzeon	**Powder, for solution:** 90 mg/vial,[a] 108 mg/vial[b]

[a]Available in the United States only.
[b]Available in Canada only.

Chemokine Receptor Type 5 Antagonist

Maraviroc is a human CCR5. It is the only agent in this class and is a novel drug for the treatment of HIV. It inhibits HIV entry into host cells.

Mechanism of Action

Maraviroc is a selective CCR5 antagonist of the G protein-coupled receptor found on the cell surface. It is associated with entry of the HIV virus into human host cells. Maraviroc binding to the CCR5 receptor prevents CCR5-tropic HIV-1 entry into cells. It does not prevent cell entry mediated by CXCR4 receptor binding of dual or mixed receptor binding.

Adverse Effects

The most common side effects of maraviroc are colds, cough, fever, rash, and dizziness. Myocardial infarction, hepatotoxicity, and increased infections or cancers have also been reported.

Chemokine Receptor Antagonist, Type 5 Antagonists Used for the Treatment of Human Immunodeficiency Virus and Acquired Immunodeficiency Syndrome

Generic Name	US Brand Name(s) Canadian Brand Name(s)	Dosage Forms and Strengths
maraviroc	Selzentry Celsentri	**Solution, oral**[a]: 20 mg/mL **Tablet:** 25 mg[a], 75 mg[a], 150 mg, 300 mg

[a]Available in the United States only.

Human Immunodeficiency Virus Integrase Strand Inhibitors

Dolutegravir, elvitegravir, bictegravir, and raltegravir are HIV integrase strand inhibitors. HIV resistance to raltegravir can develop quickly so it is indicated only in combination with other antiretroviral agents.

Human Immunodeficiency Virus Integrase Strand Inhibitors Used for the Treatment of Human Immunodeficiency Virus and Acquired Immunodeficiency Syndrome

Generic Name	US Brand Name(s) Canadian Brand Name(s)	Dosage Forms and Strengths
dolutegravir (DTG)	Tivicay Tivicay	**Tablet:** 10 mg, 25 mg, 50 mg
raltegravir (RAL)	Isentress, Isentress HD Isentress, Isentress HD	**Powder, oral**[a]: 100 mg per packet **Tablet, chewable:** 25 mg, 100 mg **Tablet:** 400 mg, 600 mg
Combination Integrase Strand Inhibitors		
dolutegravir + abacavir + lamivudine	Triumeq Triumeq	**Tablet:** 50 mg dolutegravir + 600 mg abacavir + 300 mg lamivudine
elvitegravir + cobicistat (COBI) + emtricitabine + tenofovir DF	Stribild Stribild	**Tablet:** 150 mg elvitegravir + 150 mg cobicistat + 200 mg emtricitabine + 300 mg tenofovir DF
elvitegravir + cobicistat (COBI) + emtricitabine + tenofovir AF	Genvoya Genvoya	**Tablet:** 150 mg elvitegravir + 150 mg cobicistat + 200 mg emtricitabine + 10 mg tenofovir AF
bictegravir + emtricitabine + tenofovir AF	Biktarvy Biktarvy	**Tablet:** 50 mg bictegravir + 200 mg emtricitabine + 25 mg tenofovir AF

[a]Available in the United States only.

Mechanism of Action

HIV integrase strand inhibitors block the final step in the process of human host cell infection by HIV. The HIV-1 integrase viral enzyme binds to the double-stranded viral DNA and mediates its integration into the infected host cell's DNA to produce a functional provirus.

Adverse Effects

Raltegravir side effects include headache, dizziness, diarrhea, and GI upset. Rhabdomyolysis, depression, suicide ideation, thrombocytopenia, and increased cancers have also been reported.

> **⊘ TECH ALERT!**
>
> Isentress chewable tablets and suspension are not interchangeable. Do not substitute.

TECHNICIAN'S CORNER

1. We have yet to find a cure for the common cold. Why is it difficult to find that cure?
2. HPV is spreading among teens. Why is it important to reduce the risk for HPV infection? Who should be vaccinated?

Summary of Drugs Used for the Treatment of Human Immunodeficiency Virus-Acquired Immunodeficiency Syndrome

Generic Name	Brand Name	Usual Dose and Dosing Schedule	Warning Labels
Nucleoside Reverse Transcriptase Inhibitors			
abacavir	Ziagen	300 mg bid or 600 mg once daily	TAKE EXACTLY AS DIRECTED; DON'T SKIP DOSES—All AVOID ALCOHOL—abacavir, lamivudine PROTECT FROM MOISTURE—abacavir, stavudine SWALLOW WHOLE; DON'T CRUSH OR CHEW (EXTENDED-RELEASE)—didanosine TAKE ON AN EMPTY STOMACH—didanosine DISCARD 30 DAYS AFTER RECONSTITUTION (ORAL SOLUTION)—didanosine, stavudine REFRIGERATE; DO NOT FREEZE (SOLUTION)—didanosine, emtricitabine, stavudine REFRIGERATE DILUTED IV SOLUTION (STABLE FOR 24 H AT ROOM TEMPERATURE)—zidovudine (IV); TAKE WITH FOOD—tenofovir DF TAKE WITH LOTS OF WATER—zidovudine DISCARD AFTER 48 H AFTER MIXING—zidovudine (IV)
didanosine	Videx	Varies according to body weight **Delayed-release capsule:** 400 mg once daily (>60 kg) **Oral solution:** 250 mg twice daily (<60 kg)	
emtricitabine	Emtriva	Varies according to body weight and dosage form **Capsule:** 200 mg once daily (>33 kg) **Oral solution:** 6 mg/kg up to 240 mg once daily	
lamivudine	Epivir	300 mg once daily or 150 mg twice daily	
stavudine	Zerit	**Oral solution or capsule:** 40 mg every 12 h (>60 kg) or 30 mg every 12 h (<60 kg)	
tenofovir DF	Viread	300 mg once daily	
zidovudine	Retrovir	**Oral:** 300 mg PO twice daily or 200 mg PO 3 times a day **IV:** 1 mg/kg IV given 5 or 6 times daily, around the clock	
lamivudine + zidovudine	Combivir	1 tablet twice daily	AVOID ALCOHOL—Combivir TAKE ON AN EMPTY STOMACH—didanosine, Atripla, Symfi
abacavir + lamivudine	Epzicom	1 tablet once daily	
emtricitabine + tenofovir	Truvada	1 tablet once daily	
efavirenz + emtricitabine + tenofovir	Atripla	1 tablet daily at bedtime	
efavirenz + lamivudine + tenofovir	Symfi	1 tablet daily	
abacavir + lamivudine + zidovudine	Trizivir	1 tablet twice daily	
emtricitabine + tenofovir AF	Descovy	1 tablet once daily	
emtricitabine + rilpivirine + tenofovir AF	Odefsey	1 tablet once daily	
Nonnucleoside Reverse Transcriptase Inhibitors			
delavirdine	Rescriptor	400 mg 3 times a day	TAKE EXACTLY AS DIRECTED; DON'T SKIP DOSES—All AVOID ANTACIDS WITHIN 1 H OF DOSE—delavirdine TAKE ON AN EMPTY STOMACH—efavirenz TAKE WITH FOOD—rilpivirine MAY CAUSE DIZZINESS OR DROWSINESS; ALCOHOL INTENSIFIES THIS EFFECT—efavirenz AVOID PREGNANCY.—efavirenz SHAKE GENTLY (SUSPENSION)—nevirapine
efavirenz	Sustiva	600 mg once daily	
etravirine (ETV)	Intelence	200 mg twice a day	
nevirapine	Viramune	200 mg once daily for the first 14 days, then 200 mg twice daily **Extended release:** 400 mg once daily	
rilpivirine (RIL)	Edurant	25 mg once daily	

Summary of Drugs Used for the Treatment of Human Immunodeficiency Virus-Acquired Immunodeficiency Syndrome—cont'd

Generic Name	Brand Name	Usual Dose and Dosing Schedule	Warning Labels
Protease Inhibitors			
atazanavir	Reyataz	400 mg once daily or 300 mg once daily (taken with ritonavir)	TAKE EXACTLY AS DIRECTED; DON'T SKIP DOSES—All AVOID ANTACIDS WITHIN 1 H OF DOSE—atazanavir SWALLOW WHOLE; DON'T CRUSH OR CHEW—atazanavir, Kaletra TAKE WITH FOOD—atazanavir, darunavir, fosamprenavir (peds suspension), nelfinavir, ritonavir, saquinavir, tipranavir, Kaletra TAKE ON AN EMPTY STOMACH—indinavir MAINTAIN ADEQUATE HYDRATION—indinavir PROTECT FROM MOISTURE—indinavir REFRIGERATE, DON'T FREEZE—ritonavir, tipranavir, Kaletra SHAKE WELL (SUSPENSION)—ritonavir CAPSULE STABLE FOR 30 DAYS (ritonavir), 60 DAYS (tipranavir) AT ROOM TEMPERATURE. SOLUTION STABLE FOR 60 DAYS AT ROOM TEMPERATURE—Kaletra
darunavir	Prezista	800 mg once daily or 600 mg twice daily (taken with ritonavir)	
fosamprenavir	Lexiva, Telzir	700 mg twice daily or 1,400 mg once daily (taken with ritonavir) or 1,400 mg twice daily	
indinavir	Crixivan	800 mg every 8 h or 800 mg twice daily with ritonavir	
nelfinavir	Viracept	1250 mg twice daily or 750 mg 3 times a day	
ritonavir	Norvir	600 mg twice daily (as sole PI) or 100–400 mg once daily when taken to boost the effect of other antiretrovirals	
saquinavir	Invirase	1000 mg twice daily (taken with ritonavir)	
tipranavir	Aptivus	500 mg twice daily (taken with ritonavir)	
lopinavir + ritonavir	Kaletra	Three capsules, 5 mL, or 2 tablets twice daily (400 mg lopinavir + 100 mg ritonavir) *or* Six capsules, 10 mL, or 4 tablets once daily (800 mg lopinavir + 200 mg ritonavir)	
Fusion Inhibitor			
enfuvirtide	Fuzeon	90 mg subcutaneously twice daily	TAKE EXACTLY AS DIRECTED; DON'T SKIP DOSES. REFRIGERATE DILUTED SOLUTION, DON'T FREEZE; DISCARD AFTER 24 H
CCR5 Antagonist			
maraviroc	Selzentry, Celsentri	150–600 mg twice daily	TAKE EXACTLY AS DIRECTED; DON'T SKIP DOSES. MAY CAUSE DIZZINESS OR DROWSINESS

Continued

Summary of Drugs Used for the Treatment of Human Immunodeficiency Virus-Acquired Immunodeficiency Syndrome—cont'd

Generic Name	Brand Name	Usual Dose and Dosing Schedule	Warning Labels
HIV Integrase Strand Inhibitor			
dolutegravir	Tivicay	50 mg once daily	TAKE EXACTLY AS DIRECTED; DON'T SKIP DOSES.
raltegravir	Isentress	400 mg twice	SWALLOW WHOLE; DON'T CRUSH OR CHEW— dolutegravir
			TAKE SUSPENSION WITHIN 30 MIN AFTER MIXING- raltegravir
dolutegravir + abacavir + lamivudine	Triumeq	1 tablet once daily	TAKE EXACTLY AS DIRECTED; DON'T SKIP DOSES.
elvitegravir + cobicistat (COBI) + emtricitabine + tenofovir DF	Stribild	1 tablet once daily	TAKE CALCIUM, IRON, OR ANTACIDS AT LEAST 2 H BEFORE OR 6 H AFTER DOSE—Genvoya, Stribild, Triumeq
elvitegravir + cobicistat (COBI) + emtricitabine + tenofovir AF	Genvoya	1 tablet once daily.	TAKE WITH FOOD—Genvoya, Stribild
bictegravir + emtricitabine + tenofovir AF	Biktarvy	1 tablet once daily	

Key Points

- A virus is an intracellular parasite that consists of a DNA or RNA core surrounded by a protein coat and sometimes an outer covering of lipoprotein.
- The infectious particles (virions) do not have the cellular components necessary for reproduction, so they use their host's cellular machinery to replicate.
- Viruses may cause minor illness, such as the common cold and warts, or serious infections, such as HIV infection, smallpox, and hepatitis C.
- Some viruses are linked to cancer; for example, HPV is associated with cervical cancer.
- An antiviral is a medication that is able to inhibit viral replication.
- All antiviral agents work best when the host (the individual with the infection) has a healthy immune system.
- Effective treatment of viral infections is dependent on host, virus, and antiviral agent factors.
- Some viruses can lay dormant in host cells and periodically awaken to cause recurrent disease.
- Antivirals are only effective against a specific virus.
- Antivirals inhibit virus-specific steps in the replication cycle.
- Antibiotics are not effective against viral infections.
- Viruses may become resistant to the suppressive action of antiviral agents.
- Amantadine and rimantadine inhibit viral uncoating of the influenza A virus, a necessary step in the virus replication process.
- Oseltamivir and zanamivir are indicated for the treatment of influenza A and influenza B. They are neuraminidase inhibitors. Neuraminidase inhibitors inhibit viral release.

- Interferons protect uninfected cells by promoting a resistance to virus infection.
- Interferon alfacon-1 and peginterferon alfa-2b are indicated for the treatment of hepatitis C virus.
- Interferon alfa-2b and peginterferon alfa-2a may be used for the treatment of hepatitis B and hepatitis C.
- Acyclovir, famciclovir, and valacyclovir are used for the treatment of HSV-1, the virus that causes cold sores; HSV-2, one of the viruses that cause genital warts; and VZV, the virus that causes chickenpox and shingles.
- Cidofovir, foscarnet, and ganciclovir are indicated for the treatment of CMV infections.
- Penciclovir is a metabolite of famciclovir used for the treatment of cold sores.
- Trifluridine is used to treat herpes keratoconjunctivitis of the eye.
- Ribavirin is used to treat RSV and hepatitis C when combined with interferon alfa.
- HIV is the virus that causes AIDS. The virus attacks CD4 T lymphocytes and weakens the immune system.
- The steps in the HIV life cycle are (1) binding, (2) fusion, (3) uncoating, (4) reverse transcription, (5) integration, (6) genome replication, (7) protein synthesis, (8) protein cleavage and assembly, and (9) virus release.
- Six classes of antiretrovirals are used to treat HIV infections: (1) NRTIs, (2) NNRTIs, (3) PIs, (4) fusion inhibitors, (5) CCR5, and (6) HIV integrase strand inhibitors.
- HAART, a combination of three or more medications, is prescribed in order to reduce antiretroviral resistance.

- Many NRTIs are prodrugs.
- Abacavir, DDI, emtricitabine, lamivudine, stavudine, tenofovir, and zidovudine are NRTIs that competitively inhibit reverse transcriptase, the enzyme that makes a DNA copy of the viral RNA.
- With the exception of nevirapine, NNRTIs are only used in combination therapy with NRTIs and protease inhibitors because resistance develops rapidly.
- Delavirdine, efavirenz, etravirine, nevirapine, and rilpivirine are NNRTIs.
- Nevirapine and zidovudine are used to prevent MTCT of HIV.
- Nevirapine is associated with fatal liver toxicity.
- PIs interfere with step 8 of the HIV life cycle. They block the cleavage of long-chain viral proteins into individual proteins that are assembled to make a new virus.

- PIs are administered as combination therapy.
- Atazanavir, darunavir, fosamprenavir, indinavir, nelfinavir, ritonavir, saquinavir, and tipranavir are PIs.
- Ritonavir is effective against HIV-1 and HIV-2 proteases.
- Enfuvirtide is a fusion inhibitor. It interferes with attachment of HIV to the host cell membrane (step 2 in the HIV life cycle).
- Maraviroc is a CCR5 antagonist that inhibits HIV entry into host cells.
- Dolutegravir, elvitegravir, bictegravir, and raltegravir are HIV integrase strand inhibitors that block the final step in the process of human host cell infection by HIV.
- Cobicistat inhibits the metabolism of antivirals (e.g., darunavir and atazanavir), thereby increasing systemic exposure to the antiretroviral agents.

Review Questions

1. _____is the most severe form of HIV infection.
   a. CMV
   b. AIDS
   c. HPV
   d. HSV
2. The warning label TAKE WITH FOOD should be applied to the vial of all of the following prescriptions, EXCEPT_____.
   a. Genvoya
   b. Kaletra
   c. Norvir
   d. Atripla
3. An antiviral is a medication that is able to _____ viral replication.
   a. Stimulate
   b. Inhibit
   c. Proliferate
   d. Induce
4. All of the following antivirals are combination products used to treat hepatitis C except _____.
   a. Solvadi
   b. Technivie
   c. Viekira Pak (Holkira Pak)
   d. Harvoni
5. Which of the following antivirals is indicated for the treatment of cold sores?
   a. Acyclovir
   b. Ganciclovir
   c. Cidofovir
   d. Saquinavir
6. Human immunodeficiency virus (HIV) is the virus that causes acquired immunodeficiency syndrome (AIDS). The virus attacks _____ and weakens the immune system.
   a. CD4 monocytes
   b. CD4 T lymphocytes
   c. CD2 T lymphocytes
   d. None of the above

7. All of the following antivirals and antiretrovirals liquids should be stored in the refrigerator, EXCEPT_____.
   a. Tamiflu suspension
   b. Valtrex suspension
   c. Kaletra suspension
   d. Rebetol Solution
8. Lamivudine is an NRTI that is effective against _____.
   a. HIV
   b. HBV
   c. CMV
   d. a and b
9. All of the following antiretrovirals are marketed in liquid formulations for pediatric use, EXCEPT_____.
   a. tenofovir DF (Viread), stavudine (Zerit), lamivudine (Epivir)
   b. didanosine (Videx EC), Zidovudine (Retrovir), Nevirapine (Viramune)
   c. fosamprenavir (Lexiva, Telzir), ritonavir (Norvir), lopinavir + ritonavir (Kaletra)
   d. dolutegravir (Tivicay), saquinavir (Invirase), nelfinavir (Viracept)
10. The warning label SWALLOW WHOLE; DON'T CRUSH OR CHEW should be applied to the vial of all of the following prescriptions, EXCEPT_____.
    a. True Viekira XR
    b. Videx EC
    c. Triumeq
    d. Kaletra

Bibliography

Canadian AIDS Treatment Information Exchange: HIV viral load testing, 2007. http://www.catie.ca/sites/default/files/Viral%20Load.pdf.

Centers for Disease Control and Prevention: Morbidity and mortality weekly report. In Moolenaar R, editor: *Antiviral agents for the treatment and chemoprophylaxis of influenza*, vol 60, 2011.

Center for Disease Control and Prevention: Antiviral Drug Resistance among Influenza Viruses, 2016. Retrieved October 5, 2017, from https://www.cdc.gov/flu/professionals/antivirals/antiviral-drug-resistance.htm.

Center for Disease Control and Prevention: Influenza Antiviral Drug Resistance, 2017. Retrieved October 5, 2017, from https://www.cdc.gov/flu/about/qa/antiviralresistance.htm.

Dorr P, Westby M, Dobbs S, et al: Maraviroc (UK-427,857), a potent, orally bioavailable, and selective small-molecule inhibitor of chemokine receptor CCR5 with broad-spectrum anti-human immunodeficiency virus type 1 activity, *Antimicrob Agents Chemother* 49:4721–4732, 2005.

Drug Information Handbook pp 53, 1940–1941. 24th Ed.

Erratum: Vol. 60, No. RR-1. MMWR Morb Mortal Wkly Rep 2017;66:707. DOI: http://dx.doi.org/10.15585/mmwr.mm6626a7.

Fiore AE, Fry A, Shay D, Centers for Disease Control and Prevention (CDC), et al: Antiviral agents for the treatment and chemoprophylaxis of influenza—recommendations of the Advisory Committee on Immunization Practices (ACIP), *MMWR Recomm Rep* 60:1–24, 2011.

Global AIDS update, 2017. http://www.unaids.org/.

Health Canada: Drug Product Database, 2018. Retrieved September 20, 2018, from https://health-products.canada.ca/dpd-bdpp/index-eng.jsp.

Institute for Safe Medication Practices: List of Confused Drugs, 2015. Retrieved September 9, 2017, from https://www.ismp.org/tools/confuseddrugnames.pdf.

Kalant H, Grant D, Mitchell J: *Principles of medical pharmacology*, ed 7, Toronto, 2007, Elsevier Canada, pp 739–759.

Kumar S, Jacobson IM: Antiviral therapy with nucleotide polymerase inhibitors for chronic hepatitis C, *J Hepatol* 61:S91–S97, 2014.

McColl DJ, Chen X: Strand transfer inhibitors of HIV-1 integrase: Bringing in a new era of antiretroviral therapy, *Antiviral Res* 85:101–118, 2010.

Menendez-Arias L, Alvarez M, Pacheco B: Nucleoside/nucleotide analog inhibitors of hepatitis B virus polymerase: mechanism of action and resistance, *Curr Opin Virol* 8:1–9, 2014.

Page C, Curtis M, Sutter M, et al: *Integrated pharmacology*, Philadelphia, 2005, Elsevier Mosby, pp 91–109.

Rathbun RC, Liedtke MD, Lockhart SM: Antiretroviral therapy for HIV infection, 2017. Retrieved October 27, 2017, from https://emedicine.medscape.com/article/1533218-overview.

Wong GL-H, Wong VW-S, Chan HL-Y: Combination therapy of interferon and nucleotide/nucleoside analogues for chronic hepatitis B, *J Viral Hepat* 21:825–834, 2014.

World Health Organization: Programmatic Update: Use of Antiretroviral Drugs for Treating Pregnant Women and Preventing HIV Infections in Infants, 2012. From www.who.int/hiv/PMTCT_update.pdf.

World Health Organization Implementation tool for pre-exposure prophylaxis (PrEP) of HIV infection, 2017. Module 6: Pharmacists. Geneva: World Health Organization. Licence: CC BY-NC-SA 3.0 IGO.

World Health Organization: Consolidated guidelines on the use of antiretroviral drugs for treating and preventing HIV infection: recommendations for a public health approach, 2016. Retrieved from http://www.who.int/hiv/pub/arv/arv-2016/en/.

Tech corner – HPV. Retrieved from https://www.cdc.gov/vaccines/parents/diseases/teen/hpv.html.

US Food and Drug Administration: (nd). Drugs@FDA: FDA Approved Drug Products. Retrieved September 20, 2018, from http://www.accessdata.fda.gov/scripts/cder/daf/.

US Food and Drug Administration: Hepatitis B and C Treatments, 2017. From https://www.fda.gov/forpatients/illness/hepatitisbc/ucm408658.htm.

31

Treatment of Cancers

LEARNING OBJECTIVES

1. Learn the terminology associated with cancer.
2. Identify risk factors for breast, colorectal, lung, prostate, skin, uterine, and ovarian cancer.
3. Identify causes for breast, colorectal, lung, prostate, skin, uterine, and ovarian cancer.
4. List, categorize, and describe the mechanism of action for medications used for the treatment of breast, colorectal, lung, prostate, skin, uterine, and ovarian cancer.
5. List common endings and/or beginnings for drug classes used for the treatment of breast, colorectal, lung, prostate, skin, uterine, and ovarian cancer.
6. Identify significant drug look-alike and sound-alike issues.
7. Identify warning labels and precautionary messages associated with medications used for the treatment of breast, colorectal, lung, prostate, skin, uterine, and ovarian cancer.

KEY TERMS

Benign Refers to a tumor that is not cancerous and does not spread to surrounding tissues or other parts of the body.

Cancer Term for diseases in which abnormal cells divide without control. Specific cancers are named according to the site at which the cancerous growth begins.

Chemotherapy Treatment with drugs that kill cancerous cells.

Complementary and alternative medicine Treatments that may include dietary supplements, herbal preparations, acupuncture, massage, magnet therapy, spiritual healing, and meditation.

Malignant Cancerous tumors that can invade and destroy nearby tissue and spread to other parts of the body.

Mammogram Screening examination to detect breast cancer in which a radiograph of the breast is taken.

Melanoma Form of skin cancer that arises in melanocytes, the cells that produce pigment.

Metastasis Spread of cancer from one part of the body to another.

Neoplasm An abnormal mass of tissue that results when cells divide more than they should or do not die when they should. Also called tumor.

Oncovirus Virus that is a causative agent of a cancer.

Pap test Is a procedure to detect cervical cancer that involves removal and examination of a few cells from the cervix.

Polyp Growth that protrudes from a mucous membrane.

Prostate-specific antigen test Test that measures the level of free prostate-specific antigen, a protein produced by the prostate gland. Levels are elevated in men who have prostate cancer, infection, or inflammation of the prostate gland, and benign prostatic hyperplasia.

Radiation therapy Use of high-energy radiation from X-rays, gamma rays, neutrons, and other sources to kill cancer cells and shrink tumors.

Stage Extent of a cancer within the body. Staging is based on the size of the tumor, whether lymph nodes contain cancer, and whether the disease has spread from the original site to other parts of the body.

Stem cell Undifferentiated cells that can develop into many different cell types.

Tumor marker Substance sometimes found in the blood, other body fluids, or tissues that may signal the presence of a certain type of cancer; for example, a high level of prostate-specific antigen is a signal for possible prostate cancer.

What Is Cancer?

Cancer is a disease that occurs when the normal cell renewal process fails. When old cells fail to die and new cells form more rapidly than needed, the cells may accumulate and form a mass called a *neoplasm* (also called a tumor). Tumors are caused by abnormal cell division. They may be benign or malignant. A *malignant* tumor is cancerous and can invade and destroy nearby tissue and spread via *metastasis* to other parts of the body, whereas a *benign* tumor is not cancerous and does not spread. Specific cancers are named according to the site at which the cancerous growth began. This is the site of the primary tumor. For example, with melanoma cancerous cells form in the skin; cancerous cells in blood-forming tissues lead to leukemia; in osteosarcoma bone-forming cells become cancerous; and in lymphoma cancerous cells form in the immune system.

Risk Factors for Cancer

There are many risk factors for cancer, including age, tobacco use, and exposure to ionizing radiation (Box 31.1).

Age

The risk for developing cancer increases with age. Cancers are more prevalent in persons over the age of 65 years.

• BOX 31.1   Risk Factors for Cancer

- Increasing age
- Tobacco
- Environmental pollutants
- Ionizing radiation
- Sunlight and tanning salons (UV light)
- Carcinogenic chemicals (e.g., benzene)
- Viruses (e.g., HPV, EBV)
- Bacteria (e.g., *Helicobacter pylori*)
- Hormone therapy (e.g., DES)
- Family history
- Alcohol

Tobacco

Inhalation of cigarette, cigar, and pipe tobacco smoke may increase the risk for developing cancer of the lungs, larynx, mouth, esophagus, bladder, kidney, throat, stomach, pancreas, and cervix, and acute myeloid leukemia. Smokers as well as nonsmokers exposed to second-hand tobacco smoke are at increased risk. Chewing tobacco may increase the risk for oral cancer.

Ionizing Radiation and Sunlight

X-rays, nuclear fallout (from atomic weapons testing or leaks from nuclear power plants), and radon gas are examples of ionizing radiation. Exposure increases the risk for the development of leukemia, thyroid cancer, and breast cancer. Exposure to radon gas may increase the risk for developing lung cancer.

Exposure to sunlight is necessary for the skin to make the hormone vitamin D. Excessive exposure to the sun's ultraviolet (UV) radiation can increase the risk for skin cancer (*melanoma*). The ozone layer of the atmosphere provides protection from excessive exposure to UV radiation, prompting concerns over depletion of the earth's ozone layer. UVA levels are highest during midday, whereas UVB levels are found throughout the day. Exposure to UV light from sunlamps and tanning booths also increases cancer risk.

Hazardous Chemicals and Environmental Pollutants

Cancer-causing chemicals (carcinogens) are found in the workplace, home, and environment through pollution. Industrial solvents, cleaning fluids, pesticides, and used engine oil are examples of hazardous chemicals. Known workplace carcinogens include benzene, vinyl chloride, polychlorinated biphenyls (PCBs), asbestos, cadmium, and nickel. These carcinogens may get into the environment through improper disposal or chemical spills, or they are particulates that are released into the air in the process of incineration.

Bacterial and Viral Infection

Exposure to some viruses or bacteria may increase the risk of developing certain cancers. *Helicobacter pylori* is a bacterium known to cause peptic ulcer disease (PUD). PUD is associated with stomach cancer. An *oncovirus* is a virus known to cause cancer. Epstein-Barr virus (EBV), a common virus that remains dormant in most people, has been associated with lymphomas such as Burkitt lymphoma and immunoblastic lymphoma. The virus is also linked to nasopharyngeal carcinoma. Hepatitis B virus (HBV) and hepatitis C virus (HCV) are linked to liver cancer. Human papillomavirus (HPV) is a virus that causes genital warts and cancer of the cervix.

Human immunodeficiency virus (HIV) and human herpesvirus 8 (HHV8) can cause Kaposi sarcoma. Human T cell leukemia virus-type 1 is a retrovirus that can cause leukemia and lymphoma.

Hormone Therapy

Hormone replacement therapy (HRT) and diethylstilbestrol (DES) have been linked to specific cancers. HRT, once the principal treatment for menopausal symptoms, is now limited because of the risk for the development of breast cancer, heart attack, stroke, and blood clots. DES is an estrogen-type drug that was taken by pregnant women between 1940 and 1971. Girls born to women who took DES have a higher risk for cancer of the cervix than girls born to women who did not take the drug. Women who took DES also have a higher incidence of breast cancer.

Family History

It is not known why one individual will develop cancer whereas another does not. With the exception of cancers of the breast, ovary, prostate, skin, and colon, most cancers do not run in families. For example, if a father develops stomach cancer, his children have no greater risk for stomach cancer than would a nonfamily member.

Alcohol

Chronic alcohol consumption (up to two drinks daily over a period of years) may increase the risk for cancer of the liver, mouth, throat, esophagus, larynx, and breast.

Diet, Physical Inactivity, and Obesity

A diet is that is high in fat may increase the risk of cancers of the colon, uterus, and prostate. Cancers of the breast, colon, esophagus, kidney, and uterus are higher in individuals who have little physical activity and are overweight.

Types of Cancers

In this chapter, information is provided about the most common cancers in Canada and the United States. In 2017, the seven most common cancers in the United States were breast, prostate, lung, colon and rectum (colorectal cancer), skin, and endometrium. In Canada, breast, prostate, lung, and colorectal cancer accounted for more than 51% of all cancers in 2015. Cancer of the uterus and bladder ranked within the top seven cancers.

Breast Cancer

Breast cancer is the most common cancer in the United States and Canada. In 2017, there were an estimated 252,700 new cases of breast cancer in the United States. One percent of the cases were men. Approximately 3,327,552 women were living with breast cancer. The survival rate is approximately 89.7%; however, between 2007 and 2013, nearly 40,000 individuals died from breast cancer. The median age at the time of diagnosis is 61 years. One or both breasts may be involved. The following are risk factors for breast cancer: (1) family history and inherited susceptibility (BRCA1 and BRCA2 gene); (2) nulliparity (no pregnancies); (3) early onset of menses (periods); (4) advanced age; (5) dense breast tissue; (6) history of HRT; and (7) excess alcohol intake.

Prostate Cancer

The incidence of prostate cancer increases as men grow older. The median age of diagnosis is 66 years old. Levels begin to slowly decline again after the age of 75. In 2017, there were 161,360 new cases diagnosed and 26,730 deaths in the United States. In 2014, an estimated 3,085,209 men were living with prostate cancer in the United States. In Canada, an estimated 24,000 new cases (24% of males newly diagnosed with any cancer) were diagnosed in 2015. It is estimated that one in eight males will be diagnosed with prostate cancer within their lifetime. Prostate disease, diagnosis, and treatment are described in Chapter 28.

Lung Cancer

Lung cancer is the second most common cancer in men and women. Only breast cancer and prostate cancer are more common. In the United States, the incidence of lung cancer was 55.8/100,000 cases in 2017, almost 222,500 men and women. In Canada, the incidence of lung cancer was 58/100,000 men and 48/100,000 women in 2015. Lung cancer is the leading cause of cancer-related death. The five-year survival rate is only 18.1%. There are two types of lung cancer, small cell lung cancer (SCLC) and non–small cell lung cancer (NSCLC). A history of smoking tobacco is the primary cause of SCLC. Other risk factors are increasing age, exposure to cancer-causing substances (e.g., second-hand smoke, asbestos, radon, atomic radiation), *radiation therapy* and medical imaging (e.g., x-ray to the breast or chest, computed tomography [CT] scans), air pollution, and family history.

Colorectal Cancer

Cancer of the colon and rectum affects millions of American and Canadian men and women. In the United States, there were 135,430 new cases of colorectal cancer (95,520 new cases of colon cancer and 39,910 new cases of rectal cancer). Approximately 1.3 million Americans were living with colorectal cancer in 2014. In Canada, 25,000 new cases or between 48 and 58 cases/100,000 were diagnosed in 2015. Risk factors are obesity, physical inactivity, consumption of red and processed meat, and tobacco use. The first signs of colon cancer may be the appearance of a small *polyp* and blood in the stool. Early detection through the administration of screening examinations helps reduce the numbers of deaths from the disease. Colonoscopy and a fecal occult blood test (FOBT) are screening tests for colorectal cancer.

Skin Cancer

Skin cancer is one of the top five most common cancers. Skin cancer is divided into two categories, melanoma and nonmelanoma. The most treatable form is nonmelanoma. In 2017 there were an estimated 22.3/100,000 (87,110 total) new cases of melanoma of the skin in the United States. In Canada in 2015, there were an estimated 29/100,000 new cases. The five-year survival rate for skin cancer is nearly 92%.

Nonmodifiable risk factors for developing skin cancer are having a fair complexion, personal and family history of skin cancer, or a weakened immune system. Modifiable risk factors are excessive exposure to UV light from the sun or UV lights used in tanning salons, or a history of severe blistering sunburn(s). Protection from harmful UV light is the best way to prevent skin cancer. This can be achieved by wearing protective clothing when outdoors and using sunscreen.

Cancer of the Uterus and Ovaries

The cervix is located at the neck of the uterus and the endometrium lines its inner surface (Fig. 31.1). In Canada, there were an estimated 24/100,000 new cases of cancers of uterus in 2015; the majority were cases of cancer of the endometrium. There were an estimated 25.7/100,000 (61,380 total) new cases of endometrial cancer in the United States in 2017. Endometrial cancer most commonly affects postmenopausal women.

Cancer of the cervix is linked to HPV and exposure to the drug DES while the fetus is still in the uterus. Approximately 8.1/100,000 women are diagnosed annually with cancer of the cervix, and it was estimated that in 2010 almost 12,200 women were diagnosed and 4210 women died from the disease. Cancer of the uterus, obesity, diabetes, genetic predisposition, and never having been pregnant or birthed a child are all risk factors for cancer of the cervix. Disorders of the reproductive system may also cause excessive growth of the endometrium, prevent ovulation, and produce estrogen-secreting ovarian tumors.

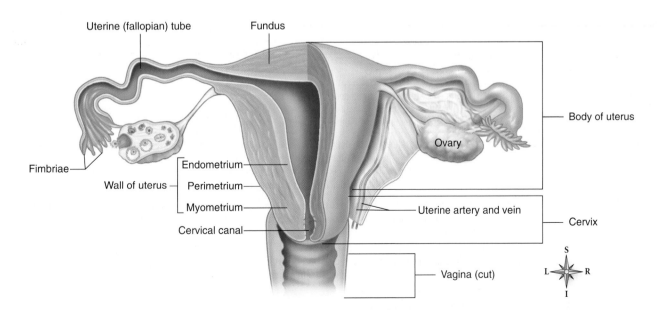

• **Fig. 31.1** Anatomy of the uterus. (From Patton KT, Thibodeau GA: *The human body in health and disease*, ed 7, St. Louis, 2018, Elsevier.)

Cancer Screening Tests

Early diagnosis is critical to successful treatment. Screening tests are recommended for the early diagnosis of breast cancer, colorectal cancer, cancer of the cervix, and prostate cancer. A *mammogram* is a screening examination used to detect breast cancer. A radiograph is taken of the breast and inspected for evidence of tumors. Sonography is an alternative method for screening for breast cancers. If a lump is found, a biopsy is performed. A biopsy is a procedure whereby the cells or tissue is (are) removed for examination by a pathologist. Regular self-examination of the breast is another important method for screening for breast cancer.

Tests to screen for colorectal cancer are the FOBT, colonoscopy, sigmoidoscopy, double-contrast barium enema, and digital rectal examination (see Chapter 28). The FOBT is a test that screens for blood in stool. Bleeding may indicate the presence of polyps or cancer. A colonoscopy and sigmoidoscopy involve the insertion of a lighted tube into the colon to inspect for abnormal growths. The procedure for X-ray screening is to administer a double-contrast barium enema to the patient in order to permit greater visualization of the bowel.

Another method of detection is to identify the presence of a *tumor marker* in the blood, other body fluids, or tissues that may signal the presence of a certain type of cancer. For example, a *prostate-specific antigen* (PSA) test is performed to screen for prostate cancer. PSA is a protein produced by the prostate gland. A high level of PSA is a signal for possible prostate cancer, although benign prostatic hypertrophy and prostate infection may also cause elevated PSA levels (see Chapter 28). A *Pap test* is a screening test for cancer of the cervix. The Pap test is a simple procedure in which cells from the cervix are removed and examined to detect cancer and changes that may lead to cancer.

Treatment of Cancer

Cancer may be treated with chemotherapy, biologic therapy, radiation therapy, and surgery. *Chemotherapy* is the use of drugs to kill or slow the growth of cancerous cells. Biologic therapy is the administration of immune system modulators to boost the body's natural defense against abnormal, invasive, and cancerous cells. Radiation therapy, the use of high-energy radiation from X-rays, gamma rays, neutrons, and other sources can be used to kill cancer cells and shrink tumors. Radiation can be administered externally or as brachytherapy, a procedure in which radioactive material sealed in needles, seeds, wires, or catheters is placed directly into or near a tumor.

Some patients may try *complementary and alternative medicine*, which may include dietary supplements, herbal preparations, acupuncture, massage, magnet therapy, spiritual healing, and meditation. *Stem cell transplantation*, another form of treatment, is a procedure that replaces cells that were destroyed by cancer treatment with stem cells. *Stem cells* are undifferentiated cells that can develop into many different cell types. For example, blood cells develop from blood-forming stem cells. Stem cells act as the body's internal repair system by replenishing cells.

The following factors influence the selection of treatment options: (1) type of cancer; (2) *stage* of cancer; (3) individual tolerance for adverse effects of treatment; (4) patient's age; (5) histological and nuclear grade of the primary tumor; and (6) capacity of the cancer to metastasize. Staging is a method used to describe how far the cancer has progressed within the body. It is based on the size of the tumor, whether lymph nodes contain the cancer, and whether the cancer has spread from the original site to other parts of the body.

This chapter focuses on chemotherapy and immunotherapy of the most common cancers. The therapeutic agents may be administered parenterally or by mouth. They work by various mechanisms to interrupt the cell replication cycle. Some agents are cell cycle–specific; they interrupt a specific stage of the cell cycle (Table 31.1). Examples include mitotic inhibitors, microtubule inhibitors, and deoxyribonucleic acid (DNA) synthesis inhibitors. Other antineoplastic agents are nonspecific. The site of action of chemotherapeutic agents is shown in Fig. 31.2.

TABLE 31.1	Summary of the Cell Life Cycle
Phase of Cell Life Cycle	**Description**
Cell Growth	Interphase
Protein synthesis	Proteins are manufactured according to the cell's genetic code; functional proteins, the enzymes, direct the synthesis of other molecules in the cells, and thus the production of more and larger organelles and plasma membrane; sometimes called the first growth phase, or the G1 phase of interphase
Deoxyribonucleic acid (DNA) replication	Nucleotides, influenced by newly synthesized enzymes, arrange themselves along the open sides of an unzipped DNA molecule, thereby creating two identical daughter DNA molecules; they produce two identical sets of the cell's genetic code, which enables the cell later to split into two different cells, each with its own complete set of DNA; sometimes called the (DNA) synthesis stage or S phase of interphase
Protein synthesis	After DNA is replicated, the cell continues to grow by means of protein synthesis and the resulting synthesis of other molecules and various organelles; this second growth phase is called the G2 phase
Cell Reproduction	M phase
Mitosis or meiosis	The parent cell's replicated set of DNA is divided into two sets separated by an orderly process into distinct cell nuclei; mitosis is subdivided into at least four phases: prophase, metaphase, anaphase, and telophase
Cytokinesis	The plasma membrane of the parent cell pinches in and eventually separates the cytoplasm and two daughter nuclei into two genetically identical daughter cells

From Patton KT, Thibodeau GA: *Anatomy and physiology*, ed 9, St. Louis, 2016, Elsevier.

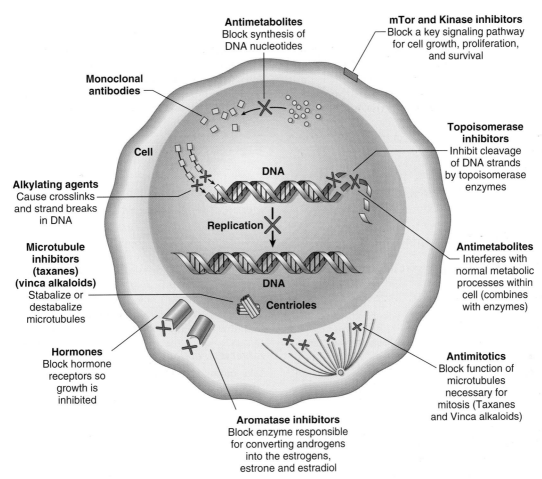

Fig. 31.2 Site of action of chemotherapeutic agents. (From Raffa RB, Rawls SM, Beyzarov EP: *Netter's illustrated pharmacology*, Philadelphia, 2005, WB Saunders.)

Pharmacotherapy for Breast Cancer

Pharmacotherapy for breast cancer includes the administration of selective estrogen receptor (ER) modulators (e.g., tamoxifen), ER downregulators (e.g., fulvestrant), aromatase inhibitors (e.g., anastrozole), and kinase inhibitors (e.g., palbociclib).

> **⚠ TECH ALERT!**
>
> All parenteral chemotherapeutic agents should be prepared in a Class II biohazard safety cabinet or a vertical flow hood containing a high-efficiency particulate air (HEPA) filter with a vertical downward flow of air. The pharmacy technician is protected by a glass front and wears a fluid-proof gown, double gloves, mask, bonnet, shoe covers, and goggles. US Pharmacopeia (USP) guidelines for safety equipment and gear are described in USP General Chapter 800 Hazardous Drugs - Handling in Healthcare Settings (https://www.usp.org/usp-chapter-800-download).

Selective Estrogen Receptor Modulators (SERMs)

The hormones estrogen and progesterone can promote the growth of ER-positive and/or progesterone receptor (PR)-positive breast cancer. The administration of a selective ER modulator (antiestrogen) can reduce the risk of breast cancer recurrence for up to five years after treatment of the primary tumor. Treatment decisions are influenced by the woman's menopausal status, the affinity of the tumor for ERs and PRs, and the human epidermal growth factor receptor 2 (HER2/neu) status (overexpression), in addition to the other factors listed earlier.

Tamoxifen and torimefene are indicated for the treatment of ER-positive breast cancer that is noninvasive or invasive (metastatic). Tamoxifen is approved for the treatment of metastatic breast cancer in premenopausal and postmenopausal women. It is also approved for the treatment of metastatic breast cancer in men. Toremifene is a derivative of tamoxifen that is indicated for the treatment of metastatic breast cancer in postmenopausal women. Raloxifene is indicated for the treatment of osteoporosis, not the treatment of breast cancer. (See Chapter 14.) It has a secondary indication to reduce the risk for invasive breast cancer in post menopausal women with osteoporosis and/or at high risk for invasive breast cancer.

> **⚠ TECH ALERT!**
>
> Tamoxifen should not be taken during pregnancy. The warning label "Avoid Pregnancy" should be applied to the prescription vial.

Mechanism of Action and Pharmacokinetics

Tamoxifen, toremifene, and raloxifene are a selective estrogen receptor modulators (SERM) that compete with estrogen for binding sites. When SERMS occupy the ERs in breast cells they block the effects of estrogen (estrogen antagonist). SERMS can have estrogenic activities in other tissues. For example, raloxifene has agonist effects on bone cell turnover (remodeling), which can decrease postmenopausal bone loss. Tamoxifen has an active metabolite and long half-life and accumulates with continued administration. It may be given once or twice daily.

Adverse Reactions

Tamoxifen and toremifene commonly produce menopause-like symptoms such as hot flashes, sweating, vaginal bleeding, vaginal itchiness, discharge or dryness, nausea, and vomiting. They may additionally cause menstrual changes. Agonist effects on the endometrium double the risks for endometrial cancer. Other adverse effects are pelvic pain, and ocular changes (e.g., cataracts). Tamoxifene and toremifene are contraindicated during pregnancy.

> **⊘ TECH ALERT!**
>
> A dangerous drug-drug interaction that may cause hemorrhage can occur when tamoxifen is taken with the anticoagulant warfarin.

Selective Estrogen Receptor Modulators

Generic Name	US Brand Name(s)	Dosage Forms and Strengths
	Canadian Brand Name(s)	
tamoxifen[a]	Soltamox	**Solution (Soltamox)**[b]: 10 mg/5 mL
	Nolvadex-D	**Tablet:** 10 mg, 20 mg
toremifene	Fareston	**Tablet:** 60 mg
	Not available	

[a]Generic available.
[b]Available in the United States only.

Estrogen Receptor Antagonist

Fulvestrant is indicated for the treatment of ER-positive, HER2-negative metastatic breast cancer in postmenopausal women with disease progression following antiestrogen therapy.

Mechanism of Action and Pharmacokinetics

Fulvestrant is an ER antagonist that produces downregulation of ER protein. It is an analogue of estradiol that acts as a competitive antagonist. When fulvestrant binds to ERs, it inhibits estrogen activity, causes changes in ER function, and triggers ER degradation. Unlike SERMS (e.g., tamoxifene) it does not have partial estrogenic activity. Fulvestrant is administered intramuscularly. Plasma concentrations are maintained at therapeutic levels for up to one month.

Adverse Reactions

Adverse effects caused by fulvestrant include pain at the injection site, generalized bone and back pain, hot flashes, headache, nausea and vomiting, diarrhea or constipation, and weakness. Fulvestrant is contraindicated during pregnancy.

Estrogen Receptor Downregulator

Generic Name	US Brand Name(s)	Dosage Forms and Strengths
	Canadian Brand Name(s)	
fulvestrant	Faslodex	**Solution, for injection:** 50 mg/mL
	Faslodex	

Aromatase Inhibitors

Anastrozole, exemestane, and letrozole are aromatase inhibitors. They may be prescribed alone or in combination with tamoxifen. They are FDA-approved for the first-line treatment of advanced or metastatic ER-positive breast cancer in postmenopausal women. They are also approved as an adjuvant for the treatment of early-stage breast cancer.

> **⊘ TECH ALERT!**
>
> A common ending for aromatase inhibitors is -trozole.

Mechanism of Action and Pharmacokinetics

The adrenal gland is the primary source of estrogen after menopause. Aromatase is an enzyme responsible for converting androgens produced by the adrenal gland into the estrogens, estrone, and estradiol in the peripheral tissues. Aromatase inhibitors block this process. Anastrozole and letrozole are nonsteroidal aromatase inhibitors and are potent inhibitors of serum estradiol levels. Exemestane is a steroidal aromatase inhibitor. It is a more potent inhibitor of estrogen than the other aromatase inhibitors.

Adverse Reactions

Like tamoxifen, aromatase inhibitors produce menopause-like symptoms, nausea, and vomiting. Additional adverse effects include dizziness, cough, headache, hair loss, constipation, mood changes, and bone pain. Administration of steroid aromatase inhibitors requires adrenal HRT to replenish depleted glucocorticoids (cortisol) and mineralocorticoids (aldosterone). Symptoms of adrenal hormone insufficiency are fatigue, weight gain, and edema.

> **⊘ TECH ALERT!**
>
> Femara and FemHRT have look-alike and sound-alike issues.

Aromatase Inhibitors

Generic Name	US Brand Name(s)	Dosage Forms and Strengths
	Canadian Brand Name(s)	
anastrozole[a]	Arimidex	**Tablet:** 1 mg
	Arimidex	
exemestane[a]	Aromasin	**Tablet:** 25 mg
	Aromasin	
letrozole[a]	Femara	**Tablet:** 2.5 mg
	Femara	

[a]Generic available.

Kinase and mTOR Inhibitors

Abemaciclib (Verzenio), palbociclib (Ibrance), ribociclib (Kisqali), lapatinib (Tykerb), and neratinib (Nerlynx) are kinase inhibitors that are indicated for the treatment of hormone receptor (HR)-positive, HER2-negative advanced, or metastatic breast cancer in postmenopausal women. Abemaciclib, palbociclib, and ribociclib are used in combination with an aromatase inhibitor (e.g., anastrozole or letrazole) as initial therapy or with fulvestrant in women with advanced metastatic breast cancer. Lapatinib is approved for the treatment of breast cancer when taken with capecitabine. Neratinib is indicated as adjuvant therapy for early stage HER2-overexpressed breast cancer following treatment the monoclonal antibody trastuzumab.

Everolimus (Afinitor) is an mTOR inhibitor that is used in combination with exemestane to treat postmenopausal women with advanced HR-positive, HER2-negative breast cancer that have already received other medicines for their cancer.

Mechanism of Action and Pharmacokinetics

Kinase inhibitors and mTOR inhibitors block a key signaling pathway for cell growth, proliferation, and survival.

Adverse Reactions

The most common adverse effects of abemaciclib, palbociclib, and ribociclib are diarrhea, anemia, increased infections, fatigue, hair loss, nausea, headache, stomatitis, and fever. Side effects of everolimus are stomatitis, infections, rash, fatigue, diarrhea, edema, abdominal pain, nausea, fever, asthenia, cough, headache, and decreased appetite.

Kinase and mTOR Inhibitors

Generic Name	US Brand Name(s) / Canadian Brand Name(s)	Dosage Forms and Strengths
abemaciclib	Verzenio	**Tablet:** 50 mg, 100 mg, 150 mg, 200 mg
	Not Available	
everolimus	Afinitor, Afinitor Disperz	**Tablet (Afinitor):** 2.5 mg, 5 mg, 7.5 mg, 10 mg **Tablet, for suspension (Afinitor Disperz):** 2 mg, 3 mg, 5 mg
	Afinitor, Afinitor Disperz	
lapatinib	Tykerb	**Tablet:** 250 mg
	Tykerb	
neratinib	Nerlynx	**Tablet:** 40 mg
	Not Available	
palbociclib	Ibrance	**Capsule:** 75 mg, 100 mg, 125 mg
	Ibrance	
ribociclib	Kisqali	**Tablet:** 200 mg
	Kisqali	
letrozole + ribociclib	Kisqali Femara Co-Pak	**Tablet:** 2.5 mg letrozole + 200 mg ribociclib
	Not Available	

Taxanes

Taxanes are cytotoxic drugs that are naturally derived from the Western yew tree (paclitaxel) and European yew tree (docetaxel). They are approved for the treatment of breast cancer.

> **① TECH ALERT!**
>
> A common ending for taxanes is -taxel.

> **① TECH ALERT!**
>
> The following drugs have look-alike and sound-alike issues:
> PACLitaxel and PACLitaxel protein-bound particles;
> Taxotere and Taxol;
> Taxol and Paxil.

Mechanism of Action and Pharmacokinetics

Taxanes interfere with the process of mitosis. Mitosis is a key step in the process of cell division and is the stage at which DNA is organized and distributed.

Adverse Reactions

Common adverse reactions produced by taxanes are diarrhea, total body hair loss, nausea, muscle pain, joint and low back pain, flushing, and sweating. They also decrease white blood cell, red blood cell, and platelet counts. When white blood cell levels drop, individuals may get infections more easily. Docetaxel may also cause discoloration of fingernails and loosening from the nail bed. Paclitaxel may cause mouth sores.

Taxanes

Generic Name	US Brand Name(s) / Canadian Brand Name(s)	Dosage Forms and Strengths
docetaxel[a]	Taxotere	**Solution, for injection:** 10 mg/mL, 20 mg/mL; 40 mg/mL
	Taxotere	
paclitaxel[a]	Taxol	**Solution, for injection:** 6 mg/mL
	Generics	
paclitaxel albumin-bound particles	Abraxane	**Powder, for suspension:** 100 mg/vial
	Abraxane	

[a]Generic available.

Microtubule Inhibitors

Ixabepilone and eribulin are microtubule inhibitors. Eribulin is isolated from the marine sponge. Both drugs are used to treat metastatic or locally advanced breast cancer.

Mechanism of Action and Pharmacokinetics

Like taxanes eribulin and ixabepilone interfere with cell mitosis. Drug action leads to cell death.

Adverse Reactions

Nausea, vomiting, constipation, neutropenia, weight loss, anorexia, and diarrhea are the most common side effects of eribulin. Muscle, joint, and bone pain may also occur.

Immunotherapy for Breast Cancer

Monoclonal Antibodies

Pertuzumab and trastuzumab are monoclonal antibodies that are used in the treatment of HER2-positive breast cancer. HER2-positive tumors are characterized by increased invasiveness and cell proliferation to other sites (metastasis), and decreased cell death.

Microtubule Inhibitors

Generic Name	US Brand Name(s)	Dosage Forms and Strengths
	Canadian Brand Name(s)	
eribulin	Halaven	Solution, for injection: 0.5 mg/mL
	Halaven	
ixabepilone	Ixempra	Powder, for injection: 15 mg/vial, 45 mg/vial
	Not available	

❶ TECH ALERT!

A common ending for monoclonal antibody immunotherapeutic agents is -*mab*.

Mechanism of Action and Pharmacokinetics

Trastuzumab is an anti-HER2/neu antibody that is effective when used as an adjuvant therapy for HER2-overexpressing breast cancer. Pertuzumab is a monoclonal antibody that reduces tumor growth and invasion by blocking epidermal growth factor receptor (EGFR) and HER2 dimerization (a process that results in joining the two proteins).

Adverse Reactions

Common side effects of pertuzumab and trastuzumab are fatigue, nausea, diarrhea, skin rash, fever, chills, infection, joint and muscle pain, anemia, and headache. Pertuzumab and trastuzumab have been linked to an increased risk for heart failure.

Monoclonal Antibodies

Generic Name	US Brand Name(s)	Dosage Forms and Strengths
	Canadian Brand Name(s)	
pertuzumab	Perjeta	Solution, for infusion: 420 mg/14 mL
	Perjeta	
trastuzumab trastuzumab-DKST ado-trastuzumab emtansine	Herceptin	Powder, for injection (Herceptin): 150 mg/vial, 440 mg/vial
	Ogivri	Powder, for injection (Kadcyla): 100 mg/vial, 160 mg/vial
	Kadcyla	
	Herceptin, Kadcyla	Powder, for injection (Ogivri): 420 mg/vial
pertuzumab + trastuzumab	Not Available	Kit[a]: 420 mg/14 mL pertuzumab + 440 mg/vial trastuzumab
	Perjeta- Herceptin	

[a]Available in Canada only.

Pharmacotherapy for Prostate Cancer

Gonadotropin-Releasing Hormone Agonists and Luteinizing Hormone-Releasing Hormone Agonists

Gonadotropin-releasing hormone (GnRH) is also known as luteinizing hormone-releasing hormone (LHRH). Goserelin is a GnRH agonist indicated for the treatment of prostate cancer in men and advanced breast cancer in premenopausal and perimenopausal women with ER-positive disease. The drug initially increases hormone levels and is followed by desensitization to the hormone's effects. When used for the treatment of prostate cancer, goserelin is given to patients with hormone-dependent advanced carcinoma of the prostate. It is used in combination with antiandrogens and radiation therapy for the management of locally advanced or bulky carcinoma of the prostate. When used for the treatment of breast cancer, GnRH agonists may be prescribed to treat premenopausal women, whereas SERMs and aromatase inhibitors are only indicated for use in postmenopausal women. GnRH and its analogues are described in depth in Chapter 27.

Gonadotropin-Releasing Hormone Agonist

Generic Name	US Brand Name(s)	Dosage Forms and Strengths
	Canadian Brand Name(s)	
goserelin	Zoladex	Implant (1 month): 3.6 mg Implant (3 months): 10.8 mg
	Zoladex, Zoladex LA	

Microtubule Inhibitors

Estramustine is an antimicrotubule agent that has antigonadotropic effects. It is approved for the treatment of hormone-refractory prostate cancer in Canada and the United States.

Mechanism of Action and Pharmacokinetics

Estramustine may also inhibit DNA synthesis and cause dose-related DNA strand breaks.

Adverse Reactions

The most common side effects of estramustine are breast tenderness, gynecomastia, elevated liver function tests, nausea, myalgia, and edema.

Microtubule Inhibitors

Generic Name	US Brand Name(s)	Dosage Forms and Strengths
	Canadian Brand Name(s)	
estramustine	Emcyt	Capsule: 140 mg
	Emcyt	

Pharmacotherapy for Lung Cancer

Lung cancer may be treated with surgery, radiation, chemotherapy, immunotherapy, and targeted agents. Drugs used in the treatment of lung cancer are typically effective against one but not both forms of the disease. Only treatments for NSCLC are covered in this chapter because chemotherapy for SCLC has limited effect of overall survival. Pharmacotherapy includes platinum-based compounds (e.g., cisplatin or carboplatin) with paclitaxel, gemcitabine, docetaxel, vinorelbine, irinotecan, protein-bound paclitaxel, pemetrexed, or etoposide. Agents used for immunotherapy are monoclonal antibodies (e.g., bevacizumab, cetuximab, or necitumumab). EGFR tyrosine kinase inhibitors (gefitinib, erlotinib, or afatinib), anaplastic lymphoma kinase (ALK) inhibitors (crizotinib and ceritinib), BRAF and MEK inhibitors (dabrafenib and trametinib), and programmed death receptor (PD-1) and programmed death ligand (PD-L1) blocking antibodies are targeted agents used to treat NSCLC.

Kinase Inhibitors

Afatinib (Gilotrif), ceritinib (Zykadia), crizotinib (Xalkiori), erlotinib (Tarceva), and gefitinib (Iressa) are kinase inhibitors that are used in the treatment of lung cancer. They block signaling pathways that are needed for tumor growth and spread to other parts of the body.

All of the kinase inhibitors may cause diarrhea, regardless of the type of cancer they are used to treat. Other adverse reactions common to the kinase inhibitor used in treating NSCLC are nausea, fatigue, and skin rashes. Additionally, Xalkori may produce vision disorders and upper respiratory infection; Tarceva can cause shortness of breath and cough. Additional details about the mechanism of action and adverse reactions of kinase inhibitors are described in this chapter under breast cancer.

Kinase Inhibitors

Generic Name	US Brand Name(s) / Canadian Brand Name(s)	Dosage Forms and Strengths
afatinib	Gilotrif / Giotrif	Tablet: 20 mg, 30 mg, 40 mg
ceritinib	Zykadia / Zykadia	Capsule: 150 mg
crizotinib	Xalkori / Xalkori	Capsule: 200 mg, 250 mg
erlotinib[a]	Tarceva / Tarceva	Tablet: 25 mg, 100 mg, 150 mg
gefitinib[ab]	Iressa / Iressa	Tablet: 250 mg

[a]Generic available.
[ab]Generic available in Canada.

Antimetabolites

Methotrexate (MTX) is the principal drug in this class. It is indicated for the treatment of lung cancer, breast cancer, bladder cancer, acute lymphocytic leukemia (ALL), cutaneous T-cell lymphoma, non-Hodgkin's lymphoma, leukemia, and osteogenic sarcoma. It is also indicated for the treatment of rheumatoid arthritis (see Chapter 13). Pemetrexed, a related compound, is indicated for the treatment of lung cancer. The purine antimetabolites 6-mercaptopurine and 6-thioguanine are primarily indicated for the treatment of ALL. Pentostatin is a structural analogue of the purine adenosine and is indicated for the treatment of hairy cell leukemia.

Mechanism of Action and Pharmacokinetics

Antimetabolites are chemotherapeutic agents that work most effectively against rapidly dividing cancerous cells. They inhibit normal DNA synthesis by forming abnormal nucleic acid base pairs, resulting in abnormal DNA. MTX is structurally similar to the vitamin folic acid and inhibits folate metabolism, which is essential to the formation of the purines. Pentostatin, 6-mercaptopurine, and 6-thioguanine are purine analogues. Purine bases, along with pyrimidine bases, make up the DNA strand. MTX also causes the depletion of thymidine, a DNA nucleoside, so DNA synthesis ceases and cells die.

Adverse Reactions

MTX and pemetrexed commonly cause hair loss, photosensitivity, loss of appetite, and nausea. They also decrease the numbers of white and red blood cells and platelets. When white blood cell levels drop, individuals may get infections more easily. Similar adverse reactions are produced by 6-mercaptopurine and 6-thioguanine, with the exception of photosensitivity. Folic acid is commonly prescribed to patients being treated for rheumatoid arthritis with MTX. It has been shown to reduce gastrointestinal (GI) side effects and risks for megaloblastic anemia. Supplementation with folic acid is controversial in patients treated for cancer with MTX. Folic acid may reduce the effectiveness of MTX by interfering with its antifolate action.

! TECH ALERT!

The warning label "Avoid aspirin, APAP, and NSAIDs" should be applied to prescription vials for MTX because these drugs may decrease MTX clearance and cause toxicity. (APAP is acetaminophen; NSAIDs are nonsteroidal anti-inflammatory drugs.)

! TECH ALERT!

The following drugs have look-alike and sound-alike issues:
purinethol and propylthiouracil;
pentostatin and Pentosan.

Immunotherapy for Lung Cancer

Monoclonal Antibodies

Atezolizumab (Tecentriq), nivolumab (Opdivo), and pembrolizumab (Keytruda) are monoclonal antibodies that are used in immunotherapy NSCLC. Keytruda and Opdivo are classified as PD-1 blocking antibodies. Tecentriq is a PD-L1 blocking antibody.

Mechanism of Action and Pharmacokinetics

The PD-1 and PD-L1 blocking antibody antitumor activity stems from their blockade of the signaling pathway that regulates late immune response and the spread of tumor-causing cells.

Adverse Reactions

The most common adverse reactions of Tecentriq, Opdiva, and Keytruda are fatigue, decreased appetite, dyspnea, cough, nausea, musculoskeletal pain, and constipation.

Antimetabolites

Generic Name	US Brand Name(s) / Canadian Brand Name(s)	Dosage Forms and Strengths
methotrexate[a] (MTX)	Otrexup, Rasuvo, Trexall, Xatmep / Generics	**Powder for injection (generics)**[b]: 1 g/vial **Solution, oral (Xatmep):** 2 mg/mL **Solution, for injection:** 10 mg/mL, 25 mg/mL **Tablet (Trexall):** 2.5 mg, 5 mg,[b] 7.5 mg,[b] 10 mg, 15 mg[b]
pemetrexed[ab]	Alimta / Alimta	**Powder for injection:** 100 mg/vial, 500 mg/vial
mercaptopurine[a]	Purinethol, Purixan / Purinethol	**Suspension, oral**[b]: 20 mg/mL **Tablet:** 50 mg
thioguanine	Thioguanine / Lanvis	**Tablet:** 40 mg
pentostatin[a]	Nipent / Not available	**Powder for injection:** 10 mg/vial

[a]Generic available.
[b]Available in the United States only.
[ab]Generic available in Canada.
Methotrexate marketed under the name of Otrexup and Rasuvo are prescribed for arthritis.

Programmed Death Receptor -1 (PD-1) and Programmed Death Ligand (PD-L1) Blocking Antibodies

Generic Name	US Brand Name(s) / Canadian Brand Name(s)	Dosage Forms and Strengths
atezolizumab	Tecentriq / Tecentriq	**Solution, for injection:** 60 mg/mL
nivolumab	Opdivo / Opdivo	**Solution, for injection:** 10 mg/mL
pembrolizumab	Keytruda / Keytruda	**Powder, for injection:** 50 mg/vial **Solution, for infusion**[a]: 25 mg/mL

[a]Available in Canada only.

Pharmacotherapy for Colorectal Cancer

Colorectal cancer is treated with surgery, radiation, chemotherapy, immunotherapy, and targeted agents. Chemotherapeutic agents include fluoropyrimidines, MTX, and platinum compounds. Bevacizumab (Avastin) is a monoclonal antibody that is used as immunotherapy. It is a biological response modifying agent.

Platinum Compounds

Carboplatin, cisplatin, and oxaliplatin are platinum compounds. Cisplatin is FDA-approved for the treatment of testicular and ovarian cancers. Carboplatin is approved for the treatment of ovarian cancer, and oxaliplatin is approved for the treatment of colorectal cancer.

> **❗ TECH ALERT!**
>
> Platinum compounds have the common ending -platin.

Mechanism of Action and Pharmacokinetics

The action of platinum compounds on purine bases (adenine and guanine) results in the formation of faulty cross-linkages and defective DNA.

Adverse Reactions

Side effects of platinum compounds are fatigue, loss of appetite, loss of hair, metallic taste, pain at the site of injection, increased infections, bleeding, bruising, and nausea. Cisplatin may also cause irreversible hearing loss and neurotoxicity. Sensory neurotoxicity produced by oxaliplatin is reversible.

> **❗ TECH ALERT!**
>
> The following drugs have look-alike and sound-alike issues:
> CARBOplatin and CISplatin;
> Platinol and Patanol.

Platinum Compounds

Generic Name	US Brand Name(s) / Canadian Brand Name(s)	Dosage Forms and Strengths
carboplatin[a]	Generics / Generics	**Solution, for infusion:** 10 mg/mL
cisplatin[a]	Generics / Generics	**Solution for injection:** 1 mg/mL
oxaliplatin[a]	Eloxatin / Generics	**Solution for infusion:** 5 mg/mL

[a]Generic available.

Fluoropyrimidines

Capecitabine, cytarabine, gemcitabine, and 5-fluorouracil (5-FU) are fluoropyrimidines, also known as fluorinated pyrimidines. These drugs are indicated for the treatment of several cancers such as colorectal cancer (capecitabine, 5-FU), leukemia (cytarabine), gastric cancer (5-FU), basal cell carcinoma (5-FU), metastatic breast cancer (capecitabine, gemcitabine, 5-FU), lung cancer (gemcitabine), ovarian cancer (gemcitabine), and pancreatic cancer (gemcitabine, 5-FU).

Mechanism of Action and Pharmacokinetics

Capecitabine and 5-FU are prodrugs. Capecitabine is converted to 5-FU by an enzyme that is present in high levels in tumors. 5-FU

• **Fig. 31.3** Deoxyribonucleic acid replication. (From Patton KT, Thibodeau GA: *Anatomy and physiology,* ed 9, St. Louis, 2016, Elsevier.)

must also be activated. Once activated, 5-FU inhibits the enzyme responsible for making thymidine (a DNA nucleoside), inhibits RNA formation, and causes mismatched DNA base pairs (Fig. 31.3).

Adverse Reactions

Adverse effects linked to capecitabine and 5-FU are stomach upset, loss of appetite, diarrhea or constipation, fatigue, muscle and bone pain, insomnia, headache, and dry, itchy skin. Additional adverse reactions include paresthesia (prickling or tingling sensation) in the hands and feet, jaundice, bone marrow suppression, fatal autoimmune anemias, increased opportunistic infections, and cardiotoxicity (capecitabine, 5-FU, and fludarabine).

Topoisomerase Inhibitors

Irinotecan (Camptosar, Onivyde) is a topoisomerase inhibitor that is indicated for the treatment of colorectal cancer. The other drugs in this class are used to treat various other cancers. Etoposide (Vepesid) is indicated for the treatment of testicular cancer, SCLC, and NSCLC. Topotecan (Hycamtin) is indicated for the treatment of ovarian cancer, cervical cancer, and SCLC. Etoposide is a semisynthetic derivative of an extract from the mandrake plant. Irinotecan and topotecan are derived from Camptotheca accuminata (a Chinese tree).

> **⊘ TECH ALERT!**
>
> Common endings for topoisomerase inhibitors are *-poside* and *-tecan.*

Mechanism of Action and Pharmacokinetics

Topoisomerases are enzymes that cleave DNA strands, a step needed for DNA replication and RNA transcription (Fig. 31.4). Topoisomerase II plays a role in mitosis. Oral absorption of the drugs is good, but penetration in the central nervous system (CNS) is poor. Irinotecan is a prodrug that has an active metabolite that is 1000 times more potent in inhibiting topoisomerase.

Adverse Reactions

Etoposide may cause diarrhea, hair loss, nausea, skin rash, fatigue, irritation at the injection site, flulike symptoms, bleeding,

or bruising. Irinotecan and topotecan produce similar side effects plus headache, gas, and weight loss. Rarely, individuals on high-dose etoposide therapy may develop acute nonlymphocytic leukemia.

Immunotherapy for Colorectal Cancer

Monoclonal Antibodies

Bevacizumab (Avastin) is used for the treatment of several cancers, including colorectal cancer with 5-FU, NSCLC in combination with carboplatin and paclitaxel, renal cancer, and glioblastoma. The mechanism of action of monoclonal antibody biological response modifiers is described in Chapter 13 and in this chapter in the sections on breast cancer.

Pharmacotherapy for Melanoma (Skin Cancer)

Melanoma is treated with chemotherapy, immunotherapy, and targeted agents (e.g., kinase inhibitors).

Kinase Inhibitors

Dabrafenib (Tafinlar), trametinib (Mekinist), and vemurafenib (Zelboraf) are kinase inhibitors that are used in the treatment of melanoma. Dabrafenib and trametinib are also indicated for the treatment of NSCLC. They block signaling pathways that are needed for tumor growth and spread to other parts of the body. Melanoma may mutate and develop alternate signaling pathways. This type of resistance quickly develops when the drugs are used as monotherapy; therefore combination therapy is often used. Mutations may lead to secondary cancers.

All of the kinase inhibitors may cause diarrhea, regardless of cancer they are used to treat. Other common adverse reactions are thickening skin, headache, and joint pain (darafenib); fatigue, fever, and skin rash (trametinib); and photosensitivity, hair loss, joint pain, and itchy skin (vermuafenib). Additional details about

Fluoropyrimidines Used in the Treatment of Colorectal Cancer

Generic Name	US Brand Name(s) / Canadian Brand Name(s)	Dosage Forms and Strengths
capecitabine	Xeloda / Xeloda	**Tablet:** 150 mg, 500 mg
fluorouracil (5-FU)[a]	Carac, Efudex, Fluroplex, Tolak / Generics	**Cream:** 0.5% (Carac),[b] 1% (Fluroplex),[b] 4% (Tolak), 5% (Efudex) **Solution, intravenous:** 50 mg/mL (5%) **Solution, topical**[b]: 2%, 5%
cytarabine[a]	Generics / Generics	**Powder, for injection**[b]: 100 mg/vial, 500 mg/vial, 1 g/vial, 2 g/vial **Solution, for injection:** 20 mg/mL, 100 mg/mL
fludarabine[a]	Generics / Fludara	**Powder, for injection**[b]: 50 mg/vial **Solution, for injection:** 25 mg/mL **Tablet:** 10 mg[c]
gemcitabine[a]	Gemzar, Infugem / Gemzar	**Powder for injection:** 200 mg, 1 g/vial, 2 g/vial[c] **Solution, for injection**[c]: 38 mg/mL, 40 mg/mL **Solution, for IV infusion (Infugem)**[b]: 1200 mg, 1300 mg, 1400 mg, 1500 mg, 1600 mg, 1700 mg, 1800 mg, 2000 mg, 2200 mg in solutions equivalent to 10 mg/mL

[a]Generic available.
[b]Available in the United States only.
[c]Available in Canada only.

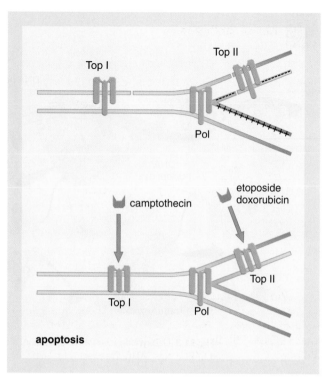

• **Fig. 31.4** Site of action of topoisomerase inhibitors. *Top I,* Topoisomerase I; *Top II,* topoisomerase II; *Pol,* DNA polymerase. (From Page C, Curtis M, Sutter M, et al: *Integrated pharmacology,* ed 3, Philadelphia, 2006, Mosby.)

Topoisomerase Inhibitors

Generic Name	US Brand Name(s) / Canadian Brand(s)	Dosage Forms and Strengths
etoposide[a]	Generics / Vepesid	**Capsule (Vepesid):** 50 mg **Solution, for injection:** 20 mg/mL
irinotecan[a]	Camptosar, Onivyde / Onivyde	**Solution, for injection:** 20 mg/mL **Suspension, for injection (Onivyde):** 43 mg/10 mL
topotecan[a]	Hycamtin / Hycamtin	**Capsule**[b]: 0.25 mg, 1 mg **Powder, injection:** 4 mg/vial **Solution, for injection:** 1 mg/mL

[a]Generic available.
[b]Available in the United States only.

Monoclonal Antibodies

Generic Name	US Brand Name(s) / Canadian Brand Name(s)	Dosage Forms and Strengths
bevacizumab	Avastin / Avastin	**Powder, for injection:** 100 mg/vial[a] 400 mg/vial[a] **Solution, for injection:** 25 mg/mL[b]
bevacizumab-AWWB	Mvasi / Not Available	**Powder, for injection:** 100 mg/vial, 400 mg/vial **Solution, for injection:** 100 mg/4 mL and 400 mg/16 mL (25 mg/mL)

[a]Available in the United States only.
[b]Available in Canada only.

the mechanism of action and adverse reactions of kinase inhibitors are described in this chapter under breast cancer.

Immunotherapy for Melanoma (Skin Cancer)

Monoclonal Antibodies

Nivolumab (Opdivo) and pembrolizumab (Keytruda) are PD-1 blocking antibodies that are indicated for metastatic melanoma and NSCLC. The mechanism of action for Keytruda and other

Kinase Inhibitors

Generic Name	US Brand Name(s)	Dosage Forms and Strengths
	Canadian Brand Name(s)	
cobimetinib	Cotellic	**Tablet:** 20 mg
	Cotellic	
dabrafenib	Tafinlar	**Capsule:** 50 mg, 75 mg
	Tafinlar	
trametinib	Mekinist	**Tablet:** 0.5 mg, 2 mg
	Mekinist	
vemurafenib	Zelboraf	**Tablet:** 240 mg
	Zelboraf	

PD-1 and PD-L1 blocking antibodies is described in this chapter in the section on lung cancer. Ipilimumab is a monoclonal antibody that blocks cytotoxic T-lymphocyte antigen 4 (CTLA-4) binding. Human CTLA-4 blocking antibodies are also called "check point" inhibitors.

Cytotoxic T-Lymphocyte Antigen 4 Blocking Antibodies

Generic Name	US Brand Name(s)	Dosage Forms and Strengths
	Canadian Brand Name(s)	
ipilimumab	Yervoy	**Solution, for injection:** 5 mg/mL
	Yervoy	

Pharmacotherapy for Cancer of the Uterus and Ovaries

Progestins

Megestrol acetate and medroxyprogesterone acetate are progestins. Megestrol is approved for the treatment of inoperable, advanced metastatic cancer of the endometrium and breast, as well as palliative treatment of advanced stage, hormone-responsive prostate cancer. Medroxyprogesterone acetate is indicated for the adjunctive and/or palliative treatment of recurrent and/or metastatic cancer of the endometrium and hormone-dependent metastatic cancer of the breast.

ⓘ *TECH ALERT!*

Megestrol suspension is prescribed to increase the appetite and combat the wasting syndrome in patients with AIDS and cancer.

Mechanism of Action

Megestrol binds to PRs where it stimulates cell maturation. It inhibits overgrowth of endometrial tissue in women who have endometrial cancer. It has androgenic properties that act on the pituitary, when taken with diethylstilbestorol, to suppress androgens in the testes that is useful for treating prostate cancer. It is not fully known how megestrol works to suppress estrogen-dependent breast tumors;

however, suppression of luteinizing hormone release from the pituitary and increased estrogen metabolism are believed to be involved.

Adverse Reactions

The most common adverse effects associated with megestrol use are hot flashes, breakthrough menstrual bleeding, and weight gain. Breast tenderness, hair loss, and hyperglycemia may also occur.

Immunotherapy for Cancer of the Uterus and Ovaries

Immunotherapeutic agents have not yet been approved for the treatments of endometrial, cervical, or ovarian cancer; however,

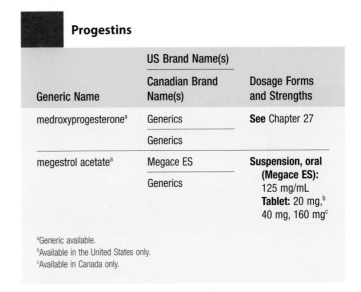

Progestins

Generic Name	US Brand Name(s)	Dosage Forms and Strengths
	Canadian Brand Name(s)	
medroxyprogesterone[a]	Generics	**See** Chapter 27
	Generics	
megestrol acetate[a]	Megace ES	**Suspension, oral (Megace ES):** 125 mg/mL
	Generics	**Tablet:** 20 mg,[b] 40 mg, 160 mg[c]

[a]Generic available.
[b]Available in the United States only.
[c]Available in Canada only.

several studies are ongoing. Clinical trials are underway evaluating the effectiveness of PD-1–blocking antibodies (nivolumab and pembrolizumab) and PD-L1 antibody (avelumab) in the treatment of ovarian cancer and endometrial cancer. Protocols for monotherapy and therapies with ipilimumab (CTLA-4–blocking antibody) or platinum compounds are being studied. The effectiveness of atezolizumab in combination with carboplatin plus cyclophosphamide is also being investigated. Studies evaluating the effectiveness of pembrolizumab, ipilimumab, and ipilimumab plus nivolumab therapies for the treatment of cervical cancer are currently underway.

Summary of Antineoplastic Agents That Treat Various Other Cancers

Alkylating Agents

Alkylating agents are one of the oldest classes of antineoplastic agents. They are related to nitrogen mustard, a lethal gas that was used for chemical warfare in World War I. Cyclophosphamide (Procytox), busulfan (Busulfex, Myleran), ifosfamide (Ifex), melphalan (Alkeran, Evomela), mechlorethamine (Mustargen), and chlorambucil (Leukeran) are all alkylating agents. Only cyclophosphamide and melphalan are approved for the treatment of one of the top six cancers described in this chapter. Cyclophosphamide is indicated for breast cancer and ovarian cancer as well as Hodgkin's disease, non-Hodgkin's lymphoma, ALL, multiple myeloma, chronic lymphocytic leukemia (CLL), mycosis fungoides, and retinoblastoma. Melphalan is indicated for ovarian cancer and multiple myeloma. The alkylating agents vary in their antitumor effects and in toxicity, but their mechanism of action is the same. All alkylating agents damage DNA and impair DNA replication and the growth phase of the cell life cycle (see Table 31.1). Alkylating agents are toxic to cancer cells and noncancerous cells, and they can cause cell mutations that lead to other cancers. Resistance can develop to the effects of cyclophosphamide and other alkylating agents.

Cyclophosphamide commonly causes hair loss, appetite and weight loss, skin discoloration, mouth sores, and fatigue. The side effects of melphalan are fatigue, diarrhea, nausea, vomiting, and anemia.

> **! TECH ALERT!**
>
> The following drugs have look-alike and sound-alike issues:
> cyclophosphamide and cycloSPORINE.

Alkylating Agents

Generic Name	US Brand Name(s) / Canadian Brand Name(s)	Dosage Forms and Strengths
cyclophosphamide[a]	Cytoxan / Procytox	**Capsule**[c]: 25 mg, 50 mg **Powder, for solution (Cytoxan, Procytox):** 200 mg/vial,[b] 500 mg/vial, 1000 mg/vial, 2000 mg/vial **Tablet**[b]: 25 mg, 50 mg
melphalan	Alkeran, Evomela / Alkeran	**Powder, for infusion:** 50 mg/vial **Tablet:** 2 mg

[a]Generic available.
[b]Available in Canada only.
[c]Available in the United States only.

Anthracyclines

Doxorubicin (Caelyx, Doxil), epirubicin (Ellence), and idarubicin (Idamycin PFS) are anthracyclines. Mitoxantrone is a related compound and is classified as an anthracenedione. Doxorubicin is indicated for the treatment of numerous cancers such as ovarian cancer, bladder cancer, lung cancer, Hodgkin's disease, leukemia, gastric cancer, soft tissue sarcoma, and thyroid cancer. Doxorubicin liposomal is approved for the treatment of ovarian cancer, Kaposi sarcoma, and multiple myeloma. Doxorubicin and epirubicin are indicated for the treatment of breast cancer, typically in combination with other antineoplastic agents. Idarubicin and mitoxantrone are approved for the treatment of acute myelogenous leukemia (AML).

Anthracyclines damage cellular DNA and inhibit the DNA and RNA enzymes that promote protein synthesis (see Fig. 31.3). This impairs DNA replication and the growth phase of the cell life cycle (see Table 31.1). Anthracyclines also inhibit the activity of the enzyme topoisomerase (see the section Topoisomerase Inhibitors), as a secondary mechanism for cellular destruction. Doxorubicin is a prodrug that is metabolized to the active metabolite idarubicin.

> **! TECH ALERT!**
>
> Doxorubicin and doxorubicin liposomal are not substitutable.

> **! TECH ALERT!**
>
> The following drugs have look-alike and sound-alike issues:
> DOXOrubicin and DOXOrubicin liposomal;
> mitoXANtrone and mitoMYcin.

Vinca Alkaloids

Vinorelbine (Navelbine), vincristine (Marqibo Kit), and vinblastine are vinca alkaloids. They are naturally derived from the periwinkle plant. Vinorelbine is used for the treatment of NSCLC. Vinblastine is indicated for the treatment of breast cancer, Kaposi sarcoma,

Anthracyclines

Generic Name	US Brand Name(s) / Canadian Brand Name(s)	Dosage Forms and Strengths
doxorubicin[a]	Generics / Adriamycin PFS	**Powder for injection:** 10 mg/vial, 20 mg/vial,[b] 50 mg/vial, 150 mg/vial[c] **Solution for injection:** 2 mg/mL
doxorubicin liposomal	Doxil / Caelyx, Myocet	**Solution, for injection:** 2 mg/mL
epirubicin[a]	Ellence / Pharmorubicin PFS	**Powder, for injection:** 50 mg/vial **Solution, for injection (Ellence, Pharmorubicin PFS):** 2 mg/mL
mitoxantrone[a]	Generics / Generics	**Solution for injection:** 2 mg/mL

[a]Generic available.
[b]Available in the United States only.
[c]Available in Canada only.

Hodgkin's disease, non-Hodgkin's lymphoma, and testicular cancer. Vincristine is indicated for the treatment of leukemia. The mechanism of action of vinca alkaloids is similar to that of taxanes. Both drugs act on microtubules to inhibit mitosis. Vinca alkaloids inhibit microtubule formation (taxanes inhibit microtubule degradation).

The side effects linked to vinca alkaloids are similar to those for taxanes, and include hair loss, nausea and vomiting, constipation, joint and muscle pain, mouth sores, increased risk for infections, and pain at the injection site.

> **! TECH ALERT!**
>
> A common beginning for vinca alkaloids is *vin-*.

> **! TECH ALERT!**
>
> VinBLAStine and vinCRIStine have look-alike and sound-alike issues.

> **! TECH ALERT!**
>
> Vincristine is usually stored in the refrigerator.

Miscellaneous Agents

Bleomycin, dactinomycin (Cosmegen), and mitomycin are antineoplastic agents approved for the treatment of various cancers. Bleomycin is indicated for the treatment of cervical, penile, testicular, and vulvar cancers, in addition to Hodgkin's disease and head and neck cancers. Dactinomycin is indicated for the treatment of testicular cancer, choriocarcinoma, and rhabdomyosarcoma. Mitomycin is approved for gastric and pancreatic cancer treatment. Mytomycin (as Mitosol) is also indicated as an adjunct to glaucoma

⚠ TECH ALERT!

The following drugs have look-alike and sound-alike issues: DACTINomycin and DAPTOmycin

Vinca Alkaloids

Generic Name	US Brand Name(s) Canadian Brand Name(s)	Dosage Forms and Strengths
vinorelbine[a]	Navelbine	Solution, for injection: 10 mg/mL
	Generics	
vinblastine[a]	Generics	Powder, for injection[b]: 10 mg/vial
	Generics	Solution, for injection: 1 mg/mL
vincristine,[a] vincristine PFS[a]	Marqibo kit	Solution, for injection: 1 mg/mL
	Generics	

[a]Generic available.
[b]Available in the United States only.

Miscellaneous Antineoplastic Agents

Generic Name	US Brand Name(s) Canadian Brand Name(s)	Dosage Forms and Strengths
bleomycin[a]	Generics	Powder, for injection: 15 units/vial, 30 units/vial[b]
	Generics	
dactinomycin[c] (actinomycin D)	Cosmegen	Powder, for injection: 500 mcg/vial
	Cosmegen	
mitomycin[a]	Mitosol	Powder, for injection: 5 mg/vial[b], 20 mg/vial, 40 mg/vial[b] Solution, topical (Mitosol): 0.2 mg/vial[b]
	Generics	
porfimer	Photofrin	Powder, for injection: 75 mg/vial
	Photofrin	

[a]Generic available.
[b]Available in the United States only.
[c]Generic available in the United States only.

surgery, where it is used to reduce scarring that might result in increased intraocular pressure. Hydroxyurea is indicated for the treatment of head and neck cancers, leukemia, and sickle cell anemia. Porifimer is used for the treatment of NSCLC.

The primary mechanism of action for bleomycin and mitomycin is to impair DNA replication by producing breaks in the DNA strands. Mitomycin also binds to DNA to form abnormal cross-links. Dactinomycin causes the DNA helix to uncoil, and inhibits DNA, RNA, and protein synthesis. Porfimer produces its cytotoxic and antitumor effects only after exposure to light. Photodynamic therapy (PDT) is administered 40 to 50 hours after administration to activate the drug.

Bleomycin, dactinomycin, and mitomycin may produce pain at the injection site, fatigue, nausea, vomiting, decreased appetite, hair loss, and darkened skin color. Mitomycin may discolor the urine and nails. Dactinomycin may cause bone marrow suppression and severe anemias, thereby increasing the risk for infection.

⚠ TECH ALERT!

Exercise precautions for handling, preparing, and administering cytotoxic drugs.

Summary of Drugs Used for the Treatment of Breast, Prostate, Lung, Colorectal, Skin, Uterine, and Ovarian Cancer

Generic Name	US Brand Name(s)	Usual Dose and Dosing Schedule	Warning Labels
Hormones			
Selective Estrogen Receptor Modulators			
tamoxifen	Soltamox	**Breast cancer:** 20–40 mg PO twice a day in divided doses	SWALLOW WHOLE (TAMOXIFEN). AVOID PREGNANCY. AVOID GRAPEFRUIT JUICE (TOREMIFENE)
toremifene	Fareston	**Breast cancer:** 60 mg PO once a day	
Estrogen-Receptor Downregulator			
fulvestrant	Faslodex	**Breast cancer:** 500 mg IM as two 5 mL injection, on day 1, 15, 29 and once monthly thereafter	AVOID PREGNANCY. REFRIGERATE; DO NOT FREEZE. STORE IN ORIGINAL CONTAINER. PROTECT FROM LIGHT

Continued

Summary of Drugs Used for the Treatment of Breast, Prostate, Lung, Colorectal, Skin, Uterine, and Ovarian Cancer—cont'd

Generic Name	US Brand Name(s)	Usual Dose and Dosing Schedule	Warning Labels
Aromatase Inhibitors			
anastrozole	Arimidex	**Breast cancer:** 1 mg PO once daily	AVOID PREGNANCY.
exemestane	Aromasin	**Breast cancer:** 25 mg PO once daily. Increase to 50 mg daily if taken with CYP3A4 inhibitor	TAKE AT THE SAME TIME EACH DAY WITH A DRINK OF WATER. TAKE WITH MEALS (EXEMESTANE).
letrozole	Femara	**Breast cancer:** 2.5 mg PO once daily	MAY CAUSE DIZZINESS OR DROWSINESS (LETROZOLE)
Gonadotropin-Releasing Hormone Agonist			
goserelin	Zoladex	**Breast cancer:** 3.6 mg subcutaneously into upper abdominal wall every 28 days **Prostate cancer (advanced):** 3.6 mg subcut implanted into upper abdominal wall every 28 days or 10.8 mg every 12 weeks	AVOID PREGNANCY. STORE AT ROOM TEMPERATURE
Progestins			
megestrol acetate	Megace	**Breast cancer:** 40 mg PO 4 times daily **Endometrial cancer:** 40–320 mg PO daily in divided doses	SHAKE WELL (SUSPENSION)
Kinase and mTOR Inhibitors			
abemaciclib	Verzenio	**Breast cancer:** Take 200 mg twice daily (monotherapy) or 150 mg twice daily with fulvestrant	SWALLOW WHOLE; DON'T CRUSH OR CHEW—abemaciclib, crizotinib, dabrafenib, everolimus, gefitinib, palbociclib, ribociclib
afatinib	Gilotrif	**Lung cancer (NSCLC):** Take 40 mg once daily	AVOID GRAPEFRUIT JUICE AND/OR POMEGRANATE JUICE—abemaciclib, lapatinib, neratinib, palbociclib, ribociclib
ceritinib	Zykadia	**Lung cancer (NSCLC):** Take 450 mg once daily	TAKE ON AN EMPTY STOMACH—afatinib, ceritinib, dabrafenib, erlotinib, lapatinib, trametinib
cobimetinib	Cotellic	**Melanoma:** Take 60 mg once daily for 21 out of a 28-day cycle	TAKE WITH FOOD—neratinib, palbociclib
crizotinib	Xalkori	**Lung cancer (NSCLC):** Take 250 mg twice daily	TAKE AS DIRECTED; DON'T SKIP DOSES—All
dabrafenib	Tafinlar	**Melanoma:** Take 150 mg twice daily	AVOID PREGNANCY—abemaciclib, afatinib, ceritinib, crizotinib, dabrafenib, erlotinib, everolimus, lapatinib, neratinib, palbociclib, ribociclib, trametinib, vemurafenib
erlotinib	Tarceva	**Lung cancer (NSCLC):** 150 mg once daily	AVOID PROLONGED EXPOSURE TO SUNLIGHT—erlotinib, vemurafenib
everolimus	Afinitor, Afinitor Disperz	**Breast cancer:** Take 10 mg once daily	DISSOLVE IN 4–8 OUNCES OF WATER; THEN DRINK SOLUTION—Afinitor Disperz, gefitinib
gefitinib	Iressa	**Lung cancer (NSCLC):** Take 250 mg once daily	AVOID ANTACIDS—lapatinib, neratinib
lapatinib	Tykerb	**Breast cancer:** Take 1250 mg once daily on days 1–21 plus capecitabine twice daily on days 1–14 in a repeating 21 day cycle	REFRIGERATE; DON'T FREEZE—trametinib
neratinib	Nerlynx	**Breast cancer:** Take 240 mg once daily	
palbociclib	Ibrance	**Breast cancer:** Take 125 mg once daily for 21 consecutive days; off 7 days then repeat	
ribociclib	Kisqali	**Breast cancer:** Take 600 mg once daily for 21 consecutive days; off 7 days then repeat	
trametinib	Mekinist	**Melanoma:** Take 2 mg once daily	
vemurafenib	Zelboraf	**Melanoma:** Take 960 mg twice daily	
letrozole + ribociclib	Kisqali Femara Co-Pak	**Breast cancer:** Take 3 Kisqali tablets (600 mg) once daily for 21 consecutive days; off 7 days. Take 1 Letrazole tablet (2.5 mg) daily for 28 days. Repeat cycle	

Summary of Drugs Used for the Treatment of Breast, Prostate, Lung, Colorectal, Skin, Uterine, and Ovarian Cancer—cont'd

Generic Name	US Brand Name(s)	Usual Dose and Dosing Schedule	Warning Labels
Anthracyclines			
doxorubicin	Generics	**Breast cancer:** 50–60 mg/m² IV bolus on day 1 of every 21 days with other agents, this is one of several dosage regimens used in combination with other agents (e.g., cyclophosphamide and fluorouracil, paclitaxel, docetaxel) **Ovarian and SCLC lung cancer:** 40–50 mg/m² per dose IV once monthly in combination with various other antineoplastics	AVOID PREGNANCY. SHAKE WELL (POWDER, FOR INJECTION). REFRIGERATE (DOXORUBICIN, EPIRUBICIN). PROTECT FROM LIGHT (DOXORUBICIN, EPIRUBICIN). MAY CAUSE DISCOLORATION OF URINE (DOXORUBICIN). STORE AT ROOM TEMPERATURE (MITOXANTRONE). SHAKE VIGOROUSLY TO DISSOLVE (EPIRUBICIN POWDER, FOR INJECTION)
epirubicin	Ellence	**Breast cancer:** 100 mg/m² IV on day 1 in combination with fluorouracil and cyclophosphamide (FEC regimen) every 21 days for 6 cycles or 60 mg/m² IV on days 1 and 8 in combination with oral cyclophosphamide and fluorouracil every 28 days for 6 cycles	
mitoxantrone	Generics	**Prostate cancer:** 12–14 mg/m² IV every 21 days in combination with prednisone or hydrocortisone	
Taxanes			
docetaxel	Taxotere	**Breast Cancer (advanced, metastatic):** 60–100 mg/m² IV over 1 h once every 3 weeks	AVOID PREGNANCY. DO NOT SHAKE (DOCETAXEL). REFRIGERATE; DON'T FREEZE (DOCETAXEL). RECONSTITUTED SOLUTION IS STABLE FOR A CERTAIN LENGTH OF TIME: DOCETAXEL (4 H); PACLITAXEL (27 H), PROTEIN-BOUND PACLITAXEL (24 H). STORE AT ROOM TEMPERATURE (PACLITAXEL). PROTECT FROM LIGHT (DOCETAXEL, PACLITAXEL). DO NOT MIX IN PVC BAGS OR USE PVC SETS (DOCETAXEL, PACLITAXEL). AVOID ASPIRIN, APAP, AND NSAIDS
paclitaxel	Taxol	**Breast Cancer (metastatic):** 175 mg/m² IV over 3 h every 3 weeks	
paclitaxel protein-bound particles	Abraxane	**Breast Cancer:** 260 mg/m² IV over 30 min once per week for 3 weeks, then 1 week off, every 28 days (dose depends on previously untreated or taxane-refractory)	
Fluoropyrimidines			
5-fluorouracil	Generics	**Breast cancer palliative:** 12 mg/kg IV daily for 4 days, if tolerated then 6 mg/kg IV daily on days 6, 8, 10, 12 (MAX dose 800 mg/day). Maintenance: If tolerated, repeat cycle evey 30 days. Regimens also for colorectal, gastric, and pancreatic cancer	ONCE THE PHARMACY BULK VIAL IS OPENED, ANY UNUSED PORTION SHOULD BE DISCARDED AFTER 1 H. AVOID PREGNANCY. AVOID PROLONGED EXPOSURE TO SUNLIGHT. AVOID ASPIRIN, APAP, AND NSAIDS. STORE AT ROOM TEMPERATURE. PROTECT DRUG FROM LIGHT
capecitabine	Xeloda	**Breast cancer:** 2500 mg/m²/day PO in 2 divided doses for 2 weeks, repeated every 3 weeks **Colorectal cancer:** 1250 mg/m² PO twice daily within 30 min for 2 weeks, repeated every 3 weeks for a total of 8 cycles	TAKE WITH FOOD (CAPECITABINE). AVOID PREGNANCY. AVOID ASPIRIN, APAP, AND NSAIDS. STORE AT ROOM TEMPERATURE (GEMCITABINE)
gemcitabine	Gemzar	**Breast cancer (metastatic):** 1250 mg/m² IV over 30 min on days 1 and 8 of a 21-day cycle in combination with paclitaxel **Lung cancer (NSCLC):** 1000 mg/m² IV on days 1, 8, 15 of a 28-day cycle or 1250 mg/m² on days 1 and 8 of a 21-day cycle. Cisplatin (100 mg/m² IV) is given following the gemcitabine infusion on day 1 of either regimen. **Ovarian cancer:** 1000 mg/m² IV over 30 min on days 1 and 8 of a 21-day cycle in combination with carboplatin on day 1 after gemcitabine infusion	

Continued

Summary of Drugs Used for the Treatment of Breast, Prostate, Lung, Colorectal, Skin, Uterine, and Ovarian Cancer—cont'd

Generic Name	US Brand Name(s)	Usual Dose and Dosing Schedule	Warning Labels
Antimetabolites			
methotrexate	Generics	**Lung cancer (SCLC): PO:** 10 mg/m² PO twice weekly ×4 doses every 3 weeks in combination with lomustine and cyclophosphamide **IV:** 20 mg/m² IV as a single dose with cisplatin, doxorubicin, and cyclophosphamide, every 28 days or numerous other regimens. **Breast cancer:** 40–60 mg/m² IV given on day 1 of every 21–28 days along with cyclophosphamide and fluorouracil. Also regimens for bladder cancer, non-Hodgkin lymphoma, and acute lymphocytic leukemia	PROTECT FROM LIGHT (METHOTREXATE). STORE AT ROOM TEMPERATURE. RECONSTITUTE POWDER IMMEDIATELY BEFORE USE AND DISCARD ANY UNUSED PORTION (METHOTREXATE). TAKE WITH A FULL GLASS OF WATER. MAY MAKE SKIN MORE SENSITIVE TO SUNLIGHT. AVOID PREGNANCY. DO NOT DRINK ALCOHOLIC BEVERAGES (METHOTREXATE).
pemetrexed	Alimta	**Lung cancer (NSCLC):** 500 mg/m² over 10 min on day 1 of each 21-day cycle	REFRIGERATE AND USE WITHIN 24 H OF RECONSTITUTION; DISCARD ANY UNUSED PORTION (PEMETREXED)
Vinca Alkaloids			
vinorelbine	Navelbine	**Breast Cancer:** 30 mg/m2 IV over 6–10 min weekly or on days 1 and 8 repeated every 21 days **Lung cancer (NSCLC):** 30 mg/m² IV over 6–10 min once weekly or 25–30 mg/m² once weekly with cisplatin	REFRIGERATE; DO NOT FREEZE (VINORELBINE) PROTECT FROM LIGHT (VINORELBINE). AVOID ASPIRIN, APAP, AND NSAIDS. SYRINGES MUST BE LABELED "FOR IV USE ONLY-FATAL IF GIVEN INTRATHECALLY"
vinblastine	Generics	**Breast Cancer:** 4.5 mg/m² IV on day 1 of every 21 days in combination with doxorubicin and thiotepa	
Platinum Compounds			
carboplatin	Generics	**Ovarian cancer:** 300 mg/m² IV on day 1 in combination with cyclophosphamide, repeated every 4 weeks for 6 cycles or 360 mg/m² IV on day 1, repeated every 4 weeks. Other regimens also recommended	AVOID PREGNANCY. AVOID ASPIRIN, APAP, AND NSAIDS. STABLE FOR 28 DAYS ONCE VIAL IS PENETRATED (CISPLATIN). PROTECT FROM LIGHT. STORE AT ROOM TEMPERATURE. RECONSTITUTED SOLUTION IS STABLE FOR 24 H IF REFRIGERATED
cisplatin	Generics	**Lung cancer (NSCLC):** 75 mg/m² IV as a single dose following administration of paclitaxel or docetaxel every 3 weeks. Other regimens also recommended	
oxaliplatin	Eloxatin	**Colorectal cancer:** Day 1, oxaliplatin 85 mg/m² IV infusion with leucovorin IV infusion given over 2 h, followed by 5-FU IV bolus over 2–4 min; then 5-FU IV infusion over 22 h. Day 2, leucovorin 200 mg/m² IV over 2 h followed by 5-FU IV bolus over 2–4 min, then 5-FU IV continuous infusion over 22 h. The 2-day regimen is repeated every 2 weeks	
Topoisomerase Inhibitors			
etoposide	Vepesid	**Lung cancer (SCLC):** 35 mg/m²/day IV for 4 days to 50 mg/m²/day IV for 5 days in combination with other antineoplastics	TAKE WITH A FULL GLASS OF WATER (ETOPOSIDE CAPSULE). SWALLOW WHOLE; DON'T CRUSH OR CHEW (ETOPOSIDE CAPSULE). AVOID PREGNANCY. RECONSTITUTED SOLUTION IS STABLE FOR 24 H AT ROOM TEMPERATURE. MAY CAUSE DIZZINESS OR DROWSINESS. AVOID ASPIRIN, APAP, AND NSAIDS
irinotecan	Camptosar	**Colorectal cancer:** 125 mg/m² IV over 90 min, once weekly for 4 weeks, every 6 weeks or 350 mg/m² by IV infusion over 90 min, once every 3 weeks. Other regimens with irinotecan followed by leucovorin and 5-FU	SWALLOW WHOLE; DON'T CRUSH OR CHEW (TOPOTECAN CAPSULES). TAKE WITH A FULL GLASS OF WATER (TOPOTECAN CAPSULES). PROTECT FROM LIGHT. AVOID ASPIRIN, APAP, AND NSAIDS. RECONSTITUTED SOLUTION IS STABLE FOR 24 H AT ROOM TEMPERATURE (TOPOTECAN)
topotecan	Hycamtin	**Ovarian cancer:** 1.5 mg/m²/day IV on days 1–5 of a 21-day course. **Cervical cancers:** 0.75 mg/m² IV on days 1–3 in combination with cisplatin IV day 1 only, every 3 weeks **Lung cancer (SCLC):** 1.5–2.3 mg/m²/day PO on days 1–5 of a 21-day course	

Summary of Drugs Used for the Treatment of Breast, Prostate, Lung, Colorectal, Skin, Uterine, and Ovarian Cancer—cont'd

Generic Name	US Brand Name(s)	Usual Dose and Dosing Schedule	Warning Labels
Microtubule Inhibitors			
eribulin	Halaven	**Breast cancer:** 1.4 mg/m² IV over 2–5 min on days 1 and 8, repeated every 21 days	AVOID PREGNANCY. AVOID ASPIRIN, APAP, AND NSAIDS. STORE AT ROOM TEMPERATURE
estramustine	Emcyt	**Prostate cancer:** 14 mg/kg/day or 600 mg/m²/day PO in 3–4 divided doses	AVOID PREGNANCY. AVOID ASPIRIN, APAP, AND NSAIDS. TAKE ON AN EMPTY STOMACH. AVOID DAIRY PRODUCTS WITHIN 2–3 H OF DOSE
ixabepilone	Ixempra	**Breast cancer:** 40 mg/m² IV over 3 h, given every 3 weeks in regimens with and without capcitabine	AVOID PREGNANCY. MAY CAUSE DIZZINESS OR DROWSINESS. AVOID ASPIRIN, APAP, AND NSAIDS. RECONSTITUTED SOLUTION IS STABLE FOR 6 H AT ROOM TEMPERATURE
Immunotherapeutic Agents			
Monoclonal Antibodies			
bevacizumab	Avastin	**Colorectal cancer:** 5 or 10 mg/kg IV every 14 days in combination with 5-FU. **Lung cancer (NSCLC):** 15 mg/kg IV every 3 weeks in combination with carboplatin and paclitaxel	REFRIGERATE; DON'T FREEZE—bevacizumab, pertuzumab, trastuzumab PROTECT FROM LIGHT- pertuzumab DO NOT SHAKE—pertuzumab AVOID PREGNANCY—bevacizumab, pertuzumab, trastuzumab
pertuzumab	Perjeta	**Breast cancer:** Initiate with 840 mg IV infusion, then 420 mg every 3 weeks thereafter	
trastuzumab	Herceptin	**Breast cancer:** 4 mg/kg IV infusion on week 1; if tolerated, at week 2, decrease to 2 mg/kg infused IV once weekly. Several other recommended regimens	
PD-1- and PD-L1-Blocking Antibodies			
atezolizumab	Tecentriq	**Lung cancer:** 1200 mg IV infusion every 3 weeks	REFRIGERATE; DON'T FREEZE—atezolizumab, nivolumab, pembrolizumab DO NOT SHAKE—atezolizumab, nivolumab, pembrolizumab AVOID PREGNANCY—atezolizumab, nivolumab, pembrolizumab PROTECT FROM LIGHT—pembrolizumab
nivolumab	Opdivo	**Melanoma and Lung cancer:** 3 mg/kg IV infusion every 2 weeks	
pembrolizumab	Keytruda	**Melanoma and Lung cancer:** Inject 200 mg every 3 weeks	
Cytotoxic T-Lymphocyte Antigen 4 Blocking Antibody			
ipilimumab	Yervoy	**Melanoma:** 3 mg/kg IV every 3 weeks for 4 doses	REFRIGERATE; DON'T FREEZE AVOID PREGNANCY PROTECT FROM LIGHT
Miscellaneous Agents			
porfimer	Photofrin	**Lung cancer (NSCLC):** 2 mg/kg IV administered over 3–5 min followed 40–50 h later by laser illumination at the site(s) of tumor involvement	AVOID PREGNANCY. PROTECT EYES FROM SUNLIGHT

TECHNICIAN'S CORNER

1. There have been many reports of the destruction of the rain forests and the possibility of losing potential cures for cancer. What can we do to prevent this from happening?
2. What are some new innovations being used to deliver chemotherapeutic agents in doses that will not harm good cells?

Key Points

- Cancer is a disease that occurs when new cells form more rapidly than needed; the cells accumulate and form a mass called a tumor.
- A malignant tumor is cancerous and can invade and destroy nearby tissue and spread to other parts of the body; a benign tumor is not cancerous and does not spread.
- Cancers are named according to the site at which the cancerous growth began. This is the site of the primary tumor.
- Age, tobacco smoking or chewing, ionizing radiation and sunlight, hazardous chemicals, environmental pollutants, bacterial and viral infection, hormone therapy, family history, alcohol consumption, and diet, obesity, and lack of physical activity are all risk factors for cancer.
- Advancing age (> 61 years) and a history of HRT increase the risk for breast cancer.
- Cancer of the cervix is linked to HPV and exposure to the drug DES.
- Endometrial cancer most commonly affects postmenopausal women.
- Skin cancer is associated with excessive exposure to UV light from the sun or UV lights used in tanning salons. Wearing protective clothing or using a sunscreen when outdoors is recommended.
- There are two types of lung cancer: SCLC and NSCLC.
- A history of smoking tobacco is almost always the cause of SCLC.
- The incidence of prostate cancer increases as men grow older.
- Staging is a method used to describe how far the cancer has progressed within the body.
- Cancer may be treated with chemotherapy, immunotherapy, radiation therapy, and surgery.
- Chemotherapy is the use of drugs to kill or slow the growth of cancerous cells.
- Immunotherapy is the administration of immune system modulators, vaccines, or synthetically generated immune components to boost the body's natural defense against abnormal, invasive, and cancerous cells.
- A common ending for monoclonal antibodies is -mab.
- Bevacizumab (Avastin) and trastuzumab (Herceptin) are monoclonal antibodies used for the treatment of metastatic breast cancer.
- Ipilimumab (Yervoy) is a immunotherapeutic antibody that works by blocking the CTLA-4. It is used to treat melanoma. PD-1– and PD-L1–blocking antibodies (atezolizumab, nivolumab, and pembrolizumab) are used to treat melanoma or lung cancer.
- The hormones estrogen and progesterone can promote the growth of ER-positive and/or PR-positive breast cancer.
- Antiestrogens are used for the treatment of ER-positive breast cancer.
- Tamoxifen and toremifene are selective ER modulators indicated for the treatment of ER-positive breast cancer.
- The warning label "Avoid Pregnancy" should be applied to the prescription vial of most antineoplastic agents.

- Fulvestrant is an ER downregulator approved for the treatment of breast cancer.
- Anastrozole, exemestane, and letrozole are aromatase inhibitors approved for the treatment of breast cancer.
- Goserelin is a gonadotropin-releasing hormone agonist indicated for the treatment of advanced breast cancer in premenopausal and perimenopausal women with ER-positive disease, and for prostate cancer in men.
- Megestrol acetate is a progestin approved for the treatment of breast cancer.
- Medroxyprogesterone acetate is approved for the treatment of inoperable metastatic endometrial cancer and renal cell cancer.
- Cyclophosphamide (Cytoxan) and melphalan (Alkeran) are alkylating agents that are used to treat ovarian cancer. Cyclophosphamide is also used to treat breast cancer.
- A common ending for taxanes is -taxel.
- Taxanes are cytotoxic drugs that are naturally derived from the Western yew (paclitaxel) and the European yew (docetaxel) trees.
- Vinorelbine, vincristine, and vinblastine are vinca alkaloids. They are naturally derived from the periwinkle plant. A common beginning for vinca alkaloids is vin-.
- A common ending for anthracyclines is -rubicin.
- Doxorubicin, epirubicin, and idarubicin are anthracyclines.
- Doxorubicin and epirubicin are indicated for the treatment of breast cancer. Doxorubicin liposomal is approved for the treatment of ovarian cancer.
- The anthracyclines may turn urine and nails red, whereas mitoxantrone causes them to turn blue-green.
- Etoposide, irinotecan, and topotecan are topoisomerase inhibitors.
- Topotecan is indicated for the treatment of ovarian, cervical, and SCLCs. Irinotecan is only indicated for the treatment of colorectal cancer.
- Platinum compounds have the common ending -platin.
- Cisplatin is approved for the treatment of testicular and ovarian cancer, carboplatin is approved for the treatment of ovarian cancer, and oxaliplatin is approved for the treatment of colorectal cancer.
- Capecitabine, cytarabine, gemcitabine, and 5-FU are fluoropyrimidines, which are also known as fluorinated pyrimidines.
- Antimetabolites are chemotherapeutic agents that work by inhibiting normal DNA synthesis.
- Bleomycin, dactinomycin, and mitomycin are antineoplastic agents approved for the treatment of various cancers. They interfere with DNA, RNA, and protein synthesis.
- Porfimer is used in the treatment of lung cancer. It produces its cytotoxic and antitumor effects only after exposure to light.
- Kinase inhibitors are used for the treatment of breast cancer, lung cancer, and melanoma. Two common ending for kinase inhibitors are -ciclib and -tinib

Review Questions

1. All of the following are agents used in the treatment of breast cancer, EXCEPT _____.
   a. palbociclib (Ibrance)
   b. letrazole (Femara)
   c. gosrelin (Zoledex)
   d. ribociclib (Kisqali)
2. Cancerous tumors that can invade and destroy nearby tissue and spread to other parts of the body are termed _____.
   a. benign
   b. malignant
   c. invasive
   d. tumors
3. Cancers are more prevalent in persons older than 65 years.
   a. True
   b. False
4. Cancer of the cervix is linked to the _____.
   a. herpes simplex virus (HSV)
   b. human immunodeficiency virus (HIV)
   c. varicella zoster virus (VZV)
   d. human papillomavirus (HPV)
5. Select the chemotherapeutic agent that must be stored in the refrigerator.
   a. Trametinib (Mekinist)
   b. Vemurafenib (Zalboraf)
   c. Palbociclib (Ibrance)
   d. Lapatinib (Tykerb)
6. Cancer may be treated with _____.
   a. chemotherapy
   b. immunotherapy
   c. radiation therapy
   d. all of the above
7. The warning label AVOID GRAPEFRUIT JUICE should be applied to each of the following chemotherapeutic agents, EXCEPT _____.
   a. torimefine (Fareston)
   b. abemaciclib (Verzenio)
   c. crizotinib (Xalkori)
   d. ribociclib (Kisqali)
8. Kinase inhibitors are used for the treatment of all of the following cancers, EXCEPT _____.
   a. prostate cancer
   b. lung cancer
   c. breast cancer
   d. skin cancer (melanoma)
9. Which one of the following is not a vinca alkaloid?
   a. Vinorelbine
   b. Vincristine
   c. Vinblastine
   d. Venlafaxine
10. _____ does NOT require the warning TAKE ON AN EMPTY STOMACH.
   a. Erlotinib (Tarceva)
   b. Capecitabine (Xeloda)
   c. Estramustine (Emcyt)
   d. Dabrafenib (Tarfinlar)

Bibliography

Gombos A, Awada A: Advances in chemical pharmacotherapy to manage advanced breast cancer, *Expert Opin Pharmacother* 18(1):95–103, 2017. doi:10.1080/14656566.2016.1269748.

Health Canada: Drug Product Database, 2017. Retrieved September 27, 2018, from https://health-products.canada.ca/dpd-bdpp/index-eng.jsp.

Institute for Safe Medication Practices: FDA and ISMP Lists of Look-Alike Drug Names with Recommended Tall Man Letters, 2016.

Iwai Y, Hamanishi J, Chamoto K, et al: Cancer immunotherapies targeting the PD-1 signaling pathway, *J Biomed Sci* 24(26):2017. doi:10.1186/s12929-017-0329-9.

Jeon M, You D, Bae SY, et al: Dimerization of EGFR and HER2 induces breast cancer cell motility through STAT1-dependent ACTA2 induction, *Oncotarget* 8(31):50570–50581, 2017.

Jinga DC, Ciuleanu T, Negru S, et al: Effectiveness and safety profile of ipilimumab therapy in previously treated patients with unresectable or metastatic melanoma—the Romanian Patient Access Program, *J BUON* 22(5):1287–1295, 2017.

Kalant H, Grant D, Mitchell J: *Principles of medical pharmacology*, ed 7, Toronto, 2007, Elsevier Canada, pp 777–790.

National Institutes of Health. National Cancer Institute. Surveillance Epidemiology and End Results Program: Cancer statistics. Cancer Stat Facts, 2017. Retrieved December 2, 2017, from https://seer.cancer.gov/statfacts/.

Page C, Curtis M, Sutter M, et al: *Integrated pharmacology*, Philadelphia, 2005, Elsevier Mosby, pp 163–185.

Thibodeau G, Patton K: Anatomy and physiology, ed 6, St. Louis, 2007, Mosby, pp 121–133.

US Food and Drug Administration: Drugs@FDA: FDA Approved Drug Products, nd. Retrieved September 27, 2018, from: http://www.accessdata.fda.gov/scripts/cder/daf/.

Ventriglia J, Paciolla I, Pisano C, et al: Immunotherapy in ovarian, endometrial and cervical cancer: state of the art and future perspectives, *Cancer Treat Rev* 59:109–116, 2017.

Wellbrock C, Arozarena I: The complexity of the ERK/MAP-kinase pathway and the treatment of melanoma skin cancer, *Front Cell Dev Biol* 4(33):2016. doi:10.3389/fcell.2016.00033.

32

Vaccines and Immunomodulators

LEARNING OBJECTIVES

1. Learn the terminology associated with vaccines and immunomodulators.
2. Describe types of vaccines and how they work.
3. Discuss the importance of the cold chain and identify vaccines requiring cold storage.
4. Provide examples of the pharmacy technician's role in maintaining the cold chain.
5. List procedures that must be followed if the cold chain is broken.
6. List and categorize immunomodulators/immunosuppressants.
7. Describe the mechanism of action for immunomodulators/immunosuppressants.
8. List common endings for selected vaccines and immunomodulators/immunosuppressants.
9. Identify warning labels and precautionary messages associated with select vaccines and immunomodulators/immunosuppressants.

KEY TERMS

Antigen Substance, usually a protein fragment, that causes an immune response.

Cold chain Set of safe handling practices ensuring that vaccines and immunologicals requiring refrigeration are maintained at the required temperature from the time of manufacture until the time of administration to patients.

Conjugate vaccine Vaccine that links antigens or toxoids to the polysaccharide or sugar molecules that certain bacteria use as a protective device to disguise themselves.

Immunomodulator Agent that modifies the immune response or the functioning of the immune system.

Immunosuppressant Agent that inhibits a rapid increase of the cells of the immune system; also known as an immunopharmacological.

Immunization Deliberate artificial exposure to disease to produce acquired immunity.

Inactivated killed vaccine Killed vaccine. It provides less immunity than a live vaccine but has fewer risks for vaccine-induced disease.

Interferons Antiviral proteins that enhance T-cell recognition of antigens (interferon-γ) and produce immune system suppression (interferon-α, interferon-β).

Live attenuated vaccine Nonvirulant, live, weakened version of the invader that does not cause disease in nonimmunocompromised individuals.

Subunit vaccine Contains an isolated part of the bacteria or its coating.

Toxoid vaccine Vaccine that stimulates the immune system to produce antibodies to a specific toxin that causes illness.

Vaccine Substance that prevents disease by taking advantage of your body's ability to make antibodies and prime killer cells to fight disease.

Overview

An *immunization* is defined as a deliberate artificial exposure to disease to produce acquired immunity. Vaccines are administered to immunize individuals against disease. They prevent disease by taking advantage of your body's ability to make antibodies and prime killer cells to disease-causing microbes and viruses. Under normal circumstances, cells of your immune system can distinguish between the cells that are part of your body, harmless bacteria normally found in your body, and harmful invaders that need to be destroyed. The first time that your body is exposed to a harmful virus or bacterium, the immune system releases macrophages, cytotoxic T cells, and B cells. The macrophages digest most parts of the virus or bacterium but not the *antigens*. B cells secrete antibodies to the antigens, and, if the person is exposed to the virus or bacteria again, the antibodies will inactivate the antigen. Cytotoxic T cells designed to destroy the virus or bacteria are also released on exposure to antigens. A *vaccine* is an altered antigen injected into your body that does not cause disease but stimulates your immune system's production of antibodies and cytotoxic T cells providing protection against the disease if you are exposed to it again.

Types of Vaccines

- *Live attenuated vaccines* are a living, but weakened, version of the invader virus and do not cause disease in healthy individuals. However, they can mutate to a virulent strain of the virus. Measles, mumps, and rubella, chicken pox, shingles, influenza nasal spray, and rotavirus vaccines are live attenuated vaccines.

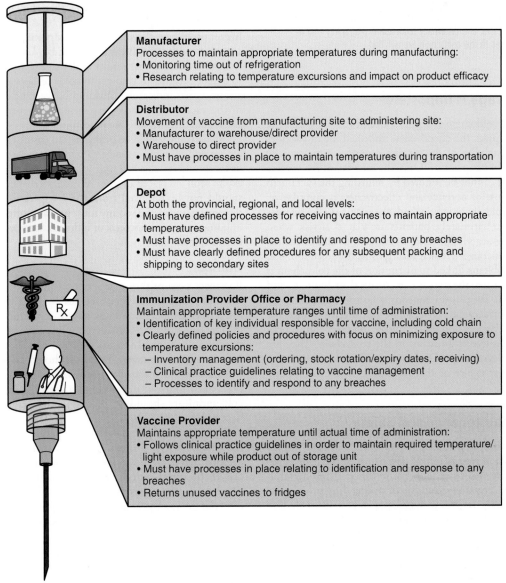

• Fig. 32.1 The cold chain. (Adapted from Public Health Agency Canada Vaccine Storage Guidelines Task Group: National Vaccine Storage and Handling Guidelines for Immunization Providers – 2015, Ottawa, 2015, Canada.)

All vaccines should be refrigerated or frozen

- *Inactivated killed vaccines* are advantageous because they cannot mutate, but they produce less immunity compared with live vaccines. Booster shots are usually required to ensure continued immunity. Flu, hepatitis A, polio (IPV), and rabies vaccines are inactivated killed vaccines.
- *Toxoid vaccines* stimulate the immune system to produce antibodies to the toxins that cause illness (e.g., tetanus and diphtheria).
- *Subunit vaccines* contain an isolated part of the bacteria or its coating. They may be genetically engineered by inserting a virus protein or gene coding into another a virus when it replicates produces the vaccine. Hepatitis B and human papillomavirus (HPV) vaccines are subunit vaccines.
- *Conjugate vaccines* link pieces of the bacteria or virus coating to a carrier protein or carbohydrate that allows the immune system to recognize and attack these disguised pathogens. *Haemophilus influenzae* type b (Hib) is a conjugate vaccine.

Special Handling Conditions for Vaccines

Cold Chain

Vaccines and immunologicals requiring refrigeration must be protected from extremes in temperature. Exposure to freezing temperatures or heat can destroy their integrity and make them unusable.

The *cold chain* (Fig. 32.1) refers to a set of safe handling practices that ensure vaccines and immunologicals requiring refrigeration are maintained at the required temperature from the time of manufacture until the time of administration to patients. This means that they must be maintained at a constant temperature from 2°C to 8°C (36°F to 46°F) throughout the transport process and placed in appropriate storage units once they are delivered to their final destination. Trained personnel, proper transportation and equipment, and efficient management procedures are key to effective maintenance of the cold chain.

❶ TECH ALERT!

Pharmacies, pharmacists, and pharmacy technicians play a key role in ensuring that breaches in the cold chain are avoided.

Why Cold Storage Is Important

Disruption of the cold chain is a public health threat. When the cold chain is disrupted, the effectiveness and shelf life of vaccines are reduced, and stability of the vaccine decreases exponentially with each increase in temperature. Once the integrity of the vaccine is compromised, it cannot be restored by returning the vaccine to the refrigerator. Loss of potency and effectiveness is cumulative, so each time the cold chain is breached, the vaccine's effectiveness is further reduced. Ultimately, patients are placed at risk when suboptimal vaccines are administered. In addition to vaccine failure, patients may experience increased reactions at the injection site. The severity of problems linked to disruption of the cold chain is dependent on whether the vaccine is chemical or biologic and whether the dosage form is an aqueous solution, suspension, or dry powder. Dry powders and chemicals are least affected by breaches in the cold chain. Vaccines and other biologic solutions and suspensions are most sensitive to breaches in the cold chain. They are more sensitive to degradation. Disruption of the cold chain is also costly. Vaccines that expire or that have been stored improperly must be destroyed.

Cold Chain Maintenance and Safety

The cold chain starts with storing the vaccines in a cold storage unit at the manufacturing plant. Maintenance of the cold chain involves appropriate selection and maintenance of refrigeration units and transport containers capable of storing drug products at required temperatures. Real-time tracking of shipments (including temperature monitoring) with technology that alerts providers that interventions are required to keep shipments safe until delivery.

Refrigeration Units

Once a vaccine is received, the pharmacy should place it in a refrigerator designated solely for vaccines. If a separate refrigerator is not feasible, vaccines should be kept separate from other refrigerated pharmaceuticals. Pharmacies that handle a large volume of vaccines should purchase a walk-in refrigeration unit. If the refrigerator is overstocked, air circulation is insufficient to maintain constant temperatures. The refrigeration unit should be equipped with a minimum-maximum thermometer to monitor temperature fluctuations and a continuous temperature-recording device. An alarm that signals when the refrigeration unit is out of range should be installed in the refrigerator. Monitors and thermometers should be calibrated routinely. It is important to place the refrigerator in a location away from a heat source because this can affect the performance of the unit.

Protocols for Receiving, Stocking, and Storing Drugs

An important component of the cold chain is establishment and adherence to protocols for receiving, stocking, storing, and transporting drugs requiring refrigeration. The pharmacy team should develop these protocols in accordance with national guidelines. Protocols for receiving vaccines should include accurate assessment of the condition of vaccines received by the pharmacy. Pharmacy personnel should be alert for warning signs that the cold chain has been broken during shipment. This might be as simple as noticing that freezer packs have thawed or that the dry ice placed in the transport container with a vaccine has evaporated. Unfortunately, exposure to heat or freezing that results in damage to the vaccine is not easy to detect because no changes in color or appearance occur. There are no visual indicators. Shaking the vaccine may reveal clumps in the vaccine that indicate freezing; however, often no clumps are visible, making this method unreliable.

A procedure should be established to ensure that stocked vaccines are rotated to avoid wastage caused by outdated supplies. Expiry dates should be checked and vaccines stocked so that those that expire soon are placed in front of vaccines that expire later. Vaccines should not be removed from the refrigerator until the time of dispensing, unless the vaccine must be transported. This is especially important for pneumococcal or influenza vaccines that are purchased in multidose vials.

Transport

Pharmacy personnel in charge of transporting vaccines are responsible for making sure that vaccines arrive at their destination at the proper temperature. How long the vaccine will be out of the refrigerator must be considered when determining the type of transport container. In most cases, vaccines should be transported in an insulated container. Protocols should be followed regarding the number of ice packs needed. Vaccines should always be positioned to avoid direct contact with the ice packs. Heat and cold monitors should be placed in the transport container, if necessary.

Vaccines should be dispensed to patients with accurate advice for transport and storage. Extremes in heat and cold must be avoided; never place vaccines in the hot glove compartment of a car. If the travel time between the pharmacy and the patient's destination, where a refrigerator is located, is less than 20 minutes, dispense the vaccine in an insulated bag. If transport time is longer than 20 minutes, the vaccine should be transported with ice packs in an insulated container. See Fig. 32.2 for a diagram explaining the importance of the pharmacy technician in cold chain management.

Immunizations

Vaccines are administered to provide immunity to a wide variety of childhood diseases, as well as influenza, hepatitis, pneumonia, viral meningitis, rabies, and other conditions. Sufficient immunity may be achieved after a single immunization; however, many vaccines must be administered as a series or require a booster shot. Epidemiologists track flu infections from sentinel sites around the globe to determine which strains of the flu virus are most virulent. Vaccines are developed for the most infectious strains of the virus. Flu vaccines must be reformulated each year. See Fig. 32.3 for age-specific immunization schedules recommended by the Centers for Disease Control and Prevention (CDC).

❶ TECH ALERT!

Pharmacists and pharmacy technicians play an important role in increasing community awareness of the importance of vaccination against vaccine-preventable illnesses. Pharmacists are authorized to administer select immunizations in community pharmacies.

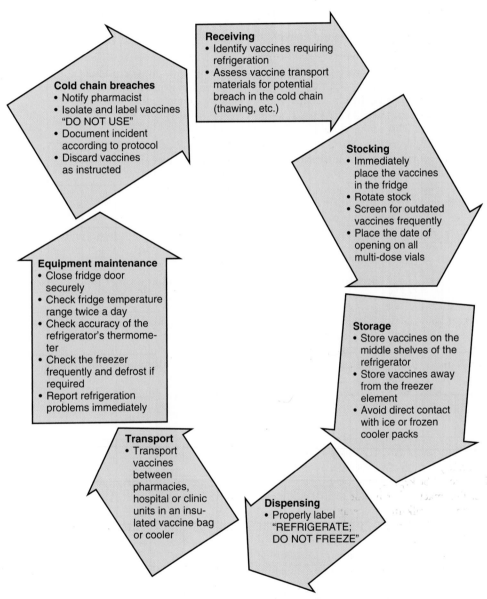

Receiving
- Identify vaccines requiring refrigeration
- Assess vaccine transport materials for potential breach in the cold chain (thawing, etc.)

Cold chain breaches
- Notify pharmacist
- Isolate and label vaccines "DO NOT USE"
- Document incident according to protocol
- Discard vaccines as instructed

Stocking
- Immediately place the vaccines in the fridge
- Rotate stock
- Screen for outdated vaccines frequently
- Place the date of opening on all multi-dose vials

Equipment maintenance
- Close fridge door securely
- Check fridge temperature range twice a day
- Check accuracy of the refrigerator's thermometer
- Check the freezer frequently and defrost if required
- Report refrigeration problems immediately

Storage
- Store vaccines on the middle shelves of the refrigerator
- Store vaccines away from the freezer element
- Avoid direct contact with ice or frozen cooler packs

Transport
- Transport vaccines between pharmacies, hospital or clinic units in an insulated vaccine bag or cooler

Dispensing
- Properly label "REFRIGERATE; DO NOT FREEZE"

• **Fig. 32.2** Pharmacy technician's role in maintaining the cold chain.

Figure 1. Recommended Immunization Schedule for Children and Adolescents Aged 18 Years or Younger—United States, 2018.
(FOR THOSE WHO FALL BEHIND OR START LATE, SEE THE CATCH-UP SCHEDULE [FIGURE 2]).

These recommendations must be read with the footnotes that follow. For those who fall behind or start late, provide catch-up vaccination at the earliest opportunity as indicated by the green bars in Figure 1. To determine minimum intervals between doses, see the catch-up schedule (Figure 2). School entry and adolescent vaccine age groups are shaded in gray.

Vaccine	Birth	1 mo	2 mos	4 mos	6 mos	9 mos	12 mos	15 mos	18 mos	19-23 mos	2-3 yrs	4-6 yrs	7-10 yrs	11-12 yrs	13-15 yrs	16 yrs	17-18 yrs
Hepatitis B¹ (HepB)	1st dose	←———— 2nd dose ————→			←——————————— 3rd dose ———————————→												
Rotavirus² (RV) RV1 (2-dose series); RV5 (3-dose series)			1st dose	2nd dose	See footnote 2												
Diphtheria, tetanus, & acellular pertussis³ (DTaP: <7 yrs)			1st dose	2nd dose	3rd dose		←————— 4th dose —————→					5th dose					
Haemophilus influenzae type b⁴ (Hib)			1st dose	2nd dose	See footnote 4		←— 3rd or 4th dose, See footnote 4 —→										
Pneumococcal conjugate⁵ (PCV13)			1st dose	2nd dose	3rd dose		←———— 4th dose ————→										
Inactivated poliovirus⁶ (IPV: <18 yrs)			1st dose	2nd dose	←——————————— 3rd dose ———————————→							4th dose					
Influenza⁷ (IIV)						Annual vaccination (IIV) 1 or 2 doses								Annual vaccination (IIV) 1 dose only			
Measles, mumps, rubella⁸ (MMR)					See footnote 8		←——— 1st dose ———→					2nd dose					
Varicella⁹ (VAR)							←——— 1st dose ———→					2nd dose					
Hepatitis A¹⁰ (HepA)							←—— 2-dose series, See footnote 10 ——→										
Meningococcal¹¹ (MenACWY-D ≥9 mos; MenACWY-CRM ≥2 mos)					See footnote 11									1st dose		2nd dose	
Tetanus, diphtheria, & acellular pertussis¹³ (Tdap: ≥7 yrs)														Tdap			
Human papillomavirus¹⁴ (HPV)														See footnote 14			
Meningococcal B¹²														See footnote 12			
Pneumococcal polysaccharide⁵ (PPSV23)												See footnote 5					

Legend:
- Range of recommended ages for all children
- Range of recommended ages for catch-up immunization
- Range of recommended ages for certain high-risk groups
- Range of recommended ages for non-high-risk groups that may receive vaccine, subject to individual clinical decision making
- No recommendation

For complete information go to https://www.cdc.gov/vaccines/schedules/downloads/child/0-18yrs-child-combined-schedule.pdf.

• **Fig. 32.3** Recommended immunization schedule for children and adolescents aged 18 years or younger, United States, 2017. (From US Department of Health and Human Services, Centers for Disease Control and Prevention (CDC), available at https://www.cdc.gov/vaccines/schedules/downloads/child/0-18yrs-child-combined-schedule.pdf.)

Selected Vaccines, Dosage Forms, and Strength

Generic Name	US Brand Name(s) / Canadian Brand Name(s)	Dosage Forms (Pediatric/Adult Use)	Storage
diphtheria and tetanus toxoids (Td)	Tenivac / TD Adsorbed	Suspension, for injection (Children 6 weeks to 6 years)	Refrigerate 2°C–8°C (35°F–46°F)
diphtheria + tetanus toxoids + acellular pertussis (DTaP)	Adacel, Boostrix, Daptacel, Infanrix / Adacel, Boostrix	Suspension, for injection: Daptacel (Children 6 weeks to 6 years); Infanrix (Children 6 weeks to 7 years); Kinrix (Children 4–6 years Suspension, for injection: Adacel, Boostrix (Booster for individuals 10 years and older)	Refrigerate 2°C–8°C (35°F–46°F)
diphtheria + tetanus toxoid + acellular pertussis + inactivated polio vaccine	Quadracel, Kinrix / Adacel-Polio, Boostrix-Polio	Suspension, for injection Adacel-Polio, Boostrix-Polio, Quadracel (Booster for individuals 4 years and older)	Refrigerate 2°C–8°C (35°F–46°F)
diphtheria toxoid + tetanus toxoid + acellular pertussis + *Haemophilus influenzae* B conjugate + poliovirus vaccine	Pentacel / Pediacel	Suspension, for injection: Pentacel (Children 6 weeks to 4 years); Pediacel (2 months to 6 years)	Refrigerate 2°C–8°C (35°F–46°F)
diphtheria toxoid + tetanus toxoid + acellular pertussis + hepatitis B surface antigen + inactivated poliovirus vaccine	Pediarix / Infanrix-Hexa	Suspension, for injection (Children 6 weeks to 6 years)	Refrigerate 2°C–8°C (35°F–46°F)
tetanus immune globulin	Hypertet S/D / Hypertet S/D	Solution, for injection	Refrigerate 2°C–8°C (35°F–46°F)
haemophilus influenzae b (Hib) conjugate vaccine (meningicoccal protein)	PedvaxHIB / Not available	Liquid, for intramuscular injection (Children 2–71 months)	Refrigerate 2°C–8°C (35°F–46°F)
haemophilus influenzae b (Hib) conjugate vaccine (tetanus protein)	ActHIB, Hiberix / ActHIB, Hiberix	Powder, for injection solution: (Children 2 months to 5 years)	Refrigerate 2°C–8°C (35°F–46°F)
inactivated polio vaccine	Ipol / Imovax Polio	Suspension, for injection, trivalent, inactivated: (Children 2 months to adult)	Refrigerate 2°C–8°C (35°F–46°F)
measles, mumps, and rubella (MMR) vaccine	M-M-R II / M-M-R II, PRIORIX	Powder, for injection solution: (12 months and older)	Keep Frozen until use. Store at –50°C to +8°C—M-M-R II ProQuad Refrigerate 2°C–8°C (35°F–46°F)—PRIORIX
measles, mumps, and rubella (MMR) vaccine + varicella zoster	ProQuad / PRIORIX-TETRA, ProQuad	Powder, for injection solution: PRIORIX-TETRA (Children 9 months to 12 years) ProQuad (Children 12 months to 12 years)	Refrigerate 2°C–8°C (35°F–46°F)—PRIORIX-TETRA Keep Frozen until use. Store at –0°C to +8°C—ProQuad
hepatitis A vaccine (inactivated)	Havrix, VAQTA / Avaxim, Avaxim Pediatric, Havrix, Havrix Jr., VAQTA	Suspension for injection: Avaxim (Individuals 12 years and older); Avaxim Pediatric (Children 12 month to 15 years), Havrix (19 years and older); Havrix Jr. (Children 12 months to 18 years)	Refrigerate 2°C–8°C (35°F–46°F)
hepatitis B vaccine surface antigen, recombinant	Energix-B, Recombivax HB / Energix-B, Recombivax HB, Recombivax HB (Dialysis)	Suspension for injection Energix-B, Recombivax HB (All ages); Recombivax HB-Dialysis (Adults only)	Refrigerate 2°C–8°C (35°F–46°F)
hepatitis B immunoglobulin	Hepagam B, Nabi-B / Hepagam B, Hyperhep B S/D	Solution, for injection (Newborn and older)	Refrigerate 2°C–8°C (35°F–46°F)

Continued

Selected Vaccines, Dosage Forms, and Strength—cont'd

Generic Name	US Brand Name(s) Canadian Brand Name(s)	Dosage Forms (Pediatric/Adult Use)	Storage
hepatitis A vaccine + hepatitis B vaccine	Twinrix Twinrix, Twinrix Jr.	Suspension for injection: (All ages)	Refrigerate 2°C–8°C (35°F–46°F)
influenza vaccine (formulated annually for selected strains each flu season)	Afluria, Fluad, Fluarix, FluMist, FluLaval, Fluvirin Fluad, Fluzone High-Dose, Fluzone Intradermal, Flublok, Fluarix, Flucelvax Flumist	Solution, nasal (Flumist), (Individuals 2–59 years) Suspension for IM injection: (Individuals 6 months and older); Fluzone high dose (65 years and older) Suspension, for intradermal injection: Fluzone Intradermal (Individuals 18–64 years)	Refrigerate 2°C–8°C (35°F–46°F)
Meningococcal (Groups A/C/Y/W-135) oligosaccharide conjugate vaccine	Menveo Menveo	Powder, for injection: (Individuals 2 months to 55 years)	Refrigerate 2°C–8°C (35°F–46°F)
meningococcal (groups A/C/Y/W-135) polysaccharide tetanus toxoid conjugate vaccine	Menomune Nimenrix	Powder, for IM injection (Individuals 12 months to 55 years-Nimenrix; older than 2 years Menomune)	Refrigerate 2°C–8°C (35°F–46°F)
meningococcal (groups A/C/Y/W-135) polysaccharide diphtheria toxoid conjugate vaccine	Menactra Menactra	Solution, for injection: (Individuals 9 months to 55 years)	Refrigerate 2°C–8°C (35°F–46°F)
Meningococcal Group B Conjugate Vaccine	Bexsero, Trumenba Not available	Suspension, for injection: (Individuals 10–25 years)	Refrigerate 2°C–8°C (35°F–46°F)
Meningococcal Group C Conjugate Vaccine	Not available Menjugate, NeisVac-C	Suspension, for injection: (Children 2 months old to adult)	Refrigerate 2°C–8°C (35°F–46°F)
pneumococcal polysaccharide 13-polyvalent vaccine	Prevnar 13 Prevnar 13	Suspension for injection: (Individuals 6 weeks and older)	Refrigerate 2°C–8°C (35°F–46°F)
pneumococcal polysaccharide 23-polyvalent vaccine	Pneumovax 23 Pneumovax 23	Solution, for injection: (Individuals 2 years and older)	Refrigerate 2°C–8°C (35°F–46°F)
rabies vaccine	Imovax rabies, RabAvert Imovax rabies, RabAvert	Powder, for injection: Imovax rabies (Adults); RabAvert (All ages)	Refrigerate 2°C–8°C (35°F–46°F)
rotavirus	RotaTeq, Rotarix RotaTeq, Rotarix	Solution, oral RotaTeq (Children 6–32 weeks old); Rotarix (Children 6–24 weeks old)	Refrigerate 2°C–8°C (35°F–46°F)
varicella vaccine (live)	Varivax Varivax III, Varilrix, Zostavax II	Powder, for injection: Varivax III, Varilrix (Individuals 12 months and older); Zostavax (Individuals 50 years and older)	Keep Frozen until use. Store at −50°C to +8°C—Varivax Ship frozen; then refrigerate at 2°C–8°C (35°F–46°F)—Varivax III; Zostavax

Immunomodulators and Immunosuppressants

Drugs that primarily act on cells of the immune system are called immunomodulators. An *immunomodulator* is an agent that modifies the immune response or the functioning of the immune system. Vaccines, corticosteroids (e.g., prednisone), antimetabolites (e.g., mycophenolate mofetil), calcineurin inhibitors (e.g., cyclosporine and tacrolimus), mTOR kinase inhibitors (e.g., everolimus and sirolimus), monoclonal antibodies (e.g., basiliximab and belatacept), and interferons and immunoglobulins (e.g., antithymocyte globulin [ATG], intravenous immunoglobulin [IVIG], Rh_o(D) immune globulin) are all categorized as immunopharmacologicals. They are used for the treatment of inflammatory autoimmune diseases, such as multiple sclerosis (see Chapter 12), rheumatoid arthritis, systemic lupus erythematosus (see Chapter 13), Crohn's disease (see Chapter 22), to prevent organ transplant (liver, heart, or kidney) rejection, and to treat specific cancers (Chapter 31). Immunomodulators that suppress,

Prograf no grapefruit

or reduce, the strength of the body's immune system and inhibit the rapid increase and spread (proliferation) of cells of the immune system are called *immunosuppressants*. Their actions may be cell specific or nonspecific.

Calcineurin Inhibitors

Cyclosporine, pimecrolimus, and tacrolimus are classified as calcineurin inhibitors. Cyclosporine is produced by a fungus (*Tolypocladium inflatum*) and is used to improve survival rates for individuals with organ transplants. It suppresses cell destruction in graft-versus-host reactions. Cyclosporine ophthalmic is used to treat chronic dry eye syndrome.

Tacrolimus and pimecrolimus are immunosuppressants. Tacrolimus is derived from a fungus (*Streptomyces tsukubaensis*). Like cyclosporine, tacrolimus is prescribed to prevent transplant rejections. Tacrolimus ointment and pimecrolimus cream are used for the treatment of mild to moderate chronic atopic dermatitis (see Chapter 36).

Mechanism of Action and Pharmacokinetics

T cells are important to the immune response. Cyclosporine reduces cellular responsiveness to inflammatory stimuli by inhibiting T-lymphocyte cell activation and suppressing interferon gamma (IFN-γ). Cyclosporine is formulated as capsules, modified and nonmodified oral solutions, and solution for injection. Cyclosporine-modified solution has greater absorption than capsules. Cyclosporine inhibits cytochrome P-450 microsomal pathways, which are responsible for several drug-drug interactions.

Tacrolimus and pimecrolimus inhibit the first phase of T-cell activation and proliferation. Pimecrolimus inhibits T-cell activation by blocking transcription of early cytokines and inhibits *interferons* and interleukins that are mediators of the inflammatory response. The exact mechanism of action for pimecrolimus effects on atopic dermatitis is unknown. Tacrolimus is more potent than cyclosporine.

Adverse Reactions

Adverse reactions of cyclosporine include acne, bleeding or tender gums, overgrowth of gum tissue, diarrhea, hirsutism, headache, leg cramps, anorexia, nausea and vomiting, and tremors. More serious adverse reactions are nephrotoxicity, neurotoxicity, and seizures. Because cyclosporine is an immunosuppressant, it can increase risk for infections. Tacrolimus may increase the risk for bacterial, fungal, protozoal, and viral infections (e.g., thrush, urinary tract infection, and upper respiratory infections). It may also produce gastrointestinal adverse reactions such as diarrhea or constipation, loss of appetite, nausea, and vomiting. Other common side effects are headache and visual disturbances. The most common side effects of tacrolimus ointment and pimecrolimus cream are burning, itching, and skin infections.

> **❶ TECH ALERT!**
>
> Cyclosporine, oral liquid nonmodified (Sandimmune), is not substitutable for cyclosporine, oral liquid modified (Neoral, Gengraf).

mTor Kinase Inhibitors

Everolimus and sirolimus are mTor kinase inhibitors that are used to prevent organ rejection in kidney transplant patients. Temsirolimus is indicated for the treatment of metastatic cancer of the kidneys.

Calcineurin Inhibitors

Generic Name	US Brand Name(s) / Canadian Brand Name(s)	Dosage Forms and Strengths
cyclosporine[a] (cyclosporin)	Cequa, Gengraf, Neoral, Restasis, Sandimmune	Capsule (Sandimmune): 25 mg, 50 mg, 100 mg
	Neoral, Restasis, Sandimmune	Capsule, modified (Gengraf, Neoral): 10 mg,[b] 25 mg, 50 mg, 100 mg Solution, for injection (Sandimmune): 50 mg/mL Solution, oral (Sandimmune): 100 mg/mL Solution, modified, oral (Gengraf, Neoral): 100 mg/mL Ophthalmic: 0.05% (Restasis), 0.09% (Cequa)
pimecrolimus	Elidel	Cream: 1%
	Elidel	
tacrolimus[a]	Astagraf XL, Envarsus XR, Prograf, Protopic	Capsule (Prograf): 0.5 mg, 1 mg, 5 mg
	Advagraf, Prograf, Protopic	Capsule, extended release (Advagraf, Astagraf XL): 0.5 mg, 1 mg, 3 mg,[b] 5 mg Intravenous solution (Prograf): 5 mg/mL Ointment (Protopic): 0.03%, 0.1% Powder, for oral suspension (Prograf)[c]: 0.2 mg/pkt, 1 mg/pkt Tablet, extended release (Envarsus XR): 0.75 mg, 1 mg, 4 mg

[a]Generic available.
[b]Available in Canada only.
[c]Available in the United States only.

Mechanism of Action and Pharmacokinetics

Sirolimus is the active metabolite of the immunosuppressant temsirolimus. Sirolimus and everolimus interfere with the second phase of T-cell activation and proliferation. Sirolimus also decreases the levels of immunoglobulins IgM, IgG, and IgA. Everolimus inhibits activation and proliferation of B lymphocytes in addition to T cells. Eating fatty foods can reduce the absorption of tacrolimus and sirolimus.

Adverse Reactions

Everolimus and sirolimus may increase the risk for bacterial, fungal, protozoal, and viral infections (e.g., thrush, urinary tract infection, or pneumonia) and produce gastrointestinal adverse reactions, such as diarrhea or constipation, nausea, and vomiting. Other side effects are mouth ulcers and stomatitis, insomnia, dizziness or drowsiness, hair loss or unusual hair growth, headache, mood changes, depression, confusion, and tremor. More serious adverse reactions include seizures, hepatitis, and hemolytic anemias.

> ⚠ **TECH ALERT!**
>
> Sirolimus tablets and oral solution are not bioequivalent and thus are not substitutable.

mTor Kinase Inhibitors

Generic Name	US Brand Name(s)	Dosage Forms and Strengths
	Canadian Brand Name(s)	
everolimus[a]	Afinitor, Afinitor Disperz, Zortress	Tablet: 0.25 mg, 0.5 mg, 0.75 mg (Zortress)[b]; 2.5 mg, 5 mg, 7.5 mg[b], 10 mg (Afinitor) Tablet, for suspension (Afinitor Disperz): 2 mg, 3 mg, 5 mg
	Afinitor, Afinitor Disperz	
sirolimus[a]	Rapamune	Solution, oral: 1 mg/mL Tablet: 0.5 mg,[b] 1 mg, 2 mg[b]
	Rapamune	
temsirolimus[a]	Torisel	Solution, for injection: 25 mg/mL
	Torisel	

[a]Generic available.
[b]Available in the United States only.

Antimetabolites

Azathioprine, mycophenolate mofetil, and mycophenolic acid are antimetabolites that are used in conjunction with corticosteroids and cyclosporine to decrease the rejection of transplanted organs.

Mechanism of Action and Pharmacokinetics

Mycophenolate mofetil is a prodrug that is metabolized to mycophenolic acid. Mycophenolic acid is an immunosuppressive agent that inhibits the enzyme required for the synthesis of purines. Purines are needed for T-cell and B-cell proliferation. Azathioprine interferes with purine metabolism, inhibiting the synthesis of cell building blocks DNA and RNA. Azathioprine is most commonly used for long-term immunosuppression rather than acute rejection episodes.

Adverse Reactions

Gastrointestinal side effects are common and include constipation, diarrhea or soft stools, gas, loss of appetite, nausea, vomiting, stomach pain, or indigestion. Mycophenolate mofetil, like other immunosuppressives, can increase the risk of bacterial and viral infections. Other serious adverse effects are leukopenia, infections, lymphomas, and other malignancies.

Monoclonal Antibodies

Monoclonal antibody immunomodulators are used in the treatment of numerous autoimmune and immune system disorders, such as multiple sclerosis (daclizumab and natalizumab), rheumatoid

Antimetabolites

Generic Name	US Brand Name(s)	Dosage Forms and Strengths
	Canadian Brand Name(s)	
azathioprine[a]	Azasan, Imuran	Powder, for injection: 50 mg/vial[c], 100 mg/vial[b] Tablet: 25 mg,[b] 50 mg, 75 mg,[b] 100 mg[b]
	Imuran	
mycophenolate mofetil,[a] mycophenolic acid[a]	CellCept	Capsule: 250 mg Powder, for injection: 500 mg/vial Powder, for oral suspension: 200 mg/mL Tablet: 500 mg Tablet, delayed-release (Myfortic): 180 mg, 360 mg
	CellCept, Myfortic	

[a]Generic available.
[b]Available in the United States only.
[c]Available in Canada only.

arthritis (adalimumab), and Crohn's disease (infliximab). Basiliximab is used to reduce transplant rejections and prolong the life of transplanted organs. Additional monoclonal antibody immunomodulators are described in Chapters 13, 14, 22, 31, and 36.

> ▪ **TECH NOTE!**
>
> A common ending for monoclonal antibody immunomodulators is -mab.

Mechanism of Action

Monoclonal antibodies act on B cells, T cells, and surface proteins important to the immune system, specifically leukocyte surface antigens, including CD3, CD4 (T helper cells), and T-cell activation markers (IL-2, IL-6, CD20, and CD25).

Adverse Reactions

Monoclonal antibodies may increase susceptibility to opportunistic infections, reactivation of dormant infections (e.g., tuberculosis), or worsening of existing infection. Other common side effects are itching at the site of infusion, nausea, and stomach pain.

Interferons

There are approximately 2000 interferon (IFN) receptors on each normal and malignant cell. These receptors recognize and bind interferons, proteins with antigenic properties. IFN-α2b is used to treat hepatitis B and C. It is also used to treat cancers such as multiple myeloma and chronic myelogenous leukemia. IFN-β1a and IFN-β1b are first line therapies for the treatment of multiple sclerosis. They alter the actions of T cells, B cells, and other cytokines that produce immune response and inflammation. They reduce the development of the brain lesions that cause disability in people who have multiple sclerosis. Adverse reactions of IFN-β1a and IFN-β1b include flulike symptoms, headache, fatigue, weight loss, anorexia, and neutropenia.

Monoclonal Antibody Immunomodulators

Generic Name	US Brand Name(s) / Canadian Brand Name(s)	Dosage Forms and Strengths
adalimumab	Humira	See Chapter 22
	Humira	
basiliximab	Simulect	Powder, for injection: 10 mg/vial,[a] 20 mg/vial
	Simulect	
certolizumab	Cimzia	See Chapter 22
	Cimzia	
daclizumab	Zinbryta	Solution, injection: 150 mg/mL
	Not available	
golimumab	Simponi	See Chapter 22
	Simponi	
infliximab	Remicade	See Chapter 22
	Remicade	
natalizumab	Tysabri	See Chapter 22
	Tysabri	
rituximab	Rituxan	See Chapter 13
	Rituxan, Rituxan SC	
tocilizumab	Actemra	See Chapter 13
	Actemra	

[a]Strength available in the United States only.

Interferons

Generic Name	US Brand Name(s) / Canadian Brand(s)	Dosage Forms and Strengths
interferon α2b	Intron A	Powder, for injection: 6 million units/mL,[a] 10 million units/mL, 18 million units/mL, 15 million units/mL, 18 million units/mL,[b] 25 million units/mL, 50 million units/mL[a]
	Intron A	
interferon β1a	Avonex, Rebif	Injection, powder for reconstitution (Avonex)[b]: 30 mcg Injection, solution (Avonex): 30 mcg/0.5 mL Injection, solution (Rebif): 22 mcg, 44 mcg (0.2, 0.5 and 1.5 mL prefilled syringe)
	Avonex, Rebif	
interferon β1b	Betaseron, Extavia	Injection, powder for reconstitution: 0.3 mg/vial
	Betaseron, Extavia	

[a]Available in Canada only.
[b]Available in the United States only.

Immunoglobulins

Antithymocyte globulin (ATG), human immune globulin (IVIG), and $Rh_o(D)$ immune globulin are immunoglobulins. ATG is primarily administered to reduce the rejection associated with organ and bone marrow transplantation. $Rh_o(D)$ immune globulin is administered to pregnant women who are Rh negative and have been exposed to blood that is Rh positive. This may occur through exposure to fetal blood, amniocentesis, ectopic pregnancy, abdominal trauma during pregnancy, or whole blood transfusions. When an Rh incompatibility exists between the pregnant woman and fetus, maternal antibodies are produced that act against the fetal red blood cells, causing erythroblastosis fetalis, a severe hemolytic disease of the fetus. Anti-D, administered within 72 hours of delivery, can prevent erythroblastosis fetalis in a subsequent pregnancy. $Rh_o(D)$ is also used in the treatment of idiopathic thrombocytopenic purpura (ITP), a condition that causes excessive bruising or bleeding. IVIG is used for the treatment of a variety of infections and chronic lymphatic leukemia.

Mechanism of Action and Pharmacokinetics

ATG is prepared by immunizing horses or rabbits with human thymocytes. The resulting horse immunoglobulin (Atgam) or rabbit immunoglobulin (Thymoglobulin) that fights against human T cells is then collected and purified. ATG reduces the number of T-cell lymphocytes. T-cell depletion persists for several days following a single dose of ATG and takes approximately two months before T-cell levels return to normal. When $Rh_o(D)$ immune globulin (anti-D) is administered to an $Rh_o(D)$ mother, antibodies contained in $Rh_o(D)$ immune globulin suppress the maternal immune system response, preventing maternal antibodies to fetal red blood cells. In the treatment of ITP, anti-D blocks platelet destruction and increases platelet count in patients with a spleen. Anti-D binding to $Rh_o(D)$ is thought to result in an anti-D–coated RBC complex. It may cause immunosuppression by stimulating cytokines. It is formulated for IM and IV administration. IVIG is collected from human plasma. It is classified as a biologic response modifier.

Adverse Reactions

Side effects associated with ATG administration are fever, chills, leukopenia, and skin rash. Additional adverse reactions are headache, dizziness, tiredness, and diarrhea. Rh_o immune globulin side effects are headache, muscle aches and pains, pain and tenderness at the injection site, chills, fever, and allergic reactions. Dizziness, weight gain, and difficulty breathing are additional side effects.

Miscellaneous Immunomodulators

Belatacept (Nulojix) is a selective, T-cell costimulation blocker that is used to prevent posttransplantation rejection in adults receiving a kidney transplant. Adverse effects include anemia, diarrhea, urinary tract infection, peripheral edema, constipation, hypertension, pyrexia, graft dysfunction, cough, nausea, vomiting, headache, hypokalemia, hyperkalemia, and leukopenia. Persons taking belatacept should not receive immunizations with live viruses. Fingolimod (Gilenya) is an immunosuppressant that is used to treat multiple sclerosis. Fingolimod is believed to reduce lymphocyte migration into the central nervous system. The most common side effects are headache, diarrhea, cough, influenza, sinusitis, back pain, abdominal pain, and pain in extremities. Glatiramer is an immunostimulant that is used for the treatment of multiple sclerosis. The most common side effects are local injection site reactions, itching, dyspnea, vasodilation, or hypersensitivity

Immunoglobulins

Generic Name	US Brand Name(s) / Canadian Brand Name(s)	Dosage Forms and Strengths
antithymocyte globulin (lymphocyte immune globulin)	Thymoglobulin	Powder, for injection (Thymoglobulin): 25 mg/vial
	Atgam, Thymoglobulin	Solution, for injection (Atgam): 50 mg/mL
immune globulin, intravenous (IVIG)	Bivigam, Carimune, Flebogmma, Gammagard, Gammaplex, Gammunex-C, Panzyga, Octagam	Powder, for injection (Gammagard S/D, Gammunex): 5 g/vial, 10 g/vial
	Gammagard S/D, Gamastan S/D, Gammunex, Octagam, Panzyga, Privigen	Solution, for IM injection: 10% (Octagam, Panzyga, Privigen), 18% (Gamastan S/D)
immune globulin (human), subcutaneous	Hizentra, Vivaglobulin Cuvitru	Solution, for injection: 20% (Cuvitru, Hizentra); 16% (Vivaglobulin)
	Hizentra, Cuvitru	
Rh₀ immune globulin	Rhophylac, WinRho SDF	Solution, for injection: 600 units/vial, 1500 units/vial, 5000 units/vial
	WinRho SDF	

reactions; however, patients should be monitored for more serious postinjection reactions.

Future of Vaccines

Scientists are researching innovative ways to deliver vaccines. Current delivery systems include nasal sprays (e.g., the flu vaccine). Future delivery forms may include food. Scientists are conducting research on "edible vaccines" made from genetically engineered foods such as potatoes and bananas. They have engineered a potato-based vaccine against hepatitis and are also modifying bananas to prevent norovirus. Other food-based vaccines are also being researched.

Miscellaneous Immunomodulators

Generic Name	US Brand Name(s) / Canadian Brand Name(s)	Dosage Forms and Strengths
belatacept	Nulojix	Powder, for injection: 250 mg/vial
	Not available	
fingolimod	Gilenya	Capsule: 0.25 mg[b], 0.5 mg
	Gilenya	
glatiramer[a]	Copaxone, Glatopa	Solution, for injection: 20 mg/mL, 40 mg/mL
	Copaxone, Glatect	

[a]Generic available.
[b]Available in the United States only.

Summary of Selected Immunomodulators

Generic Name	Brand Name	Use	Warning Labels
Calcineurin Inhibitors			
cyclosporine	Neoral, Sandimmune	Heart and kidney transplantation prophylaxis	AVOID PREGNANCY. DILUTE ORAL SOLUTION IN LIQUID. SWALLOW CAPSULES WHOLE, DON'T CRUSH OR CHEW. AVOID GRAPEFRUIT JUICE. DO NOT REFRIGERATE. ORAL SOLUTION MUST BE USED WITHIN 2 MONTHS OF OPENING. DISCARD DISCOLORED OR CLOUDY SOLUTION FOR INJECTION.
pimecrolimus	Elidel	Atopic dermatitis, see Chapter 36.	See Chapter 36
tacrolimus	Prograf, Protoptic	Heart and kidney transplantation prophylaxis Atopic dermatitis, see Chapter 36.	AVOID GRAPEFRUIT JUICE. TAKE ON AN EMPTY STOMACH.
mTor Kinase Inhibitors			
everolimus	Afinitor	Kidney transplantation prophylaxis	AVOID PREGNANCY. AVOID PROLONGED EXPOSURE TO SUNLIGHT; USE SUNSCREEN. AVOID ASPIRIN, ACETAMINOPHEN, AND NSAIDS. AVOID GRAPEFRUIT JUICE.
sirolimus	Rapamune	Kidney transplantation prophylaxis	AVOID PREGNANCY. AVOID GRAPEFRUIT JUICE. AVOID PROLONGED EXPOSURE TO SUNLIGHT; USE SUNSCREEN. DILUTE ORAL SOLUTION WITH WATER OR ORANGE JUICE. REFRIGERATE; DISCARD WITHIN 30 DAYS OF OPENING (ORAL SOLUTION).

Summary of Selected Immunomodulators—cont'd

Generic Name	Brand Name	Use	Warning Labels
Immunoglobulins			
antithymocyte globulin	Atgam	Bone marrow and kidney transplant prophylaxis	GENTLY ROTATE SOLUTION; DO NOT SHAKE. REFRIGERATE DILUTED SOLUTION.
intravenous immunoglobulin (IVIG)	Gammagard	Primary immunodeficiency	PROTECT FROM LIGHT DO NOT FREEZE
Rh$_0$ immune globulin	WinRho	Rh isoimmunization prophylaxis	REFRIGERATE; DO NOT FREEZE. PROTECT FROM LIGHT.
Antimetabolites			
azathioprine	Imuran	Treatment of Rheumatoid Arthritis, see Chapter 13	See Chapter 13
mycophenolate mofetil	CellCept	Heart, kidney, and liver transplant prophylaxis	SHAKE WELL (SUSPENSION). SWALLOW WHOLE; DON'T CRUSH OR CHEW. TAKE ON AN EMPTY STOMACH. STORE RECONSTITUTED SUSPENSION AT ROOM TEMPERATURE AND DISCARD IN 60 DAYS.
Monoclonal Antibody Immunomodulators			
adalimumab	Humira	Crohn, RA, ulcerative colitis, see Chapter 22	REFRIGERATE; DO NOT FREEZE. MIX GENTLY; DO NOT SHAKE—golimumab, infliximab, rituximab, toclizumab
basiliximab	Simulect	Prevent kidney transplant rejection	
certolizumab	Cimzia	Crohn, RA, ulcerative colitis, see Chapter 22	
daclizumab	Zinbryta	Multiple sclerosis, see Chapter 12	
golimumab	Simponi	Crohn, RA, ulcerative colitis, see Chapter 22	
infliximab	Remicade	Crohn, RA, ulcerative colitis, see Chapter 22	
natalizumab	Tysabri	Crohn, RA, ulcerative colitis, see Chapter 22	
rituximab	Rituxan	RA See Chapter 13	
toclizumab	Actemra	RA See Chapter 13	
Miscellaneous			
belatacept	Nujolix	Kidney transplantation prophylaxis	AVOID PROLONGED EXPOSURE TO SUNLIGHT. REFRIGERATE; DON'T FREEZE. PROTECT DRUG FROM LIGHT.
fingolimod	Gilenya	Multiple Sclerosis	AVOID PREGNANCY
glatiramir	Copaxone	Multiple Sclerosis	REFRIGERATE; DON'T FREEZE. PROTECT DRUG FROM LIGHT.

TECHNICIAN'S CORNER

1. If a patient receives a vaccine, can that patient still become ill with the disease related to the vaccine?
2. Why does the body reject transplanted organs and not manufactured parts?

Key Points

- An immunization is defined as a deliberate artificial exposure to disease to produce acquired immunity.
- Vaccines prevent disease by taking advantage of your body's ability to make antibodies and prime killer cells to combat disease-causing microbes and viruses.
- Live attenuated vaccines are a living, but weakened, nonvirulent version of the invader microbe or virus.
- Inactivated killed vaccines are advantageous because they cannot mutate but they produce less immunity than live vaccines.
- Toxoid vaccines stimulate the immune system to produce antibodies to the toxins that cause illness.
- Conjugate vaccines link antigens or toxoids to the polysaccharide or sugar molecules that certain bacteria use as a protective device to disguise themselves.
- The cold chain refers to a set of safe handling practices that ensure vaccines and immunologicals requiring refrigeration are maintained at the required temperature from the time of manufacture until the time of administration to patients.
- When the cold chain is disrupted, the effectiveness and shelf life of vaccines are reduced.
- Loss of potency and effectiveness is cumulative. Each time the cold chain is breached, the vaccine's effectiveness is further reduced.
- Patients are placed at risk when suboptimal vaccines are administered.
- Vaccines and other biologic solutions and suspensions are most sensitive to breaches in the cold chain.
- Vaccines should be placed in a refrigerator designated solely to vaccines or, if a separate refrigerator is not feasible, vaccines should be separated from other refrigerated pharmaceuticals.
- An important component of the cold chain is establishment and adherence to protocols for receiving, stocking, storing, and transporting drugs requiring refrigeration.
- Pharmacy personnel should be alert for warning signs that the cold chain has been broken during shipment. This might be as simple as noticing that freezer packs have thawed or that dry ice placed in the transport container with a vaccine has evaporated.
- Vaccine stock should be rotated to avoid wastage because of outdated supplies. Expiration dates should be checked frequently.

- Vaccines should not be removed from the refrigerator until the time of dispensing or until the vaccine must be transported.
- In most cases, vaccines should be transported in an insulated container.
- Extremes in heat and cold must be avoided; vaccines should never be placed in the hot glove compartment of a car.
- Vaccines are administered to provide immunity to a wide variety of childhood diseases, influenza, hepatitis, pneumonia, viral meningitis, rabies, and other conditions.
- Immunosuppressants inhibit proliferation of cells of the immune system.
- Drugs that have their primary action on cells of the immune system are used to treat autoimmune diseases, such as multiple sclerosis, rheumatoid arthritis, systemic lupus erythematosus, and Crohn's disease; prevent tissue or organ rejection after transplantation surgery; and treat cancer.
- Corticosteroids, antimetabolites, calcineurin inhibitors, mTor kinase inhibitors, immunoglobulins, and monoclonal antibodies are all immunopharmacologicals.
- Cyclosporine is used to improve survival rates for individuals with organ transplants.
- Everolimus and sirolimus are mTor kinase inhibitors that are used to prevent transplant rejection.
- Tacrolimus interferes with the first phase of T-cell activation, and sirolimus interferes with a key enzyme that regulates the second phase of T-cell activation and proliferation.
- T-cell depletion persists for several days following a single dose of ATG and takes approximately two months before T-cell levels return to normal.
- Mycophenolate mofetil is a prodrug. It inhibits T-cell and B-cell proliferation.
- Basiliximab, daclizumab, and muromonab are monoclonal antibody immunomodulators that are used to reduce transplant rejections and prolong the life of transplanted organs.
- IVIG is collected from human plasma. It is used for the treatment of a variety of infections and chronic lymphatic leukemia.
- $Rh_o(D)$ immune globulin is administered to pregnant women who are Rh negative and have been exposed to blood that is Rh positive.

Review Questions

1. A living but weakened version of an invader that does not cause disease (nonvirulent) is called a _____.
   a. live attenuated vaccine
   b. dead attenuated vaccine
   c. live encapsulated vaccine
   d. live strengthened vaccine
2. All of the following immunosuppressants are used to prevent organ transplant rejection, EXCEPT: _____.
   a. cyclosporine
   b. mycophenolate mofetil
   c. tacrolimus
   d. pimecrolimus

3. Immunization is not always achieved by administering vaccines.
   a. True
   b. False
4. Examples of inactivated killed vaccine(s) are _____ vaccines.
   a. flu
   b. hepatitis A
   c. polio
   d. all of the above

5. These vaccines stimulate the immune system to produce antibodies to the toxins that cause illnesses such as tetanus and diphtheria.
   a. Conjugated vaccine
   b. Live attenuated vaccines
   c. Toxoid vaccines
   d. Inactivated killed vaccines

6. Which of the following statements is FALSE?
   a. Pharmacy technicians must protect against breaches in the cold chain by assessing integrity of refrigerated items received in the pharmacy.
   b. Pharmacy technicians must protect against breaches in the cold chain by placing vaccines directly on ice packs or cold packs during transport
   c. Pharmacy technicians must protect against breaches in the cold chain by checking the refrigerator temperature up to twice daily.
   d. Pharmacy technicians must protect against breaches in the cold chain by selecting the appropriate transport containers/packaging for vaccines that must be stored between 2°C and 8°C.

7. Which of the following drugs are not categorized as immunopharmacologicals?
   a. Corticosteroids
   b. Antineoplastics
   c. Antivirals
   d. Intravenous immunoglobulin

8. Select the immunosuppressant that is available as a topical dosage form.
   a. CellCept
   b. Imuran
   c. Protoptic
   d. Rapimune

9. A common ending for monoclonal antibody immunomodulators is _____.
   a. -tan
   b. -mab
   c. -ine
   d. -olol

10. $Rh_o(D)$ immune globulin is administered to pregnant women who are Rh _____ who have been exposed to blood that is Rh _____.
   a. negative; positive
   b. positive; negative
   c. both a and b
   d. $Rh_o(D)$; negative

Bibliography

Centers for Disease Control and Prevention: List of Vaccines. November 22, 2016. Retrieved August 16, 2017, from https://www.cdc.gov/vaccines/vpd/vaccines-list.html.

Childhood Immunization Division, Bureau of Communicable Disease Epidemiology, Laboratory Centre for Disease Control, Canada: National guidelines for vaccine storage and transportation, *Can Commun Dis Rep* 21:93–97, 1995.

Collins BH: Renal Transplantation Medication. 2015. Retrieved August 27, 2017, from http://emedicine.medscape.com/article/430128-medication#showall.

Different Types of Vaccines: 2013. Retrieved August 15, 2017, from https://www.historyofvaccines.org/content/articles/different-types-vaccines.

Dimayuga R, Scheifele D, Bell A: Effects of freezing on DPT and DPT-IPV vaccines, adsorbed, *Can Commun Dis Rep* 21:101–103, 1995.

Health Canada: Drug Product Database. 2018. Retrieved September 30, 2018, from https://health-products.canada.ca/dpd-bdpp/index-eng.jsp.

Institute for Safe Medication Practices: FDA and ISMP Lists of Look-Alike Drug Names with Recommended Tall Man Letters. 2016.

Kalant H, Grant D, Mitchell J: *Principles of medical pharmacology*, ed 7, Toronto, 2007, Elsevier Canada, pp 546–552.

Moscou K: Tech Talk CE: The Vaccine Cold-Chain. 2007. Retrieved from http://www.canadianhealthcarenetwork.ca/files/2009/10/tt_ce_e_jan_feb07.pdf.

Murdoch J: Chill out: what pharmacists need to know about the room temperature stability of refrigerated pharmaceutical products, *Pharm Pract* 22:32–42, 2006.

National Institute of Allergy and Infectious Diseases: Vaccines of the Future. 2008. Retrieved August 16, 2017.

Patil US, Jaydeokar AV, Bandawane DD: Immunomodulators: pharmacological review, *Int J Pharm Pharm Sci* 4(S1):2012.

Seto J, Marra F: Keeping it cool: A pharmacist's guide. Executive summary, University of British Columbia, Continuing Pharmacy Professional Development, Home Study Program, 2005, Rogers, pp 1–7.

US Food and Drug Administration: Drugs@FDA: FDA Approved Drug Products. nd. Retrieved September 30, 2018, from http://www.accessdata.fda.gov/scripts/cder/daf/.

US Food and Drug Administration: Licensed Biological Products with Supporting Documents, 2018. Retrieved September 28, 2018, from US Food and Drug Administration: https://www.fda.gov/BiologicsBloodVaccines/ucm133705.htm#I.

Weir E, Hatch K: Preventing cold-chain failure: vaccine storage and handling, *JAMC* 171:2004.

UNIT **XI**

Drugs Affecting the Integumentary System

The integumentary system or skin is classified as a cutaneous membrane. The primary layers are the epidermis, a superficial thin layer composed of squamous tissue; the dermis, a deep, thicker layer of connective cells; and the hypodermis, a layer of loose subcutaneous tissue, rich in fat and areolar tissue beneath the dermis. The skin forms a self-repairing and protective boundary between the internal environment of the body and the outside elements that could potentially damage vital, life-sustaining organs. The epidermis has the ability to create new cells and repair itself after injury or disease. The dermis is sometimes called the true skin because it protects against mechanical injury and compression. Additional functions of the skin are sensation detection, growth, synthesis of important chemicals and hormones (vitamin D), excretion, temperature regulation, and immunity.

In Unit XI, the various types of medications used to treat diseases of the integumentary systems, such as fungal infections, decubitus ulcers, burns, atopic dermatitis, psoriasis, acne lice, and scabies are described. A brief description of each disorder is provided, followed by a description of the drugs indicated for treatment that includes mechanisms of action, adverse reactions, strength(s), and dosage forms. Pharmacy technicians need to familiar with various types of skin products applied to treat skin conditions, because customers may ask questions about OTC skin, hair products, and lice treatments sold in the pharmacy.

33

Treatment of Fungal Infection

LEARNING OBJECTIVES

1. Learn the terminology associated with fungal infections.
2. Identify risk factors for fungal infections.
3. List and categorize medications used for the treatment of fungal infections.
4. Describe the mechanism of action for drugs used for the treatment of fungal infections.
5. List common endings for drug classes used for the treatment of specific fungal infections.
6. Identify significant drug look-alike and sound-alike issues, warning labels, and precautionary messages associated with medications used for the treatment of fungal infections.

KEY TERMS

Antifungal Drug used to treat a fungal infection.
Candida Genus of a type of fungus. It is also called yeast.
Fungus (*pl.,* fungi) Organism similar to plants but lacking chlorophyll and capable of producing mycotic (fungal) infections.
Mycosis General term for a fungal infection.

Onychomycosis Fungal infection involving the fingernails or toenails, also known as tinea unguium.
Ringworm Group of tinea infections involving the body or scalp that have a characteristic ring-like shape. Ringworm is spread person to person and animal to person.
Vulvovaginal candidiasis Yeast vaginitis.

What Are Fungi and Yeast?

Fungi are organisms similar to plants but lacking chlorophyll and capable of producing mycotic (fungal) infections. Thousands of different fungi exist. Mold, mildew, yeast, and mushrooms are all types of fungi. Many fungi are beneficial and do not cause disease. For example, some mushrooms and fungi are edible. The antibiotic penicillin is derived from a mold, and yeast causes bread to rise. Other fungi can cause severe illness. *Pneumocystis jiroveci* is a fungus that can cause pneumonia in individuals who have a decreased immune system response (are immunocompromised); *Aspergillus fumigatus* is a mold that also causes serious respiratory infection.

Fungal Infections of the Skin and Nails

The general term used to describe a fungal infection is *mycosis.* Most fungal infections of the skin are caused by a group of fungi called dermatophytes. Dermatophyte infections are common and affect up to 20% to 25% of the global population. This is because fungi are ubiquitous (found everywhere). They are found in the air, soil, plants, and water. They are also found on surfaces in the home, office, schools, and gyms and even occur normally on our bodies. Fungi that are part of the normal body flora may become pathogenic (cause infection) only when the normal balance of flora is upset. For example, women who take broad-spectrum antibiotics may get a yeast infection because the bacteria and fungi that keep the yeast that are normally present in the vagina from overgrowing are killed by the antibiotic. Dermatophytes thrive on

dead keratin, a tough protein substance found in the top layer of skin, nails, and hair.

Fungal infections caused by the dermatophyte tinea are named for the site of the infection. For example, tinea manus is a fungal infection on the hands, tinea corporis is an infection on the body, and tinea capitis is located on the head (hence cap). Tinea infections are also commonly called *ringworm.*

> **❶ TECH ALERT!**
>
> Ringworm is caused by a fungus, not a worm, as the name implies!

Athlete's Foot

Athlete's foot (tinea pedis) (Fig. 33.1) is a common fungal infection that affects athletes and nonathletes. Symptoms are peeling, flaking skin between the toes, redness, itchiness, burning or stinging, and blisters and thickening of skin on the soles of the feet and heels. It may be accompanied by a foul odor. If severe, it may cause cracking of the skin, oozing, and secondary bacterial infection.

Individuals who have abrasions on the feet, as caused by improperly fitted shoes that rub against the skin, are more susceptible to athlete's foot. Tips for prevention of athlete's foot are listed in Box 33.1.

"Ringworm"

Ringworm infections are caused by tinea fungi (*Tinea mentagrophytes, Tinea rubrum,* and *Microsporum canis*) and may occur on the scalp,

• **Fig. 33.1** Athlete's foot. (From Callen JP, Greer KE, Hood A, et al: *Color atlas of dermatology*, Philadelphia, 1993, WB Saunders.)

• **BOX 33.1** **Prevention of Athlete's Foot**

- Keep your feet clean and dry.
  - Dry between your toes after swimming or bathing.
  - Wear leather shoes or sandals that allow your feet to breathe.
  - When indoors, wear socks without shoes.
  - Wear cotton socks to absorb sweat. Change your socks twice a day. (White socks do not prevent athlete's foot, as some people believe.)
  - Use talcum or antifungal powder on your feet.
- Allow your shoes to air for at least 24 h before you wear them again.
- Wear shower sandals in public pools and showers.

• **Fig. 33.2** Tinea corporis. (From Zitelli BJ, McIntire S, Nowalk AJ: *Zitelli and Davis' atlas of pediatric physical diagnosis*, ed 6, Philadelphia, 2012, Elsevier.)

• **Fig. 33.3** Ringworm of the scalp. (From Callen JP, Greer KE, Paller LJ, et al: *Color atlas of dermatology*, ed 2, Philadelphia, 2000, Saunders.)

body, feet, fingernails, or toenails. Ringworm is contagious and is spread person to person by physical contact with infected surfaces or lesions. Ringworm can also spread between humans and animals. Cats and dogs may be carriers of the fungus.

Ringworm of the body is also known as tinea corporis. Patches and plaques appear pink to red, with raised scaly borders. They form in a distinctive circular pattern that gives the name of "ring" worm (Fig. 33.2).

Tinea capitis is also called ringworm of the scalp. It occurs more frequently in children than in adults and is spread by sharing contaminated hats, combs, clothing, bedding, and linens. It may also be spread from animal to person. The fungus can cause bald patches on the scalp (Fig. 33.3).

Tinea manus affects the hands, and tinea unguium affects the nails. A fungal infection of the nails is also called *onychomycosis*. Infected nails become discolored and thick and may crumble or fall off. Onychomycosis is hard to treat with topically applied *antifungals* because it is difficult for drugs to penetrate the nails and nail bed (Fig. 33.4).

TECH NOTE!

Frequent removal and replacement of artificial nails can cause thinning of the nail bed, increasing susceptibility to onychomycosis.

• **Fig. 33.4** Onychomycosis.

• BOX 33.2 Risk Factors for Vulvovaginal Candidiasis

- Age
- Decreased immune status
- Diabetes
- Drug therapy (e.g., hormone replacement therapy, oral contraceptives, antibiotics, immunosuppressives, corticosteroids)
- Douching
- Diet
- Menses
- Pregnancy
- Sexual activity
- Stress
- Tight-fitting clothing and synthetic underwear

• BOX 33.3 Signs of Vulvovaginal Candidiasis

- Itching
- Cottage cheese–like vaginal discharge
- Burning
- Pain during intercourse

• **Fig. 33.5** Thrush.

Candidiasis

Candida, also called "yeast," is a type of fungus that thrives in warm moist areas and can cause fungal infections in the vagina, groin, penis, skin folds, corners of the mouth, and nail beds. *Candida* is normally present in the gastrointestinal tract and vagina but causes infection only when conditions are favorable for the overgrowth of yeast.

Vulvovaginal candidiasis is also known as yeast vaginitis. The risk for getting yeast vaginitis increases with age. Changes in hormone levels, such as occurs during pregnancy or when taking oral contraceptives or hormone replacement therapy, can also increase the risk of infection. When the body's ability to fight infection is suppressed because of infections such as human immunodeficiency virus (HIV) or if taking immunosuppressive drugs (e.g., corticosteroids, antineoplastic agents), fungal infections may flourish. Risk factors of vulvovaginal candidiasis are listed in Box 33.2. Signs and symptoms of vulvovaginal candidiasis are shown in Box 33.3.

Candida can also cause infections in the oral cavity and in the area surrounding the mouth. A *Candida* infection in the oral cavity is termed *thrush* (Fig. 33.5). Thrush is most common in infants. A thrush infection in adults is a sign that the immune system is compromised. Thrush is an opportunistic infection that occurs in individuals with diseases that affect the immune system (such as HIV), persons who take immunosuppressive medicines for cancer treatment or after stem cell and organ transplantation, and individuals taking broad-spectrum antiinfective agents.

Treatment of Fungal and Yeast Infections

There are three primary mechanisms of action for antifungal agents. Most antifungal agents act by destroying the fungus's cell membrane. The cell membrane of fungi differs from the cell membrane of human cells, so destruction of fungi does not destroy human cells. A second mechanism is interference with the synthesis of nucleic acids needed for replication. A third mechanism is inhibiting the synthesis of the fungal cell wall. Some fungal infections can be treated with nonprescription antifungal agents. Ringworm, vulvovaginal candidiasis, jock itch, and athlete's foot are examples of fungal infections that are cured using over-the-counter (OTC) drugs. Onychomycosis and systemic fungal infections must be treated with prescription antifungals.

Imidazoles and Triazoles

Imidazoles and triazoles are formulated for the treatment of cutaneous (skin) fungal infections and systemic infections. Clotrimazole and miconazole are topical imidazoles that are available without prescription (OTC) in the United States and Canada. Butoconazole, ketoconazole, and tioconazole are OTC antifungals that treat athlete's foot, vulvovaginal candidiasis, jock itch, ringworm, and oral candidiasis. The remaining imidazoles (econazole, oxiconazole, sulconazole, sertaconazole) are restricted to prescription use in both countries. Fluconazole, itraconazole, posaconazole, terconazole, and voriconazole are triazoles. All require a prescription in the United States. Fluconazole is available without prescription in Canada.

> **❶ TECH ALERT!**
>
> The following drugs have look-alike and sound-alike issues:
> Diflucan and Diprivan

Mechanism of Action and Pharmacokinetics
The imidazoles and triazoles interfere with ergosterol, an essential component needed for the synthesis of the fungal cell membrane. This causes cellular contents to leak out, and the cell dies. Topical azoles are formulated for application to the skin (creams, gel, lotion), mucous membranes (vaginal creams, suppositories), and scalp (shampoo).

Adverse Effects
The most common adverse effects for topical imidazoles and triazoles are stinging or burning at the application site, redness, itchiness, or blistering. Nausea and vomiting, skin rash, liver toxicity, and photophobia are adverse reactions linked to oral use of ketoconazole.

Imidazoles and Triazoles

Generic Name	US Brand Name(s) / Canadian Brand Name(s)	Dosage Forms and Strengths	Prescription/OTC Status
butoconazole[a]	Gynezole-1	Cream, vaginal: 2%	OTC
	Not available		
clotrimazole[a]	Fungicure Intensive, Lotrimin AF Jock Itch, Lotrimin AF, Mycelex, Trivagizole 3	**Cream, topical**: 1% **Solution, Topical**: 1% **Cream, vaginal**: 1%, 2%, 10%[b] **Tablet, vaginal tab**: 100 mg, 200 mg, 500 mg **Vaginal tab + cream (Combipak):** 500-mg vaginal tab + 1% cream, 200-mg vaginal tab + 1% cream **Troche:** 10 mg	OTC and prescription
	Canasten, Canesten Cream 1, Canesten Cream 3, Canesten Cream 6, Canesten Comfortab 1, Canesten Comfortab 3, Canasten Comfortab Combi-Pak-1, Canasten Comfortab Combi-Pak-3, Clotrimaderm Cream, Clotrimaderm Vaginal Cream		
econazole[a]	Ecoza, Spectazole	**Cream (Spectazole):** 1% **Foam, topical (Ecoza):** 1%	Prescription
	Not available		
fluconazole[a]	Diflucan	**Capsule (Canesoral, Diflucan One, Monicure)**[b]**:** 150 mg **Powder, for oral suspension:** 10 mg/mL; 40 mg/mL[c] **Solution, for injection:** 2 mg/mL **Tablet:** 50 mg, 100 mg, 150 mg[c], 200 mg[c]	OTC and prescription (Canada) Prescription only (United States)
	Canesoral, Diflucan, Diflucan One, Monicure		
itraconazole[a]	Sporonox, Onmel	**Capsule:** 100 mg **Tablet (Onmel):** 200 mg **Solution, oral:** 10 mg/mL	Prescription
	Sporonox		
ketoconazole[a]	Extina, Nizoral, Nizoral A-D, Xolegel, Ketozole	**Cream (Ketoderm, Ketozole, Nizoral):** 2% **Foam, topical (Extina):** 2% **Gel (Xolegel):** 2% **Shampoo:** 1% (Nizoral A-D),[c] 2% **Tablet:** 200 mg	OTC—Cream and shampoo Prescription—Other formulations
	Ketoderm, Nizoral Cream		
miconazole[a]	Desenex AF, Lotrimin AF, Micatin, Monistat 3, Monistat 7, Monistat 1 Combination Pack, Monistat 1 Triple Action System Combination Pack, Monistat 1 Day or Night Combination Pack, Monistat 3 combination pack, M-Zole 3 Combination Pack, Oravig, Ting, Zeasorb	**Cream (Micatin Derm, Monistat Derm):** 2% **Lotion (Zeasorb):** 2% **Ointment:** 2% **Buccal tablet (Oravig):** 50 mg **Powder, topical (Lotrimin AF, Micatin, Desenex, Zeasorb AF):** 2% **Spray, solution (Lotrimin AF):** 2% **Spray, powder (Cruex, Desenex Jock Itch, Lotrimin AF Deodorant, Ting):** 2% **Vaginal cream:** 2% (Monistat-7), 4% (Monistat-3) **Vaginal suppository:** 100 mg[c] (Monistat 7), 200 mg[c] (Monistat 3), 400 mg[b] (Monistat 3), 1200 mg (Monistat 1) **Vaginal suppository + cream:** 100-mg suppository + 2% cream (Monistat 7 Dual-Pak); 200-mg suppository + 2% cream (Monistat 3 combination pack, M-Zole 3 combination); 400-mg suppository + 2% cream (Monistat 3 Dual-Pak); 1200-mg suppository + 2% cream (Monistat 1 combination pack) **Vaginal cream 2% + topical cream 2%:** (Monistat 7 Triple Action Pack	OTC and Prescription
	Micatin, Micoderm, Monistat 7, Monistat Derm, Monistat 1 Combination Pack, Monistat 3 Dual-Pak, Monistat 7 Dual-Pak, Monistat 1 Vaginal Ovule, Monistat 3 Vaginal Ovules, Monistat 3 Vaginal cream,		

Imidazoles and Triazoles—cont'd

Generic Name	US Brand Name(s) / Canadian Brand Name(s)	Dosage Forms and Strengths	Prescription/OTC Status
miconazole + zinc oxide + petrolatum	Vusion / Not available	**Ointment**: 0.25% miconazole + 15% + zinc oxide + 81.35% petrolatum	Prescription
oxiconazole	Oxistat / Not available	**Cream**: 1% **Lotion**: 1%	Prescription
posaconazole	Noxafil / Posanol	**Solution, IV**: 18 mg/mL **Suspension, oral**: 40 mg/mL **Tablet, delayed release**: 100 mg	Prescription
sertaconazole	Ertaczo / Not available	**Cream**: 2%	Prescription
sulconazole	Exelderm / Not available	**Cream**: 1% **Topical solution**: 1%	Prescription
terconazole[a]	Generic / Generic	**Vaginal cream**: 0.8%,[c] 0.4% **Vaginal suppository**[c]: 80 mg	Prescription
tioconazole[a]	Vagistat-1 / Not available	**Vaginal ointment**: 6.5%	OTC
voriconazole[a]	Vfend / Vfend	**Powder, for injection**: 200 mg per vial **Powder, for oral suspension**: 40 mg/mL **Tablet**: 50 mg, 200 mg	Prescription
clotrimazole + fluconazole	Not available / Canesoral Combipak, Clotrimaderm-Fluconazole Combipak	**Vaginal cream + capsule**: 1% clotrimazole cream + 150 mg fluconazole	OTC
clotrimazole + betamethasone	Lotrisone / Lotriderm	**Cream**: 1% clotrimazole cream + betamethasone 0.05% **Lotion**[c]: 1% clotrimazole cream + betamethasone 0.05%	Prescription

[a]Generic available.
[b]Available in Canada only.
[c]Available in the United States only.
OTC, Over-the-counter.

---

❶ TECH ALERT!

Fluconazole, itraconazole, ketoconazole, and posaconazole interact with numerous drugs (e.g., macrolide antibiotics, quinidine, protease inhibitors, statins, cimetidine, and calcium channel blockers).

❶ TECH ALERT!

Fungicure, Zeasorb, Lotrimin, Lamisil, and other antifungal products are marketed in formulations that contain clotrimazole, terbinafine, tolnaftate, or undecylenic acid. Read labels carefully to select the desired product.

Allylamine Antifungals

Butenafine, naftifine, and terbinafine are classified as allylamine antifungals. Lamisil (terbinafine) is effective for treating fungal infections involving the nails.

Mechanism of Action and Pharmacokinetics

Allylamine antifungals inhibit the synthesis of the cell membrane of susceptible fungi by blocking an enzyme needed for the synthesis of ergosterol. Butenafine and naftifine are only available for topical application. Terbinafine is formulated for topical and oral use. Terbinafine is fungicidal (kills fungi), whereas "azole" antifungals (e.g., clotrimazole and miconazole) are only fungistatic (slow the growth of fungi). When administered orally, therapeutic levels are reached within 3 to 18 weeks. Therapeutic levels persist in the skin for 2 to 3 weeks after terbinafine has been discontinued.

Adverse Effects

Orally administered terbinafine may produce nausea, vomiting, altered taste, headache, and tiredness. Topical application of terbinafine, butenafine, or naftifine may produce burning, stinging, redness, itchiness, and drying of the skin.

Allylamines

Generic Name	US Brand Name(s) Canadian Brand Name(s)	Dosage Form and Strength	Prescription/OTC Status
butenafine[a]	Mentax, Lotrimin Ultra	**Cream:** 1%	Prescription (Mentax)
	Not available		OTC (all Lotrimin Ultra)
naftifine[a]	Naftin	**Cream:** 1%, 2%	Prescription
	Not available	**Gel:** 1%, 2%	
terbinafine[a]	Lamisil, Lamisil AT	**Cream:** 1%	Prescription
	Lamisil	**Tablet:** 250 mg	OTC (all Lamisil AT formulations)[b]
		Spray: 1%	
		Topical solution[b]: 1%	

[a]Generic available.
[b]Available in the United States only.
OTC, Over-the-counter.

Polyene Class of Antifungals

Nystatin, natamycin, and amphotericin B are derived from the fungi-like bacteria *Streptomyces*. They belong to the class of antifungals called polyenes. Nystatin is used for the treatment of *Candida* infections on the skin and mucous membranes. Nystatin suspension is commonly prescribed for the treatment of thrush. Amphotericin B is prescribed for systemic infections caused by various fungi, including candidiasis, histoplasmosis, and aspergillosis. Natamycin is used to treat fungal infections in the eye (e.g., blepharitis, conjunctivitis, keratitis). These infections are described in Chapter 15.

Mechanism of Action and Pharmacokinetics

Nystatin, natamycin, and amphotericin B inhibit the synthesis of the fungal cell membrane by binding irreversibly to ergosterol. Nystatin is available only for oral and topical use. Oral absorption of amphotericin B is low so the drug is administered parenterally. Natamycin is formulated for ophthalmic use.

Adverse Effects

Systemic absorption of nystatin is low when administered topically and orally, so adverse effects are minimal. Oral administration may produce nausea or diarrhea. Amphotericin B may produce nausea, vomiting, kidney damage, fever, chills, headache, and thrombophlebitis when administered intravenously. Amphotericin B may also cause potassium loss (hypokalemia).

Thiocarbamates

Tolnaftate is the only antifungal belonging to the thiocarbamate class. It is approved for the treatment and prevention of athlete's foot. It is also indicated for the treatment of ringworm and jock itch. Tolnaftate is available without prescription.

Mechanism of Action and Pharmacokinetics

The mechanism of action for tolnaftate is similar to that of terbinafine and naftifine.

Adverse Effects

Adverse reactions are mild; they include irritation at the site of application, itching, or burning.

Echinocandins

Anidulafungin, caspofungin, and micafungin belong to a class of antifungal agents called echinocandins. They are effective for treating infections caused by *Candida* and *Aspergillus*.

> **⊘ TECH ALERT!**
>
> A common ending for echinocandin antifungals is *-fungin.*

Mechanism of Action and Pharmacokinetics

Echinocandins interfere with the synthesis of the fungal cell wall. They are not toxic to human cells because their target is a cell wall component that does not exist in human cells. Oral absorption is poor, so echinocandins are formulated for parenteral use.

Adverse Effects

Echinocandins have fewer adverse effects and drug interactions than other oral or parenterally administered antifungals. They can cause elevated liver enzyme levels, diarrhea, and hypokalemia.

Miscellaneous Agents

The remaining antifungal agents work by various mechanisms of action. Ciclopirox and undecylenic acid are effective for treating athlete's foot and jock itch. Ciclopirox is a broad-spectrum antifungal agent and is also approved for the treatment of ringworm and mild onychomycosis. Griseofulvin is an orally administered drug used to treat onychomycosis. Povidone-iodine is used to treat thrush and is also used as an antiseptic wash (orally and topically).

Mechanism of Action and Pharmacokinetics

Ciclopirox, povidone-iodine, and undecylenic acid are topical antifungal agents. Ciclopirox interferes with DNA and RNA

Polyenes

Generic Name	US Brand Name(s) / Canadian Brand Name(s)	Dosage Form and Strength	Prescription/OTC Status
amphotericin B[a]	Abelcet, Ambisome / Abelcet, Ambisome, Fungizone	**Powder, for injection (Ambisome, Fungizone):** 50 mg/vial / **Suspension, for IV (Abelcet):** 5 mg/mL	Prescription
natamycin	Natacyn / Not available	**Ophthalmic suspension:** 5%	Prescription
nystatin[a]	Generic / Nyaderm	**Cream:** 100,000 units/g / **Tablet, oral[b]:** 500,000 units / **Ointment:** 100,000 units/g / **Powder, topical[b]:** 100,000 units / **Suspension, oral:** 100,000 units/mL / **Vaginal cream:** 25,000 units/g	Prescription OTC (topical)[c]
nystatin + triamcinolone acetonide[a]	Mykacet / Not available	**Cream:** 100,000 U nystatin + 1% triamcinolone / **Ointment:** 100,000 U nystatin + 1% triamcinolone	Prescription

[a]Generic available.
[b]Available in the United States only.
[c]Available in the Canada only.
OTC, Over-the-counter.

Thiocarbamates

Generic Name	US Brand Name(s) / Canadian Brand Name(s)	Dosage Forms and Strengths	Prescription/OTC status
tolnaftate[a]	Lamisil AF Defense, Myocide Clinical NS, Pro Clerz Fungi-Cide PM, Tinactin, Tinactin Jock Itch / Dr. Scholl's Athlete's Foot, Odor Eaters, Tinactin, Tinactin Chill, Zeasorb AF, Pro Clerz Antifungal Liquid	**Cream (Pro Clerz Fungi-Cide PM, Tinactin, Tinactin Jock Itch):** 1% / **Spray (Lamisil Defense AF, Odor Eaters, Tinactin, Tinactin Liquid Chill):** 1% / **Topical powder (Dr. Scholl's Athlete's Foot, Lamisil AF, Tinactin Aerosol Powder, Zeasorb AF):** 1% / **Topical solution (Pro Clerz Fungi-Cide):** 1%	OTC

[a]Generic available.
OTC, Over-the-counter.

Echinocandins

Generic Name	US Brand Name(s) / Canadian Brand Name(s)	Dosage Forms and Strengths	Prescription/OTC status
anidulafungin	Eraxis / Eraxis	**Powder, for IV infusion:** 50 mg/vial,[a] 100 mg/vial	Prescription
caspofungin[b]	Cancidas / Cancidas	**Powder, for IV infusion:** 50 mg/vial, 70 mg/vial	Prescription
micafungin	Mycamine / Mycamine	**Powder, for IV infusion:** 50 mg/vial, 100 mg/vial	Prescription

[a]Strength available in the United States only.
[b]Generic available.
OTC, Over-the-counter.

synthesis. Undecylenic acid and zinc undecylate are combined to produce a drug that decreases the spread of susceptible fungi. Formulations must contain at least 10% undecylenate to be effective (between 10% and 27% undecylenate). In addition, zinc undecylenate is an astringent and reduces irritation.

Griseofulvin interferes with fungal mitosis. This disrupts the ability of the fungus to replicate. Griseofulvin formulations made with ultramicronized crystals (Gris-PEG) offer the best absorption. Absorption is also increased when the drug is taken with a fatty meal.

❶ TECH ALERT!

Griseofulvin microsize and griseofulvin ultramicrosize have look-alike and sound-alike issues.

Adverse Effects

Topically applied antifungals may produce mild burning, stinging, itching, swelling, or other signs of skin irritation. Common adverse effects caused by the administration of griseofulvin are nausea, vomiting, headache, dizziness, gas, and heartburn.

Miscellaneous Antifungal Agents

Generic Name	US Brand Name(s) / Canadian Brand Name(s)	Dosage Forms and Strengths	Prescription/ OTC Status
ciclopirox[a]	Loprox, Penlac / Loprox, Penlac, Steiprox	**Cream:** 0.77%,[b] 1%[c] **Lotion:** 0.77%,[b] 1%[c] **Nail lacquer (Penlac):** 8% **Shampoo:** 1% (Loprox), 1.5% (Steiprox)	Prescription
griseofulvin[a]	Gris-PEG / Not available	**Suspension:** 125 mg/5 mL **Tablet, ultramicrosize:** 125 mg, 250 mg	Prescription
povidone-iodine[a]	Betadine First Aid Spray, E-Z Scrub / Generics	**Douche:** 0.3% **Ophthalmic solution:** 5% **Scrub, cleanser:** 7.5% **Solution:** 1%, 5%, 10% **Spray:** 5% **Sponge (E-Z Scrub):** 10%, 20%	Prescription—ophthalmic OTC—all other formulations
undecylenic acid[a]	Desenex, Fungicure Liquid, Fungi Nail Antifungal / Fungicure Liquid	**Solution, topical:** 25% **Ointment:** 25% **Pen brush:** 25%	OTC

[a]Generic available.
[b]Available in the United States only.
[c]Available in Canada only.
OTC, Over-the-counter.

Summary of Drugs Used for the Treatment of Fungal and Yeast Infections

Generic Name	US Brand Name(s)	Usual Dose and Dosing Schedule[a]	Warning Labels
Imidazoles and Triazoles			
butoconazole	Gynezole-1	**Vaginal cream:** One applicatorful vaginally at bedtime for 3–7 days depending on product formulation	COMPLETE THE FULL COURSE OF THERAPY—ALL
clotrimazole	Canasten Mycelex	**Vaginal Cream:** One applicatorful at bedtime for 3–14 days depending on product formulation **Vaginal tablet:** Insert once daily for 1–3 days depending on product formulation **Topical cream** Apply twice daily.	
econazole	Ecoza Spectazole	**Topical:** Apply twice daily.	

Summary of Drugs Used for the Treatment of Fungal and Yeast Infections—cont'd

	Generic Name	US Brand Name(s)	Usual Dose and Dosing Schedule[a]	Warning Labels
	fluconazole	Diflucan	**Oral or IV:** 200 mg on day 1, then 100 mg daily for 2 weeks (esophageal or oropharyngeal candidiasis) *or* 150–200 mg as a single dose or three doses for 3 days each (vulvovaginal candidiasis)	SHAKE WELL (SUSPENSION)— fluconazole, posaconazole
	itraconazole	Sporonox, Onmel	**Oral:** 100–400 mg once daily **Topical:** Apply 1–2 times daily	TAKE WITH FOOD (CAPSULES) AVOID GRAPEFRUIT JUICE (CAPSULES)—itraconazole vorconazole
	ketoconazole	Nizoral	**Oral:** 200–400 mg once daily **Topical:** Apply daily for up to 6 weeks **For dandruff:** Use shampoo every 3–4 days for up to 8 weeks	TAKE WITH FOOD (TABLETS)— ketoconazole, posaconazole AVOID ALCOHOL—ketoconazole, voriconazole
	miconazole	Monistat	**Vaginal:** One applicatorful or one suppository at bedtime for 1–14 days depending on product formulation **Topical:** Apply twice a day.	
	oxiconazole	Oxistat	**Topical:** Apply once or twice daily	
	posaconazole	Noxafil	**Oral:** 200 mg 3 times a day	
	sulconazole	Exelderm	**Topical:** Apply once or twice daily	
	terconazole	Generic	**Vaginal:** One applicatorful or one suppository at bedtime for 3–7 days depending on product formulation	
	tioconazole	Vagistat-1	**Vaginal:** One applicatorful as a single dose	
	sertaconazole	Ertaczo	Apply a thin layer of 2% cream to cleansed, dry, infected area twice daily for 4 weeks	
	voriconazole	Vfend	**Parenteral:** 6 mg/kg IV every 12 h **Oral:** 400 mg every 12 h loading dose on day 1, followed by 200 mg every 12 h	TAKE ON AN EMPTY STOMACH—vorconazole
Allylamines				
	butenafine	Mentax	**Topical:** Apply once daily for 2–4 weeks	COMPLETE THE FULL COURSE OF THERAPY—ALL
	naftifine	Naftin	**Topical:** Apply cream once daily and apply gel twice daily.	TAKE WITH FOOD (TABLETS)— terbinafine
	terbinafine	Lamisil AF	**Topical:** Apply cream twice daily and apply gel once daily for 1–4 weeks **Oral:** 250 mg once daily for 6–12 weeks	
Polyenes				
	amphotericin B	Fungizone	**IV:** 0.25–1.5/kg/day (max, 1.5 mg/day)	PROTECT FROM LIGHT (IV SOLUTION)—amphotericin B REFRIGERATE. amphotericin B
	natamycin	Natacyn	**Ophthalmic:** See Chapter 15	SHAKE WELL—natamycin
	nystatin	Generics	**Capsule:** 1 cap 3 times a day **Suspension:** 4–6 mL swished in mouth 4 times a day **Topical:** Apply twice daily. **Vaginal:** One insert nightly for 14 days	COMPLETE THE FULL COURSE OF THERAPY—natamycin SHAKE WELL (SUSPENSION)— natamycin
Thiocarbamates				
	tolnaftate	Tinactin	**Topical:** Apply twice daily for 2–4 weeks	COMPLETE THE FULL COURSE OF THERAPY

Continued

Summary of Drugs Used for the Treatment of Fungal and Yeast Infections—cont'd

Generic Name	US Brand Name(s)	Usual Dose and Dosing Schedule[a]	Warning Labels
Echinocandins			
anidulafungin	Eraxis	100-mg IV loading dose on day 1, followed by 50 mg IV daily for 7 days after symptoms resolve	REFRIGERATE; DON'T FREEZE—anidulafungin, caspofungin
caspofungin	Cancidas	70-mg IV infusion as a loading dose on day 1, followed by 50- mg IV infusion once daily for at least 14 days	TO MIX, GENTLY SWIRL; DO NOT SHAKE—micafungin
micafungin	Mycamine	150 mg IV daily for 10–30 days	MAY BE STORED AT ROOM TEMPERATURE FOR 24 H—micafungin
Miscellaneous Agents			
griseofulvin	Gris-PEG	375–750 mg daily or in 1 or 2 divided doses	COMPLETE THE FULL COURSE OF THERAPY—ALL
ciclopirox	Loprox	**Topical:** Apply twice daily	TAKE WITH FOOD—griseofulvin SHAKE WELL (LOTION)—ciclopirox

[a]Usual dose for candidiasis or tinea.

TECHNICIAN'S CORNER

1. There are many reports of onychomycosis caused by artificial nails. What is causing these infections, and how can they be prevented?
2. How did the term *athlete's foot* come about?

Key Points

- Some fungi are beneficial to humans, whereas others cause serious infections.
- The general term used to describe a fungal infection is *mycosis*.
- Fungal infections caused by the dermatophyte tinea are named for the site of the infection. For example, tinea manus is a fungal infection on the hands, tinea corporis is an infection on the body, and tinea capitis is located on the head (cap).
- Athlete's foot (tinea pedis) is a common fungal infection that affects athletes and nonathletes.
- Athlete's foot can be prevented by the following: (1) keeping feet clean and dry; (2) wearing open sandals to permit feet to breathe; (3) not walking barefoot across the floor of public facilities; (4) wearing cotton socks and changing socks daily; and (5) using antifungal powders to prevent recurrent infections.
- Tinea infections are also called *ringworm*. Ringworm has a characteristic ring-like shape and may affect the body, scalp, nails, or feet.
- Ringworm is contagious and is spread via person-to-person and animal-to-person contact.
- Women who take broad-spectrum antiinfectives may get a yeast infection because the bacteria and fungi that keep the yeast that are normally present in the vagina from overgrowing are killed by the antibiotic.
- *Candida,* also called yeast, is a type of fungus that thrives in warm moist areas that causes fungal infections in the vagina, groin, and mouth.
- Vulvovaginal candidiasis is also known as yeast vaginitis.
- A *Candida* infection in the oral cavity is called thrush.
- Fungal infections such as vulvovaginal candidiasis, jock itch, and athlete's foot can be cured using OTC drugs. Some of these drugs can also be used as prophylaxis.
- There are three primary mechanisms of action for antifungal agents: (1) destroy the cell membrane of the fungus; (2) interfere with the synthesis of nucleic acids needed for replication; and (3) inhibit the synthesis of the fungal cell wall.
- Topical antifungal agents are formulated for application to the skin (creams, gel, lotion), mucous membranes (vaginal creams, suppositories), and scalp (shampoo).
- Butenafine, naftifine, and terbinafine are classified as allylamine antifungals.
- Nystatin, natamycin, and amphotericin B are all derived from the fungi-like bacteria *Streptomyces* and belong to the class of antifungals called polyenes.
- Nystatin, natamycin, and amphotericin B inhibit the synthesis of the fungal cell membrane.
- Tolnaftate is the only antifungal belonging to the thiocarbamate class. It is approved for the treatment and prevention of athlete's foot.
- Anidulafungin, caspofungin, and micafungin belong to a class of antifungal agents called echinocandins.
- Echinocandins interfere with the synthesis of the fungal cell wall.

Review Questions

1. *Candida* is a type of _____. It is also called yeast.
   a. virus
   b. bacteria
   c. fungus
   d. protozoan
2. Select the antifungal that is not an OTC product applied or inserted vaginally to treat vaginal yeast infections.
   a. Gynezole-1
   b. Canesten Comfortab 1
   c. Diflucan
   d. Monistat-3
3. Ringworm is caused by a _____.
   a. worm
   b. fungus
   c. bacteria
   d. insect
4. Fungal infections of the _____ are called onychomycosis.
   a. hair
   b. skin
   c. scalp
   d. nails
5. Which of the following is the primary mechanism of action for antifungal agents?
   a. Destroying the cell membrane of the fungus
   b. Interfering with the synthesis of nucleic acids needed for replication
   c. Inhibiting the synthesis of the fungal cell wall
   d. All of the above

6. _____ is effective for treating fungal infections involving the nails.
   a. terbinafene
   b. tioconazole
   c. nystatin
   d. clotrimazole
7. Nystatin suspension is commonly prescribed for the treatment of thrush.
   a. True
   b. False
8. All of the following antifungal are marketed as OTC formulations EXCEPT _____.
   a. povidone
   b. clotrimazole
   c. miconazole
   d. itraconazole
9. Echinocandins are formulated for oral use.
   a. True
   b. False
10. Sporonox may be administered _____.
    a. topically
    b. orally
    c. parenterally
    d. a and b

Bibliography

Aaron DM: Candidiasis (Mucocutaneous Moniliasis). 2017a. From: http://www.merckmanuals.com/professional/dermatologic-disorders/fungal-skin-infections/candidiasis-mucocutaneous#v964306. (Retrieved 28 October 2017).

Aaron DM: Overview of Dermatophytoses. 2017b. From: http://www.merckmanuals.com/professional/dermatologic-disorders/fungal-skin-infections/overview-of-dermatophytoses?qt=ringwormandalt=sh. (Retrieved 29 October 2017).

Cappelletty D, Eiselstein-McKitrick K: The echinocandins, *Pharmacotherapy* 27:369–388, 2007.

FDA: Drugs@FDA: FDA Approved Drug Products. nd. From: http://www.accessdata.fda.gov/scripts/cder/daf/. (Retrieved 20 September 2018).

Health Canada: Drug Product Database. 2017. From: https://health-products.canada.ca/dpd-bdpp/index-eng.jsp. (Retrieved 20 September 2018).

Institute for Safe Medication Practices: List of Confused Drugs. 2015. From: https://www.ismp.org/tools/confuseddrugnames.pdf. (Retrieved 9 September 2017).

Jaulim Z, Salmon N, Fuller C: Fungal skin infections: current approaches to management, *Prescriber* 26(19):31–35, 2015.

Kalant H, Grant D, Mitchell J: *Principles of medical pharmacology*, ed 7, Toronto, 2007, Elsevier Canada, p 688, 691–695.

Lance L, Lacy C, Armstrong L, et al: *Drug information handbook for the allied health professional*, ed 12, Hudson, OH, 2005, APhA Lexi-Comp.

MedlinePlus: Cutaneous candidiasis, 2017. http://www.nlm.nih.gov/medlineplus/ency/article/000880.htm.

MedlinePlus: Tinea infections (ringworm), 2016. http://www.nlm.nih.gov/medlineplus/tineainfections.html.

Merck Manual Online Professional Library: Dermatophytoses, 2017. http://www.merck.com/mmpe/sec10/ch120/ch120c.html?qt=ringwormandalt=sh.

National Institute of Allergy and Infectious Diseases: *Understanding Microbes in Sickness and in Health*, Bethesda, 2006, US Department of Health and Human Services. National Institutes of Health. NIH Publication No. 06-4914.

Pray W: *Nonprescription product therapeutics*, Baltimore, 1999, Lippincott Williams and Wilkins, pp 542–551.

US National Library of Medicine: Sexually transmitted diseases (STDs), 2017. https://medlineplus.gov/sexuallytransmitteddiseases.html.

34

Treatment of Pressure Injuries and Burns

LEARNING OBJECTIVES

1. Learn the terminology associated with pressure injures and burns.
2. Describe the stages of pressure injuries and degrees of burns.
3. List and categorize medications used to treat pressure injuries and burns.
4. Describe the mechanism of action for each class of drugs used to treat pressure injuries and burns.
5. Identify significant drug look-alike and sound-alike issues.
6. Identify warning labels and precautionary messages associated with medications used to treat pressure injuries and burns.

KEY TERMS

Blister Collection of fluid below or within the epidermis.
Debridement Surgical removal of foreign material and dead tissue from a wound in order to prevent infection and promote healing.
Pressure injury Pressure sore or "bedsore."
Dehiscent wound A wound that has reopened after it has been closed surgically.
Eschar Blackened necrotic tissue of a pressure injury.
Escharotomy Removal of necrotic skin and underlying tissue.
First-degree burn Minor discomfort and reddening of the skin.
Fourth-degree burn Burn that involves underlying muscles, fasciae, or bone.

Full-thickness burn Third-degree burn where the epidermis and dermis are destroyed.
Partial-thickness burns First- and second-degree burns.
Rule of palms Rule for determining the extent of a burn surface area. A palm size of a burn victim is about 1% of total body surface area.
Rule of nines Formula for estimating the percentage of adult body surface covered by burns dividing the body into 11 areas, each representing 9% of the body surface area.
Second-degree burn Burn that involves deep epidermal layers and causes damage to the upper layers of dermis.
Third-degree burn Burn that is characterized by destruction of the epidermis and dermis.

Pressure Injuries

A *pressure injury* (formerly termed "decubitus ulcers") is commonly called a "bedsore" (Fig. 34.1). A common cause of pressure injuries is lying in a prone position for long periods. Pressure injuries typically occur in patients who are confined to a bed or chair. Patients with sensory or mobility deficits such as spinal cord injury, stroke, coma, multiple sclerosis, peripheral vascular disease, or diabetes; hospitalized older patients; nursing home residents; and malnourished patients are all at risk.

All pressure injuries have a course of injury similar to a burn and are classified in stages according to severity. Pressure injuries can range from a mild pink coloration of the skin, which disappears in a few hours after pressure is relieved on the area, to a deep wound extending to and sometimes through a bone into internal organs. Burns can cause a mild redness of the skin and/or blistering (*first-degree burn*) or produce a deep open wound with blackened tissue (eschar), such as with a *third-degree burn*.

Nonpharmacological Management of Pressure Injuries and Burns

A pressure injury typically forms from continuous pressure to an area; however, it can also occur from friction caused by rubbing against something, such as a bedsheet, cast, or brace, or prolonged exposure to cold. The most common places for pressure injuries to form are over bones close to the skin, such as the elbows, heels, hips, sacrum, ankles, shoulders, back, and back of the head. The weight of a body presses on the bone, and the bone presses on the tissue and skin that it covers. This tissue begins to decay from lack of blood circulation.

The Norton or Braden scale is a simple assessment tool used to determine a patient's risk for developing a pressure injury. The patient is rated on a scale of 1 to 4 on five risk factors (physical condition, mental state, level of activity, mobility, and incontinence). Patients with the lowest score are at the highest risk for pressure injuries.

(A) Stage 1 Pressure Injury – Edema

(B) Stage 2 Pressure Injury

(C) Stage 3 Pressure Injury

(D) Stage 4 Pressure Injury

(E) Unstageable Pressure Injury - Slough and Eschar

• **Fig. 34.1** Pressure Injury. (A) Stage 1. (B) Stage 2. (C) Stage 3. (D) Stage 4. (E) Unstageable. (From National Pressure Ulcer Advisory Panel: Pressure injury staging illustrations, available at http://www.npuap.org/resources/educational-and-clinical-resources/pressure-injury-staging-illustrations/.)

The most important principle is to prevent initial skin damage, which promotes ulceration. In at-risk patients, aggressive nursing practices, such as frequent turning of immobile patients (changing position every two hours or more frequently if needed) and the application of skin protection to bony body parts, can be effective. This two-hour time frame is generally accepted as the maximum interval that the tissue can tolerate pressure without damage. Range-of-motion exercises and early ambulation are encouraged along with the use of low-pressure mattresses and special beds.

Wound Stages

Pressure injuries and burns are often categorized according to stages of severity.

Stage 1: Nonblanchable Erythema of Intact Skin

This stage is characterized by a surface reddening of the skin. The skin is unbroken, and the wound is superficial. Examples of stage 1 wounds are a light sunburn, a first-degree burn, or a pressure injury. The burn heals spontaneously or the pressure injury quickly fades when pressure is relieved on that area. Changes in sensation, temperature, or firmness may precede visual changes. The key factors to consider in a stage 1 wound are the causes of the wound, how to alleviate the pressure on the area to prevent it from worsening, and improving the nutritional status of the individual. The presence of a stage 1 wound is an indication or early warning of a problem and a signal to take preventive action.

Stage 2: Partial-Thickness Skin Loss With Exposed Dermis

This stage is characterized by a *blister*, either broken or unbroken. A partial layer of the skin is injured and the dermis is exposed. The goal of care is to cover, protect, and clean the area. Coverings are designed to insulate, absorb, and protect. Close attention to prevention, protection, nutrition, and hydration is also important. With quick attention, a stage 2 wound can heal rapidly. In general, pressure wounds developing beyond stage 2 are the result of lack of aggressive intervention when first noted at stage 1.

Stage 3: Full-Thickness Skin Loss

In stage 3, the wound has extended through all layers of the skin. It is the primary site for a serious infection to occur. The depth of tissue damage varies by the part of the body that is affected. The goal of treatment is to alleviate pressure, cover and protect the wound, and place an increased emphasis on nutrition and hydration. Medical care is necessary to promote healing and to treat and prevent infection. If left unattended, this type of wound will worsen rapidly. Infection is a grave concern.

Stage 4: Full-Thickness Skin and Tissue Loss

Stage 4 wounds extend through the skin and involve underlying muscle, tendons, and bone. The diameter of the wound is not as important as the depth. Stage 4 wounds are very serious and can produce life-threatening infections. Treatment involves protecting, cleaning, and alleviating pressure on the area. Nutrition and hydration are now critical, because without adequate nutrition, this wound will not heal.

Anyone with a stage 4 wound requires medical care by someone skilled in wound care. A skilled wound care physician, physical therapist, or nurse can sometimes successfully treat a smaller diameter wound without surgery. Surgical removal of the necrotic or decayed tissue (*escharotomy*) is often necessary for wounds of larger diameter.

Drug Therapy for Pressure Injuries

The treatment for a pressure injury involves keeping the area clean and removing necrotic (dead) tissue, which can form a breeding ground for infection. There are many procedures and products available for this purpose. Topical treatments aid the healing of partial-thickness sores (Box 34.1).

• BOX 34.1 Topical Treatment of Decubitus Ulcers

- Occlusive hydrocolloid dressings
- Polyurethane films
- Absorbable gelatin sponges
- Karaya gum patches
- Antiseptic irrigations
- Antibiotic ointments
- Air-permeable occlusive clear dressings (allow aspiration of collected fluids)
- Supportive adhesive-backed foam padding
- Absorptive dextranomer beads

Recombinant Platelet-Derived Growth Factor

Becaplermin is a biologically engineered platelet-derived growth factor. It promotes wound repair by increasing the recruitment and proliferation of cells involved in wound healing and formation of granulation tissue. It is indicated for the treatment of diabetic neuropathic ulcers.

Collagenase

Collagenase is used to promote *debridement* (removal of foreign material and dead tissue from a wound) in dermal ulcers and severe burns. Collagenase is a water-soluble proteinase that specifically breaks down collagen into gelatin, allowing less specific enzymes to act. Commercially available preparations of collagenase (e.g., Santyl) are derived from the bacterium *Clostridium histolyticum*. There is evidence that elastin and fibrin are also degraded by collagenase, but to a lesser degree.

Papain and Urea

Papain/urea an enzymatic debriding ointment is used to slough off necrotic tissue from pressure injuries, varicose and diabetic ulcers, burns, and miscellaneous postoperative and traumatic wounds. Papain is derived from the carica papaya fruit. Papain works by attaching to and breaking down any proteins containing cysteine residues. Collagen contains no cysteine residues and is therefore unaffected by papain. In 2015, the FDA ordered manufacturers to stop producing and marketing papain containing products unless approved by the FDA. There are currently no products approved by the FDA, however sales of existing stock is permitted until depleted.

Trypsin, Balsam Peru, and Castor Oil

Trypsin, balsam Peru, and castor oil are used in the treatment of pressure injuries, varicose ulcers, sunburns, *dehiscent wounds* that have come apart, and for debridement of eschar. Trypsin is used to debride necrotic tissue, balsam Peru increases blood flow to the wound site and may be mildly bactericidal, and castor oil prevents skin cells from breaking down, acts as a protectant covering, and helps reduce pain. Local application may produce temporary stinging at the application site.

Antibacterials

Antibacterial drugs may be used if the pressure injury is not healing or it continues to ooze after two weeks of proper cleansing and bandage changes. Some antibacterial preparations can be applied

---

ⓘ TECH ALERT!

The following drugs have look-alike and sound-alike issues: Granulex and Regranex.

Topical Drugs Used for the Treatment of Pressure Injuries

Generic Name	US Brand Name(s) Canadian Brand Name(s)	Dosage Forms and Strengths
becaplermin	Regranex	Gel: 100 mcg/g (0.01%)
	Not available	
collagenase	Santyl, Xiaflex	**Ointment (Santyl):** 250 units/g
	Santyl	
trypsin, balsam Peru, and castor oil	Granulex, Vasolex	**Aerosol (Granulex):** trypsin 0.1 mg, balsam Peru 72.5 mg, castor oil 650 mg
	Not available	**Ointment (Vasolex):** balsam Peru 87 mg/g, castor oil 788 mg/g, trypsin 90 USP units/g
Topical Antibacterials		
bacitracin zinc[a]	Not available	**Ointment:** 500 units/g
	Bacitin	
gentamicin[a]	Generics	**Cream:** 0.1% **Ointment:** 0.1%
	Not available	
mupirocin[a]	Centany	**Cream:** 2% **Ointment:** 2%
	Bactroban, Bactroban Cream	
Combination Topical Antibacterials		
bacitracin + hydrocortisone + neomycin+ polymixin	Cortisporin	**Ointment:** 400 IU bacitracin + 1% hydrocortisone + 3.5 mg neomycin+ 5000 units polymixin
	Not Available	
bacitracin + gramacidin + polymixin	Not available	**Cream:** 500 IU bacitracin, 0.25 mg gramicidin + 10,000u polymixin
	Polysporin	
bacitracin + polymixin	Not available	Ointment: 500 g bacitracin + 10,000 units polymixin per gram
	Bioderm, Polyderm, Polytopic, Sterisporin	
Antiseptics		
povidone-iodine[a]	Betadine	**Scrub, cleanser:** 7.5%, 10%, 20% **Solution:** 1%, 5%, 10% **Spray:** 5% **See Chapter 33 for additional dosage forms**
	Generics	

[a]Generic available.

directly to the skin. Anti-infectives given by mouth or injection are needed for those who have sepsis or infections in the skin or underlying bone. Anti-infectives are also given to prevent diseased heart valves from getting infected, or when the injury needs surgical repair.

Burns

Typically we think of a burn as a thermal injury or lesion caused by contact of the skin with some hot object or fire. In addition, overexposure to ultraviolet (UV) light (sunburn) or contact with an electric current, corrosive chemical, or radioactive agents causes injury or death to skin cells. The injuries that result can be classified as burns; the effects may be local or systemic, involving primary shock (which occurs immediately after injury and rarely is fatal) or secondary shock (which develops insidiously following severe burns and is often fatal). Worldwide, more than 11 million people

are burned annually (WHO). More than 450,000 people in the United States and Canada receive medical treatment for burns annually; more than 50,000 of these burn victims require hospitalization.

Estimating Burn Surface Area

When burns involve large areas of skin, treatment and the prognosis for recovery depend in large part on the total area involved and severity of the burn. The severity of a burn is determined by the depth and extent (percentage of body surface area [BSA]) of the lesion. There are several ways to estimate the extent of BSA burned. The *rule of palms* method is based on the assumption that the palm size of a burn victim is about 1% of the total BSA. Therefore estimating the number of palms that are burned approximates the percentage of BSA involved.

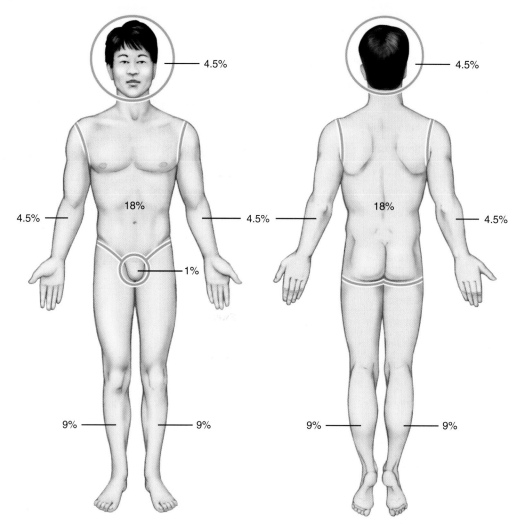

• **Fig. 34.2** Rule of 9s. (From Patton KT, Thibodeau GA: *The human body in health and disease*, ed 6, St. Louis, 2014, Elsevier.)

Another method is the *rule of 9s* (Fig. 34.2). In this technique, the body is divided into 11 areas of 9%, with the area around the genitals, called the perineum, representing the additional 1% of BSA (see Fig. 34.2). The rule of 9s works well with adults, but does not reflect the differences of BSA in small children. Special tables called Lund-Browder charts, which take the large surface area of certain body areas (e.g., the head) in a growing child into account, are used by physicians to estimate burn percentages in children.

The depth of a burn injury depends on the tissue layers of the skin that are involved (Fig. 34.3). A first-degree burn (typical sunburn) causes minor discomfort and some reddening of the skin. Although the surface layers of the burned area may peel in one or two days, no blistering occurs, and the actual tissue destruction is minimal. It can be treated with lidocaine and aloe vera gel or cream. First- and second-degree burns are called *partial-thickness burns*.

Second-degree burns involve the deep epidermal layers and always cause injury to the upper layers of the dermis. In deep second-degree burns, damage to sweat glands, hair follicles, and sebaceous glands may occur, but tissue death is not complete. Blisters, severe pain, generalized swelling, and edema characterize this type of burn. Scarring is common. It is treated with over-the-counter pain medications and antibiotic cream.

Third-degree, or *full-thickness burns* are characterized by destruction of both the epidermis and dermis. Tissue death extends below the follicles and sweat glands. If the burn involves underlying muscles, fasciae, or bone, it may be called a *fourth-degree burn*. A distinction between a second- and third- or fourth-degree burn is that a third- or fourth-degree lesion is insensitive to pain immediately after injury because of destruction of the nerve endings. Scarring is a serious problem. Third- and fourth-degree burns are best managed in specialized burn centers.

Complications

Sloughing of skin, gangrene, scarring, erysipelas (skin infection caused by group A staphylococci), nephritis (kidney infection), pneumonia, immune system impairment, and intestinal disturbances are possible complications. The risk for infection and dehydration is greatest when more than 25% of the body surface is burned.

Signs of infection are as follows:
- Change in color of the burned area or surrounding skin
- Purplish discoloration, particularly if swelling is also present
- Change in thickness of the burn
- Greenish discharge or pus
- Fever

Capillary

Sebaceous
gland

Epidermis

Dermis

Subcutaneous
tissue

Muscle

Bone

Blood vessel

Nerve endings

Hair follicle

Sweat gland

FIRST
DEGREE

SECOND
DEGREE
(partial
thickness)

THIRD
DEGREE
(full
thickness)

FOURTH
DEGREE
(full
thickness—
reaching
muscle or
bone)

• **Fig. 34.3** Classification of burns. (From Patton KT, Thibodeau GA: *The human body in health and disease,* ed 6, St. Louis, 2014, Elsevier.)

Signs of dehydration are as follows:
- Thirst
- Lightheadedness or dizziness (when moving from lying or sitting to standing)
- Weakness
- Dry skin
- Urinating less often than usual

Precautions

Sunburn can be prevented by using sunscreen or sunblock and avoiding excess exposure to UV radiation. Chemical-related skin burns can be prevented by avoiding strong chemicals. "Stop, drop, and roll" should be the first actions if a person is on fire. A rug, blanket, or anything within reach can be used to smother flames. Care must be taken so that the individual does not inhale the smoke. Clothing must be carefully cut away so that skin is not pulled away. Blisters should not be opened, because this will increase the chance for infection. All burned patients must receive appropriate tetanus prophylaxis.

Treatment of Burns

Treatment involves the administration of antibiotics, analgesics, and fluid replacement. Nonpharmacological management includes monitoring cardiac output, tissue perfusion, urinary output, blood

• **BOX 34.2** **Management of Severe Burns**

- Check for airway injury or impaired breathing. Airway injury is most likely to occur after facial burns or smoke inhalation in closed spaces.
- Remove overlying clothing and irrigate affected tissues. Avoid excessive cooling of the body.
- Pharmacologic therapy: antibiotics, IV analgesics, volume replenishment with crystalloid intravenous fluids to ensure adequate hydration
- Gentle debridement of tissues followed by the application of nonadherent dressings, skin substitutes, topical antiseptics, or autografts, as dictated by circumstances
- Nutritional and emotional support

pressure and pulse, body weight, and renal function. Fluid balance is carefully monitored, as well as nutritional therapy (Box 34.2).

Silver Sulfadiazine

Silver sulfadiazine is the most frequently used topical agent for burns. It is used to prevent and treat infections in second- and third-degree burns. The drug is bactericidal against gram-positive and gram-negative organisms, but resistance has occasionally been reported.

Adverse Effects

Local skin reactions such as pain, burning, itching, and hypersensitivity are occasionally reported. Transient leukopenia occurs in

5% to 15% of patients, but there is no increased incidence of infectious complications.

Mafenide

Mafenide is an adjunctive antibacterial agent used for the treatment of first- and second-degree burns. It appears to act on bacterial cellular mechanisms. It interferes with bacterial folic acid synthesis through competitive inhibition of para-aminobenzoic acid. With topical application, mafenide is bacteriostatic against gram-positive and gram-negative bacteria.

Adverse Effects

Pain or a burning sensation following mafenide application is the most frequently reported adverse effect. Mafenide may cause alkaline diuresis, leading to acid-base abnormalities. It also inhibits epithelial regeneration (growth of new tissue).

Silver Nitrate

Silver nitrate is a broad-spectrum agent. It is bacteriostatic at a concentration of 5%. The effects of silver nitrate may result from silver ions readily combining with several biologically important chemical groups.

Adverse Effects

Silver nitrate is prepared with distilled water. The hypotonic solution may lead to electrolyte imbalance.

Povidone-Iodine

Povidone-iodine acts by destroying microbial protein and DNA. This drug has excellent in vitro antimicrobial activity but is inactivated by wound exudates. In vitro refers to a test that is done in glass or plastic vessels in the laboratory. More information about povidine-iodine is found in Chapter 33.

Adverse Effects

Systemic absorption of iodine results in renal and thyroid dysfunction.

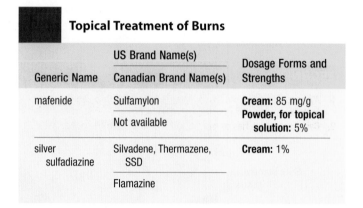

Topical Treatment of Burns

Generic Name	US Brand Name(s)	Dosage Forms and Strengths
	Canadian Brand Name(s)	
mafenide	Sulfamylon	**Cream:** 85 mg/g
	Not available	**Powder, for topical solution:** 5%
silver sulfadiazine	Silvadene, Thermazene, SSD	**Cream:** 1%
	Flamazine	

Rehabilitation

During rehabilitation, individually fitted elastic garments are used to prevent hypertrophic scar formation, and joints are exercised to promote a full range of motion. Referrals for occupational therapy, psychological counseling, support groups, or social services are often necessary to assist the patient with life adjustments.

Summary of Drugs Used in the Treatment of Decubitus Ulcers and Burns

Generic Name	Brand Name	Usual Dose and Dosing Schedule	Warning Labels
Debriding Agents			
Collagenase	Santyl	Apply once daily (more if dressing becomes soiled).	DO NOT TOUCH THE TIP OF THE TUBE TO ANY SURFACE, INCLUDING A FINGER, THE WOUND, OR STERILE GAUZE PAD.
trypsin, balsam peru, and castor oil	Granulex	Apply a minimum of 2 times a day or as often as necessary.	FLAMMABLE—Aerosols
Topical Antibacterials			
0.25 pt	Baciguent	Apply 1–5 times daily for up to 7 days.	NOT TO BE USED FOR LONGER THAN 1 WEEK UNLESS PRESCRIBED.
gentamicin[a]		**Topical:** Apply 3 or 4 times daily to affected area.	REPORT ANY DIZZINESS OR SENSATIONS OF RINGING OR FULLNESS IN EARS.
mupirocin	Bactoban	Apply small amount to affected area 3 times a day for 7 to 14 days.	FOR TOPICAL USE ONLY. DISCONTINUE IF RASH, ITCHING, OR IRRITATION OCCURS.
silver sulfadiazine	Silvadene	Apply bid with a sterile-gloved hand; apply to thickness of $\frac{1}{16}$ inch.	FOR EXTERNAL USE ONLY
mafenide	Sulfamylon	Apply once or twice daily with a sterile-gloved hand; apply to thickness of $\frac{1}{16}$ inch. The burned area should be covered with cream at all times.	DISCONTINUE AND REPORT IMMEDIATELY IF RASH, BLISTERS, OR SWELLING APPEAR WHILE USING CREAM. FOR EXTERNAL USE ONLY
silver nitrate	Generics	Apply a cotton applicator dipped in solution on the affected area 2 or 3 times/week for 2–3 weeks.	DISCONTINUE IF REDNESS OR IRRITATION DEVELOPS.

Summary of Drugs Used in the Treatment of Decubitus Ulcers and Burns—cont'd

Generic Name	Brand Name	Usual Dose and Dosing Schedule	Warning Labels
Antiseptics			
povidone-iodine	Betadine	Apply as needed for treatment and prevention of susceptible microbial infections.	DO NOT SWALLOW. FOR EXTERNAL USE AVOID CONTACT WITH THE EYES.

ᵃGeneric available.

TECHNICIAN'S CORNER

1. Aloe vera is widely used to treat minor burns. Which active ingredient in the aloe vera promotes healing of burns?
2. Can pressure injuries be prevented from developing? If so, how?

Key Points

- Pressure injuries can be very mild, disappearing in a few hours after pressure is relieved, or very serious, extending into bone and internal organs.
- Pressure injuries form in areas exposed to continuous pressure, friction, or prolonged exposure to cold.
- The treatment for a pressure injury involves keeping the area clean and removing necrotic (dead) tissue, which can form a breeding ground for infection.
- Collagenase is used to promote debridement of necrotic tissue in dermal ulcers and severe burns.
- Trypsin, balsam Peru, and castor oil are used for the treatment of decubitus ulcers, varicose ulcers, debridement of eschar, dehiscent wounds, and sunburns.
- Antibacterial drugs may be used if the pressure injury is not healing or it continues to ooze after two weeks of proper cleansing and bandage changes.
- Fire, sun, electricity, chemicals, and radioactive agents can cause burns.
- The severity of a burn is determined by the depth and extent (percentage of BSA) of the lesion.
- One method of estimating the extent of BSA burned is called the rule of palms. It is based on the assumption that the palm size of a burn victim is approximately 1% of the total BSA.

- The rule of 9s is another and more accurate method of determining the extent of a burn injury. With this method, the body is divided into 11 areas of 9%, with the area around the genitals, called the perineum, representing the additional 1% of BSA.
- A first-degree burn (typical sunburn) causes minor discomfort and some reddening of the skin.
- Second-degree burns involve the deep epidermal layers and always cause injury to the upper layers of the dermis.
- Third-degree, or full-thickness, burns are characterized by destruction of both the epidermis and dermis.
- Fourth-degree burns involves underlying muscles, fasciae, or bone.
- Two common complications of burns are infection and dehydration.
- Silver sulfadiazine is the most frequently used topical agent for burns. It is thought to act via the inhibition of DNA replication and modification of the cell membrane and cell wall.
- Mafenide appears to act on bacterial cellular mechanism. It interferes with bacterial folic acid synthesis through competitive inhibition of para-aminobenzoic acid.
- Silver nitrate is a broad-spectrum agent. It is bacteriostatic at a concentration of 5%.

Review Questions

1. Pressure sores typically occur in patients who are _____.
   a. confined to the bed
   b. chair-bound
   c. ambulatory
   d. a and b
2. The usual mechanism of forming a pressure injury is from _____.
   a. immobilization
   b. infection
   c. inflammation
   d. laceration

3. In stage _____ of a pressure injury, the wound has extended through all layers of the skin.
   a. 1
   b. 2
   c. 3
   d. 4
4. Frequent turning is optional to alleviate pressure on the wound and to promote healing.
   a. True
   b. False

5. The severity of a burn is determined by the _____ (percentage of body surface area) of the lesion.
   a. depth
   b. width
   c. extent
   d. a and c

6. The rule of 9s is a more accurate method of determining the extent of a burn injury than the rule of palms.
   a. True
   b. False

7. Third-degree, or _____, burns are characterized by destruction of both the epidermis and dermis.
   a. partial-thickness
   b. full-thickness
   c. total thickness
   d. all of the above

8. Common complications of burns are _____ and _____.
   a. infection, dehydration
   b. infection, stroke
   c. dehydration, stroke
   d. stroke, shock

9. _____ is the most frequently used topical agent for burns.
   a. Gentamycin
   b. Silver sulfadiazine
   c. Silver nitrate
   d. Mupirocin

10. The removal of necrotic skin and underlying tissue from a burn or decubitus ulcer is termed _____.
    a. escharectomy
    b. escharotomy
    c. necrotomy
    d. ulcerectomy

Bibliography

Health Canada: Drug Product Database, 2018. Retrieved September 20, 2018, from https://health-products.canada.ca/dpd-bdpp/index-eng.jsp.

Khan A, Solan M: Burns: Types, Treatments, and More, 2016. Retrieved October 4, 2017, from https://www.healthline.com/health/burns?m=0#outlook9.

MedLinePlus: Pressure Sores, 2017. Retreived from https://vsearch.nlm.nih.gov/vivisimo/cgi-bin/query-meta?v%3Aproject=medlineplus&v%3Asources=medlineplus-bundle&query=pressure+sores&_ga=2.34949153.1844835335.1501108504-1627283694.1501108504.

National Pressure Ulcer Advisory Panel: National Pressure Ulcer Advisory Panel (NPUAP) announces a change in terminology from pressure ulcer to pressure injury and updates the stages of pressure injury, 2016. Retrieved October 4, 2017, from http://www.npuap.org/national-pressure-ulcer-advisory-panel-npuap-announces-a-change-in-terminology-from-pressure-ulcer-to-pressure-injury-and-updates-the-stages-of-pressure-injury/.

https://www.accessdata.fda.gov/scripts/cder/daf/index.cfm?event=BasicSearch.process. 2017.

Noronha C, Almeida A: Local burn treatments, 1999. Retrieved from http://www.medbc.com/annals/review/vol_13/num_4/text/vol13n4p216.htm.

Sussman C, Bates-Jensen B: *Wound care*, Gaithersburg, MD, 1998, Aspen Publishers.

Thibodeau G, Patton K: *Anatomy and physiology*, ed 6, St. Louis, 2007, Mosby.

US Food and Drug Administration: Drugs@FDA: FDA Approved Drug Products, nd. Retrieved September 20, 2018, from http://www.accessdata.fda.gov/scripts/cder/daf/.

Wolf SE: Burns, 2017. Retrieved October 4, 2017, from http://www.merckmanuals.com/home/injuries-and-poisoning/burns/burns?qt=burns&alt=sh.

35

Treatment of Acne

LEARNING OBJECTIVES

1. Learn the terminology associated with acne.
2. Describe the types and causes of acne.
3. List and categorize medications used to treat acne.
4. Describe mechanism of action for each class of drugs used to treat acne.
5. Identify significant drug look-alike and sound-alike issues.
6. Identify warning labels and precautionary messages associated with medications used to treat acne.

KEY TERMS

Acne Disorder resulting from the action of hormones and other substances on the skin's oil glands (sebaceous glands) and hair follicles.
Acne vulgaris Most common form of acne.
Blackhead Trapped sebum and bacteria partially open to the surface that turn black because of changes in sebum as it is exposed to air; also called an open comedone.
Comedone Enlarged and plugged hair follicles; the most characteristic sign of acne.
Cysts Deep, painful, pus-filled lesions that can cause scarring.
Keratolytic A peeling agent that causes the softening and shedding of the horny outer layer of the skin.

Milia Tiny little bumps that occur when normally sloughed skin cells become trapped in small pockets on the surface of the skin.
Nodule Large, painful, solid lesions that are lodged deep within the skin.
Papule Obstructed follicle that becomes inflamed.
Pustule Larger lesions that are more inflamed than papules and can be superficial or deep.
Whitehead Trapped sebum and bacteria that stay below the skin surface; may show up as tiny white spots, or they may be so small that they are invisible to the naked eye; also called a closed comedone.

Acne

Acne is a disorder that causes plugged pores and outbreaks of lesions, commonly called pimples or "zits." Acne lesions usually occur on the face, neck, back, chest, and shoulders (Fig. 35.1). Severe acne can lead to permanent scarring. It is a disease of the pilosebaceous units (PSUs). Found over most of the body, PSUs consist of sebaceous glands connected to canals, called follicles that contain fine hairs (Fig. 35.2). These units are most numerous on the face, upper back, and chest. The sebaceous glands make sebum (an oily substance) that normally empties onto the skin surface through the opening of the follicle or pore.

When hair, sebum, and keratinocytes (the cells that line the follicle) fill the narrow follicle and produce a plug, it prevents sebum from reaching the surface of the skin through the pores. The mixture of oil and cells allows the bacteria *Propionibacterium acnes*, which normally live on the skin, to grow in the plugged follicles. These bacteria produce chemicals and enzymes and attract white blood cells that cause inflammation (swelling, redness, heat, and pain). When the wall of the plugged follicle breaks down, it spills sebum, shedding skin cells and bacteria into the nearby skin, leading to lesions or pimples.

Common acne, or *acne vulgaris*, occurs most frequently during adolescence because the rate of sebum secretion increases more

than fivefold between 10 and 19 years of age. An estimated 80% of all people between the ages of 11 and 30 years have acne outbreaks at some point. For most people, acne tends to go away by the time they reach their 30s; however, some people in their 40s and 50s continue to experience this skin problem.

People with acne frequently have a variety of lesions. The basic acne lesion (*comedone*) is simply an enlarged and plugged hair follicle and is the most characteristic sign of acne. If the plugged follicle, or comedone, stays beneath the skin, it is called a closed comedone and produces a white bump called a *whitehead*. A comedone that reaches the surface of the skin and opens up is called an open comedone or *blackhead* because it looks black on the skin's surface (Fig. 35.3). This black discoloration is caused by changes in sebum as it is exposed to air. It is not caused by dirt. Whiteheads and blackheads may stay in the skin for a long time and are considered to be noninflammatory acne.

Blackheads and whiteheads normally release their contents at the surface of the skin and then heal. If the follicle wall ruptures, inflammatory acne can ensue. This rupture can be caused by random occurrence or by picking or touching the skin. This is why it is important to leave acne-prone skin relatively untouched. Troublesome acne lesions can develop, including the following:

- *Papules*—inflamed lesions that usually appear as small pink bumps on the skin; can be tender to the touch.

• **Fig. 35.1** Adult acne. (From Callen JP, Paller AS, Greer KE, Swinyer LF: *Color atlas of dermatology*, ed 2, Philadelphia, 2000, WB Saunders.)

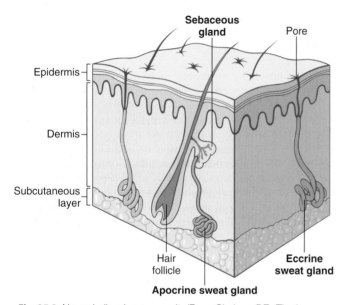

• **Fig. 35.2** Normal pilosebaceous unit. (From Chabner DE: *The language of medicine*, ed 10, St. Louis, 2014, Elsevier.)

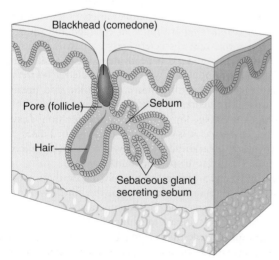

• **Fig. 35.3** Open comedone. (From Chabner DE: *The language of medicine*, ed 10, St. Louis, 2014, Elsevier.)

• BOX 35.1 Medications That Trigger or Exacerbate Acne

More Common
- Anabolic steroids (e.g., danazol [Danocrine], testosterone)
- Bromides
- Corticosteroids (e.g., prednisone [Deltasone])
- Corticotropin (H.P. Acthar)
- Isoniazid
- Lithium
- Phenytoin (Dilantin)

Less Common
- Azathioprine (Imuran)
- Cyclosporine (Sandimmune, Neoral)
- Disulfiram (Antabuse)
- Phenobarbital
- Quinidine
- Tetracycline
- Vitamins B_1, B_6, B_{12}, and D

- *Pustules* (pimples)—papules topped by white or yellow pus-filled lesions that may be red at the base. The pus-filled pimples result from secondary infections within or beneath the epidermis, often in a hair follicle or sweat pore.
- *Nodules*—large, painful, solid lesions that are lodged deep within the skin.
- *Cysts*—deep, painful, pus-filled lesions that can cause scarring.

Milia are tiny little bumps that occur when normally sloughed skin cells get trapped in small pockets on the surface of the skin. They are common in newborns across the nose and upper cheeks, and can also be seen on adult skin. The bumps disappear as the surface is worn away and the dead skin is sloughed. In newborns, the bumps usually disappear within the first few weeks of life. However, for adults, milia may persist indefinitely. Treatment is not indicated for children. Adults can have them removed by a physician for cosmetic reasons.

Causes of Acne

The exact cause of acne is unknown; however, it is believed to result from several related factors. One important factor is an increase in androgens (sex hormones). The hormones increase in boys and girls during puberty, and cause the sebaceous glands to enlarge and make more sebum. Hormonal changes related to pregnancy or starting or stopping birth control pills can also cause acne.

Another factor is heredity or genetics. Researchers believe that the tendency to develop acne can be inherited from parents. For example, studies have shown that many school-age boys with acne have a family history of the disorder. Other risk factors for acne are the use of certain drugs, including androgens and lithium (Box 35.1), and the use of greasy cosmetics. They may alter the cells of the follicles and make them stick together, producing a plug. Other factors that make acne worse are shown in Box 35.2.

Myths About the Causes of Acne

There have been many theories concerning the causes of acne. Because adolescents commonly suffer from acne and indulge in

• BOX 35.2 Factors That Can Worsen Acne

- Changing hormone levels in adolescent girls and adult women two to seven days before their menstrual period starts
- Oil from skin products (moisturizers or cosmetics) or grease encountered in the work environment (e.g., a kitchen with fry vats)
- Pressure from sports helmets or equipment, backpacks, tight collars, or tight sports uniforms
- Environmental irritants (e.g., pollution, high humidity)
- Squeezing or picking at blemishes and hard scrubbing of the skin
- Stress

fast food, junk food, and sweets, these food items are often blamed as the causes of acne. Not keeping one's skin clean is also blamed for causing blackheads, but that also is a myth. Another supposed cause of acne is stress. Stress in itself does not cause acne but can make existing acne worse.

Treatment of Acne

The goals of treatment are to heal existing lesions, stop new lesions from forming, prevent scarring, and minimize the psychological stress and embarrassment caused by this disease. Drugs used to treat acne act by breaking down comedones (comedolytics), increasing cell turnover, destroying bacteria causing acne, and reducing hormones that increase acne.

Depending on the severity of the acne, one or more topical medicines may be used (over-the-counter [OTC] and/or prescription), or combined therapy with oral and topical medicines may be recommended. Mild cases of acne can sometimes be controlled at home by gently washing the affected area(s) with warm water and a mild soap twice daily to remove dead skin cells and excess oil and use of the products described below.

Treatment of Mild Acne With Over-the-Counter Medications

Topical OTC medicines are available in many forms, such as lotions, creams, washes, kits, scrubs, brushes, and devices, gels, soaps, or pads. Treatment with OTC topical medicines may take up to eight weeks before noticeable improvement can be seen. Common active ingredients found are OTC acne products are benzoyl peroxide (2.5% to 10%), salicylic acid (0.5% to 5%), alpha hydroxy acids, and sulfur.

Once acne clears, treatment must be continued to prevent new lesions from forming. If the acne does not respond to at-home treatment, a dermatologist can assess the situation and determine an appropriate alternative therapy. In these cases, combination therapy of two or more treatments may be used. Combination therapy may include the use of a prescription topical antimicrobial or topical retinoid. These prescription topical products can be effective for clearing mild acne.

Antimicrobials

Benzoyl Peroxide

Mechanism of Action and Pharmacokinetics. Benzoyl peroxide is the most effective and widely used nonprescription medication currently available for the treatment of noninflammatory acne. It causes irritation and desquamation (skin peeling) that prevents closure of the pilosebaceous duct. Its irritant effects cause increased turnover of epithelial cells lining the follicular duct, which then increases sloughing and promotes resolution of the comedones. When benzoyl peroxide combines with proteins in the comedones, oxygen is released. *P. acne* is anaerobic and is destroyed in the presence of oxygen. Pharmacokinetic data for benzoyl peroxide are limited. Approximately 5% of a topical dose is absorbed systemically.

Adverse Effects. The adverse effects are dryness and irritation of the skin. Benzoyl peroxide may also bleach clothing or hair that it comes in contact with.

Keratolytics

Salicylic Acid

Mechanism of Action and Pharmacokinetics. Salicylic acid is a mild comedolytic agent, and surface *keratolytic* (peeling agent) helps break down blackheads and whiteheads and cuts down the shedding of cells lining the hair follicles. In cleansing preparations, salicylic acid is considered an adjunctive treatment. Absorption of topically applied salicylates is variable and depends on the dosage formulation (range, 9% to 25%). The absorbed drug is 95% eliminated in urine, and treatment for 8 to 12 weeks is needed before improvement.

Adverse Effects. The adverse effects are burning, redness, and peeling of skin.

Sulfur-Resorcinol Combination

Mechanism of Action and Pharmacokinetics. Combinations of sulfur 3% to 8% with resorcinol 2%, which enhances the effects of the sulfur, are available without prescription. The combination is a keratolytic, fostering cell turnover and desquamation, and helping break down blackheads and whiteheads. Sulfur is a weak keratolytic and antibacterial agent. Resorcinol primarily acts as an adjuvant boosting the effectiveness of sulfur. Pharmacokinetic data for the sulfur-resorcinol combination (Acnomel) are unavailable.

Adverse Effects. The adverse effects are redness and peeling of skin. The odor of sulfur limits its use. Resorcinol may produce brown, scaly areas, which is reversible.

Treatment of Moderate to Moderately Severe Acne

In moderate to moderately severe acne, numerous whiteheads, blackheads, papules, and pustules appear to cover from 25% to 75% of the face and/or other affected area(s). Up to 100 comedones may be visible with 15 to 50 inflammatory lesions. Moderate to moderately severe acne usually requires the help of a dermatologist and combination therapy. Treatments used for moderate to moderately severe acne are as follows:

- Physical methods, such as comedone extraction or ultraviolet (UV) light therapy
- Oral antibiotics—help stop or slow the growth of bacteria and reduce inflammation
- Vitamin A derivatives (retinoids) unplug existing comedones (plural of comedo), allowing other topical medicines, such as antibiotics, to enter the follicles. Some may also help decrease the formation of comedones.
- Prescription-strength topical keratolytics
- Oral contraceptives

Antibiotics

Oral and topical antibiotics may be prescribed for the treatment of acne and are initial therapy for patients with moderate to severe inflammatory acne. Systemic antibiotics decrease *P. acnes* colonization and have intrinsic antiinflammatory effects. First-line oral

Over-the-Counter Acne Products

Generic Name	US Brand Name(s) / Canadian Brand Name(s)	Dosage Forms and Strengths
benzoyl peroxide[a] (there are more than 95 OTC brands)	Acne Clear, Benzac AC, Benzac W, Benzagel, BenzEFoam, Benziq, Brevoxyl-8, Clearasil Daily Acne Cream, Clearasil Ultra Rapid Action, Clearskin, DesQuam-E, DesQuam X, NeoBenz Micro, Neutrogena On-The-Spot, Oxy Acne, Oxy Rapid Treatment, PanOxyl, Persa-Gel-10, Proactiv, Seba-Clear, SoluCLENZ Rx, Triaz, Zapzyt Acne Treatment Gel	**Cream:** 3.5%, 5.5%, 8.5%, 10% **Foam (BenzEFoam):** 5.3%, 9.8% **Gel:** 2.5%, 2.75%, 3%, 4%, 5%, 5.25%, 6%, 7%, 8%, 9%, 10% **Lotion:** 2.5%, 4%, 5%, 10%, 20% **Ointment (Eraser):** 5% **Pad:** 3%, 4%, 4.25%, 6%, 7%, 8%, 9% **Wash/Soap:** 2.5%, 3%, 3.5%, 4%, 4.25%, 4.5%, 5%, 5.25%, 7%, 8%, 10%
	Adasept B.P.5, Benzagel 5, Benzac W, Clean & Clear Persagel, Clearasil Daily Clear Acne Treatment, Clinique Acne Solutions, Eraser, Proactiv, Spectro Acne Clear Wash, Stubborn Acne Cleanser, Stubborn Spot Gel	
resorcinol and sulfur	Acnomel Adult Acne, Clearasil Daily Clear, Rezamid	**Cream:** resorcinol 2% + sulfur 8%, resorcinol 2% + sulfur 5%
	Acnomel Cream	
salicylic acid[a]	Clean & Clear Advantage Spot Treatment, Clearasil Ultra Daily Face Wash Clearasil Ultra-Rapid Action Treatment Lotion Neutrogena Acne Wash Oil-Free, ZapZyt Acne Wash	**Cleanser:** 2% **Cream:** 2% **Cloths/Pads:** 2% **Gel:** 2% **Lotion:** 2%
	Bioré Blemish Fighting Ice Cleanser, Bioré Blemish Fighting Astringent, Clean and Clear Advantage Acne Spot treatment Clearasil Ultra Exfoliating Scrub, Clearasil Daily Clear Pore Cleansing Pads, Neutrogena Naturals Acne, Neutrogena Acne Stress Control, Oxy Deep Daily Cleaning Pads, Oxy Deep Pore Daily Facial, Oxy Clarifying Medicated Acne Pads,	

[a]Generic available.

antibiotics have included tetracycline, doxycycline, and minocycline. Clindamycin, sulfonamides, and erythromycin are less commonly used for the treatment of acne. Because the resistance of *P. acne* to erythromycin has increased, it has become a second-line agent used when treatment with tetracycline antibiotics fails or is not tolerated. The mechanism of action and adverse effects produced by these antibiotics are described in Chapter 29.

Oral antibiotics must be taken for six to eight weeks before results are evident, and treatment should be given for six months to prevent the development of microbial resistance. Oral antibiotics may be discontinued after inflammation has resolved; however, topical antibiotics may be continued for prophylaxis. Some patients may require long-term oral antibiotic therapy to control their acne and prevent scarring.

Topical antiinfective agents are used for the treatment of acne to reduce inflammation caused by bacteria rather than having a direct bactericidal effect. Topical antiinfectives used for the treatment of acne are clindamycin, dapsone, and erythromycin.

Retinoids

Retinoids include vitamin A and its derivatives. Adapalene, tretinoin, and tazarotene are retinoids. Topical retinoids are effective in treating non-inflammatory acne because they reduce the number of comedones and prevent comedone formation and have mild antiinflammatory properties.

Adapalene

Mechanism of Action and Pharmacokinetics. Adapalene is a retinoid-type drug that affects the growth of skin cells and thereby reduces the formation of pimples. It is available for topical use only. Adapalene modulates cell differentiation and keratinization, which is responsible for the drug's ability to break down comedones.

It is also a potent anti-inflammatory. The absorption, distribution, and metabolism of topically applied adapalene are unknown. Excretion appears to be primarily by the biliary route.

Adverse Effects. The adverse effects are irritation, redness, dryness, itching, peeling, and burning. It is also a photo irritant.

Tretinoin

Mechanism of Action and Pharmacokinetics. Tretinoin is a retinoid. It is used for the treatment of mild to moderate acne. Tretinoin increases cell turnover in the follicular wall and decreases the cohesiveness of cells, leading to the extrusion of comedones and inhibition of the formation of new comedones. The rapid turnover of cells prevents new pimples from forming. Tretinoin is administered topically and orally. The effects of topical administration appear approximately two to three weeks after initiation of therapy. When applied for cosmetic use to reduce wrinkles, the beneficial effects may take up to six months to be achieved. Tretinoin is well absorbed orally, but protein binding is greater than 95%. Tretinoin is metabolized by the cytochrome P450 hepatic enzyme system, and the drug appears to induce its own metabolism.

Adverse Effects. Common adverse effects of topical tretinoin are dry skin, peeling, itching, burning, stinging, redness, and photosensitivity.

Clindamycin-Tretinoin

Mechanism of Action and Pharmacokinetics. Clindamycin and tretinoin are combined as a topical formulation for the treatment of acne. Clindamycin belongs to the lincomycin antibiotics class and works by slowing or stopping the growth of bacteria. Topical clindamycin has minimal systemic absorption. Tretinoin is minimally absorbed following topical application.

Adverse Effects. Common adverse effects are redness, scaling, dryness, itching, burning, and stinging, and sunburn.

> **⚠ TECH ALERT!**
>
> The following drugs have look-alike and sound-alike issues:
> Dynacin and DynaCirc;
> tretinoin and ISOtretinoin.

Tazarotene

Mechanism of Action and Pharmacokinetics. Tazarotene is a retinoid prodrug that modulates the differentiation and proliferation of epithelial tissue and has some antiinflammatory and immunological activity. Absorption is minimal when applied topically. It is metabolized rapidly via esterase hydrolysis in the skin to tazarotenic acid, an active metabolite. The topical half-life ($t_{1/2}$) of tazarotenic acid is approximately 18 hours.

Adverse Effects. Common adverse effects are itching burning, stinging, redness, irritation, swelling, dryness of the skin, and pain.

Azelaic Acid

Mechanism of Action and Pharmacokinetics. Azelaic acid occurs naturally and is found in whole-grain and animal products. It reduces redness and inflammatory papules and pustules associated with rosacea and acne. It works by killing the bacteria that infect pores and by decreasing the production of keratin, a natural substance that could lead to the development of acne. Approximately 4% of topically applied azelaic acid is absorbed systemically. Azelaic acid is mainly excreted unchanged in the urine; the $t_{1/2}$ is approximately 12 hours after topical application.

Adverse Effects. Azelaic acid may cause slight stinging or burning, tingling, and redness, and drying of the skin may occur.

Treatment of Severe Acne

Severe acne is characterized by deep cysts, inflammation, extensive damage to the skin, and scarring. Severe acne is characterized by more than 100 comedones, inflammatory lesions, and cysts. It requires an aggressive treatment regimen and should be treated by a dermatologist. Severe disfiguring forms of acne can require years of treatment, and individuals may experience one or more treatment failures. Almost every case of acne can be successfully treated. Treatment involves nonpharmaceutical methods and medications (isotretinoin, antibiotics, oral contraceptives). The pharmacology of oral contraceptives is described in Chapter 27.

Isotretinoin

For patients with severe inflammatory acne that does not improve with the medications discussed earlier, the physician may prescribe isotretinoin, a retinoid (vitamin A derivative). Isotretinoin is an oral drug that is usually taken once or twice daily with food for 15 to 20 weeks. Isotretinoin decreases the size and output of sebaceous glands, and makes the cells that are sloughed off into the sebaceous glands less sticky and therefore less able to form comedones.

Adverse Reactions. Isotretinoin can produce fetal abnormalities. Women must use two separate, effective forms of birth control at the same time for one month before treatment begins, during the entire course of treatment, and for one full month after stopping the drug.

Other possible side effects of isotretinoin include dry eyes, mouth, lips, nose, or skin (very common), itching, nosebleeds, muscle aches, sensitivity to the sun, poor night vision, changes in mood, depression, suicidal thoughts, changes in the blood lipids (e.g., an increase in fat levels in the blood [triglycerides, cholesterol]), and changes in liver function. Blood tests to determine baseline liver function are taken before isotretinoin is started and periodically during treatment. Side effects usually cease after the medicine is stopped. Oral administration of isotretinoin may produce hyperglycemia.

> **⚠ TECH ALERT!**
>
> Isotretinoin must be dispensed in the manufacturer's original packaging with the warning label "Avoid Pregnancy."

FDA iPLEDGE Program for Isotretinoin

To make sure that women do not become pregnant while taking isotretinoin, the FDA requires wholesalers, prescribers, pharmacies, and patients to participate in the iPLEDGE risk minimization program. Only prescribers registered and activated in iPLEDGE can prescribe isotretinoin, and only patients registered and qualified in iPLEDGE can be given isotretinoin.

See the following website for more details on the iPLEDGE program: https://www.ipledgeprogram.com.

Treatment of Hormonally Influenced Acne in Women

In some women, acne is caused by an excess of androgen hormones. They may exhibit hirsutism (excessive growth of hair on the face or body), premenstrual acne flares, irregular menstrual cycles, and elevated blood levels of certain androgens. The physician may prescribe one of several drugs to treat women with this type of acne.

Oral Contraceptives

Oral contraceptives (OCs) help suppress androgens produced by the ovaries. Side effects are nausea, weight gain, menstrual spotting, and breast tenderness. OCs used to treat acne typically have estrogen and progestins with a low androgen level. OCs that produce low androgenic effects include drospirenone, desogestrel, or norgestimate. The choice of OC is typically based on tolerability.

Nonpharmaceutical Treatment of Acne

Physicians may use other types of procedures in addition to drug therapy to treat patients with acne. For example, the physician may remove the patient's comedones during an office visit. Sometimes the physician will inject corticosteroids directly into lesions to help reduce the size and pain of inflamed cysts and nodules.

If scarring has occurred, dermabrasion (or microdermabrasion), which is a form of sanding down scars, is sometimes used. Another treatment option for deep scars caused by cystic acne is the transfer of fat from another part of the body to the scar. Alternatively, a synthetic filling material may be injected under the scar to improve its appearance.

> **TECHNICIAN'S CORNER**
>
> 1. There are many OTC and prescription medications available for the treatment of acne. Are there any natural/herbal remedies available?
> 2. What advice can one give to a teenager with acne?

Drug Treatment for Moderate to Moderately Severe Acne

Generic Name	US Brand Name(s) / Canadian Brand Name(s)	Dosage Forms and Strengths
adapalene[a]	Differin[b]	**Cream:** 0.1%
	Differin, Differin XP	**Gel:** 0.1%,[bc] 0.3% **Lotion**[c]**:** 0.1% **Solution**[c]**;** 0.1%
adapalene + benzoyl peroxide	Epiduo, Epiduo Forte	**Gel:** 0.1% adapalene + 2.5% benzoyl peroxide (Epiduo, Tactupump); 0.3% adapalene + 2.5% benzoyl peroxide (Epiduo Forte, Tactupump Forte)
	Tactupump, Tactupump Forte	
alitretinoin	Panretin	**Capsule (Toctino)**[d]**:** 10 mg, 30 mg
	Toctino	**Gel (Panretin)**[c]**:** 0.1%
azelaic acid	Azelex, Finacea	**Cream (Azelex)**[c]**:** 20%
	Finacea	**Foam (Finacea)**[c]**:** 15% **Gel (Finacea):** 15%
benzoyl peroxide[a]	See earlier table for OTC acne products.	See earlier table for OTC acne products.
	See earlier table for OTC acne products.	
clindamycin (topical)[a]	Cleocin, Cleocin T, Clinda-derm, Clindagel, Clindets, Evoclin	**Foam:** 1% **Gel:** 1%
	Clinda-T, Dalacin T	**Solution:** 1% **Swab:** 1%
erythromycin base,[a] topical	Erygel	**Gel:** 2%
	Not available	**Solution, topical**[c]**:** 2%
benzoyl peroxide and erythromycin[a]	Benzamycin	**Gel:** benzoyl peroxide 5%, erythromycin 3%
	Benzamycin	
benzoyl peroxide and clindamycin[a]	Acanya, Benzaclin, Duac, Neuac, Onexton	**Gel:** benzoyl peroxide 2.5% + clindamycin phosphate 1.2% (Acanya); benzoyl peroxide 3% + clindamycin 1% (Clindoxyl ADV); benzoyl peroxide 3.75 % + clindamycin 1.2% (Onexton); benzoyl peroxide 5% + clindamycin phosphate 1.2% (Duac; benzoyl peroxide 5% + clindamycin phosphate 1% (Benzaclin, Clindoxyl)
	Benzaclin, Clindoxyl, Clindoxyl ADV	
dapsone	Aczone	**Gel:** 5%, 7.5%
	Aczone	
doxycycline hyclate[a]	Acticlate, Doryx, Vibramycin, (Apprilon, Atridox, LymePak, Oracea)[e]	**Capsule:** 50 mg, 100 mg, 150 mg **Tablet:** 20 mg, 100 mg, 150 mg
	Doxycin, Doxytab, (Apprilon, Atridox, Periostat)[e]	**Tablet, delayed-release (Doryx):** 75 mg, 100 mg, 150 mg, 200 mg
doxycycline monohydrate	Monodox, Avidoxy	**Capsule (Monodox):** 50 mg, 75 mg, 100 mg
	Not available	**Tablet (Avidoxy):** 100 mg
minocycline[a]	Dynacin, Minocin, Minolira, Soladyn, Ximino	**Capsule (Dynacin, Minocin):** 50 mg, 75 mg,[c] 100 mg **Capsule, extended release (Ximino)**[c]**:** 45 mg, 90 mg, 135 mg
	Generics	**Tablet**[c]**:** 50 mg, 75 mg, 100 mg **Tablet ER**[c]**:** 55 mg, 65 mg, 80 mg, 105 mg, 115 mg (Solodyn); 105 mg, 135 mg (Minolira)
tetracycline[a]	Achromycin V	**Capsule:** 250 mg, 500 mg[c]
	Generics	
tazarotene	Avage, Fabior, Tazorac	**Cream:** 0.05%, 0.1%
	Tazorac	**Foam (Fabior):** 0.1% **Gel:** 0.05%, 0.1%

Drug Treatment for Moderate to Moderately Severe Acne—cont'd

Generic Name	US Brand Name(s) / Canadian Brand Name(s)	Dosage Forms and Strengths
tretinoin[a]	Altreno, Atralin, Avita, Renova, Retin-A, Retin-A Micro, Tretin-X Retin-A, Retin-A Micro, Stieva-A	**Cream:** 0.01% (Stieva-A), 0.02% (Renova), 0.025% (Retin-A, Avita, Stieva-A), 0.05%, 0.1% (Avita, Retin-A, Stieva-A) **Gel:** 0.01%, 0.025% (Avita, Retin-A), 0.04% (Retin-A Micro), 0.05% (Atralin), 0.1% (Retin-A, Retin-A Micro) **Lotion:** 0.05% **Solution:** 0.05% (Retin A)
tretinoin + clindamycin[a]	Veltin, Ziana Biacna	**Gel:** tretinoin 0.025% + clindamycin phosphate 1.2%

[a]Generic available.
[b]*OTC*, Over-the-counter.
[c]Available in the United States only.
[d]Available in Canada only.
[e]Indicated for treatment of periodontal disease or Lyme's disease. See Chapter 29.
[bc]OTC in the United States only.

Treatment for Severe Acne

Generic Name	US Brand Name(s) / Canadian Brand Name(s)	Dosage Forms and Strengths
isotretinoin	Absorica, Amnesteem, Claravis, Myorisan, Zenatane Accutane, Clarus, Epuris	**Capsule:** 10 mg, 20 mg, 25 mg,[a] 30 mg, 35 mg,[a] 40 mg
oral antibiotics	See Chapters 29.	See Chapter 29.

[a]Available in the United States only.

Treatment of Hormonally Induced Acne in Women

Generic Name	US Brand Name(s) / Canadian Brand Name(s)	Dosage Forms and Strengths
oral contraceptives[a]	See Chapter 27.	See Chapter 27.

[a]A complete listing of oral contraceptives is given in Chapter 27.

Summary of Drugs Used for the Treatment of Acne

Generic Name	Brand Name	Usual Dose and Dosing Schedule	Warning Labels
Topical			
adapalene	Differin	Apply once daily at bedtime.	FOR EXTERNAL USE ONLY—all
azelaic acid	Azelex	Apply and massage a thin film into affected area twice daily.	KEEP AWAY FROM EYES, EARS, AND MOUTH—azelaic acid, benzoyl peroxide + clindamycin, salicylic acid
benzoyl peroxide	Various OTC and Rx brands and generics	**Cleansers:** Wash once or twice daily. **Topical:** Apply sparingly once daily; increase to two or three times daily if needed.	BLEACHING AGENT; AVOID CONTACT WITH FABRIC AND HAIR—benzoyl peroxide DO NOT USE IF PREGNANT—tazarotene, tretinoin
benzoyl peroxide + clindamycin	BenzaClin, Duac	**BenzaClin:** Apply bid. **Duac:** Apply once daily in the evening.	MAY CAUSE SENSITIVITY TO SUNLIGHT—tretinoin, tretinoin + clindamycin
benzoyl peroxide + erythromycin	Benzamycin	Apply bid, morning and evening.	

Continued

Summary of Drugs Used for the Treatment of Acne—cont'd

Generic Name	Brand Name	Usual Dose and Dosing Schedule	Warning Labels
dapsone	Aczone	Apply a small amount twice daily.	
resorcinol + sulfur	Acnomel	Apply a small amount to affected area as directed by physician.	
salicylic acid	Clean and Clear Advantage Acne Spot treatment	**Cream, cloth, foam, liquid, Gel:** Apply to skin once or twice daily and rinse thoroughly. **Pads:** Apply to affected area one to three times daily. **Wash:** Wash once daily,	
tazarotene	Avage, Tazorac	Apply thin film once daily in the evening to the affected area.	
tretinoin	Renova, Retin-A	Apply to acne lesions once daily before bedtime or on alternate days.	
tretinoin + clindamycin	Ziana, Veltin	Apply to entire face every night at bedtime.	
Systemic			
doxycycline	Vibramycin	50–100 mg twice daily or 40 mg (Oracea) once daily	AVOID PROLONGED SUNLIGHT—doxycycline, minocycline, isotretinoin AVOID TAKING ANTACIDS, IRON, AND DAIRY PRODUCTS—minocycline TAKE WITH FOOD—isotretinoin AVOID PREGNANCY—doxycycline, minocycline, isotretinoin AVOID USE OF VITAMIN A PRODUCTS—isotretinoin
erythromycin	Various brands and generics	**Oral:** 250–500 mg twice daily	
isotretinoin	Accutane, Clarus, Clavaris	0.5–1 mg/kg/day PO given in two divided doses for 15–20 weeks	
minocycline	Solodyn ER	Take dose (1 mg/kg) once daily	
tetracycline	Generics	250–500 mg/dose every 6 h	

Key Points

- Acne is a disorder resulting from the action of hormones and other substances on the skin's oil glands (sebaceous glands) and hair follicles.
- Common acne, or acne vulgaris, occurs most frequently during adolescence as a result of overactive secretion by the sebaceous glands, accompanied by blockages and inflammation of their ducts.
- Pus-filled pimples, or pustules, that erupt on the skin are caused by secondary infections within or beneath the epidermis, often in a hair follicle or sweat pore.
- The goals of treatment for acne are to heal existing lesions, stop new lesions from forming, prevent scarring, and minimize the psychological stress and embarrassment caused by this disease.
- Benzoyl peroxide is the most effective and widely used non-prescription medication currently available for the treatment of noninflammatory acne.
- Salicylic acid is a mild comedolytic agent (keratolytic) that provides a milder, less effective alternative to the prescription agent tretinoin.
- Topical OTC medicines are available in many forms, such as gels, lotions, creams, soaps, and pads. In some people, OTC acne medicines may cause side effects such as skin irritation, burning, or redness, which often get better or go away with continued use of the medicine.
- Adapalene is believed to affect the growth of skin cells and thereby reduce the formation of pimples.
- Azelaic acid works by killing the bacteria that infect pores and by decreasing the production of keratin, a natural substance that could lead to the development of acne.
- Tazarotene modulates the differentiation and proliferation of epithelial tissue and has some antiinflammatory and immunological activity.
- Tretinoin increases cell turnover in the follicular wall and decreases the cohesiveness of cells.
- Severe acne is characterized by deep cysts, inflammation, extensive damage to the skin, and scarring. It requires an aggressive treatment regimen and should be treated by a dermatologist.
- For patients with severe inflammatory acne a physician may prescribe isotretinoin, a retinoid (vitamin A derivative).
- Early treatment is the best way to prevent acne scars. Once scarring has occurred, dermabrasion may be used to treat irregular scars.

Review Questions

1. An enlarged and plugged hair follicle, the most characteristic sign of acne, is called a _____.
   a. milia
   b. pustule
   c. comedone
   d. papule

2. The warning label "Avoid Pregnancy" should be applied to prescription containers for _____.
   a isotretinoin
   b erythromycin
   c salicylic acid
   d benzoyl peroxide

3. _____ is the most effective and widely used nonprescription medication currently available for the treatment of noninflammatory acne.
   a. Salicylic acid
   b. Benzoyl peroxide
   c. Sulfur
   d. Doxycycline

4. At-home treatment for acne requires _____ to see improvement.
   a. 2 to 4 weeks
   b. 4 to 8 weeks
   c. 6 to 10 weeks
   d. 8 to 10 weeks

5. When acne is resistant to topical therapies, intravenous antibiotics may be used.
   a. True
   b. False

6. Which of the following oral antibiotics is less commonly used for the treatment of moderate to severe acne?
   a. Doxycycline
   b. Tetracycline
   c. Clindamycin
   d. Minocycline

7. _____ works by killing the bacteria that infect pores and by decreasing the production of keratin, a natural substance that could lead to the development of acne.
   a. Azelaic acid
   b. Adapalene
   c. Benzoyl peroxide
   d. a and c

8. _____ is an effective medicine that can help prevent scarring.
   a. Tretinoin
   b. Isotretinoin
   c. Retinoin
   d. All of the above

9. Oral contraceptives are used to treat which type of acne?
   a. Mild
   b. Moderate
   c. Severe
   d. Hormonally induced

10. Which of the following drugs are used for treating hormonally influenced acne?
    a. Corticosteroids
    b. Antiandrogens
    c. Progestins
    d. All of the above

Bibliography

American Pharmacists Association: *Handbook of nonprescription drugs*, ed 16, Washington DC, 2009, American Pharmacists Association.

Decker A, Graber EM: Over-the-counter acne treatments: a review, *J Clin Aesthet Dermatol* 5(5), 2012. Retrieved from https://www.ncbi.nlm.nih.gov/pmc/articles/PMC3366450/.

Dlugosz CK, OTC Advisor: Self care for dermatologic disorder, monograph 6. 2010, American Pharmacists Association.

Health Canada, 2018. Drug Product Database. Retrieved September 21, 2018, from https://health-products.canada.ca/dpd-bdpp/index-eng.jsp.

Mayo Clinic Staff: Over-the-counter acne products: What works and why, 2018. Retrieved September 21, 2018, from https://www.mayoclinic.org/diseases-conditions/acne/in-depth/acne-products/art-20045814?pg=2&p=1.

National Institute of Arthritis and Musculoskeletal and Skin Diseases: Acne. NIH Publication No. 15-4998, 2016. Retrieved June 8, 2017 from http://www.niams.nih.gov/Health_Info/Acne/default.asp.

Repchinsky C: *Patient self-care: helping your patients make therapeutic choices*, ed 2, 2010, Canadian Pharmacists Association, pp 577–596.

Repchinsky C: *Compendium of self care products*, ed 2, 2010, Canadian Pharmacists Association, pp 173–174.

Thibodeau G, Patton K: *Anatomy and physiology*, ed 6, St. Louis, 2007, Mosby.

Titus S, Hodge J: Diagnosis and Treatment of Acne, *Am Fam Physician* 86(8):734–740, 2012.

US Food and Drug Administration, nd. Drugs@FDA: FDA Approved Drug Products. Retrieved September 21, 2018, from https://www.accessdata.fda.gov/scripts/cder/daf/index.cfm.

36

Treatment of Atopic Dermatitis and Psoriasis

LEARNING OBJECTIVES

1. Learn the terminology associated with atopic dermatitis and psoriasis.
2. Describe the causes of atopic dermatitis and psoriasis.
3. List the symptoms of atopic dermatitis and psoriasis.
4. List and categorize medications used to treat atopic dermatitis and psoriasis.
5. Describe the mechanism of action for drugs used to treat atopic dermatitis and psoriasis.
6. Identify significant drug look-alike and sound-alike issues.
7. Identify warning labels and precautionary messages associated with medications used to treat atopic dermatitis and psoriasis.

KEY TERMS

Atopic dermatitis Chronic inflammatory disease of the skin.
Cutaneous Pertaining to the skin.
Dermatitis Inflammation of the skin.
Eczema General term used to describe several types of inflammation of the skin.
Phototherapy Treatment for atopic dermatitis that involves exposing the skin to ultraviolet A or B light waves.

Plaque psoriasis Most common form of psoriasis. It is characterized by raised, inflamed (red) lesions covered with a silvery white scale.
Psoriasis Chronic disease of the skin characterized by itchy red patches covered with silvery scales.

Overview

Eczema is a general term used to describe several types of inflammation of the skin. It is a common condition affecting millions of Americans and Canadians. There are several types of eczema—atopic dermatitis, allergic contact eczema, contact eczema, dyshidrotic eczema, neurodermatitis, nummular eczema, seborrheic eczema, and stasis dermatitis.

Atopic refers a group of diseases in which there is an inherited tendency to develop other allergic conditions. *Atopic dermatitis* is the most common form of eczema, affecting more than 15 million Americans and 25% of school-aged children and 10% of adults globally. It is a chronic disease of the skin that often develops in infancy and may continue throughout adulthood. It is a forerunner to asthma and food allergies. Up to 40% of individuals that have eczema (atopic dermatitis) also have allergies, asthma, and food allergies.

Unlike contact *dermatitis* (inflammation of the skin), in which symptoms appear after exposure to an allergen, the cause of atopic dermatitis is unknown. Atopic dermatitis is characterized by autoimmune-mediated inflammatory response that produces abnormal changes in epidermal skin cells and a hyperactive dermal response to irritants. Common irritants are listed in Box 36.1.

Psoriasis is another autoimmune, chronic inflammatory condition of the skin. It affects 2% to 5% of the global population. *Psoriasis* is a condition associated with the rapid turnover of skin cells.

Whereas the normal rate of cell turnover is approximately 30 days, the cell turnover rate may be as short as three to four days in people who have psoriasis.

Symptoms of Atopic Dermatitis and Psoriasis

Atopic dermatitis commonly produces symptoms of intense itching, redness (from scratching), skin irritation, and inflammation (Box 36.2). Eczematous patches may form that are flaky and crusting and may even ooze a clear fluid (Fig. 36.1). Individuals with psoriasis have thick silvery scaly patches; this is the most common type, known as *plaque psoriasis*. They may also have some redness and swelling. Itchy psoriatic patches may be found on the neck, elbows, genitals, scalp, hands, and feet.

Individuals with atopic dermatitis and psoriasis may experience periods when their symptoms worsen (exacerbation) and periods when they get better or go away completely (remission). It is not uncommon for eczema that has gone into remission in childhood to return with the onset of puberty. Factors that exacerbate symptoms of atopic dermatitis and psoriasis are as follows:
- Stress
- Contact with environmental pollutants and household cleaning products

• **Fig. 36.1** Eczema. (A) Infantile phase. (B) Childhood phase. (A and B from Fitzpatrick JE, Morelli JG: *Dermatology secrets in color*, ed 3, Philadelphia, 2007, Mosby.)

• BOX 36.1 **Common Irritants**

- Wool or synthetic fibers
- Soaps and detergents
- Perfumes and cosmetics
- Cleaning solvents, mineral oil, and chlorine
- Dust
- Sand

• BOX 36.2 **Signs and Symptoms of Eczema**

- Dry, rectangular scales on the skin
- Small rough bumps and papules on arms, legs, face
- Thickened, leathery patches of skin
- Inflammation around the corners of the mouth and face rash
- Darkened eyelids and skin around the eyes
- Extra skin fold under the eye
- Excess creases in the palms of the hands
- Hives (urticaria)
- Intense itching
- Redness

• BOX 36.3 **Recommended Skin Care for Persons with Eczema**

- Avoid hot baths or showers
- Air-dry or gently pat skin dry after bathing (avoid vigorous rubbing)

- Food allergy (e.g., to eggs, peanuts, milk, fish, soy products, wheat)
- Wearing wool or clothing that rubs and irritates skin
- Factors that cause dry skin (e.g., low-humidity environments, not applying moisturizer, hot baths)
- Scratching

Scratching can break down the protective layer of the skin and increase the risk of developing secondary bacterial or viral infections.

Nonpharmaceutical Treatment of Atopic Dermatitis and Psoriasis

Nonpharmaceutical treatment for atopic dermatitis and other forms of eczema involves using skin care regimens that reduce irritation as well as avoiding allergens and known irritants (Box 36.3). Nonpharmaceutical treatment of psoriasis may also include the use of phototherapy. *Phototherapy* involves exposing the skin to ultraviolet (UV) A or B light waves. It may be used alone or in combination with drug therapy. Phototherapy is only recommended for those older than 12 years. Adverse reactions to the use of UV light therapy are premature aging of the skin and increased risk for skin cancer.

Dietary supplements and nutraceuticals have been promoted to benefit atopic dermatitis. They include probiotics, prebiotics, vitamin D, fish oil, evening primrose oil, borage seed oil, and Chinese herbal medicine. To date, only the combination of pre- and probiotics (symbiotics) have shown some benefit over placebo in randomized controlled trials. More studies are needed.

Pharmaceutical Treatment of Eczema and Psoriasis

The use of topical agents is a first line treatment strategy for the treatment of atopic dermatitis, psoriasis, seborrhea, and other inflammatory skin conditions. Absorption of drugs across psoriatic skin is poor because thick, scaly plaques and dry skin reduce penetration of topically applied drugs. This may limit the effectiveness of topical treatments.

---

❶ TECH ALERT!

The following drugs have look-alike and sound-alike issues:
fluocinolone and fluocinonide;
hydrocortisone, hydrocortisone butyrate, and hydrocortisone valerate;
betamethasone dipropionate and betamethasone valerate;
betamethasone dipropionate augmented formula and betamethasone dipropionate regular.

Corticosteroids

The use of topical corticosteroids continues to be a mainstay of therapy for the treatment of atopic dermatitis and psoriasis. The use of oral corticosteroids is reserved for severe symptoms.

Topical corticosteroids are categorized into seven groups based on potency (Box 36.4). Class I agents (e.g., diflorasone diacetate)

• BOX 36.4 Potency Classification of Selected Topical Corticosteroids (Generic Names)

Class I: Super–High Potency
- Clobetasol propionate
- Diflorasone diacetate

Class II: Super Potent
- Betamethasone dipropionate (optimized vehicle)
- Halobetasol propionate

Class III: Very Potent
- Amcinonide
- Desoximetasone
- Halcinonide
- Fluocinonide
- Mometasone furoate
- Diflorasone diacetate (cream)
- Triamcinolone (>0.5%)

Class IV: Potent
- Betamethasone dipropionate (regular vehicle)
- Flurandrenolide (ointment)
- Mometasone furoate

Class V: Medium Potency
- Beclomethasone
- Betamethasone valerate
- Diflucortolone valerate
- Fluocinolone acetonide
- Flurandrenolide (cream)
- Fluticasone propionate (cream)
- Hydrocortisone butyrate (cream)
- Hydrocortisone valerate (cream)
- Triamcinolone acetonide (>0.5%)

Class VI: Mild Potency
- Alclometasone dipropionate (cream, ointment)
- Desonide (cream)
- Prednicarbate

Class VII: Mildest Potency
- Dexamethasone
- Hydrocortisone base

Adapted from Raymond G, Houle M.-C: A review of corticosteroids for the treatment of psoriasis. Skin Ther Lett 2, 2007 [last updated 2016] (http://www.skintherapyletter.com/pharmacist-edition/corticosteroids-psoriasis-pharm/).

are superhigh potency. Class VII agents include hydrocortisone, which is mild enough for over-the-counter (OTC) use. The vehicle (base) in which the corticosteroid is suspended may influence the potency. For example, betamethasone dipropionate, augmented is formulated in a base that is superpotent (class II), whereas the same drug in a non-augmented base is less potent (class IV). Higher potency corticosteroids have more adverse reactions. Only the mildest potency agents, such as hydrocortisone, should be used on the face.

Mechanism of Action and Pharmacokinetics
Topical corticosteroids possess antiinflammatory and immunosuppressive properties and produce vasoconstriction. They reduce the permeability of the cells to T lymphocytes and eosinophils, thereby decreasing the release of mediators of the inflammatory response (e.g., cytokines). They also reduce the number of inflammatory cells, which decreases redness, swelling, and inflammation.

Adverse Effects
Long-term use of topical corticosteroids can result in thinning of the skin, stretch marks (striae), spider veins, acne, milia, rosacea (enlarged blood vessels, especially on the nose), bruising, atrophy, lacerations, and poor wound healing when applied topically. Adverse reactions are more extensive when high-potency corticosteroids are used, and they are applied to a large body surface area.

Immunomodulators: Calcineurin Inhibitors

Calcineurin inhibitors are immunomodulators. They control inflammation and reduce the immune system response to allergens. Pimecrolimus is indicated for the treatment of mild to moderate atopic dermatitis. It is approved for short-term and intermittent long-term therapy. Tacrolimus is approved for the treatment of moderate to severe atopic dermatitis that has failed to respond to corticosteroid treatment. Pimecrolimus and tacrolimus are not effective in treating plaque psoriasis.

Mechanism of Action and Pharmacokinetics
Pimecrolimus and tacrolimus inhibit T-cell activation and the production of cytokines, interleukins, and interferons that mediate the inflammatory response. Pharmacokinetic data on pimecrolimus are limited. Absorption through the skin is minimal and *cutaneous* metabolism is negligible. Pimecrolimus is marketed as a cream for topical application to affected areas. Tacrolimus ointment (Protopic) is used for the treatment of atopic dermatitis. Tacrolimus capsules and solution for injection (Avagraf and Prograf) are used to reduce organ transplant rejection (see Chapter 32).

Adverse Effects
Common adverse reactions associated with topical application are local burning and itching of the skin. The US Food and Drug Administration (FDA) and Health Canada require manufacturers to include a boxed warning in the package insert, advising health care providers that pimecrolimus and tacrolimus may increase the risk for the development of lymphoma.

⚠ TECH ALERT!
Prograf and PROzac have look-alike and sound-alike issues.

Vitamin D Analogues
Calcitriol is an active form of vitamin D_3. Calcipotriene is a synthetic analogue of vitamin D. Its generic name is calcipotriol in Canada. Calcitriol and calcipotriene (calcipotriol) are approved for the treatment of psoriasis. Signs of improvement can be seen in approximately two weeks after calcipotriene administration; however, maximum effects may take four to eight weeks.

■ TECH NOTE!
Calcitriol capsules and oral solution (Rocaltrol) as well as solution for injection (Calcijex) are used in the treatment of hypocalcemia caused by dialysis and vitamin D resistant rickets.

Topical Corticosteroids

Generic Name	US Brand Name(s) / Canadian Brand Name(s)	Dosage Forms and Strengths
alclometasone dipropionate[a]	Generics	**Cream:** 0.05%
	Not available	**Ointment:** 0.05%
amcinonide[a]	Generics	**Cream:** 0.1%
	Generics	**Lotion:** 0.1%
		Ointment: 0.1%
betamethasone dipropionate[a]	Diprolene, Diprolene AF, Sernivo	**Cream:** 0.05%
	Diprolene, Diprosone, Topilene, Topisone	**Gel, augmented:** 0.05%[b]
		Lotion: 0.05%
		Lotion, augmented: 0.05%
		Ointment: 0.05%
		Ointment, augmented: 0.05%
		Spray, topical (Sernivo): 0.05%
betamethasone valerate[a]	Beta-Val, Dermabet, Luxiq, Valnac	**Cream:** 0.05%[c], 0.1%
	Betaderm, Celestoderm V, Celestoderm V/2, Luxiq, Ratio-Ectosone-Mild, Ratio-Ectosone Regular, Valisone G	**Lotion:** 0.05%[c], 0.1%
		Ointment: 0.05%[c], 0.1%
		Topical foam (Luxiq): 0.12%
clobetasol propionate[a]	Clobex, Cormax, Embeline, Embeline E, Impoyz, Olux, Olux-E	**Cream:** 0.025%[b], 0.05%
	Clobex, Dermovate, Olux-E	**Foam (Olux, Olux-E):** 0.05%
		Gel: 0.05%[b]
		Lotion: 0.05%
		Ointment: 0.05%
		Shampoo: 0.05%
		Spray: 0.05%
		Solution: 0.05%
clocortolone	Cloderm	**Cream:** 0.1%
	Not available	
desonide[a]	Desonate, Desowen, Verdeso	**Cream:** 0.05%
	Tridesilon	**Foam (Verdeso)[b]:** 0.05%
		Gel (Desonate)[b]: 0.05%
		Lotion[b]: 0.05%
		Ointment: 0.05%
desoximetasone[d]	Topicort	**Cream:** 0.05% (Topicort Mild), 0.25% (Topicort)
	Topicort, Topicort Mild	**Gel:** 0.05%
		Ointment: 0.25%, 0.05%[b]
		Spray[b]: 0.25%
diflorasone diacetate[a]	ApexiCon E	**Cream:** 0.05%
	Not available	**Ointment:** 0.05%
fluocinolone acetonide[d]	Capex, DermaSmoothe/FS, Synalar	**Cream:** 0.01%, 0.025%
	DermaSmoothe/FS, Synalar	**Oil, topical (DermaSmoothe/FS):** 0.01%
		Ointment: 0.025%
		Shampoo (Capex): 0.01%
		Solution: 0.01%
fluocinonide[d]	Lidex, Vanos	**Cream:** 0.05%, 0.1%[b]
	Lidemol, Lidex, Lyderm, Tiamol	**Cream, emulsified (Lidemol):** 0.05%
		Gel: 0.05%
		Ointment: 0.05%
		Solution: 0.05%[b]

Continued

Topical Corticosteroids—cont'd

Generic Name	US Brand Name(s) Canadian Brand Name(s)	Dosage Forms and Strengths
flurandrenolide[a]	Cordran, Cordran SP, Cordran Tape	Cream: 0.025%, 0.05% Lotion: 0.05% Ointment: 0.05% Tape: 4 mcg/sq cm
	Not available	
fluticasone propionate[a]	Cutivate	Cream: 0.05% Lotion: 0.05% Ointment: 0.005%
	Not available	
halcinonide	Halog	Cream: 0.1% Ointment: 0.1%
	Not available	
halobetasol propionate[a]	Ultravate	Cream: 0.05% Foam: 0.05% Lotion: 0.05% Ointment: 0.05%
	Ultravate	
hydrocortisone base[a] (only Rx trade names listed)	Ala-cort, Ala-Scalp, Stie-cort, Texacort	Cream: 1%, 2.5% Lotion: 1%, 2%, 2.5% Ointment: 1% Solution: 2.5%
	OTC (1% or less)	
hydrocortisone acetate[a] (only Rx trade names listed)	Micort HC	Cream: 2.5%
	OTC (1% or less)	
hydrocortisone butyrate[a]	Locoid	Cream: 0.1% Cream, lipocream: 0.1% Lotion: 0.1% Ointment: 0.1% Solution: 0.1%
	Not available	
hydrocortisone probutate	Pandel	Cream: 0.1%
	Not available	
hydrocortisone valerate[d]	Generics	Cream: 0.2% Ointment: 0.2%
	Hydroval	
mometasone furoate[a]	Elocon	Cream: 0.1% Lotion: 0.1% Ointment: 0.1%
	Elocom	
prednicarbate[d]	Dermatop, Dermatop E	Cream, emollient: 0.1% Ointment: 0.1%
	Dermatop	
triamcinolone acetonide[a]	Kenalog, Triderm	Cream: 0.025%[b], 0.1%, 0.5% Lotion: 0.025%[b], 0.1% Ointment: 0.1% Topical spray: 0.147 mg/g
	Aristocort C, Aristocort R, Triaderm	

[a]Generic available.
[b]Available in the United States only.
[c]Available in Canada only.
[d]Generic available in the United States only.

Mechanism of Action and Pharmacokinetics

Calcipotriene (calcipotriol) inhibits the rapid and repeated production of new skin cells (proliferation). It inhibits the proliferation of T cells and inhibits the release of mediators of inflammation (e.g., cytokines, interleukins, interferons). The mechanism of action for topical calcitriol is unknown. When applied to skin with psoriasis, approximately 6% of the drug is absorbed. Absorption is slightly less through intact skin (5%). Calcipotriene is rapidly metabolized to vitamin D_3, in the liver.

Adverse Effects

Most adverse reactions are localized to the site of application. Irritation and redness are common. When large areas of the body are covered with the drug, some systemic absorption may occur.

Calcineurin Inhibitors

Generic Name	U.S. Brand Name(s)	Dosage Forms and Strengths[b]
	Canadian Brand Name(s)	
pimecrolimus	Elidel	**Cream:** 1%
	Elidel	
tacrolimus[a]	Protopic	**Ointment (Protoptic):** 0.03%, 0.1%
	Protopic	

[a]Generic available.
[b]Only topical dosage forms listed in table.

Vitamin D Analogues

Generic Name	US Brand Name(s)	Dosage Forms and Strengths[c]
	Canadian Brand Name(s)	
calcipotriene[a] (calcipotriol in Canada)	Dovonex, Sorilux	**Cream**[b]: 0.005% **Foam (Sorilux)**[b]: 0.005% **Solution, scalp**[b]: 0.005% **Ointment:** 0.005%
	Dovonex	
calcipotriene + betamethasone dipropionate[a]	Enstilar, Taclonex, Taclonex Scalp	**Foam (Enstilar):** 0.064% betamethasone + 0.005% calcipotriol **Gel (Dovobet):** 0.05% betamethasone + 0.005% calcipotriol **Ointment:** 0.05% betamethasone + 0.005% calcipotriol (Dovobet), 0.064% betamethasone + 0.005% calcipotriene (Taclonex) **Suspension (Taclonex):** 0.064% betamethasone + 0.005% calcipotriene
	Dovobet, Enstilar	
calcitriol	Vectical	**Ointment:** 3 mcg/g
	Silkis	

[a]Generic available in the United States only.
[b]Available in the United States only.
[c]Only topical dosage forms listed in table.

Vitamin D plays an important role in calcium absorption. Calcipotriene (calcipotriol) can raise calcium levels in the blood and urine.

Furanocoumarins

The psoralens are a class of drugs that increase photosensitivity and are classified as furanocoumarins. Methoxsalen, the only drug in this class is derived from a naturally occurring photoactive substance that is found in the seeds of the Ammi majus (Umbelliferae) plant. It is approved for the treatment of atopic dermatitis and psoriasis, along with UV light therapy. Methoxsalen and UV light work synergistically. Methoxsalen increases the skin's sensitivity to UV light and UV light activates methoxsalen. Psoralen plus UVA light therapy is also known as PUVA.

> **TECH NOTE!**
> Methoxsalen solution for injection (UVADEX) is used for the treatment of cutaneous T-cell lymphoma (see Chapter 31).

Mechanism of Action and Pharmacokinetics

The action of methoxsalen on pyrimidine bases of the DNA molecule results in the suppression of DNA synthesis, which decreases cell replication and proliferation. DNA photo damage produces cutaneous immunosuppression by affecting leukocyte regulatory mechanisms. Psoralens may be administered orally, topically, or parenterally. Oxsorelan-Ultra should be taken with low-fat food or milk. Methoxsalen is extensively metabolized in the liver and 90% to 95% is eliminated in urine. The elimination half-life is approximately two hours.

Adverse Effects

Adverse reactions produced by oral methoxsalen therapy are photosensitivity, insomnia, headache, dizziness, leg cramps, itching, dry skin, nausea, and vomiting. Topical application can cause burning, blistering, and swelling at the site of application.

Furanocoumarins Used to Treat Psoriasis

Generic Name	US Brand Name(s)	Dosage Forms and Strengths
	Canadian Brand Name(s)	
methoxsalen	Oxsoralen Ultra	**Capsule (Oxsoralen Ultra):** 10 mg
	Not available	

Immunosuppressives and Immunomodulators

Atopic dermatitis is believed to be an autoimmune disease; therefore immune system modulation and immunosuppression can downregulate the body's response to allergens and other irritants. Cyclosporine and methotrexate are immunosuppressants used for the treatment of psoriasis. Both drugs are used to treat other conditions such as cancer (Chapter 31) and methotrexate is also used to treat rheumatoid arthritis (Chapter 13). Cyclosporine is FDA-approved for the short-term treatment of severe atopic dermatitis and psoriasis. Methotrexate is an antimetabolite that is indicated for the treatment of moderate to severe chronic psoriasis and psoriatic arthritis. Apremilast (Otezla) is approved for moderate-to-severe plaque psoriasis.

Etanercept, infliximab, and adalimumab are biologics that are indicated for the treatment of psoriasis. They are classified as tumor necrosis factor (TNF)-α inhibitors. TNF-α inhibitors are genetically engineered drugs that block the inflammatory process triggered by high concentrations of TNF. Psoriasis is a condition that is linked to high levels of TNF-α. TNF-α inhibitors decrease inflammation and epidermal thickness. Ixekizumab, secukinumab, and ustekinumab are interleukin inhibitors. Interleukins are proinflammatory substances that are released as part of the immune response. They are approved for the treatment of moderate to severe plaque psoriasis.

Mechanism of Action and Pharmacokinetics

Cyclosporine selectively interferes with T cell proliferation and interleukin production. The result is a decreased immune system response. Methotrexate also interferes with normal DNA synthesis. Apremilast improves psoriasis and thickening skin by reducing the release of substances that produce an inflammatory response. It is one of a few agents that is taken orally.

The absorption of modified cyclosporine (Neoral) is decreased by food. The absorption of methotrexate is dose-dependent. Absorption from the GI tract occurs by active transport. Absorption decreases at higher doses. Food also delays absorption. Metabolism occurs in the liver, gut, and cells, and methotrexate is subject to first pass metabolism. Because methotrexate is primarily eliminated in the kidney, high dose therapy can cause high urine concentrations and crystalluria, leading to kidney damage. TNF-α inhibitors (e.g., etanercept) prevent cell lysis (destruction) and release of the substances that cause inflammation. Secukinumab and ixekizumab are antibodies that work by inhibiting specific interleukins. The effectiveness of some of the biologics used in treating psoriasis (e.g., etanercept, infliximab, and adalimumab) may decrease over time. See Chapters 13 and 31 for additional pharmacokinetic information.

Adverse Effects

Cyclosporine and methotrexate may produce nausea and vomiting. All of the drugs may also increase the risk for infection. Cyclosporine and methotrexate can cause kidney toxicity. Weight gain and hypertension are other side effects of cyclosporine therapy. Adverse reactions of etanercept are nausea, stomach pain, and headache. Adalimumab, etanercept, and infliximab are also associated with unspecified rashes and possible new-onset psoriasis. All of the biologics may increase risk for infections. Parenterally administered agents can cause redness and itching at the injection site. See Chapters 13 and 31 for a complete listing of adverse reactions.

> ● **TECH NOTE!**
>
> Folic acid is commonly prescribed to patients being treated with methotrexate.

Retinoids

Retinoid analogues are used to treat psoriasis. Acitretin is a synthetic retinoid and tazarotene is a retinoid prodrug (see Chapter 35). Acitretin is used as monotherapy or used concurrently with phototherapy to increase its effectiveness.

Mechanism of Action and Pharmacokinetics

When acitretin binds to retinoic acid receptors it modifies epithelial cell growth and differentiation. Tazarotene inhibits epidermal hyperproliferation in treated plaques. The absorption of tazarotene is minimal when applied topically. Metabolism occurs in the skin and results in the active metabolite tazarotenic acid. Tazarotenic acid is systemically absorbed and metabolized further. The half-life ($t_{1/2}$) of tazarotenic acid is approximately 18 hours. A drug interaction with alcohol may convert acitretin to a new molecule that can take up to three years to fully eliminate from the body.

Adverse Reactions

Itching, burning, stinging, redness, and worsening of psoriasis occur in up to 30% of people using tazarotene. Up to 10% may experience eczema, contact dermatitis, fissures, and/or bleeding. Tazarotene is contraindicated in pregnancy, and a negative pregnancy test should be obtained prior to use. Acitretin use may produce hypervitaminosis A. In addition, up to 75% of people using acitretin develop cheilitis (inflammation of the lips), alopecia, and peeling skin. Redness, itching and dry skin, and a nail disorder may also occur.

Immunosuppressants and Immunomodulators

Generic Name	US Brand Name(s) / Canadian Brand Name(s)	Dosage Forms and Strengths
cyclosporine[a]	Gengraf, Neoral	**Capsule, modified (Gengraf, Neoral):** 10 mg[b], 25 mg, 50 mg, 100 mg
	Neoral	**Solution, oral, modified (Gengraf, Neoral):** 100 mg/mL (See Chapters 13 and 31 for additional dosage forms and brand names.)
Antimetabolites (DMARDs)		
methotrexate[a] (MTX)	Methotrexate	**Tablet:** 2.5-mg (See Chapters 13 and 31 for additional dosage forms and brand names.)
	Methotrexate	
Immunomodulators (Biologics)		
adalimumab	Humira	**Prefilled pen kit:** 40 mg/0.8 mL, 40 mg/0.4 mL[b]
	Humira	
adalimumab-ATTO[c]	Anjevita	20 mg/0.4mL, 40 mg/0.8 mL
adalimumab-ADBM[c]	Cyltezo	40 mg/0.8 mL
etanercept	Enbrel, Elrezi	**Injection, powder for reconstitution:** 25 mg/vial
	Brenzys, Enbrel, Elrezi	**Injection, solution:** 50 mg/ (prefilled syringe)
infliximab	Inflectra, Remicade	**Injection, powder for reconstitution:** 100-mg/ vial
	Remicade	
infliximab-ABDA	Renflexis	
infliximab-DYYB	Inflectra	
infliximab-QBTX	Xifi	
	Inflectra, Remicade	
ixekizumab	Taltz	**Solution, for injection:** 80 mg/mL
	Taltz	
secukinumab	Cosentyx	**Solution, for injection:** 150 mg/mL
	Cosentyx	
ustekinumab	Stelara	**Solution, for injection:** 45 mg/0.5 mL, 90 mg/mL, 5 mg/mL[c]
	Stelara	
Miscellaneous		
apremilast	Otezla	**Tablets:** 10 mg, 20 mg, 30 mg
	Otezla	

[a]Generic available.
[b]Available in Canada only.
[c]Available in the United States only.

Retinoids

Generic Name	US Brand Name(s)	Dosage Forms and Strengths
	Canadian Brand Name(s)	
acitretin[a]	Soriatane	**Capsule:** 10 mg, 17.5 mg[b], 22.5 mg[b], 25 mg
	Soriatane	
tazarotene	Avage, Fabior Tazorac	**Cream:** 0.05%, 0.1%
	Tazorac	**Foam (Fabior):** 0.1%
		Gel: 0.05%, 0.1%

[a]Generic available
[b]Available in the United States only.

TECHNICIAN'S CORNER

1. Because atopic dermatitis is allergy-related, how can one prevent flare-ups from occurring?
2. How well do calamine lotion and oatmeal soap (both OTC products) work in decreasing the symptoms of atopic dermatitis?

Summary of Drugs Used for the Treatment of Eczema and Psoriasis

Generic Name	Brand Name	Usual Dose and Dosing Schedule	Warning Labels
Topical Corticosteroids			
alclometasone dipropionate[a]	Generics	**Cream or ointment:** Apply a thin film two or three times daily.	FOR EXTERNAL USE.
amcinonide[a]	Generics	**All dosage forms:** Apply a thin film two or three times daily.	FOR EXTERNAL USE.
betamethasone dipropionate[a]	Diprolene AF	**Cream, lotion, ointment:** Apply a thin film two to four times daily.	FOR EXTERNAL USE.
	Diprosone		
betamethasone valerate[a]	Betaderm, Luxiq, Valisone	**Foam:** Apply twice a day. **Cream, lotion, ointment:** Apply a thin film two to four times daily.	FOR EXTERNAL USE. SHAKE WELL (FOAM, LOTION).
clobetasol propionate[a]	Clobex, Olux	**All dosage forms:** Apply twice a day.	SHAKE WELL—(FOAM) FOR EXTERNAL USE.
desonide[a]	Desowen, Verdeso	**Foam:** Apply twice a day. **Cream, lotion, ointment:** Apply a thin film two to four times daily.	FOR EXTERNAL USE. SHAKE WELL—(FOAM).
	Tridesilon		
desoximetasone[a]	Topicort	**Cream, gel, ointment:** Apply a thin film twice a day.	FOR EXTERNAL USE.
diflorasone diacetate[a]	Generics	**Nonemollient dosage forms:** Apply a thin film one to four times daily. **Emollient dosage forms:** Apply a thin film one to three times daily.	FOR EXTERNAL USE.
fluocinolone acetonide[a]	Synalar	**Cream, ointment, solution:** Apply a thin film two to four times daily. **Oil:** Apply a thin film three times a day.	FOR EXTERNAL USE.
	Derma-Smoothe/FS		
halcinonide	Halog	**Cream, ointment, solution:** Apply a thin film two to four times daily.	FOR EXTERNAL USE.
halobetasol propionate[a]	Ultravate	**Cream or ointment:** Apply a thin film once or twice daily.	FOR EXTERNAL USE.
hydrocortisone, acetate[a]	Micort HC	**All dosage forms:** Apply three or four times daily.	FOR EXTERNAL USE.
hydrocortisone butyrate[a]	Locoid	**All dosage forms:** Apply once or twice daily.	FOR EXTERNAL USE.
hydrocortisone valerate[a]	Generics	**All dosage forms:** Apply two to four times daily.	FOR EXTERNAL USE.
mometasone furoate[a]	Elocon	**Topical dosage forms:** Apply once daily.	FOR EXTERNAL USE.

Continued

Summary of Drugs Used for the Treatment of Eczema and Psoriasis—cont'd

Generic Name	Brand Name	Usual Dose and Dosing Schedule	Warning Labels
prednicarbate[a]	Dermatop	**Cream or ointment:** Apply a thin film twice daily.	FOR EXTERNAL USE.
triamcinolone acetonide[a]	Generics	**Cream, lotion, ointment:** Apply a thin film two to four times daily.	FOR EXTERNAL USE.
Calcineurin Inhibitors			
pimecrolimus	Elidel	**Atopic dermatitis:** Apply a thin layer twice a day.	AVOID EXCESS EXPOSURE TO SUNLIGHT. AVOID GRAPEFRUIT JUICE (CAPSULE).
tacrilimus	Protopic	**Atopic dermatitis:** Apply a thin layer twice a day.	
Immunosuppressants			
cyclosporine	Neoral	**Psoriasis:** 1.25 mg/kg orally bid up to 4 mg/kg daily	TAKE WITH FOOD. AVOID PREGNANCY. AVOID ALCOHOL. SWALLOW WHOLE; DON'T CRUSH OR CHEW.
methotrexate	Generics	**Psoriasis:** 10–25 mg PO, IV, or IM given as a single weekly dose or 2.5–5 mg PO every 12 h for 3 doses every week	AVOID ALCOHOL. AVOID PROLONGED EXPOSURE TO SUNLIGHT. AVOID PREGNANCY. EXERCISE PRECAUTIONS FOR HANDLING, PREPARING, AND ADMINISTERING CYTOTOXIC DRUGS.
Vitamin D Analogues			
calcipotriene	Dovonex	**Psoriasis:** Apply a thin layer twice a day.	FOR EXTERNAL USE. AVOID EXCESS EXPOSURE TO SUNLIGHT. AVOID FACE.
calcipotriene + betamethasone	Taclonex	**Psoriasis:** Apply a thin layer once daily.	
calcitriol	Vectical	**Mild to moderate psoriasis:** Apply twice a day.	
Furanocoumarins			
methoxsalen	Oxsoralen Ultra	**Psoriasis:** 1 cap 1.5–2 h before UVA therapy	TAKE WITH FOOD OR MILK. AVOID SUN EXPOSURE FOR 24 H BEFORE AND 48 H AFTER TREATMENT.
Immunomodulators			
adalimumab	Humira	**Chronic plaque psoriasis:** 80 mg subcutaneously in two injections on day 1, then 40 mg every other week	REFRIGERATE; DO NOT FREEZE.— adalimumab, etanercept, infliximab, ixekizumab, secukinumab, ustekinumab PROTECT FROM LIGHT.—etanercept, ixekizumab, secukinumab, ustekinumab GENTLY SWIRL RECONSTITUTED PRODUCT— infliximab DO NOT SHAKE.—infliximab, ixekizumab, secukinumab, ustekinumab DISCARD ANY UNUSED PORTION—infliximab, ixekizumab, secukinumab, ustekinumab
etanercept	Enbrel	**Psoriasis:** 50 mg subcutaneously weekly given as one 50-mg injection or as two 25-mg injections 3–4 days apart	
infliximab	Remicade	**Psoriasis:** 5 mg/kg IV given at week 0, 2, and 6 and repeated every 8 wk thereafter	
ixekizumab	Taltz	Inject subcutaneously, 160 mg followed by 80 mg every 2 weeks on weeks 2, 4, 6, 8, 10, and 12; then 80 mg every 4 weeks.	
secukinumab	Cosentyx	**Plaque Psoriasis:** 300 mg By subcutaneous injection at Weeks 0, 1, 2, 3, and 4 followed by 300 mg every 4 weeks.	
ustekinumab	Stelara	**Plaque psoriasis (Moderate to Severe)** (100 kg or less), 45 mg subcutaneously initially and at week 4; then 45 mg every 12 weeks (Greater than 100 kg), 90 mg subcutaneously initially and at week 4; then 90 mg every 12 weeks	

Summary of Drugs Used for the Treatment of Eczema and Psoriasis—cont'd

Generic Name	Brand Name	Usual Dose and Dosing Schedule	Warning Labels
apremilast	Otezla	**Plaque psoriasis, Moderate to severe** Begin: 10 mg orally in AM; Day 2, 10 mg twice daily; Day 3, 10 mg in AM, 20 mg in PM; Day 4, 20 mg twice daily; Day 5, 20 mg in AM, 30 mg in PM Maintenance: Day 6 and thereafter, 30 mg orally twice daily	SWALLOW WHOLE; DON'T CRUSH OR CHEW.
Retinoids			
acitretin	Soriatane	**Recalcitrant psoriasis:** 25–50 mg PO once daily	TAKE WITH MAIN MEAL. AVOID ALCOHOL.
tazarotene	Tazorac	**Psoriasis:** Apply once daily, in the evening, to psoriatic lesions (max, 12 weeks).	PROTECT SKIN FROM THE SUN. AVOID PREGNANCY.

ᵃGeneric available.

Key Points

- Atopic diseases are an autoimmune disorder.
- Atopic dermatitis is the most common form of eczema.
- Atopic dermatitis is a chronic disease of the skin that often develops in infancy and may continue throughout adulthood.
- Atopic dermatitis commonly produces symptoms of intense itching, redness (from scratching), skin irritation, and inflammation. Eczematous patches may form that are flaky and crusting, and may even ooze a clear fluid.
- Psoriasis is a condition associated with the rapid turnover of skin cells and is caused by hyperactivity of the T cells.
- Individuals with psoriasis have thick, silvery, scaly patches. They may also have some redness and swelling.
- Individuals with atopic dermatitis and psoriasis may experience periods when their symptoms worsen (exacerbation) and periods when they get better or go away completely (remission).
- Nonpharmaceutical treatment for eczema involves using skin care regimens that reduce irritation and avoiding allergens and irritants, and may include the use of phototherapy.
- Phototherapy involves exposing the skin to ultraviolet A or B light waves.
- UV light therapy may cause premature aging of the skin and increase the risk for skin cancer.
- The use of topical corticosteroids continues to be a mainstay of therapy for the treatment of atopic dermatitis and psoriasis.
- Topical corticosteroids are categorized into seven groups based on potency.
- The vehicle (base) in which the corticosteroid is suspended may influence the potency.
- Higher potency corticosteroids cause more adverse reactions.
- Only the mildest potency agents, such as hydrocortisone, should be used on the face.
- Long-term use of topical corticosteroids can produce thinning of the skin, stretch marks (striae), spider veins, acne, milia, rosacea (enlarged blood vessels, especially on the nose), bruising,

atrophy, lacerations, poor wound healing, and growth suppression (in children).
- Pimecrolimus and tacrolimus are calcineurin inhibitor immunomodulators that control inflammation and reduce the immune system response to allergens.
- Pimecrolimus is indicated for the treatment of mild to moderate eczema (atopic dermatitis).
- Tacrolimus is approved for the treatment of moderate to severe atopic dermatitis that has failed to respond to corticosteroid treatment.
- Calcipotriene is a synthetic analogue of vitamin D. It is known as calcipotriol in Canada.
- Calcipotriene (calcipotriol) inhibits the rapid and repeated production of new skin cells and is used for the treatment of psoriasis.
- Calcitriol is an active form of vitamin D that is used topically for the treatment of psoriasis.
- Psoralens are a class of drugs that increase photosensitivity and are classified as furanocoumarins. Methoxsalen is the only drug in this class.
- Psoralens plus ultraviolet light A therapy is also known as PUVA.
- Cyclosporine is FDA-approved for the short-term treatment of severe atopic dermatitis and psoriasis. It decreases immune system hyperactivity.
- Methotrexate is an antimetabolite indicated for the treatment of moderate to severe chronic psoriasis and psoriatic arthritis.
- Methotrexate slows the rapid rate of skin cell turnover that occurs with eczema and psoriasis.
- The retinoids acitretin and tazarotene are used for the treatment of psoriasis.
- Adalimumab, etanercept, and infliximab are TNF-α inhibitors indicated for the treatment of plaque psoriasis.
- Ixekizumab, secukinumab, and ustekinumab are interleukin inhibitors that are approved for the treatment of moderate to severe plaque psoriasis. They block proinflammatory substances that are release as part of the immune response.

Review Questions

1. A chronic disease of the skin characterized by itchy red patches covered with silvery scales is known as _____.
   a. eczema
   b. psoriasis
   c. dermatitis
   d. rosacea

2. All of the following treatments for psoriasis are applied topically, except _____.
   a. Dovonex
   b. Taclonex
   c. Neoral
   d. Tazorac

3. When symptoms worsen, it is called _____, and periods when they get better or go away completely are called _____.
   a. exacerbation; metastasis
   b. exacerbation; remission
   c. metastasis; inflammation
   d. allergic; nonallergic

4. Phototherapy reduces the risk for skin cancer.
   a. True
   b. False

5. A mainstay of therapy for the treatment of eczema is the use of _____.
   a. antibiotics
   b. corticosteroids
   c. antihistamines
   d. none of the above

6. Pimecrolimus (Elidel) is indicated for the treatment of moderate to severe eczema.
   a. True
   b. False

7. All of the following treatments for psoriasis are administered by injection, except:
   a. Humira
   b. Soriatane
   c. Enbrel
   d. Remicade

8. All of the following products must be stored in the refrigerator, except_____.
   a. Stelara
   b. Taltz
   c. Cosentyx
   d. Otezla

9. _____ is an antimetabolite indicated for the treatment of moderate to severe chronic psoriasis and psoriatic arthritis.
   a. Anthralin
   b. Cyclosporine
   c. Methotrexate
   d. Calcipotriene

10. Select the Class VII corticosteroid that is safe for use on the face.
    a. Hydrocortisone
    b. Betamethasone
    c. Clobetasol
    d. Mometasone

Bibliography

Brown S: Molecular mechanisms in atopic eczema: insights gained from genetic studies, *J Pathol* 241:140–145, 2017. doi:10.1002/path.4810.

Health Canada. 2018. Drug Product Database. Retrieved September 22, 2018, from https://health-products.canada.ca/dpd-bdpp/index-eng.jsp.

Institute for Safe Medication Practices. 2016. FDA and ISMP Lists of Look-Alike Drug Names with Recommended Tall Man Letters.

Hoffman MB, Hill D, Feldman SR: Current challenges and emerging drug delivery strategies for the treatment of psoriasis, *Expert Opin Drug Deliv* 13(10):1461–1473, 2016. doi:10.1080/17425247.2016.1188801.

Kalant H, Grant D, Mitchell J: *Principles of medical pharmacology*, ed 7, Toronto, 2007, Elsevier Canada, pp 891–898.

Khandpur S, Sharma VK, Sumanth K: Topical immunomodulators in dermatology, *J Postgrad Med* 50:131–139, 2004.

Lance L, Lacy C, Armstrong L, et al: *Drug information handbook for the allied health professional*, ed 12, Hudson, OH, 2005, APhA Lexi-Comp.

National Institute of Arthritis and Musculoskeletal and Skin Diseases: Atopic dermatitis. Retrieved 2016 from https://www.niams.nih.gov/health-topics/atopic-dermatitis.

National Institute of Arthritis and Musculoskeletal and Skin Diseases: Psoriasis. Retrieved 2017 from https://www.niams.nih.gov/health-topics/psoriasis.

Page C, Curtis M, Sutter M, et al: *Integrated pharmacology*, Philadelphia, 2005, Elsevier Mosby, pp 506–508, 512–514.

Raymond GP, Houle M-C: A Review of Corticosteroids for the Treatment of Psoriasis, *Skin Therapy Letter-Pharmacist Edition* 2(1):2007. [updated May 2016]. http://www.skinpharmacies.ca/2_1_2.html.

Sala M, Elaissari A, Fessi H: Advances in psoriasis physiopathology and treatments: Up to date of mechanistic insights and perspectives of novel therapies based on innovative skin drug delivery systems (ISDDS), *J Control Release* 239:182–292, 2016.

Schlichte MJ, Vandersall A, Katta R: Diet and eczema: a review of dietary supplements for the treatment of atopic dermatitis, *Dermatol Pract Concept* 6(3):6, 2016. doi:10.5826/dpc.0603a06.

US Food and Drug Administration. nd. Drugs@FDA: FDA Approved Drug Products. Retrieved September 22, 2018, from http://www.accessdata.fda.gov/scripts/cder/daf/.

Wawrzyniak P, Akdis CA, Finkelman FD, et al: Advances and highlights in mechanisms of allergic disease in 2015, *J Allergy Clin Immunol* 137:1681–1696, 2016.

37

Treatment of Lice and Scabies

LEARNING OBJECTIVES

1. Learn the terminology associated with lice and scabies.
2. Describe the epidemiology of lice and scabies infestation.
3. List the symptoms of lice and scabies infestation.
4. List prevention strategies.
5. List and categorize medications used to treat lice and scabies.
6. Describe mechanism of action for drugs used to lice and scabies.
7. Identify warning labels and precautionary messages associated with medications used to treat lice and scabies.

KEY TERMS

Lice Group of parasites (*Pediculus humanus capitis, Pediculus humanus corporis, Phthirus pubis*) that can live on the body, scalp, or genital area of humans.
Nits Head lice eggs.
Nymph Baby louse.
Ovicidal Kills eggs.

Parasite Organism that benefits by living in, with, or on another organism.
Pediculicide Drug that kills lice.
Scabicide Drug that kills the scabies mite.
Scabies Parasitic infection caused by the mite *Sarcoptes scabiei*.

Epidemiology of Lice and Scabies Infestation

Lice and *scabies* infestations affect people worldwide without regard for social status or race. They are caused by parasites and are readily spread person to person. A *parasite* is an organism that benefits by living in, with, or on another organism (host), usually to the detriment of the host.

Lice

Head Lice

Head lice most commonly infests children aged 3 to 11 years and their families, but anyone can become infested (Fig. 37.1A and B). The parasite *Pediculus humanus capitis* is spread between individuals through head-to-head contact, as occurs during children's play and sports. Less commonly, transmission occurs by sharing personal items such as combs, brushes, hats, towels, scarves, pillows, and coats with someone who has head lice.

The life cycle of a head louse is approximately four to six weeks. The adult females lay eggs, also called *nits*, at the base of the hair shaft (see Fig. 37.1C) within 24 hours of mating. In approximately seven days, the nits hatch and a nymph emerges. A *nymph* is a baby louse. The nymph becomes an adult in approximately seven days; and the adult lives for approximately 30 days.

Lice are parasites that feed on blood. This is why eggs are laid close to the base of the hair shaft and nits that are found within $\frac{1}{4}$ inch of the scalp are typically viable eggs. Newly hatched nymphs must be close to a blood source. Nit shells found farther than a fingertip away from the base of the scalp (2 to 5 cm) are likely remains of an earlier infestation; treatment is not necessary. An adult louse can live for up to three days away from a human host. Head lice are a nuisance but are not a health risk.

> **❶ TECH ALERT!**
> It is a myth that head lice infestation is caused by poor hygiene (lack of cleanliness).

> **● TECH NOTE!**
> Head lice do not live on pets, there is no human-to-pet transmission, and pets need not be treated with pediculicides.

> **● TECH NOTE!**
> Pharmacy technicians may have customers coming into the pharmacy asking about head lice treatments. Because these products are available over the counter (OTC), they will be able to direct customers to the pharmacy shelves where available products are located.

Body Lice

Body lice infestations are caused by the parasite *Pediculus humanus corporis*. Infestations are a serious public health concern because body lice may cause epidemics of typhus and louse-borne relapsing fever. Body lice thrive in crowded environments with chronic

• **Fig. 37.1** (A) Adult head louse. (B) Head lice infestation. (C) Nit attached to hair shaft. ([A], Courtesy of Dr. Dennis D. Juranek, Centers for Disease Control and Prevention; [B], From Callen J, Greer K, Hood A, et al: *Color atlas of dermatology*, Philadelphia, 1993, WB Saunders; [C], from Kumar V, Abbas AK, Fausto M: *Robbins and Cotran pathologic basis of disease*, ed 7, Philadelphia, 2005, Saunders.)

poverty and unsanitary conditions, such as refugee camps, temporary housing from natural disasters, and prisons. In the United States and Canada, body lice infestations rarely occur except in populations without access to bathing facilities (e.g., homelessness).

Like head lice, body lice infestation is spread person to person through direct contact with a person who has body lice. Another mode of transmission is through shared bedding or clothes. Body lice can live in the seams of the clothing of infested individuals.

The life cycle of body lice is similar to that of head lice and begins with laying eggs. The nits hatch and nymphs mature to adults in seven days. Adults can only survive away from a human host for 10 days.

Pubic Lice

Pubic lice, or "crabs," is sometimes classified as a sexually transmitted infection (STI) because it is usually spread through sexual contact (Fig. 37.2). It is rare for lice to be spread through contact with bedding, linens, or clothes. Although the life cycle of pubic lice is the same as that of head lice, pubic lice and head lice are different species. Head lice do not inhabit the genitalia, and pubic lice do not live in the hair. Lice infestation in the pubic region is caused by the parasite *Phthirus pubis*.

> **⚠ TECH ALERT!**
>
> It is a myth that individuals can get pubic lice from sitting on a public toilet seat.

• **Fig. 37.2** Pubic lice. (From Mahon CR, Lehman DC, Manuselis G: *Textbook of diagnostic microbiology*, ed 3, St. Louis, 2007, Saunders.)

Scabies

Scabies infestations are caused by a parasitic mite called *Sarcoptes scabiei*. The mite flourishes and spreads by person-to-person contact in environments in which the population density is high, such as hospitals, nursing homes, child care facilities, and schools. Transmission occurs through close contact and sharing bedding, linen, clothing, or sexual relations. Infestations are common and can affect anyone.

• **BOX 37.1** **Symptoms of Lice and Scabies Infestation**

Head and Pubic Lice
- Itching
- Feeling of something moving in hair or genital area
- Sores (from scratching)

Body Louse
- Itching
- Rash
- Thickening and discoloration of skin

Scabies
- Intense itching
- Pimple-like rash

• **BOX 37.2** **Strategies to Prevent Reinfestation**

- Treat all infested and probably infested household members simultaneously.
- Use a nit comb to remove eggs. Use daily lice combing between pediculicidal treatments.
- Don't wash the hair for one to two days after the treatment is rinsed from the hair.
- Vacuum the floor and furniture in infested household.
- Wash clothing, linens, and bedding in hot water (130°F [54°C]).
- Dry-clean clothing that is not washable.
- Place stuffed toys, clothing, and bedding that cannot be washed or dry-cleaned in a large plastic bag and seal the bag for 2 weeks.

The scabies mite burrows beneath the skin. Sites of infestation can be seen in the webbing between fingers and toes; skin folds of the breast, penis, and shoulder blades; and in the bends of the elbows, knees, and wrists. Like lice, *S. scabiei* feeds on blood and dies if away from a human host for longer than 48 to 72 hours. The adult mite can live for approximately 30 days.

Symptoms of Lice and Scabies Infestation and Prevention of Lice Reinfestation

Symptoms of lice and scabies infestation are listed in Box 37.1. Methods for the prevention of lice reinfestation are listed in Box 37.2.

> **❗ TECH ALERT!**
> Shaving the head is not necessary to treat head lice!

Treatment of Head Lice, Pubic Lice, and Scabies

Head lice may be treated with nonprescription and prescription *pediculicides*. The Centers for Disease Control and Prevention (CDC) and Nova Scotia Public Health Services recommend that all family members with active infestations, as well as those with probable infestations (nits but no live lice), be treated. Treatment is more effective if a fine-toothed nit comb is used to remove eggs from the hair shaft. OTC and prescription agents are effective treatments for head lice and pubic lice. OTC products are more

effective and have a lower risk of toxicity than lindane. Drug resistance is a growing problem for OTC and prescription pediculicides, especially permethrin, because of the residue left after treatment.

> **● TECH NOTE!**
> There is no proof that lice sprays are any more effective than vacuuming. Lice transmission is via person-to-person contact; the risk of transmission by sitting on a piece of furniture is very low.

Pediculicides

Pediculicides that treat lice and/or scabies are crotamiton, benzoyl alcohol, isopropyl myristate and ivermectin, lindane, malathion, pyrethrins (plus piperonyl butoxide), permethrin, and spinosad. They are formulated in various dosage forms, such as shampoo, cream rinse, lotion, and household spray. Pyrethrins (plus piperonyl butoxide), permethrin, and isopropyl myristate are marketed for OTC use. Crotamiton is marketed as an OTC product in Canada and prescription access only in the United States.

Pyrethrins and Permethrin

Pyrethrins are naturally derived from the chrysanthemum flower. Their effectiveness is boosted by the addition of piperonyl butoxide, a petroleum distillate. Pyrethrins are indicated for the treatment of head lice, pubic lice, and body lice. Permethrin is a mixture of synthetic isomers of pyrethrins. It is more effective for the treatment of head lice but less effective against pubic lice (as low as 57% efficacy). It is also effective against the scabies mite.

Pyrethrins are not *ovicidal* (do not kill the eggs), so retreatment is necessary in 7 to 10 days to kill newly hatched nymphs. Permethrin is ovicidal.

Mechanism of Action and Pharmacokinetics

Pyrethrins and permethrin paralyze and kill. Their action is discontinued once the drug is washed off. Permethrin leaves a residue on the hair that can destroy eggs and newly hatched nymphs. Absorption of pyrethrins and permethrin through the skin is minimal. Both drugs are rapidly metabolized in the liver.

Adverse Effects

The most common adverse effects caused by topical application of pyrethrins are redness, itching and stinging, tingling, and minor swelling.

> **❗ TECH ALERT!**
> Pharmacy technicians must apply the warning label "For External Use Only" to prescription vials containing lindane lotion and shampoo.

> **● TECH NOTE!**
> Permethrin is approved for use in children three months of age and older; however, the CDC recommends that manual removal of nits and lice in children younger than two years be tried first.

Benzoyl Alcohol

Benzoyl alcohol 5% is used to treat head lice. It is marketed in the United States only.

Pyrethins and Permethrin

Generic Name	US Brand Name(s)	Dosage Forms and Strengths	Prescription/OTC status
	Canadian Brand Name(s)		
pyrethrins + piperonyl butoxide	R&C II, RID Step 1 Lice-Killing shampoo, RID Home Lice, Bedbug & Dust Mite Spray R&C Shampoo + Conditioner	**Shampoo:** pyrethrins 0.33% + piperonyl butoxide 4% (RID); pyrethrins 0.33% + piperonyl butoxide 3% (R&C) **Spray (R&C II):** pyrethrins 0.3% + piperonyl butoxide 1.5%	**OTC**
permethrin[a]	Nix, Elimite Cream Kwellada-P Cream Rinse, Kwellada-P Lotion, Nix Cream Rinse, Nix Dermal Cream	**Cream rinse:** 1% **Lotion:** 1%, 5%[b] **Cream:** 5%	**All strengths OTC (Canada)** **5% Prescription (US)**

[a]Generic available.
[b]Available in Canada only.

Mechanism of Action and Pharmacokinetics

Benzoyl alcohol 5% asphyxiates the louse. It is not effective in killing the eggs, so a second treatment is required seven days after the primary treatment (after the eggs hatch). Topical application is approved for persons over the age of six months.

Adverse Reactions

Topical application may cause redness and skin irritation.

Benzoyl Alcohol

Generic Name	US Brand Name(s)	Dosage Forms and Strengths	Prescription/OTC status
	Canadian Brand Name(s)		
benzoyl alcohol	Ulesfia Not available	**Solution:** 5%	**Prescription**

Isopropyl Myristate

Isopropyl myristate 50% is available in Canada for the OTC treatment of head lice. It is not available in the United States.

Mechanism of Action and Pharmacokinetics

Isopropyl myristate purportedly dissolves the louse exoskeleton, resulting in dehydration and death. It is not ovicidal, so nit removal and retreatment in 10 days are required. Evidence of the effectiveness of isopropyl myristate is lacking. Pharmacokinetic information is unavailable.

Adverse Effects

Adverse effects caused by topical application of isopropyl myristate are redness, itching, and mild skin irritation.

Ivermectin

Ivermectin has been used for more than 20 years worldwide as a treatment for filarial worm infections. It is also an effective head lice treatment. Ivermectin lotion, 0.5%, is approved for treatment of infested persons six months of age and older. It kills newly hatched lice but not the eggs. It is used as a single application on dry hair. A health care provider should be consulted before retreatment.

Isopropyl Myristate

Generic Name	US Brand Name(s)	Dosage Forms and Strengths	Prescription/OTC status
	Canadian Brand Name(s)		
isopropyl myristate	Not available Resultz	**Solution:** 50%	**OTC**

Mechanism of Action

Ivermectin is a member of the avermectin class of pediculicides that kill parasites. It increases the permeability of the cell membrane to chloride ions, causing hyperpolarization and paralysis of invertebrate nerve and muscle cells. Ivermectin does not readily cross the blood–brain barrier in humans.

Adverse Reactions and Precautions

The most common side effects are eye redness, burning of the skin, and dryness. Ivermectin should not be used in children weighing less than 15 kg or in pregnant women.

Ivermectin

Generic Name	US Brand Name(s)	Dosage Forms and Strengths	Prescription/OTC status
	Canadian Brand Name(s)		
ivermectin	Sklice, Soolantra Rosiver	**Cream:** 1% **Lotion:** 0.5%	**Prescription**

Lindane

Lindane is an organochlorine pesticide. It is both a *scabicide* and pediculicide, killing all type of lice, scabies, and their eggs. It is a second line treatment for head lice due to toxicity.

Mechanism of Action and Pharmacokinetics

Lindane is absorbed through into the body of the scabies mite and lice, where it paralyzes and kills the parasite. Lindane is highly lipid-soluble and absorption through the skin is variable. Absorption of lindane through intact human skin increases with repeated applications; the half-life is long ($t_{1/2}$ = 18 hours). Lindane is stored in body fats and is significantly metabolized in the liver. Repeated use causes accumulation and increases the risk for neurotoxicity.

Adverse Effects

Lindane is neurotoxic and can cause illness, vomiting, seizures, and death if accidentally swallowed. The US Food and Drug Administration (FDA) has required manufacturers to place a boxed warning in the package insert to alert health care providers of the following:

- Lindane is not a first-line therapy, and repeat applications should be avoided.
- Lindane should not be used by infants, young children, elders, adults weighing less than 110 lb [50 kg], and breast feeding women.
- The drug should be dispensed in 1- to 2-ounce single-application vials, the maximum amount needed for a treatment.
- The FDA recommends that Lindane shampoo only be used when you have already been treated with other products that did not work or you cannot use other safer medications.

■ Lindane

Generic Name	US Brand Name(s) / Canadian Brand Name(s)	Dosage Forms and Strengths	Prescription/ OTC status
lindane[a]	Generics	Lotion: 1%	Prescription
	Not available	Shampoo: 1%	

[a]Generic available.

Malathion

Malathion is an organophosphate pesticide used in agriculture to control pests and medically to kill head lice and their eggs. It was withdrawn from the US market and then reintroduced in 1999 following labeling changes. It remains withdrawn from the market in Canada.

Mechanism of Action and Pharmacokinetics

Malathion is a prodrug that must be metabolized to its active metabolite malaoxon. It paralyzes the central nervous system of parasites by causing an accumulation of acetylcholine (ACh). The pharmacokinetics of malathion are dependent on the dose and route of exposure. Less than 10% of the applied dose is absorbed systemically. Absorption through the scalp of infants is greater, and the use of malathion is contraindicated in this age group. Safety in children less than six years old has not been established. The onset of action is three seconds to one hour. The elimination half-life ranges between 8 and 48 hours.

Adverse Effects

The most common adverse effects linked to malathion use are stinging, redness, minor swelling, itching, and tingling.

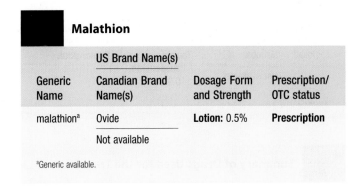

⚠ TECH ALERT!

Malathion is flammable, and those using the product should stay away from open flames, hair dryers, curling irons, and lit cigarettes, cigars, and pipes.

■ Malathion

Generic Name	US Brand Name(s) / Canadian Brand Name(s)	Dosage Form and Strength	Prescription/ OTC status
malathion[a]	Ovide	Lotion: 0.5%	Prescription
	Not available		

[a]Generic available.

Crotamiton

Crotamiton is a scabicide. Its mechanism of action is unknown. It is an alternative to lindane that can be used during pregnancy. The pharmacokinetics and degree of systemic absorption of crotamiton after topical application have not been determined.

Adverse Effects

Crotamiton has few adverse reactions. Reactions are linked to drug allergy and include itchiness, minor swelling, and redness.

■ Crotamiton

Generic Name	US Brand Name(s) / Canadian Brand Name(s)	Dosage Forms and Strengths	Prescription/ OTC status
crotamiton	Eurax, Crotan	Cream: 10%	OTC: Canada
	Eurax	Lotion[a]: 10%	Prescription: United States

[a]Available in United States only.

Spinosad

Spinosad is a pediculicide indicated for the topical treatment of head lice infestations in patients 4 years of age and older. It is derived from *Saccharopolyspora spinosa*, a bacterium found in soil.

Mechanism of Action and Pharmacokinetics

Spinosad produces neuronal excitation in lice, resulting in hyper-excitation, paralysis, and death. The pharmacokinetics and degree of systemic absorption of spinosad after topical application have not been determined. Systemic exposure is not expected.

Adverse Effects

Most common adverse reactions are application site redness (3%), redness and irritation of the eyes (2%), and application site irritation (1%).

Spinosad

Generic Name	US Brand Name(s) / Canadian Brand Name(s)	Dosage Forms and Strengths	Prescription/OTC Status
spinosad	Natroba / Not available[a]	**Topical suspension:** 0.9%	Prescription

[a]Marketed as a chewable tablet for veterinary use only in Canada.

TECHNICIAN'S CORNER

1. Resistance to head lice treatments is a growing concern. Can drug resistance be limited? What are treatment options when drug resistance is encountered?
2. Why is a boxed warning put on some drugs, such as lindane?

Summary of Drugs Used for the Treatment of Lice and Scabies

Generic Name	Brand Name	Usual Dose and Dosing Schedule	Warning Labels
Over-the-Counter			
crotamiton	Eurax	Apply after bathing to the skin over the entire body from the chin to the toes. Repeat in 24 h. Bathe 48 h *after* second dose. Treatment may be repeated in 7–10 days if needed.	SHAKE WELL.
pyrethrins + piperonyl butoxide	RID, R&C various	**Lice, shampoo, cream rinse:** Apply to dry hair. Saturate hair with product. Leave on for as long as instructed on product label. Rinse hair. Use nit comb to remove eggs. **Scabies, lotion, cream:** Apply after bathing to the skin over the entire body from the chin to the toes. Leave on overnight (or 8 h). Wash off. Repeat treatment in 7–10 days if needed.	SHAKE WELL (LOTION, CREAM RINSE).—All DO NOT REWASH HAIR FOR 1–2 DAYS AFTER TREATMENT. TREAT ALL INFESTED AND PROBABLY INFESTED HOUSEHOLD MEMBERS. DO NOT OVERUSE PRODUCT. SHAKE WELL.
permethrin	Kwellada, NIX	**Lice, cream rinse:** Apply to dry hair. Apply a sufficient amount of product to saturate the hair and scalp thoroughly. Let set for 10 min; then rinse hair with water and towel-dry. Use lice comb to remove dead lice and nits. Retreat in 10 days.	
isopropyl myristate	Resultz	**Cream rinse:** Apply to dry hair. Apply a sufficient amount of product to saturate the hair and scalp thoroughly. Let set for 10 min; then rinse hair with water and towel dry. Use lice comb to remove dead lice and nits. Retreat in 10 days.	SHAKE WELL.
Prescription Only			
benzoyl alcohol	Ulesfia	Apply to dry hair. Saturate hair completely with product. Leave on for 10 min. Rinse hair. Use nit comb to remove eggs. Repeat in 7 days.	SHAKE WELL.
crotamiton	Eurax	See product description under OTC. Prescription only in the United States.	
ivermectin	Sklice	Apply to dry hair. Saturate hair completely with product. Leave on for 10 min. Rinse hair. Use nit comb to remove eggs.	SHAKE WELL. WASH HANDS AFTER APPLYING.
lindane	Generics	**Shampoo:** Saturate hair with product. Leave on for 4 min; rub until a lather is formed, then rinse hair. Use nit comb to remove eggs. **Lotion, cream:** Apply 1 h after bathing to the skin over the entire body from the chin to the toes. Leave on 8–12 h. Wash off.	SHAKE WELL. DO NOT REWASH HAIR FOR 1–2 DAYS AFTER TREATMENT. TREAT ALL HOUSEHOLD MEMBERS. RETREAT IN 7–10 DAYS IF CRAWLING BUGS ARE EVIDENT. DO NOT OVERUSE PRODUCT.
malathion	Ovide	Saturate hair with product. Leave on 8–12 h; then wash hair. Use nit comb to remove eggs.	FLAMMABLE; AVOID FLAMES.
spinosad	Natroba	Apply a sufficient amount of spinosad suspension to cover dry scalp and hair, up to one bottle (120 mL). Leave on for 10 min and then rinse thoroughly. If live lice are still seen 7 days after the first treatment, apply a second treatment.	WASH HANDS AFTER APPLYING.

Key Points

- Lice and scabies infestations affect people worldwide.
- Head lice, body lice, pubic lice, and scabies are spread through direct person-to-person contact.
- Lice and scabies infestations are caused by parasites.
- A parasite is an organism that benefits by living in, with, or on another organism (host), usually to the detriment of the host.
- Head lice most commonly affects children aged 3 to 11 years and their families, but anyone can become infested.
- Head lice infestation is caused by the parasite *Pediculus humanus capitis*; it is not caused by poor hygiene (lack of cleanliness).
- Body lice infestations are caused by the parasite *Pediculus humanus corporis*.
- Body louse infestations are a serious public health concern because body lice may cause epidemics of typhus and louse-borne relapsing fever.
- Pubic lice, or "crabs," is sometimes classified as an STI because it is most commonly spread through sexual contact.
- Lice infestation in the pubic region is caused by the parasite *Phthirus pubis*.
- Scabies infestations are common and are caused by a parasitic mite called *Sarcoptes scabiei*.
- The mite flourishes and spreads via person-to-person contact in environments in which the population density is high, such as hospitals, nursing homes, child care facilities, and schools.
- Like lice, *S. scabiei* feeds on blood and dies if away from a human host for longer than 48 to 72 hours.
- Strategies to prevent lice and scabies reinfestation include the following: (1) treat all household members; (2) use a nit comb to remove eggs (lice); (3) wash clothing, linens, and bedding in hot water (130°F [54°C]); (4) dry-clean clothing that is not washable; and (5) place stuffed toys, clothing, and bedding that cannot be washed or dry-cleaned in a large plastic bag and seal the bag for 2 weeks.
- Head lice and pubic lice may be treated with nonprescription and prescription pediculicides.
- A pediculicide is a drug that kills lice.
- Drug resistance is a growing problem for OTC and prescription pediculicides, especially permethrin, because of the residue left after treatment.
- Pyrethrins are indicated for the treatment of head lice, body lice, and pubic lice, whereas permethrin is only approved for the treatment of head lice.
- Permethrin is ovicidal (kills eggs)
- Benzoyl alcohol 5% is used to treat head lice. It asphyxiates the louse but does not kill the eggs.
- Ivermectin is applied topically to treat head lice and orally to treat worm infections..
- Repeated use of lindane causes accumulation and increases the risk for neurotoxicity.
- Pharmacy technicians must apply the warning label "For External Use Only" to prescription vials containing lindane lotion and shampoo.
- Malathion is flammable; those using it should stay away from open flames, hair dryers, curling irons, and lit cigarettes, cigars, and pipes.
- Crotamiton is a scabicide that can be used during pregnancy.
- Spinosad is a pediculicide indicated for the topical treatment of head lice infestations in patients four years of age and older.

Review Questions

1. A _____ is an organism that benefits by living in, with, or on another organism (host); usually to the detriment of the host.
   a. parasite
   b. protozoan
   c. proteus
   d. bacteria
2. The life cycle of a head louse is approximately _____.
   a. 1 to 2 weeks
   b. 2 to 3 weeks
   c. 3 to 5 weeks
   d. 4 to 6 weeks
3. Select the pediculicide that is OTC in Canada but prescription only in the United States.
   a. Eurax
   b. Resultz
   c. NIX
   d. R&C shampoo
4. _____, or crabs, is sometimes classified as a sexually transmitted infection.
   a. Scabies
   b. Head lice
   c. Pubic lice
   d. Body lice
5. Select the pediculicide that is used to treat head lice that is marketed as an OTC product.
   a. Ulesfia
   b. Sklice
   c. Natroba
   d. NIX
6. _____ may be treated with nonprescription and prescription pediculicides.
   a. Scabies
   b. Head lice
   c. Pubic lice
   d. b and c
7. Pyrethrins are naturally derived from the _____ flower.
   a. passion
   b. chrysanthemum
   c. periwinkle
   d. cone
8. Lindane _____.
   a. is neurotoxic
   b. should not be used by anyone weighing less than 100 lb (50 kg)
   c. in only dispensed in 1- or 2-oz applicator bottles
   d. all of the above

9. Malathion, an organophosphate pesticide used in agriculture to control pests and as an agent to kill head lice and their eggs, is sold in the US market and in Canada.
   a. True
   b. False

10. Crotamiton is a(n) _____ can be used during pregnancy and is an alternative to lindane.
   a. scabicide
   b. pediculicide
   c. insecticide
   d. pesticide

Bibliography

Burgess I: Head lice: resistance and treatment options, *Pharm J* 297, 2016. (September 7, 2016) https://www.pharmaceutical-journal.com.

Centers for Disease Control and Prevention: 2016. Head Lice Treatment. Retrieved November 2, 2017, from https://www.cdc.gov/parasites/lice/head/treatment.html.

Centers for Disease Control and Prevention: 2015. Pubic Lice Treatment. Retrieved November 2, 2017, from https://www.cdc.gov/parasites/lice/pubic/treatment.html.

Centers for Disease Control and Prevention: 2016. Scabies Treatment. Retrieved November 2, 2017, from https://www.cdc.gov/parasites/scabies/treatment.html.

Centers for Disease Control and Prevention (CDC): Unintentional topical lindane ingestions—United States, 1998–2003, *MMWR Morb Mortal Wkly Rep* 54:533–535, 2005.

Health Canada: 2018. Drug Product Database. Retrieved September 28, 2018, from https://health-products.canada.ca/dpd-bdpp/index-eng.jsp.

US Food and Drug Administration: nd. Drugs@FDA: FDA Approved Drug Products. Retrieved September 28, 2018, from http://www.accessdata.fda.gov/scripts/cder/daf/.

Glossary

Absorption Process involving movement of drug molecules from the site of administration into the circulatory system.

Acetylcholinesterase Enzyme that degrades acetylcholine and reverses acetylcholine-induced depolarization.

Acne vulgaris Most common form of acne.

Acne Disorder resulting from the action of hormones and other substances on the skin's oil glands (sebaceous glands) and hair follicles.

Acupuncture Nonpharmacological treatment for pain that involves the application of needles to precise points on the body.

Acute pain Sudden pain that results from injury or inflammation; usually self-limiting.

Additive effect Increased drug effect produced when a second similar drug is added to therapy that is greater than the effects produced by either drug alone.

Adenosine triphosphate Nucleotide that supplies the energy required for muscle contraction.

Adjunct Drug used to complement the effects of another drug.

Affinity Attraction that the receptor site has for the drug.

Agonist Drug that binds to its receptor site and stimulates a cellular response.

AIDS (acquired immunodeficiency syndrome) Most severe form of human immonodeficiency virus (HIV) infection. HIV-infected patients are diagnosed with AIDS when their CD4 cell count falls below 200 cells/mm^3 or develop an AIDS-defining illness (an illness that is very unusual in someone who is not HIV-positive).

Aldosterone Hormone that promotes sodium and fluid reabsorption.

Allergen Substance that produces an allergic reaction.

Allergic asthma Asthma symptoms induced by a hypersensitivity reaction caused by overexpression of immunoglobulin E antibodies on exposure to environmental allergens.

Allergic conjunctivitis Inflammation of the tissue lining the eyelids caused by the reaction to an allergy-causing substance.

Allergic rhinitis Seasonal condition characterized by inflammation and swelling of the nasal passageways (rhinitis) accompanied by a runny nose (rhinorrhea).

Allergy Hypersensitivity reaction by the immune system on exposure to an allergen.

Alzheimer's disease Neurodegenerative disease that causes memory loss and behavioral changes.

Amenorrhea Absence of normal menstruation.

Amyotrophic lateral sclerosis Degenerative disease that causes muscle wasting and muscle weakness; also known as Lou Gehrig's disease.

Analgesic Drug that reduces pain.

Anaphylactic shock Acute, life-threatening allergic reaction that produces peripheral vasodilation.

Anaphylaxis Life-threatening allergic reaction.

Aneurysm Weakened spot of the artery wall that has stretched or burst, filling the area with blood.

Angina pectoris Symptomatic manifestation of ischemic heart disease characterized by a severe squeezing or pressure-like chest pain; brought on by exertion or stress.

Angioedema Allergic skin disease characterized by patches of circumscribed swelling involving the skin and its subcutaneous layers, the mucous membranes, and sometimes the viscera.

Angiotensin-converting enzyme Enzyme that catalyzes the conversion of angiotensin I to angiotensin II.

Angiotension II Potent vasoconstrictor that is produced when the renin-aldosterone-angiotensin system is activated.

Angle-closure glaucoma Sudden increase in intraocular pressure caused by obstruction of the drainage portal between the cornea and iris (angle); can rapidly progress to blindness.

Anion Negatively charged particle.

Anoxia Absence of oxygen supply to cells that results in cell damage or death.

Antagonism Drug-drug interaction or drug-food interaction that causes decreased effects (e.g., when a pharmacological antagonist is administered to block the effect of another drug).

Antagonist Drug that binds to the receptor site and does not produce an action. An antagonist prevents another drug or natural body chemical from binding and activating the receptor site.

Antibiotic Naturally occurring substance produced by a microorganism or semisynthetic substance derived from a microorganism capable of destroying or inhibiting the growth of another microorganism.

Anticoagulant Drug that prolongs coagulation time and is used to prevent clot formation.

Antidiarrheal Drug that prevents or relieves diarrhea.

Antifungal Drug used to treat a fungal infection.

Antigen Substance, usually a protein fragment, that causes an immune response.

Antimicrobial Substance capable of destroying or inhibiting the growth of a microorganism.

Antinuclear antibody Autoantibody or abnormal antibody that attacks the nucleus of normal cells.

Antiplatelet drug Drug that prevents accumulation of platelets, thereby blocking an important step in the clot formation process.

Antiretroviral Medication that interferes with the replication of retroviruses (e.g., HIV is a retrovirus).

Antithrombotic Drug that inhibits clot formation by reducing the coagulation action of the blood protein thrombin.

Antiviral resistance Ability of a virus to overcome the suppressive action of antiviral agents.

Antiviral Medication that is able to inhibit viral replication.

Anxiety Condition associated with tension, apprehension, fear, or panic.

Anxiolytic Drug used to treat anxiety.

ApoE4 allele Defective form of apolipoprotein E associated with Alzheimer's disease.

Aqueous humor Portion of anterior cavity that lies in front of the lens and is filled with a clear watery liquid.

Arterial plaque Hardened lipid streak within an artery formed by deposits of cholesterol, lipid material, and lipophages.

Arteriosclerosis Loss of elasticity (hardening) of the arteries. Thickening and loss of elasticity of arterial walls; sometimes called hardening of the arteries.

Arthritis Condition that is associated with joint pain.

Asthma Chronic disease that affects the airways and causes irritation, inflammation, and difficulty breathing.

Atheromas Hard plaque formed within an artery.

Atherosclerosis Process in which plaques (atheromas) containing cholesterol, lipid material, and lipophages are formed within arteries, impeding the flow of blood and oxygen.

Atherothrombosis Formation of a blood clot in an artery.

Atopic dermatitis Chronic inflammatory disease of the skin.

Atrial fibrillation Rapid and uncoordinated contractions during which the heart may beat from 300 to 400 beats/min.

Atrial flutter Irregular heart beat in which contractions in the atrium exceed the number of contractions in the ventricle. The heart rate is from 160 to 350 beats/min.

Atrophic vaginitis Postmenopausal thinning and dryness of the vaginal epithelium related to decreased estrogen levels.

Aura Unusual sensation and/or auditory, visual, or olfactory hallucination experienced just before the onset of a seizure.

Autoantibody Abnormal antibody that attacks healthy cells and tissue.

Autoimmune disease Disease that occurs when the immune system turns against the parts of the body it is designed to protect.

Automaticity Spontaneous depolarization (contraction) of heart cells.

Autonomic nervous system (ANS) Division of nervous system that controls involuntary body functions; consists of sympathetic and parasympathetic divisions.

Bactericidal Able to destroy bacteria.

Bacteriostatic Able to inhibit bacterial proliferation; host defense mechanisms destroy the bacteria.

Benign prostatic hyperplasia Noncancerous growth of cells in the prostate gland.

Benign Tumor that is not cancerous and does not spread to surrounding tissues or other parts of the body.

Bicarbonate Substance used as a buffer to maintain the normal levels of acidity (pH) in blood and other fluids in the body.

Bioavailability Fraction of administered drug dose that enters the systemic circulation and is available to produce a drug effect.

Bioequivalent drug Drug that shows no statistical differences in the rate and extent of absorption when it is administered in the same strength, dosage form, and route of administration as the brand name product.

Biofeedback Nonpharmacological treatment for pain that involves relaxation techniques and gaining self-control over muscle tension, heart rate, and skin temperature.

Biopharmaceutical Pharmaceutical derived from biological sources (e.g., proteins, gene sequences) and manufactured using biotechnology methods such as recombinant DNA technology.

Biotransformation Process of drug metabolism in the body that transforms a drug to a more active, equally active, or inactive metabolite.

Bipolar disorder Mental illness associated with sudden swings in mood between depression and periods of mania, racing thoughts, distractibility, and increased goal-directed behavior.

Blackhead (open comedone) Trapped sebum and bacteria partially open to the surface that turn black due to changes in sebum as it is exposed to air.

Blepharitis Chronic disease of the eye that produces distinctive flaky scales that form on the eyelids and eyelashes.

Blister Collection of fluid below or within the epidermis.

Bone mineral density test Test carried out to measure the degree of bone loss.

Bone resorption Process during which bone is broken down into mineral ions (e.g., calcium).

Botulinum toxin Toxin produced by the bacterium *Clostridium botulinum* that causes muscle paralysis.

Bradykinesia Slowness in initiating and carrying out voluntary movements.

Breakthrough pain Pain that occurs in between scheduled doses of analgesics.

Broad-spectrum antibiotic Antimicrobial capable of destroying a wide range of bacteria.

Bronchodilator Drug that relaxes tightened airway muscles and improves air flow through the airways.

Cancer Term for diseases in which abnormal cells divide without control. Specific cancers are named according to the site where the cancerous growth begins.

Candida Type of fungus; also called yeast.

Cardiac output Volume of blood ejected from the left ventricle in 1 minute.

Cardioglycosides Class of drugs, generally derived from the foxglove plant, that can alter cardiovascular function. Digitalis is representative of this class of drugs.

Cardiomyopathy Heart disease that causes abnormal enlargement of the heart.

Catatonia Symptom of schizophrenia associated with unresponsiveness and immobility.

CD4 T lymphocyte White blood cell that fights infection.

Central nervous system (CNS) Consists of the brain and spinal cord.

Central-acting muscle relaxant Drug that produces relaxation of muscles through central nervous system depression blocking nerve transmission between the spinal cord and muscles.

Cephalgia Head pain.

Cerebral palsy Neurologic disorder that affects muscle movement and coordination.

Cerumen Waxlike substance secreted by modified sweat glands in the ear.

Chemotherapy Treatment with drugs that kill cancer.

Cholesterol Naturally occurring waxy substance produced by the liver and found in foods that maintain cell membranes; needed for vitamin D production. Excess cholesterol can cause atherosclerosis.

Chronic obstructive pulmonary disease Progressive disease of the airways that produces gradual loss of pulmonary function.

Chronic pain Pain that persists for a long period that is worsened by psychological factors and is resistant to many medical treatments.

Circadian rhythms Biological changes that occur according to time cycles.

Clonus Involuntary rhythmic muscle contraction that causes the feet and wrists to flex and relax involuntarily.

Cluster headache Intensely painful vascular headache that occurs in groups and produces pain on one side of the head.

Cognitive function Ability to take in information via the senses, process the details, commit the information to memory, and recall it when necessary.

Cold chain Set of safe handling practices that ensure that vaccines and immunologicals requiring refrigeration are maintained at the required temperature from the time of manufacture until the time of administration to patients.

Colloids Proteins or other large molecules that remain suspended in the blood for a long period and are too large to cross membranes.

Colonoscopy Examination of the colon for signs of inflammation and damage; performed by inserting a thin tube with a small light and camera at the end (i.e., endoscope) into the anus.

Comedone Enlarged and plugged hair follicle; the most characteristic sign of acne.

Complementary and alternative medicine (CAM) Treatments that may include dietary supplements, herbal preparations, acupuncture, massage, magnet therapy, spiritual healing, and meditation.

Complex focal seizure Seizure disorder that produces a blank stare, disorientation, repetitive actions, and memory loss.

Computed tomography (CT) Diagnostic examination in which a series of detailed pictures are taken of areas inside the body; created by a computer linked to an x-ray machine.

Condom Thin, flexible, penile sheath made of synthetic or natural material that is placed over the penis; used to prevent pregnancy and some sexually transmitted infections.

Conduction impairment Blocking of air waves as they are conducted through the external and middle ears to the sensory receptors of the inner ear.

Conjugate vaccine Vaccine that links antigens or toxoids to polysaccharide or sugar molecules; used by certain bacteria as a protective device to disguise themselves.

Conjunctivitis (pink eye) Common, self-limiting ailment that causes itching, burning, and teary outflow.

Constipation Abnormally delayed or infrequent passage of dry hardened feces.

Controlled substance Drug whose possession and distribution is restricted because of its potential for abuse as determined by federal or state law. Controlled substances are placed in schedules according to their abuse potential and effects if abused.

Convulsions Sudden contraction of muscles caused by seizures.

Cornea Clear part of the eye located in front of the iris.

Coronary artery disease Condition that occurs when the arteries that supply blood to the heart muscle become hardened and narrowed.

Crohn's disease Irritable bowel disease that produces inflammation and damage anywhere along the gastrointestinal tract.

Cross-resistance Development of resistance to one drug in a particular class that results in resistance to other drugs in that class.

Crystalloid Intravenous solution that contains electrolytes in concentrations similar to those of plasma.

Cutaneous Pertaining to the skin.

Cyclooxygenase-2 inhibitor Analgesic antiinflammatory drug that preferentially blocks cyclooxygenase-2, an enzyme that produces prostaglandin, which is a substance involved in mediating pain.

Cysts End products of pustules or nodules.

Cytomegalovirus retinitis Viral opportunistic infection of the eye that can cause pain and blindness.

Débridement Surgical removal of foreign material and dead tissue from a wound to prevent infection and promote healing.

Decubitus ulcer Pressure sore, or bed sore.

Dehiscent wound A wound that has reopened after it has been closed surgically.

Delusion Irrational thoughts or false beliefs that dominate a person's behavior and viewpoint and do not change, even when evidence is provided that these beliefs are not valid.

Dementia Condition associated with loss of memory and cognition.

Deoxyribonucleic acid (DNA) DNA is the repository of hereditary characteristics; it is a nucleic acid that contains the genetic blueprint.

Depolarization Process during which the heart muscle conducts an electrical impulse, causing a contraction.

Depolarizing neuromuscular blocker Drug that acts as an agonist at acetylcholine receptor sites and produces sustained depolarization, causing the receptors to convert to an inactive state.

Dermatitis Inflammation of the skin.

Desquamation Shedding of the outer layers of the skin.

Diabetes mellitus Chronic condition in which the body is unable to use glucose (sugar) as energy effectively.

Diabetic neuropathy Nerve disorder caused by uncontrolled diabetes. It leads to pain or a loss of feeling in the toes, feet, legs, hands, and/or arms.

Diaphragm Rubber or plastic cup that fits over the cervix; used for contraception.

Diarrhea Abnormally frequent passage of loose and watery stools.

Diastolic blood pressure Blood pressure measured when the heart is at rest (diastole).

Diffusion Passive movement of molecules across cell membranes from an area of high drug concentration to an area of lower concentration.

Digestion Complete process of altering the physical and chemical composition of ingested food materials so they can be absorbed and used by the body's cells.

Digital rectal examination Screening examination involving palpation of the prostate gland; conducted by insertion of a gloved lubricated finger into the rectum.

Disinhibition Opposite of inhibited.

Distribution Process of movement of the drug from the circulatory system across barrier membrane(s) to the site of drug action.

Diuretic Drug that produces diuresis (urination).

Dosage form Drug formulation (e.g., capsule, tablet, solution).

Dose Amount of a drug required for one application or administration.

Dosing schedule How frequently a drug dose is administered (e.g., "four times a day").

Double-contrast barium enema Diagnostic test to examine the colon and rectum in which an individual is administered a barium-containing enema and then radiographs are taken.

Drug delivery system Dosage form or device designed to release a specific amount of drug.

Drug dependence Occurs when a person taking a drug does not continue to take it and suffers from physical or psychological withdrawal symptoms, or both.

Drug resistance testing Laboratory test to determine whether an individual's HIV strain is resistant to any anti-HIV medications.

Drug Substance used to diagnose, treat, cure, prevent, or mitigate disease in humans or other animals.

Drug-disease contraindication No rationale for drug use; drug administration should be avoided because it may worsen the patient's medical condition.

Drug-drug interaction Reaction that occurs when two or more drugs are administered at the same time.

Drug-food interaction Altered drug response that occurs when a drug is administered with certain foods.

Dry eye disease Occurs when the eye does not produce tears properly, or when the tears are not of the correct consistency and evaporate too quickly.

Duodenal ulcer Ulcer located in the upper portion of the small intestine or duodenum.

Duration of action Time between the onset of drug action and discontinuation of drug action.

Dysfunctional uterine bleeding Irregular or excessive uterine bleeding that results from a structural problem or hormonal imbalance.

Dysmenorrhea Difficult or painful menstruation.

Dysphoria Feeling of emotional or mental discomfort, restlessness, and depression; the opposite of euphoria.

Eclampsia Life-threatening condition that can develop in pregnant women that causes high blood pressure and seizures.

Ectopic Occurring in an abnormal location.

Eczema General term used to describe several types of inflammation of the skin.

Efficacy Measure of a drug's effectiveness.

Ejaculation Release of semen from the penis during orgasm.

Ejection fraction Percentage of blood ejected from the left ventricle with each heartbeat.

Electrical cardioversion Process of applying an electrical shock to the heart with a defibrillator to convert the heart to a normal rhythm.

Electrolytes Small charged molecules essential for homeostasis that play an important role in body chemistry.

Elimination Process that results in the removal of drug from the body.

Embolic stroke Stroke caused by an emboli obstructing the flow of blood through an artery.

Embolus Moving blood clot.

Endometriosis Presence of functioning endometrial tissue outside the uterus.

Endorphins, enkephalins, and dynorphin Substances released by the body in response to painful stimuli that act as natural painkillers.

Endoscope Thin flexible tube with a small video camera and light attached to one end.

Endoscopy Test used to look for ulcers inside the stomach and small intestine using an endoscope.

Endotracheal intubation Process of inserting a tube into the trachea or windpipe to facilitate mechanical ventilation.

Endplate Projection extending off the end of a motor neuron where the neurotransmitter acetylcholine is released.

Enteral Refers to a drug dosage form that is administered orally.

Enuresis Bedwetting or uncontrollable urination during sleep.

Enzyme Protein capable of causing a chemical reaction. Enzymes are involved in the metabolism of some drugs.

Epilepsy Recurrent seizure disorder characterized by a sudden, excessive, disorderly discharge of cerebral neurons.

Equilibrium Steadiness or balance accompanied by a sense of knowing where the body is in relationship to surroundings.

Erectile dysfunction Persistent inability to achieve and/or maintain an erection sufficient for satisfactory sexual intercourse.

Erythrocytes Red blood cells.

Erythropoiesis Formation of red blood cells.

Eschar Blackened necrotic tissue of a decubitus ulcer.

Escharotomy Removal of necrotic skin and underlying tissue.

Euphoria State of intense happiness or well-being; the opposite of dysphoria.

Exacerbation Aggravation of symptoms or increase in the severity of the disease.

Extrapyramidal symptoms Excessive muscle movement (motor activity) associated with the use of neuroleptics; includes muscular rigidity, tremor, bradykinesia (slow movement), and difficulty in walking.

Fasting blood glucose Blood glucose level after a person has not eaten for 8 to 12 hours (usually overnight).

Febrile seizure Seizure associated with a sudden spike in body temperature.

Fecal occult blood test (FOBT) Test to check for blood in stool.

Fertility Being fertile; able to reproduce.

First-degree burn Minor discomfort and reddening of the skin.

First-pass effect Process whereby only a fraction of an orally administered drug reaches the systemic circulation because much of the drug is metabolized in the liver to an inactive metabolite before entering the general circulation.

Fistula Ulcer that tunnels from the site of origin to surrounding tissues.

Fontanels Soft spots found in a baby's skull.

Forced expiratory volume (FEV) The maximum volume of air that can be breathed out in 1 second; also called forced vital capacity.

Fourth-degree burn Burn that involves underlying muscles, fasciae, or bone.

Full-thickness burn Third-degree burn in which the epidermis and dermis are destroyed.

Fungus (pl., fungi) Organism similar to a plant but lacking chlorophyll; capable of producing mycotic (fungal) infection.

Fusarium keratitis Rare fungal infection that occurs in soft contact lens wearers; can result in blindness.

Gastric ulcer Ulcer located in the stomach.

Gastroenteritis Inflammation of the lining membrane of the stomach and intestines.

Gastroesophageal reflux disease (GERD) Motility disorder associated with impaired peristalsis that results in the backflow of gastric contents into the esophagus.

Generalized anxiety disorder Condition associated with excessive worrying and tension that is experienced daily for more than 6 months.

Generalized seizures Seizures that spread across both cerebral hemispheres; include tonic-clonic seizures.

Gestational diabetes Diabetes that may be caused by the hormones of pregnancy or a shortage of insulin.

Gingival hyperplasia Excess growth of gum tissue that could grow over the teeth.

Glial cells Cells that form the blood-brain barrier and support function of the neurons.

Gout Disease associated with deposits of urate crystals in the joints that produces inflammation; caused by hyperuricemia.

Graves' disease Autoimmune disorder that causes hyperthyroidism.

Gynecomastia Painful breast enlargement in men.

Half-life ($t_{1/2}$) Length of time it takes for the plasma concentration of an administered drug to be reduced by 50%.

Hallucination Visions or voices that exist only in a person's mind and cannot be seen or heard by others.

Hashimoto's disease Autoimmune disorder that causes hypothyroidism.

Heart failure Clinical syndrome in which the heart is unable to pump blood at a rate necessary to meet the body's metabolic needs.

Helminthes Group of parasitic worms that can cause eye infection and blindness.

Hemoglobin A1c test Blood test that measures a person's average blood glucose level over a period of 2 to 3 months.

Hemoglobin Red pigment made up of iron atoms; transports oxygen and carbon dioxide in the body.

Hemorrhagic stroke Sudden bleeding into or around the brain.

Hemostasis Process of stopping the flow of blood.

Hepatoxicity Serious adverse reaction that occurs in the liver.

Herpes simplex keratitis Painful eye infection caused by a herpesvirus that can lead to blindness.

Herpes zoster ophthalmicus Painful eye infection caused by a herpesvirus that can lead to blindness.

Hiatal hernia Condition in which the lower esophageal sphincter shifts above the diaphragm.

High-density lipoprotein Lipoprotein that transports cholesterol, triglycerides, and other lipids from blood to body tissues; known as good cholesterol.

Highly active antiretroviral therapy (HAART) Combination of three or more antiretroviral medications taken in a regimen.

Hirsutism Excessive hair growth in women.

Histamine Organic nitrogen compound involved in local immune responses; has a regulating physiological function in the gut and acts as a neurotransmitter.

Homeopathic medicine Medical field in which drugs are administered in minute quantities to stimulate natural body healing systems.

Host Individual infected with a virus.

Huntington's disease Progressive and degenerative disease of neurons that affects muscle movement, cognitive functions, and emotions.

Hydrophilic Having a strong affinity for water; water-loving; able to dissolve in and absorb water.

Hydrophobic Lacking an affinity for water; water-hating; resistant to wetting.

Hyperalgesia Heightened sensitivity to pain that can result from treatment of chronic pain with high-dose opioids.

Hyperglycemia Condition of elevated blood glucose levels.

Hyperkalemia Condition in which the serum potassium level is higher than 5.5 mEq/L.

Hyperlipidemia Increased concentration of cholesterol and triglycerides in the blood associated with the development of atherosclerosis.

Hyperopia Farsightedness.

Hyperplasia Abnormal increase in the number of cells in an organ or tissue.

Hypertension High blood pressure; elevated diastolic or systolic blood pressure, or both.

Hyperthyroidism Condition in which there is an excessive production of thyroid hormones.

Hyperuricemia Condition in which urate levels build up in the blood.

Hypnotic Drug that induces sleep.

Hypoglycemia Low blood glucose levels.

Hypogonadism Inadequate production of sex hormones.

Hypothyroidism Condition in which there is insufficient production of thyroid hormones.

Hysterectomy Surgical removal of the uterus.

Idiosyncratic reaction Unexpected drug reaction.

Immunization Deliberate artificial exposure to disease to produce acquired immunity.

Immunoglobulin E Antibody associated with allergies.

Immunomodulator Chemical agent that modifies the immune response or functioning of the immune system.

Immunosuppressant Drug that inhibits proliferation of the cells of the immune system; also known as an immunopharmacological.

Implant radiation Procedure, also known as brachytherapy, in which radioactive material sealed in needles, seeds, wires, or catheters is placed directly into or near a tumor in the body.

Inactivated killed vaccine Killed vaccine; provides less immunity than live vaccines but has fewer risks for vaccine-induced disease.

Incontinence Loss of bladder or bowel control.

Infarction Sudden loss of blood supply to an area that results in cell death. A myocardial infarction (MI) is known as a heart attack. A cerebral infarction is also known as a stroke.

Infertility Inability to achieve pregnancy during 1 year or more of unprotected intercourse.

Inflammation Response to tissue irritation or injury marked by signs of redness, swelling, heat, and pain.

Inflammatory bowel disease (IBD) Chronic disorder of the gastrointestinal tract characterized by inflammation of the intestines; results in abdominal cramping and persistent diarrhea.

Insomnia Condition characterized by difficulty falling asleep, staying asleep, or both.

Insulin resistance Condition in which the body does not respond to insulin; contributes to the development of type 2 diabetes.

Interferon Antiviral protein that enhances T cell recognition of antigens (interferon-γ) and produce immune system suppression (interferon-α, interferon-β).

Intraocular pressure Inner pressure of the eye. Normal intraocular pressure ranges from 12 to 22 mm Hg.

Intrauterine device (IUD) Device inserted in the uterus to prevent pregnancy.

Inverse agonist Drug that has affinity and activity at the receptor site. The drug can turn off a receptor that is activated or turn on a receptor that is not currently active.

Ionization Chemical process involving the gain or release of a proton (H⁺). Ionized drug molecules may have a positive or negative charge.

Ionizing radiation Type of high-frequency radiation produced by x-ray procedures, radioactive substances, and ultraviolet (UV) light that can lead to health risks, including cancer, at certain doses.

Iris Colored part of the eye that can expand or contract to allow the correct amount of light to enter the eye.

Iritis Condition associated with inflammation of the iris.

Irritable bowel syndrome Condition that causes abdominal distress and erratic movement of the contents of the large bowel resulting in diarrhea and/or constipation.

Ischemia Reduction of blood supplied to tissues; typically caused by blood vessel obstruction due to atherosclerosis, stenosis, or plaque.

Ischemic heart disease Any condition in which heart muscle is damaged or works inefficiently because of an absence or relative deficiency of its blood supply.

Ischemic stroke Ischemia in the brain.

Isolated systolic hypertension Condition involving only elevated systolic blood pressure. Diastolic blood pressure is within the normal range.

Kallman's syndrome Congenital disorder that causes hypogonadism and loss of the sense of smell.

Keratitis Severe infection of the cornea that may be caused by bacteria or fungi.

Keratolytic Pertains to keratolysis, the softening and shedding of the horny outer layer of the skin. A keratolytic agent is a peeling agent.

Klinefelter's syndrome A chromosomal disorder in males. People with this condition are born with at least one extra X chromosome.

Labyrinth Bony structure in the inner ear consisting of three parts (vestibule, cochlea, and semicircular canals) involved in balance.

β-Lactamase Enzyme secreted by some microbes that has the ability to destroy β-lactam antibiotics.

Laryngopharyngeal reflux Reflux of gastric contents into the larynx and pharynx.

Laxative Medicine that induces evacuation of the bowel.

Legend drugs Drugs required by state or federal law to be dispensed by a prescription only. Prescriptions must be written for a legitimate medical condition and issued by a practitioner authorized to prescribe.

Leukemia Cancer that starts in blood-forming tissue such as the bone marrow.

Leukocytes White blood cells (WBCs).

Leukocytosis Abnormally high WBC count.

Leukopenia Abnormally low WBC count.

Leukotriene Proinflammatory mediator released as part of the allergic inflammatory response. Leukotrienes also trigger contractions in the smooth muscles of airways.

Lice Group of parasites (*Pediculus humanus capitis, Pediculus humanus corporis, Phthirus pubis*) that can live on the body, scalp, or genital area of humans.

Lipid Fatlike substance.

Lipophilic Having an affinity for lipids; lipid-loving.

Lipoprotein Small globules of cholesterol covered by a layer of protein.

Live attenuated vaccine Living, but weakened, version of an invader that does not cause disease in nonimmunocompromised individuals (nonvirulent).

Low-density lipoprotein Compound consisting of a lipid and protein that carries most of the total cholesterol in the blood and deposits the excess along the inside of arterial walls; also known as bad cholesterol.

Lower esophageal sphincter Sphincter separating the esophagus and stomach.

Lower motor neurons Neurons that branch out from the spinal cord to the muscles and tissues of the body.

Lymphoma Cancer that begins in cells of the immune system.

Major depression Mental illness associated with persistent feelings of sadness, emptiness, or hopelessness that lasts for several weeks.

Malignant Cancerous tumors that can invade and destroy nearby tissue and spread to other parts of the body.

Mammography Screening examination to detect breast cancer in which a radiograph is taken of the breast.

Mast cells Granule-containing cells found in connective tissue. They contain many granules rich in histamine, which are released during allergic reactions.

Mastication Chewing.

Materia medica Medicinal materials.

Mechanism of action Manner in which a drug produces its effect.

Medication error Error made in the process of prescribing, preparing, dispensing, or administering drug therapy.

Melanoma Form of skin cancer that arises in melanocytes, the cells that produce pigment.

Melatonin Hormone released by the pineal gland that makes a person feel drowsy.

Ménière's disease Chronic inner ear disease associated with intermittent buildup of fluid in the inner ear that causes hearing loss and vertigo.

Menopause Termination of menstrual cycles; an event usually marked by the passage of at least 1 year without menstruation.

Menorrhagia Excessive menstrual bleeding.

Metabolic syndrome Important risk factor of hypertension that promotes the development of atherosclerosis and cardiovascular disease.

Metabolism Biochemical process involving transformation of active drugs to a compound that can be easily eliminated, or the conversion of prodrugs to active drugs.

Metabolite Product of drug metabolism. Metabolites may be inactivated drugs or active drugs with equal or greater activity than the parent drug.

Metastasis Spread of cancer from one part of the body to another.

Metered-dose inhaler Device used for delivering a dose of inhaled medication. A solution or powder is delivered as a mist and inhaled.

Microbial resistance Ability of bacteria to overcome the bactericidal or bacteriostatic effects of an anti-infective. Resistance traits are encoded on bacterial genes and can be transferred to other bacteria.

Microvilli Brushlike border of each villus in the small intestine; increases the surface area for absorption.

Migraine Vascular headache that is often accompanied by nausea and visual disturbances.

Milia Tiny little bumps that occur when normally sloughed skin cells get trapped in small pockets on the surface of the skin.

Mitral valve stenosis Disease of the mitral valve involving the buildup of plaquelike material around the valve.

Monoamine oxidase Enzyme found in the liver, intestine, and terminal neurons; responsible for degradation of monoamine neurotransmitters and dietary amines.

Mother to child transmission Transmission of a substance or virus (e.g., HIV from an HIV-infected mother) to her baby during pregnancy or delivery, or through breast milk (also called perinatal transmission).

Motor neuron Neuron that connects to the sarcolemma to form a neuromuscular junction.

Multiple sclerosis Autoimmune disease that causes progressive damage to nerves resulting in spasticity, pain, mood changes, and other physical symptoms.

Myasthenia gravis Autoimmune disease in which the immune system attacks the muscle cells at the neuromuscular junction and is characterized by muscle weakness.

Mycosis General term for a fungal infection.

Myelin Fatty covering that insulates nerve cells in the brain and spinal cord.

Myocardial infarction Condition that results in heart muscle tissue death; caused by the occlusion (blockage) of a coronary artery; also referred to as a heart attack.

Myoclonic seizure Seizure characterized by jerking muscle movements; caused by contraction of major muscle groups.

Myopia Nearsightedness.

Myositis Autoimmune disease that causes chronic inflammation of the muscles.

Natriuretic peptides Hormones that play a role in cardiac homeostasis.

Nebulizer Device that creates a mist out of a liquid inhalant solution, making drug delivery easier.

Necrosis Cell death that may be caused by lack of blood and oxygen to the affected area(s).

Negative symptoms Spasticity symptoms, which may indicate schizophrenia, that can produce muscle weakness, decreased endurance, and reduction in the ability to make voluntary muscle movements.

Neoplasm Tumor.

Nephrotoxicity Serious adverse effect that occurs in the kidneys.

Neurodegeneration Destruction of nerve cells.

Neurodegenerative disease Disorder that results in progressive destruction of neurons.

Neuroleptic malignant syndrome Potentially fatal reaction to administration of neuroleptics. Symptoms include stupor, muscle rigidity, and high temperature.

Neuroleptic Drug used to treat schizophrenia and psychoses.

Neuromuscular junction Space between motor neuron endplate and muscle sole plate that neurotransmitters must cross.

Neuron Functional unit of the nervous system, which includes the cell body, dendrites, axon, and terminals.

Neuropathic pain Type of pain associated with nerve injury caused by trauma, infection, or chronic diseases such as diabetes.

Neuroprotective Protects nerve cells from damage.

Neurotransmitter Protein that transmits nerve signals from one neuron to another.

Nigrostriatal pathway Pathway located in the substantia nigra that stimulates and inhibits movement.

Nits Head lice eggs.

Nociceptors Thin nerve fibers in the skin, muscle, and other body tissues that carry pain signals.

Nocturia Nighttime urination.

Nodule Ruptured pustules that form abscesses.

Noncompetitive antagonist Drug that binds to an alternative receptor site that prevents the agonist from binding to and producing its desired action.

Nondepolarizing competitive blockers Drugs that compete with acetylcholine for binding sites.

Non–rapid eye movement (REM) sleep Stages 1 through 4 of the sleep cycle.

NSAID Nonsteroidal anti-inflammatory drug.

Nymph Baby louse.

Obsessive-compulsive disorder Condition associated with the inability to control or stop repeated unwanted thoughts or behaviors.

Oncovirus Virus that is a causative agent in a cancer.

Onset of action Time it takes for drug action to begin.

Onychomycosis Fungal infection involving the fingernails or toenails; also known as tinea unguium.

Open-angle glaucoma Disorder characterized by elevated pressure in the eye that can lead to permanent blindness.

Opiate-naïve Refers to a person who has no current exposure to opioids.

Opioid Naturally occurring or synthetically derived analgesic with properties similar to those of morphine.

Optic nerve Bundle of nerve fibers located in the back of the eye that connects the retina to the brain.

Orthostatic hypotension Sudden drop in blood pressure that occurs when arising from lying down or sitting to standing.

Osmosis Movement of water across a semipermeable membrane from an area of higher concentration to an area of lower concentration.

Osteoblast Cell responsible for bone formation, deposition, and mineralization of the collagen matrix of bone.

Osteoclast Cell responsible for bone resorption.

Osteolysis Dissolution or degradation of bone.

Osteopenia Decrease in bone mineral density that places people at increased risk of developing osteoporosis.

Osteoporosis Chronic progressive disease of bone characterized by loss of bone density and bone strength; results in increased risk for fractures.

Otitis Inflammation of the ear.

Otitis externa Inflammation of the ear canal or external ear.

Otitis media Infection of the middle ear; typically caused by viral or bacterial infection.

Otoliths Calcium carbonate crystals found in the utricle and saccule of the inner ear.

Otorrhea Discharge coming from the external auditory canal or inside the canal.

Otosclerosis Hardening of the bones of the middle ear.

Ototoxicity Damage or toxicity to the ear or eighth cranial nerve (associated with hearing).

Over-the-counter (OTC) drugs Drugs that can be obtained without a prescription.

Ovicidal Able to destroy eggs.

Panic disorder Condition associated with repeated sudden onset of feelings of terror.

Pap test (Pap smear) Screening test in which cells from the cervix are examined to detect cancer and changes that may lead to cancer.

Papule Obstructed follicle that becomes inflamed.

Parasite Organism that benefits by living in, with, or on another organism.

Parasympathetic nervous system Division of the autonomic nervous system (ANS) that functions during restful situations; the "rest and digest" part of the ANS.

Parenteral Refers to a drug dosage form administered by injection or infusion.

Parkinson's disease Progressive disorder of the nervous system involving degeneration of dopaminergic neurons and causing impaired muscle movement.

Partial agonist Drug that behaves like an agonist under some conditions and acts like an antagonist under different conditions.

Partial thromboplastin time Blood test that determines the effectiveness of heparin in reducing antithrombotic activity; measures how long it takes for blood to clot.

Partial-thickness burns First- and second-degree burns.

Pathophysiology Study of structural and functional changes produced by disease.

PCA Patient-controlled analgesia.

Peak effect Maximum drug effect produced by a given dose of drug after the drug has reached its maximum concentration in the body.

Peak flow meter Handheld device used to measure the volume of air exhaled and how rapidly the air is moved out.

Pediculicide Drug that kills lice.

Pelvic inflammatory disease Infection of the uterus, fallopian tubes, and adjacent pelvic structures that is not associated with pregnancy or surgery.

Peptic ulcer disease Term used to describe ulcers located in the duodenum or stomach.

Peripheral nervous system (PNS) Division of the nervous system outside the brain and spinal cord.

Peripheral vascular resistance Resistance to the flow of blood in peripheral arterial vessels that is associated with blood vessel diameter, vessel length, and blood viscosity.

Peripheral vision Sometimes called side vision, this is usually the first area of vision to be lost with glaucoma.

Peripheral-acting muscle relaxants Drugs that block nerve transmission between the motor endplate and skeletal muscle receptors.

Peristalsis Forceful wave of contractions in the esophagus that moves food and liquids from the mouth to the stomach.

Petit mal seizure Absence seizure in which the person experiences a brief period of unconsciousness and stares vacantly into space.

Pharmaceutical alternative Drug that contains the same active ingredient as the brand name drug; however, the strength and dosage form may be different.

Pharmaceutical equivalent Drug that contains identical amount of active ingredient as a brand name drug but may have different inactive ingredients, be manufactured in a different dosage form, and exhibit different rates of absorption.

Pharmacodynamics Study of drugs and their actions on a living organism.

Pharmacognosy Science dealing with the biologic and biochemical features of natural drugs and their constituents. It is the study of drugs of plant or animal origin.

Pharmacokinetics Science dealing with what the body does to a drug; includes the study of absorption, distribution, metabolism, and elimination.

Pharmacology Study of drugs and their interactions with living systems, including chemical and physical properties, toxicology, and therapeutics.

Pharmacotherapeutics Use of drugs in the treatment of disease. It is the study of factors that influence patient response to drugs.

Pharmacotherapy Use of drugs in the treatment of disease.

Phenylketonuria Disease marked by failure to metabolize the amino acid phenylalanine to tyrosine; results in severe neurological deficits in infancy if untreated.

Phobia Irrational fear of things or situations that produce symptoms of intense anxiety.

Phosphodiesterase type 5 inhibitor Drug used to relax smooth muscle and blood vessels that supply the corpus cavernosum and control penile engorgement.

Photopsia Condition similar to floaters; associated with flashes of light.

Phototherapy Treatment for atopic dermatitis that involves exposing the skin to ultraviolet A or B light waves.

Pilosebaceous units (PSUs) These consist of a sebaceous gland connected to a canal, called a follicle; contain fine hairs.

Plaque psoriasis Most common form of psoriasis characterized by raised inflamed (red) lesions covered with a silvery white scale.

Plaque Fatty cholesterol deposits; patchy areas of inflammation and demyelination that disrupt nerve signals between the brain and the rest of the body.

Plasticity Ability of the brain to restructure itself and adapt to injury.

Platelets Structures found in the blood involved in the coagulation process.

Polycystic ovary disease Condition characterized by ovaries twice the normal size that contain fluid-filled cysts.

Polymyositis Form of myositis that affects multiple muscles, particularly the muscles closest to the trunk.

Polyp Growth that protrudes from a mucous membrane.

Positive inotropic effect Increase in the force of myocardial contractions.

Positive symptoms Hallucinations, delusions, or other unusual thoughts or perceptions that are symptoms of schizophrenia; also, spasticity symptoms that cause muscle spasms and hyperexcitable reflexes.

Positron emission tomography (PET) Diagnostic examination used to detect cancer cells in the body in which a small amount of radioactive glucose (sugar) is injected into a vein and a scanner is used to make detailed, computerized pictures of areas inside the body where the glucose is used.

Postprandial After eating.

Post-traumatic stress disorder Stress disorder that develops in persons who have participated in, witnessed, or been a victim of a terrifying event.

Postural hypotension Drop in blood pressure caused by a change in posture.

Potency Measure of the amount of drug required to produce a response. It is the effective dose concentration.

Potentiation Process whereby one drug, acting at a separate site or via a different mechanism of action, increases the effect of another drug but produces no effect when administered alone. Food can also potentiate the effects of a drug.

Prediabetes Condition of impaired fasting glucose and impaired glucose tolerance in which the body consistently has elevated glucose levels.

Pregnancy Condition of having a developing embryo or fetus in the body after successful conception.

Prehypertension Systolic blood pressure ranging between 120 and 139 mm Hg and diastolic blood pressure ranging between 80 and 89 mm Hg.

Premenstrual dysphoric disorder Disorder characterized by symptoms such as depression, anxiety, hopelessness, sad feelings, and self-depreciation.

Premenstrual syndrome Condition involving a group of symptoms (e.g., headache, irritability, depression, fatigue, sleep changes, weight gain) that occur before the start of the menstrual cycle.

Pressure injury Pressure sore or "bedsore."

Primary tumor Original tumor or initial tumor.

Prodrug Drug administered in an inactive form that is metabolized in the body to an active form.

Prolactinoma Pituitary tumor that produces an excessive amount of prolactin.

Prostate gland Gland in the male reproductive system just below the bladder, surrounding the urethra.

Prostate-specific antigen (PSA) Protein produced by the prostate gland. Levels are elevated in men who have prostate cancer, infection, or inflammation and tumors of the prostate gland and benign prostate hyperplasia.

Prostate-specific antigen (PSA) test Blood test to measure PSA. A free PSA test result reports the percentage of PSA that is not attached to another chemical compared with the total amount in a man's blood. Free PSA is linked to benign prostate hyperplasia but not to cancer.

Prostatitis Inflammation of the prostate gland.

Prothrombin time Test given to determine the effectiveness of warfarin in reducing clotting time.

Pseudoparkinsonism Adverse reaction to the administration of neuroleptics; characterized by symptoms mimicking those of Parkinson's disease.

Psoriasis Chronic disease of the skin characterized by itchy red patches covered with silvery scales.

Psychosis Mental state characterized by disorganized behavior and thought, delusions, hallucinations, and loss of touch with reality.

Purine One of two nitrogen-containing bases found in DNA and RNA. Purine bases are metabolized.

Pustule Larger lesions that are more inflamed than papules; can be superficial or deep.

Radiation therapy Use of high-energy radiation from x-rays, gamma rays, neutrons, and other sources to kill cancer cells and shrink tumors.

Radioactive iodine uptake Test using radioactive iodine to screen for thyroid disease.

Radionuclide scan Diagnostic test in which an individual is administered a small amount of radioactive material. A scanner is used to take pictures of the internal parts of the body to detect where the radiation concentrates.

Radon Radioactive gas that if inhaled in sufficient quantity can lead to lung cancer.

Rapid eye movement (REM) sleep Stage of sleep when dreaming occurs.

Rebound hypersomnia Condition associated with excessive sleep that follows long-term insomnia or the use of drugs that depress REM and non-REM sleep.

Receptor site Location of drug-cell binding.

Reflux Backflow of gastric contents into the esophageal or laryngopharyngeal region.

Refractory period Time between contractions that it takes for repolarization to occur.

Remission Lessening in severity or abatement of symptoms.

Remodeling Process of continual turnover of bone.

Renin–aldosterone–angiotensin system System that is activated when there is a drop in renal blood flow. Activation increases blood volume, blood flow to the kidneys, vasoconstriction, and blood pressure.

Repolarization Period of time when the heart is recharging and preparing for another contraction.

Rh factor Antigen present in the red blood cells of Rh-positive individuals.

Rhabdomyolysis Breakdown of muscle fibers and release of muscle fiber contents into the circulation.

Rheumatoid arthritis Chronic disease characterized by inflammation and remodeling of the joints.

Rheumatoid factor Immunoglobulin (antibody) present in many people who have rheumatoid arthritis.

Ribonucleic acid (RNA) Nucleic acid involved in protein synthesis that carries and transfers genetic information and assembles proteins.

Ringworm Group of tinea infections involving the body or scalp that have a characteristic ringlike shape. Ringworm is spread by person to person and animal to person contact.

Rule of nines Formula for estimating the percentage of adult body surface covered by burns; divides the body into 11 areas, each representing 9% of the total body surface area.

Rule of palms Rule for determining the extent of a burn surface area. A palm size of a burn victim is about 1% of the total body surface area.

Saccule Saclike inner ear structure that senses vertical motion of the head.

Salpingitis Inflammation of the fallopian tube, usually as a result of a sexually transmitted infection.

Sarcomere Basic contractile unit of the muscle cell.

Sarcoplasmic reticulum (SR) Networks of tubules and sacs contained in muscle cells.

Scabicide Drug that kills the scabies mite.

Scabies Parasitic infection caused by the mite *Sarcoptes scabei.*

Schizophrenia Type of psychosis characterized by delusions of thought, visual or auditory hallucinations (or both), and speech disturbances. Paranoid schizophrenia is characterized by delusions of persecution.

Second-degree burn Burn that involves deep epidermal layers and causes damage to the upper layers of the dermis.

Sedative Drug that causes relaxation and promotes drowsiness.

Seizure threshold Measure of a person's susceptibility to seizures.

Semen Fluid containing sperm and secretions from glands of the male reproductive tract.

Serotonin syndrome Potentially life-threatening adverse drug reaction that produces symptoms of confusion, agitation, diarrhea, tremors, and increased blood pressure; caused by excessive serotonin.

Shingles Recurring and painful skin rash caused by the herpes zoster virus.

Simple focal seizures Seizure that affects only one part of the brain; causes the person to experience unusual sensations or feelings.

Sinus cavity Mucous-lined, air-filled space found in the frontal bone (frontal sinuses), sphenoid, ethmoid, maxillae (paranasal sinuses), and middle and inner ear (mastoid sinuses).

Soleplate Portion of the membrane of muscle cells that receives messages transmitted by motor neurons.

Somatic nervous system Division of the nervous system that carries information to the somatic effectors or skeletal muscles.

Sonogram Computer image of internal organs and tissues produced by ultrasound.

Spacer Device attached to the end of a metered-dose inhaler that facilitates drug delivery into the lungs (rather than to the back of the throat).

Spasticity Motor disorder that causes increased muscle tone, exaggerated tendon jerks, and hyperexcitable muscles.

Spirometry Test that measures the volume of air that is expired (blown out of the lungs) after taking a deep breath and how rapidly the volume of air is expired.

Stage Refers to the extent of a cancer within the body. Staging is based on the size of the tumor, whether lymph nodes contain cancer, and whether the disease has spread from the original site to other parts of the body (metastasis).

Status epilepticus Medical emergency brought on by repeated generalized seizures that can deprive the brain of oxygen.

Stem cell Type of cell from which other types of cells develop; for example, blood cells develop from blood-forming stem cells.

Stem cell transplantation Procedure used to replace cells that were destroyed by cancer treatment.

Stimulant Drug that increases activity in the brain and is used to treat ADHD and narcolepsy.

Stroke volume Equal to the volume of blood ejected by the left ventricle during each cardiac contraction minus the volume of blood in the ventricle at the end of systole.

Stye Painful lump located on the eyelid margin caused by an acute self-limiting infection of the oil glands of the eyelid.

Substance P Peptide involved in the production of pain sensations; controls pain perception.

Substantia nigra Part of the basal ganglia containing clusters of dopamine-producing neurons.

Supraovulation Simultaneous rupture of multiple mature follicles.

Supraventricular tachycardia Heart rate up to 200 beats/min that originates in an area above the ventricles.

Sympathetic nervous system Division of the ANS that functions during stressful situations; fight-or-flight part of the ANS.

Synapse Gap between neurons where nerve information is transmitted from one neuron to another.

Synarthrosis Immovable joint (skull).

Synergistic effect Drug-drug or drug-food interaction that produces an effect greater than the effect that would be produced if either drug were administered alone.

Synovium Thin layer of tissue that lines the joint space.

Systemic lupus erythematosus (SLE) Autoimmune disease that affects almost all body systems.

Systolic blood pressure Measure of the pressure when the heart's ventricles are contracting (systole).

Tangles Twisted fibers made up of clumps of a protein called tau that interfere with nerve signal transmission.

Tardive dyskinesia Inappropriate postures of the neck, trunk, and limbs accompanied by involuntary thrusting of the tongue.

Tear deficiency Also known as dry eyes.

Tetanus Potentially fatal condition characterized by a continuous muscle spasm caused by exposure to the nerve toxin produced by the bacterium *Clostridium tetani.* It is also known as lockjaw.

Tetraiodothyronine (T$_4$) Most abundant thyroid hormone; contains four atoms of iodine; also known as thyroxine.

Tetraiodothyronine test Test to measure the level of free circulating thyroid hormone.

Therapeutic alternative Drug that contains different active ingredient(s) than the brand name drug but produces the same desired therapeutic outcome.

Therapeutic duplication Administration of two drugs that produce similar effects and side effects.

Therapeutic index (TI) Ratio of the effective dose to the lethal dose.

Third-degree burn Burn characterized by destruction of the epidermis and dermis.

Thrombocytes Platelets.

Thrombocytopenia Condition that results from a deficiency in the platelet count.

Thrombolytic Drug used to dissolve blood clots.

Thrombosis Formation of a blood clot.

Thrombotic stroke Stroke caused by thrombosis.

Thrombus Stationary blood clot.

Thyroid antibody test Diagnostic test used to measure levels of thyroid antibodies; diagnostic for autoimmune thyroid disease.

Thyroid-releasing factor Hormone released by the hypothalamus that stimulates the pituitary gland to release thyroid-stimulating hormone.

Thyroid-stimulating hormone (TSH) Hormone released by the pituitary gland that stimulates the thyroid gland to produce and release thyroid hormones.

Thyroid-stimulating hormone test Diagnostic test used to measure the level of TSH in the blood; low level signals hyperthyroidism.

Tinnitus Intermittent or continuous whistling, crackling, squeaking, or ringing noise in the ears.

Tissue plasminogen activator Naturally occurring thrombolytic substance.

Tolerance Increasing doses of a drug are required to achieve the same effects as were achieved previously at lower doses.

Tonic-clonic (grand mal) seizure Generalized seizure that causes stiffening of the limbs, difficulty breathing, and jerking movements; is followed by disorientation and limbs that become limp.

Tonometry Use of a device to measure the pressure in the eye.

Toxic megacolon Life-threatening condition characterized by a very inflated colon, abdominal distention, and sometimes fever, abdominal pain, or shock.

Toxic shock syndrome Rare disorder caused by certain *Staphylococcus aureus* strains that occurs in women using tampons.

Toxicology Science dealing with the study of poisons.

Toxoid vaccine Vaccine that stimulates the immune system to produce antibodies to a specific toxin that causes illness.

Trabecular meshwork Small openings around the outer edge of the iris that form meshlike drainage canals surrounding the iris; sometimes referred to as the canal of Schlemm.

Transient ischemic attack (TIA) Stroke that typically lasts for a few minutes; also known as a ministroke.

Trigeminal neuralgia Painful condition that produces intense stabbing pain in areas of the face innervated by branches of the trigeminal nerve.

Triglycerides Storage form of energy found in fat tissue muscle; metabolize to very low-density lipoproteins.

Triiodothyronine (T$_3$) Hormone secreted by the thyroid gland; contains three atoms of iodine.

Tumor marker Substance sometimes found in the blood, other body fluids, or tissues that may signal the presence of a certain type of cancer; for example, a high level of PSA is a signal for possible prostate cancer.

Tumor necrosis factor (TNF) Inflammatory cytokine released as part of the immune response; found in the synovial fluid of people with rheumatoid arthritis.

Tumor Abnormal mass of tissue that results from excessive cell division. Tumors may be benign (not cancerous) or malignant (cancerous).

Turner's syndrome Congenital endocrine disorder caused by failure of the ovaries to respond to pituitary hormone (gonadotropin) stimulation.

Tympanic membrane Eardrum.

Type 1 diabetes Autoimmune disease that results in high blood glucose levels. Pancreatic beta cells are destroyed and insufficient amounts of insulin are produced.

Type 2 diabetes Condition that results in high blood glucose levels. People with type 2 diabetes have insulin resistance.

Ulcer Open wound or sore.

Ulcerative colitis Irritable bowel disease that results in inflammation, ulcers, and damage to the colon.

Upper esophageal sphincter Sphincter separating the pharynx and esophagus. It relaxes to permit passage of food and liquids during swallowing, prevent air from entering the esophagus during breathing, and prevent gastric secretions from entering the pharynx.

Upper motor neurons Neurons that carry messages from the brain down to the spinal cord.

Urate Product of purine metabolism. Urate crystals may accumulate in joints and produce inflammation and pain.

Uricosuric Drug that increases the renal clearance of urates.

Urinalysis Microscopic and chemical examination of a fresh urine sample.

Urinary frequency Need to urinate more often than is normal.

Urticaria Hives.

Uveitis Serious eye condition that produces inflammation of the uvea; can cause scarring of the eye and blindness if untreated.

Vaccine Substance that prevents disease by taking advantage of the body's ability to make antibodies and prime killer cells to fight disease.

Vaginitis Inflammation of the vagina.

Vasospasm Spasms that constrict blood vessels and reduce the flow of blood and oxygen.

Ventricular fibrillation Life-threatening arrhythmia during which the heart beats up to 600 beats/min.

Ventricular tachycardia Condition in which ventricles beat faster than 200 beats/min.

Vertigo Feeling of spinning in space (dizziness and loss of balance).

Viral load Amount of materials from the virus that get released into the blood when HIV reproduces.

Virion Infectious particles of a virus.

Virostatic Able to suppress viral proliferation.

Virus Intracellular parasite that consists of a DNA and RNA core surrounded by a protein coat and sometimes an outer covering of lipoprotein.

Vitreous floaters Particles that float in the vitreous and cast shadows on the retina; these appear as spots, cobwebs, or spiders.

Vulvovaginal candidiasis Yeast vaginitis.

Wheal Raised blister-like area on the skin.

Whitehead (closed comedo) Trapped sebum and bacteria that stay below the skin surface; may show up as tiny white spots or may be so small that they are invisible to the naked eye.

Index

Page numbers followed by "*f*" indicate figures, "*t*" indicate tables, and "*b*" indicate boxes.